# MIND/BODY HEALTH

# MIND/BODY HEALTH

## The Effects of Attitudes, Emotions, and Relationships

**THIRD EDITION**

Keith J. Karren

Brent Q. Hafen

N. Lee Smith

Kathryn J. Frandsen

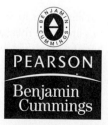

PEARSON

Benjamin Cummings

San Francisco  Boston  New York
Cape Town  Hong Kong  London  Madrid  Mexico City
Montreal  Munich  Paris  Singapore  Sydney  Tokyo  Toronto

Senior Acquisitions Editor: Deirdre Espinoza
Development Manager: Claire Alexander
Assistant Editor: Alison Rodal
Managing Editor: Deborah Cogan
Production Supervisor: Beth Masse
Copy Editor: Cheryl Adam
Cover Designer: Yvo Riezebos Design
Cover Image: Getty Images
Senior Manufacturing Buyer: Michael Early
Senior Marketing Manager: Sandra Lindelof
Project Coordination and Composition: WestWords, Inc.

**Library of Congress Cataloging-in-Publication Data**

Mind/body health : the effects of attitudes, emotions, and relationships / Keith Karren ...
   [et al.].— 3rd ed. p. ; cm.
 Includes bibliographical references and index.
 ISBN 0-8053-7886-3
1. Medicine, Psychosomatic. 2. Emotions—Health aspects. 3. Psychoneuroimmunology.
4. Mind and body.
  [DNLM: 1. Psychosomatic Medicine. 2. Attitude to Health. 3. Emotions. 4. Personality.
5. Social Support. WM 90 M662 2006] I. Karren, Keith J.
 RC49.M522 2006
 616'.001'9—dc22

2005007989

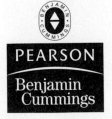

PEARSON

Benjamin
Cummings

ISBN 0-8053-7886-3

1 2 3 4 5 6—DOC—08 07 06 05

**www.aw-bc.com**

# Contents

Preface . . . . . . . . . . . . . . . . . . . . . . . . . . . . . . . . . . . . . . xiii

**PART I**  THE MIND/BODY CONNECTION . . . . . . . . . . . . . . . . . 1

Chapter 1:  **Psychoneuroimmunology: The Connection Between the Mind and the Body** . . . . . . . . . . . . . . . . . . . . . . . . . . 3
A Definition . . . . . . . . . . . . . . . . . . . . . . . . . . . . . . . . . 4
A Brief History . . . . . . . . . . . . . . . . . . . . . . . . . . . . . . . 6
The Mind-Body Connection Today . . . . . . . . . . . . . . . . . . 8
PNI: The Major Components . . . . . . . . . . . . . . . . . . . . . . 9
The Immune System. . . . . . . . . . . . . . . . . . . . . . . . . . . 14
The Immune System in Action. . . . . . . . . . . . . . . . . . . . 16
Malfunctions. . . . . . . . . . . . . . . . . . . . . . . . . . . . . . . . 17
The Brain-Immune System Connection. . . . . . . . . . . . . . 18
The Immune System and Emotion. . . . . . . . . . . . . . . . . 20
The Role of Religion . . . . . . . . . . . . . . . . . . . . . . . . . . 23
The Emotion-Immunity Connection in Heart Disease, Cancer, and Other Conditions. . . . . . . . . . . . . . . . . . . . . 24
The Mind and Longevity . . . . . . . . . . . . . . . . . . . . . . . 34
Criticisms of the Mind-Body Approach . . . . . . . . . . . . . 36
The Challenge for the Twenty-first Century. . . . . . . . . . . 37
Endnotes. . . . . . . . . . . . . . . . . . . . . . . . . . . . . . . . . . 38

Chapter 2:  **The Impact of Stress on Health** . . . . . . . . . . . . . . . . 42
Definitions of Stress . . . . . . . . . . . . . . . . . . . . . . . . . . 42
The Stress Response . . . . . . . . . . . . . . . . . . . . . . . . . . 45
Costs and Outcomes of Stress. . . . . . . . . . . . . . . . . . . . 48
Factors Leading to Stress . . . . . . . . . . . . . . . . . . . . . . . 49
Job Stress and Health . . . . . . . . . . . . . . . . . . . . . . . . . 56
Factors That Influence How We Cope with Stress . . . . . . . . 64
Self-Perceptions of Stress . . . . . . . . . . . . . . . . . . . . . . . 76
How to Protect Yourself from Stress. . . . . . . . . . . . . . . . 76
Keys for Handling Job Stress . . . . . . . . . . . . . . . . . . . . 78
Endnotes. . . . . . . . . . . . . . . . . . . . . . . . . . . . . . . . . . 80

**PART II**   PERSONALITY STYLES AND HEALTH . . . . . . . . . . . . . . . . 85

Chapter 3:   **The Disease-Prone Personality** . . . . . . . . . . . . . . . . . . . 87
 Definitions and Foundation . . . . . . . . . . . . . . . . . . . . . 87
 Disease and Personality: Exploring the Connection . . . . . . . . . . . . . . 90
 Type A Personality: The Coronary Artery Disease–Prone Personality . . 95
 Type D Personality . . . . . . . . . . . . . . . . . . . . . . . . . 114
 The Controversy . . . . . . . . . . . . . . . . . . . . . . . . . . 115
 Type C Personality: The Cancer-Prone Personality . . . . . . . . . . . . . 116
 The Rheumatoid Arthritis–Prone Personality . . . . . . . . . . . . . . . 123
 The Ulcer-Prone Personality . . . . . . . . . . . . . . . . . . . . . 127
 An Asthma-Prone Personality . . . . . . . . . . . . . . . . . . . . 128
 Reducing Your Risks . . . . . . . . . . . . . . . . . . . . . . . . 129
 Endnotes . . . . . . . . . . . . . . . . . . . . . . . . . . . . . . 131

Chapter 4:   **Anger, Hostility, and Health** . . . . . . . . . . . . . . . . . . 139
 The Definitions of Anger and Hostility . . . . . . . . . . . . . . . . . 140
 Manifestations of Anger and Hostility . . . . . . . . . . . . . . . . . 142
 The Significance of Anger and Hostility . . . . . . . . . . . . . . . . . 144
 Causes of Hostility . . . . . . . . . . . . . . . . . . . . . . . . . . 145
 The Need to Express Anger . . . . . . . . . . . . . . . . . . . . . . 146
 How the Body Reacts: The Health Effects of Anger and Hostility . . . . . 149
 Anger: The Cancer Connection . . . . . . . . . . . . . . . . . . . . 156
 An Angry/Hostile Heart, an Ill Heart . . . . . . . . . . . . . . . . . 157
 Hostility and Mortality . . . . . . . . . . . . . . . . . . . . . . . . 162
 What to Do if Anger Is a Problem . . . . . . . . . . . . . . . . . . . 165
 Endnotes . . . . . . . . . . . . . . . . . . . . . . . . . . . . . . 166

Chapter 5:   **Worry, Anxiety, Fear, and Health** . . . . . . . . . . . . . . . . 172
 Definitions of Worry . . . . . . . . . . . . . . . . . . . . . . . . . 173
 Generalized Anxiety Disorder . . . . . . . . . . . . . . . . . . . . . 174
 Panic Disorder . . . . . . . . . . . . . . . . . . . . . . . . . . . . 175
 Other Common Anxiety Disorders . . . . . . . . . . . . . . . . . . . 175
 Somaticizing . . . . . . . . . . . . . . . . . . . . . . . . . . . . . 176
 Effects on the Body . . . . . . . . . . . . . . . . . . . . . . . . . . 178
 The Association of Anxiety with Common Medical Illnesses . . . . . . . 179
 Worry and the Circulatory System . . . . . . . . . . . . . . . . . . . 181
 Worry and Asthma . . . . . . . . . . . . . . . . . . . . . . . . . . 182

The Effects of Uncertainty. . . . . . . . . . . . . . . . . . . . . . . . . . . 183
The Health Consequences of Fear. . . . . . . . . . . . . . . . . . . . . 184
What to Do About Worry and Anxiety. . . . . . . . . . . . . . . . . 187
Endnotes. . . . . . . . . . . . . . . . . . . . . . . . . . . . . . . . . . . . . . 188

Chapter 6: **Depression, Despair, and Health**. . . . . . . . . . . . . . . . . 192
A Definition . . . . . . . . . . . . . . . . . . . . . . . . . . . . . . . . . . . 192
Prevalence and Manifestations. . . . . . . . . . . . . . . . . . . . . . 194
Causes of Depression . . . . . . . . . . . . . . . . . . . . . . . . . . . . 196
Characteristics of Depression . . . . . . . . . . . . . . . . . . . . . . 200
Depression and Premenstrual Syndrome . . . . . . . . . . . . . . 202
Seasonal Affective Disorder . . . . . . . . . . . . . . . . . . . . . . . 203
The Physiological Changes of Depression. . . . . . . . . . . . . . 205
Depression and Longevity. . . . . . . . . . . . . . . . . . . . . . . . . 208
Depression and the Heart . . . . . . . . . . . . . . . . . . . . . . . . . 210
Depression and the Immune System . . . . . . . . . . . . . . . . . 214
Depression and Cancer. . . . . . . . . . . . . . . . . . . . . . . . . . . 218
Feeling Sad, Feeling Bad. . . . . . . . . . . . . . . . . . . . . . . . . . 219
What to Do About Depression . . . . . . . . . . . . . . . . . . . . . 220
Endnotes. . . . . . . . . . . . . . . . . . . . . . . . . . . . . . . . . . . . . . 221

Chapter 7: **Insomnia and Sleep Deprivation: Health Effects
and Treatment**. . . . . . . . . . . . . . . . . . . . . . . . . . . . . . . . . 228
Types and Causes of Insomnia . . . . . . . . . . . . . . . . . . . . . 231
Factors in the Development of Chronic Insomnia . . . . . . . . 232
Why Do We Sleep?. . . . . . . . . . . . . . . . . . . . . . . . . . . . . . 234
Behavioral and Psychological Effects of Insomnia . . . . . . . 235
Physiological Effects of Insomnia . . . . . . . . . . . . . . . . . . . 237
Treatment of Insomnia . . . . . . . . . . . . . . . . . . . . . . . . . . . 239
Specific Behavioral Strategies for Treating Insomnia . . . . . 240
Using Medication to Treat Insomnia. . . . . . . . . . . . . . . . . . 244
Primary Medical Sleep Disorders . . . . . . . . . . . . . . . . . . . 245
Conclusions. . . . . . . . . . . . . . . . . . . . . . . . . . . . . . . . . . . . 246
Endnotes. . . . . . . . . . . . . . . . . . . . . . . . . . . . . . . . . . . . . . 247

Chapter 8: **The Disease-Resistant Personality** . . . . . . . . . . . . . . . 251
The Role of Stress in Health . . . . . . . . . . . . . . . . . . . . . . . 252
The Mechanisms of Stress. . . . . . . . . . . . . . . . . . . . . . . . . 253

Stress Buffers. . . . . . . . . . . . . . . . . . . . . . . . . . . . . . . . . . . 255
Gender Differences . . . . . . . . . . . . . . . . . . . . . . . . . . . . . . 256
Personality Traits That Keep Us Well . . . . . . . . . . . . . . . . 258
Endnotes. . . . . . . . . . . . . . . . . . . . . . . . . . . . . . . . . . . . . . 268

**PART III**   SOCIAL SUPPORT AND HEALTH. . . . . . . . . . . . . . . . . . 273

Chapter 9:   **Social Support, Relationships, and Health** . . . . . . . . . . . . . 275
Social Support Defined. . . . . . . . . . . . . . . . . . . . . . . . . . . 277
Sources of Social Support . . . . . . . . . . . . . . . . . . . . . . . . 278
How Does Social Support Protect Health? . . . . . . . . . . . . . 280
The Ties That Bind . . . . . . . . . . . . . . . . . . . . . . . . . . . . . 284
Love Stronger, Live Longer. . . . . . . . . . . . . . . . . . . . . . . . 291
Social Connections and the Heart. . . . . . . . . . . . . . . . . . . 295
The Best Health Bet—Good Social Ties. . . . . . . . . . . . . . . 299
Touch: A Crucial Aspect of Social Support . . . . . . . . . . . . . 303
Endnotes. . . . . . . . . . . . . . . . . . . . . . . . . . . . . . . . . . . . . 305

Chapter 10:   **Loneliness and Health** . . . . . . . . . . . . . . . . . . . . . . . . . . 310
What Is Loneliness? . . . . . . . . . . . . . . . . . . . . . . . . . . . . . 311
Loneliness Versus Aloneness. . . . . . . . . . . . . . . . . . . . . . . 312
Trends in Being Alone. . . . . . . . . . . . . . . . . . . . . . . . . . . . 313
Reasons for Loneliness . . . . . . . . . . . . . . . . . . . . . . . . . . 314
Causes of Loneliness. . . . . . . . . . . . . . . . . . . . . . . . . . . . 315
Risk Factors for Loneliness . . . . . . . . . . . . . . . . . . . . . . . 317
The Health Consequences of Loneliness. . . . . . . . . . . . . . . 319
The Importance of Good Friends . . . . . . . . . . . . . . . . . . . . 327
The Importance of Pets . . . . . . . . . . . . . . . . . . . . . . . . . . 331
Endnotes. . . . . . . . . . . . . . . . . . . . . . . . . . . . . . . . . . . . . 335

Chapter 11:   **Marriage and Health** . . . . . . . . . . . . . . . . . . . . . . . . . . . 340
The Health Hazards of Divorce . . . . . . . . . . . . . . . . . . . . . 340
The Divorced Versus the Unhappily Married . . . . . . . . . . . . 346
The Health Benefits of a Happy Marriage. . . . . . . . . . . . . . 349
Marriage and Life Expectancy. . . . . . . . . . . . . . . . . . . . . . 357
Endnotes. . . . . . . . . . . . . . . . . . . . . . . . . . . . . . . . . . . . . 358

Chapter 12: **Families and Health** . . . . . . . . . . . . . . . . . . 362
    What Is a Family? . . . . . . . . . . . . . . . . . . . . . . 362
    The Early Influence of Parents . . . . . . . . . . . . . . . 363
    Traits of Weak or Stressed Families . . . . . . . . . . . . . 369
    Health Problems in Weak or Stressed Families . . . . . . . . 372
    Traits of Strong Families . . . . . . . . . . . . . . . . . . 376
    The Health Benefits of Strong Families . . . . . . . . . . . 380
    Family Reunions: More than a Good Time . . . . . . . . . . . 384
    Endnotes . . . . . . . . . . . . . . . . . . . . . . . . . . 385

Chapter 13: **Grief, Bereavement, and Health** . . . . . . . . . . . 388  √
    The Loss That Leads to Grief . . . . . . . . . . . . . . . . 389
    Grief: The Natural Effect of Loss . . . . . . . . . . . . . . 391
    The Health Consequences of Bereavement . . . . . . . . . . . 393
    General Mortality Rates . . . . . . . . . . . . . . . . . . . 407
    Cutting the Risk . . . . . . . . . . . . . . . . . . . . . . 409
    Endnotes . . . . . . . . . . . . . . . . . . . . . . . . . . 411

**PART IV**   SPIRITUALITY AND HEALTH . . . . . . . . . . . . . . . 415  √

Chapter 14: **The Healing Power of Spirituality** . . . . . . . . . . 417
    What Is Spirituality and Spiritual Health? . . . . . . . . . 420
    Influences on Health . . . . . . . . . . . . . . . . . . . . 425
    Crisis as a Growth Experience . . . . . . . . . . . . . . . . 429
    The Power of Prayer on Health . . . . . . . . . . . . . . . . 431
    The Healing Power of Forgiveness . . . . . . . . . . . . . . 434
    Church Affiliation and Health . . . . . . . . . . . . . . . . 437
    The Essence of Spirituality and Spiritual Well-Being . . . . 444
    Endnotes . . . . . . . . . . . . . . . . . . . . . . . . . . 446

Chapter 15: **The Healing Power of Altruism** . . . . . . . . . . . . 452
    How Altruism Boosts Health . . . . . . . . . . . . . . . . . 453
    The Altruistic Personality . . . . . . . . . . . . . . . . . 457
    The Health Benefits of Volunteerism . . . . . . . . . . . . . 460
    Love: The Emotion Behind It . . . . . . . . . . . . . . . . . 466
    Endnotes . . . . . . . . . . . . . . . . . . . . . . . . . . 469

Chapter 16:  **The Healing Power of Faith and Religion** . . . . . . . . . . . . . . . 471
The Impact of Faith. . . . . . . . . . . . . . . . . . . . . . . . . . . . . . . . . . 475
The Influence of Spirituality, Religion, and Faith on Health . . . . . . . . 476
The Healing Power of Faith. . . . . . . . . . . . . . . . . . . . . . . . . . . . . 480
Faith and the Placebo Effect . . . . . . . . . . . . . . . . . . . . . . . . . . . 486
Endnotes . . . . . . . . . . . . . . . . . . . . . . . . . . . . . . . . . . . . . . . . 498

Chapter 17:  **The Healing Power of Optimism** . . . . . . . . . . . . . . . . . . . . . 502
Who Are Optimists? . . . . . . . . . . . . . . . . . . . . . . . . . . . . . . . . . 502
How Optimism Influences Health. . . . . . . . . . . . . . . . . . . . . . . . . 505
Optimism and Healing . . . . . . . . . . . . . . . . . . . . . . . . . . . . . . . 510
Optimism: A Boost to Immunity. . . . . . . . . . . . . . . . . . . . . . . . . 514
Optimism's Effect on Mental Health and Performance. . . . . . . . . . . . 515
Optimists and Longevity . . . . . . . . . . . . . . . . . . . . . . . . . . . . . . 517
Endnotes . . . . . . . . . . . . . . . . . . . . . . . . . . . . . . . . . . . . . . . . 519

**PART V**  PERCEPTION AND HEALTH . . . . . . . . . . . . . . . . . . . . . . . . 521

Chapter 18:  **Explanatory Style and Health** . . . . . . . . . . . . . . . . . . . . . . 523
What Is Explanatory Style? . . . . . . . . . . . . . . . . . . . . . . . . . . . . 523
How Permanent Is Explanatory Style? . . . . . . . . . . . . . . . . . . . . . 525
What Are the Effects of Explanatory Style? . . . . . . . . . . . . . . . . . . 525
The Influence of Explanatory Style on Health . . . . . . . . . . . . . . . . 526
A Healthy Style, a Healthy Immune System. . . . . . . . . . . . . . . . . . 531
Endnotes . . . . . . . . . . . . . . . . . . . . . . . . . . . . . . . . . . . . . . . . 532

Chapter 19:  **Locus of Control and Health** . . . . . . . . . . . . . . . . . . . . . . . 534
What Does Locus of Control Mean? . . . . . . . . . . . . . . . . . . . . . . . 534
A Brief History of Control. . . . . . . . . . . . . . . . . . . . . . . . . . . . . 536
What is the Source of Control? . . . . . . . . . . . . . . . . . . . . . . . . . . 536
Hardiness and Control . . . . . . . . . . . . . . . . . . . . . . . . . . . . . . . 537
The Influence of Control on Health . . . . . . . . . . . . . . . . . . . . . . . 538
The Stress-Buffering Power of Control. . . . . . . . . . . . . . . . . . . . . . 542
The Influence of Control on Immunity and Healing . . . . . . . . . . . . . 543
Endnotes . . . . . . . . . . . . . . . . . . . . . . . . . . . . . . . . . . . . . . . . 545

Chapter 20:  **Self-Esteem and Health** . . . . . . . . . . . . . . . . . . . . . . . . . . 547
What Is Self-Esteem? . . . . . . . . . . . . . . . . . . . . . . . . . . . . . . . . 548
Where Does Self-Esteem Come From? . . . . . . . . . . . . . . . . . . . . . 550

The Impact of Self-Esteem on the Body . . . . . . . . . . . . . . . . . . . . . . . 551
Self-Efficacy: Believing in Yourself . . . . . . . . . . . . . . . . . . . . . . . . 552
Endnotes . . . . . . . . . . . . . . . . . . . . . . . . . . . . . . . . . . . . . . . . . . 556

Chapter 21:  **The Healing Power of Humor and Laughter** . . . . . . . . . . . . . . . 559
Professional Trends Toward Humor . . . . . . . . . . . . . . . . . . . . . . . 561
The Impact of Humor on Health . . . . . . . . . . . . . . . . . . . . . . . . . . 563
Laughter: The Best Medicine . . . . . . . . . . . . . . . . . . . . . . . . . . . 570
The Health Benefits of Laughter . . . . . . . . . . . . . . . . . . . . . . . . . 573
Endnotes . . . . . . . . . . . . . . . . . . . . . . . . . . . . . . . . . . . . . . . . . . 580

PART VI  THE INTERVENTION OF BEHAVIORAL MEDICINE . . . . . . . . 583

Chapter 22:  **The Importance of Nutrition to Mind and Body Health** . . . . . . 585
The Basic Principles of Nutrition . . . . . . . . . . . . . . . . . . . . . . . . . 586
The Typical American Diet . . . . . . . . . . . . . . . . . . . . . . . . . . . . . 589
How Nutrition Affects the Brain . . . . . . . . . . . . . . . . . . . . . . . . . . 590
How Nutrition Affects Physical and Mental Health . . . . . . . . . . . . . 595
Obesity . . . . . . . . . . . . . . . . . . . . . . . . . . . . . . . . . . . . . . . . . . . 596
Insulin Resistance . . . . . . . . . . . . . . . . . . . . . . . . . . . . . . . . . . . 597
The "Second Brain": The Gastrointestinal Tract . . . . . . . . . . . . . . . 600
The Impact of Wheat Allergies on the Brain . . . . . . . . . . . . . . . . . 604
Conclusion . . . . . . . . . . . . . . . . . . . . . . . . . . . . . . . . . . . . . . . . 604
Endnotes . . . . . . . . . . . . . . . . . . . . . . . . . . . . . . . . . . . . . . . . . . 605

Chapter 23:  **Behavioral Medicine Treatment: Effects on Medical
and Health Outcomes and Costs** . . . . . . . . . . . . . . . . . . . . . . . 610
The Connection Between Mental Stress and Medical Symptoms . . . . 613
Outcome Data from Behavioral Medicine Interventions . . . . . . . . . . 615
High-Volume Users of Medical Care and Resources . . . . . . . . . . . . . 617
Outcomes for Specific Medical Illnesses . . . . . . . . . . . . . . . . . . . . 620
Cost and Medical Care Utilization Issues . . . . . . . . . . . . . . . . . . . 628
Endnotes . . . . . . . . . . . . . . . . . . . . . . . . . . . . . . . . . . . . . . . . . . 635

Chapter 24:  **Methods of Intervention and the Principles
of Stress Resilience** . . . . . . . . . . . . . . . . . . . . . . . . . . . . . . . . 642
Lessons from Cancer Studies . . . . . . . . . . . . . . . . . . . . . . . . . . . 643
Four Core Principles Underlying Stress Resilience and Well-Being . . . 645
A Sense of Empowerment and Personal Control . . . . . . . . . . . . . . . 648

Cognitive Structuring and Therapy. . . . . . . . . . . . . . . . . . . . . . . . . . . . 651
Basic Elements of Behavior Change . . . . . . . . . . . . . . . . . . . . . . . . . . 654
Methods of Eliciting the Relaxation Response . . . . . . . . . . . . . . . . . . . 654
Methods of Changing Behavior . . . . . . . . . . . . . . . . . . . . . . . . . . . . 657
Other Ways to Change Behavior . . . . . . . . . . . . . . . . . . . . . . . . . . . . 658
Mind-Body Treatment: Can It Change the Course of Disease? . . . . . . 660
The Spiritual Connection . . . . . . . . . . . . . . . . . . . . . . . . . . . . . . . . . 662
Endnotes . . . . . . . . . . . . . . . . . . . . . . . . . . . . . . . . . . . . . . . . . . . . . 664

**Epilogue** . . . . . . . . . . . . . . . . . . . . . . . . . . . . . . . . . . . . . . . . . 666

Appendix A  **The Elements of Human Fulfillment** . . . . . . . . . . . . . . . . . . . 675

Appendix B  **The Seven Habits of Highly Effective People** . . . . . . . . . . . . . . 678

Appendix C  **The Misunderstood Alternative: Effective Type B
Characteristics That Can Protect from Heart Disease** . . . . . . . . . 679

**Name Index** . . . . . . . . . . . . . . . . . . . . . . . . . . . . . . . . . . . . . . 681

**Subject Index** . . . . . . . . . . . . . . . . . . . . . . . . . . . . . . . . . . . . 688

# *Preface*

*The body is the shadow of the soul.*

—Marsilio Ficino

Take your mind back 300 years to a simple, rough-hewn dinner table somewhere in colonial North America. Spread out across the table were the bounties of hunt and harvest—the succulent browned flesh of the pheasant, the savory goodness of carrot and parsnip, the robust sweetness of carmelized onions. Plump berries exploded from crusts glazed with milk and sugar, staining the folds of thick muslin used to carry the steaming dishes to the table.

Everywhere was evidence of the gardens, plotted in neat rows between the brick houses, shaded by the towering elms that lined the streets. Their harvest might have looked much like yours and mine—except that no one was eating tomatoes. Tomatoes were "poisonous." Everyone knew they were poisonous. After all, they were a member of the nightshade family, and members of the nightshade family were poisonous.

The fact that the French and Italians were eating plenty of tomatoes without any harmful effects did not encourage colonial Americans to try them. The very thought was an outrage: It simply did not make sense to eat poisonous food. And so America's tables, set by the warm yellow glow of lantern and lamp, peppered the colonies of New England without even a crimson hint of a ripened tomato. It took a rebel to turn the tide. Not until 1820, when Robert Gibbon Johnson ate a tomato on the steps of the court-house in Salem, New Jersey, and survived, did the people of America slowly start to eat tomatoes. Centuries later, the tomato is prized not only for its flavor, but also for its versatility and nutritional value.

The history of the tomato in colonial America gave rise to what scientists call *the tomato effect.* It happens when something beneficial is ignored or rejected because it doesn't make sense in light of what we already "know." It gives us tacit permission to turn away from new ideas because they don't fit neatly into the framework we have already constructed with materials we have grown comfortable with. But consider this: We are tethered to that comfortable framework. Its comfort, at once secure and predictable, comes at a heavy price.

Today, the vestiges of colonial America survive only in the villages preserved as museums along the eastern seaboard. In those townships, curators work pits of clay into bricks with their bare feet and spin dense curls of wool into lengths of soft thread. They sit on needlepoint stools and stitch the tucked bodices of aprons by hand, or work the supple reeds that grow along the ditch into a basket for gathering the eggs. They drag thick-bristled brushes through the manes of chestnut horses and repair splintering carriage wheels. In those villages, you will see horehound candy and fresh-brewed ale. You will see cobbled walks and windows of thick-paned glass. You will see muskets and tin toys. But you will not see any tomatoes.

Not so in the rest of this nation—or the world. You've undoubtedly savored the rich pungency of a juicy tomato—either fresh from the garden, sliced and lightly sprinkled with salt, or cooked until thick and ladled over a steaming plate of firm spaghetti noodles. There's nothing poisonous there.

So we ask you to savor the evidence presented in this book. It may challenge notions you have held for a long time. It may ask you to step outside the comfortable framework you have constructed. It may seem to fly in the face of what you have "known" to be true. But, just like the warm tomato you pluck from the vine along the back fence on a languid late August afternoon, there's no poison here. Nothing here will hurt you. On the contrary, you may find information that will change your life, enhance your health, and help you live a richer, fuller existence.

What you find here comes from a new field of medicine that has shattered traditional ideas about sickness—and wellness. For hundreds of years, we have been mired in the paradigm that disease is all about organisms: bacteria and viruses and parasites invade our body, overpower our immunity, and make us sick. For hundreds of years, scientists focused on that premise. As a result, we made giant inroads in the war against communicable disease. Today, smallpox has been virtually wiped out. Polio is unknown in all but third world countries. The diseases that once killed people the world over in epidemic proportions are now controlled by simple antibiotics. We have waged war on the bacteria and viruses and parasites, and it's a war we are winning by increasing margins.

Even then, however, we had precious little information on the human immune system. We knew how to stimulate it with vaccinations and immunizations, how to make it recognize a previously encountered enemy and how to raise the armaments. But we did not know what made it strong. We could not explain why one of two children exposed to the influenza virus remained robust and healthy while the other huddled under layers of patchwork quilts, chattering with the chills of relentless fever.

Nor did we understand how to confront our nation's new killers: chronic maladies like heart disease and cancer that, for the most part, were not caused by microorganisms. These were caused instead by some inherent weakness in the complex physical structure. Just as we could not explain the child who scampered happily through the crackling autumn leaves while his brother lay weakened with the flu, we could not explain why one executive in the office suite had a heart attack—or why one member of the golf foursome was ravaged by cancer. Why not all the executives in all the offices along the winding corridor? And why not all—or none—of the golfers?

Researchers who clamored for the answers did a good job of identifying risk factors. You can probably name most of them. Cigarettes. Obesity. High blood pressure. Lack of exercise. A high-fat diet. Valid as they are, they paint only a small part of the picture. Why? Because they concern themselves with only a small part of the person: the body.

Look in the mirror. What you see is an intricate body composed of complex physical systems that work together to sustain life. What you *don't* see—but what you know is there, just as surely as if you could see it in the mirrored reflection—is a mind that is marked by eagerness and curiosity, emotions that can change in an instant, a spirit that yearns for meaning, and a personality that sets you apart from every other person on this earth. And thanks to the work of a growing army of researchers, we know that your mind, your emotions, your spirit, and your personality have a profound impact on your body—and are powerful determinants in who stays well and who gets sick.

What started out as a few radical pioneers has swelled into a respected body of scientists who are bringing us the information we need to live longer, healthier lives. You may recognize some of their names: Deepak Chopra, an endocrinologist who has synthesized ancient and modern medicine, physics, and philosophy, teaches that mental awareness results in physical chemistry—and that our reality is a result of our perception. His is a world of "infinite possibilities." Physician Larry Dossey argues that the emotional and mental currency of *meaning* actually enters the body and alters its cells. His provocative research on the power of prayer has led to large-scale studies that are influencing the direction of medicine. Medical psychologist Joan Borysenko demonstrates how the mind, body, and spirit are inseparably linked—and are at work in the intricacies of human immunity. These ideas at first seem surreal; even Dossey, who has pioneered many of them, admits that they are "stretching our conceptual paradigms to the breaking point."

With that stretch, however, comes discovery. With that stretch comes compelling research and irrefutable scientific evidence that proves that we are all the product of a mind, body, and spirit—and that all three play a critical role in health and wellness.

Some of the evidence is simple: The hormones that are pumped into your bloodstream when you're angry literally corrode the lining of your arteries. Could it be, then, that anger and hostility are as important in the development of heart disease as too many fat-laden meals? Some of the evidence seems to boggle the mind: Every emotion you experience literally creates a chain of molecules that subsequently attaches to immune system cells. Could it be, then, that attitudes of hope and optimism may physically boost immunity?

Scientific studies say so. Researchers who follow thousands of people for a dozen or more years draw inescapable conclusions about how the closeness of their community protects them from heart disease—even in the presence of hearty Italian cooking. Anecdotal evidence says so, too. Renowned researcher Henry Dreher remembers Michael Callen, an intelligent, gritty, compassionate man who lived for twelve years after being diagnosed with AIDS because he rejected its death sentence and concentrated instead on searching for meaning in his life. "I couldn't help but wonder if his personality had contributed to his unexpected survival," Dreher wrote. "The passage of time would only reinforce my suspicion that it had."

What started as a preposterous notion—that the brain and the immune system are interconnected—is now irrefutable fact. What started out as a "fringe" group of eccentric but courageous pioneers has swelled into a burgeoning army of researchers from the fields of medicine, psychology, immunology, endocrinology, and neurology. Because of their careful scientific work, spanning two decades, we know that the nervous, endocrine, and immune systems "talk" to each other in a language that consists of cell products—and that they take their direction from the mind. As Dreher writes, "We can no longer carve up our biological systems into separate work forces based on a false division of labor."

In the pages that follow, you'll read about their amazing discoveries. You'll learn what we know about how emotions and attitudes affect health. Drawing on landmark scientific studies by many distinguished scientists, many of whom are now at the forefront of medical research, we build a solid foundation of evidence that shows the undeniable connection between the mind and the body. You'll see how "negative" emotions such as worry, anxiety, depression, hostility, and anger, when nurtured, can increase susceptibility to disease. You'll discover how "positive" emotions such as optimism, humor, and a fighting spirit can protect your health and help to heal. In exploring the powerful connection between your mind and body, we discuss:

- How your body responds to the way you see yourself and your circumstances
- Why social support, friendship, and strong, stable relationships protect your health
- How different personalities are either prone to, or able to resist, disease

- The scientifically proven changes in your body chemistry, heart rate, and hormones that accompany various attitudes and emotions
- How attitudes and emotions actually affect your immunity from disease

We hope you will be able to see a little bit of yourself in these pages and will be able to make some affirmations about what you will do with the emotions you experience in the course of everyday living. Above all, what is written here may help you learn to appreciate the tremendous healing power of your mind and your heart, and may help you focus both on an appreciation of life itself. Perhaps former *Saturday Review* editor Norman Cousins said it best in these words:

*An appreciation of life can be a prime tonic for mind and body. Being able to respond to the majesty of the way nature fashions its art—the mysterious designs in the barks of trees, suggesting cave paintings or verdant meadows interrupted by silvery streams; the rich and luminous coloring of carp fish with blues and yellows and crimsons seemingly lit up from within; the bird of paradise flower, an explosion of colors ascending to a triumphant and jaunty crest of orange and purple; the skin of an apple, so thin it defies measurement but supremely protective of its precious substance; they say the climbing trunk of a tree will steer its growth around solid objects coming between itself and the sun; the curling white foam of an ocean wave advancing on the shore, and the way sand repairs and smooths itself by the receding water; the purring of a kitten perched on your shoulder, or the head of a dog snuggling under your hand; the measured power of Beethoven's Emperor Concerto, the joyous quality of a Chopin nocturne, the serene and stately progression of a Bach fugue, the lyrical designs in a Mozart composition for clarinet and strings; the sound of delight in a young boy's voice on catching his first baseball; and, most of all, the expression in the face of someone who loves you—all these are but a small part of a list of wondrous satisfactions that come with the gift of awareness and that nourish even as they heal.*

# Acknowledgments

Our lives have collectively been blessed with many wonderful individuals who have made contributions to this third edition of Mind/Body Health. We were incredibly blessed to have the help of Rilla Leckie, our research assistant, and Hugo Rodier, M.D., our colleague who developed the original nutrition chapter.

A special thanks goes to our dear friend and colleague, Kathy Frandsen, whose writing and editing expertise have made this revision a success.

We also express much gratitude to Deirdre Espinoza and Alison Rodal of Benjamin Cummings for positive prodding and requesting excellence. Though this was a challenging process, they kept us on track, helping us keep our goals in sight.

Lastly, we pay tribute to our dear, departed friend and colleague, Dr. Brent Hafen, whose foresight envisioned the importance of this book.

Finally, the many reviewers of this book gave us excellent direction and played an integral part of the revision. Many thanks to Anna Tacon, Texas Tech University; Michael Olpin, Weber State University; Mel Minarik, University of Nevada, Reno; Stanley Snegroff, Adelphi University; Kelly Glazer, University of Utah; David Holtzman, State University of New York, Brockport; Carlos Escoto, Eastern Connecticut State University; Nancy Barone-Sevigny, Johnson State College; Jane Marie Clipman, Penn State University; Susan Rivers, Skidmore College; Sandra Sperling, Ivy Tech State College; and Justin Laird, State University of New York, Brockport.

# Part I

# The Mind/Body Connection

This introductory section of the book presents information to acquaint the reader with psychoneuroimmunology, proof of the connection between mind and body and the effects of distress on health. The chapters and topics presented in this section are:

**Chapter 1**   *Psychoneuroimmunology: The Mind/Body Connection*

**Chapter 2**   *Impact of Stress on Health*

# Psychoneuroimmunology: The Connection Between the Mind and the Body

*Great men are they who see that spiritual force is stronger than any material force, that thoughts rule the world.*

—Ralph Waldo Emerson

## Learning Objectives

- Define psychoneuroimmunology.
- Understand the major historical milestones in the development of mind-body medicine.
- Define the role of and connection between the brain and the immune system.
- Understand the role of emotions and immunity in major diseases, such as heart disease and cancer.
- Understand the criticisms of mind-body medicine.
- Understand the challenges for mind-body medicine in the next century.

In a pronouncement that at first surprised the medical community, if not the lay public, one practitioner proclaimed that an estimated 90 percent of all physical problems have emotional roots. He followed up by saying that his estimate was, at best, conservative. A growing body of evidence now indicates that virtually every illness—from arthritis to migraine headaches, from the common cold to cancer—is influenced, for good or bad, by how we think and feel. Solid research is now confirming what many physicians have long observed: The state of the mind directly affects physical illness.[1]

There are compelling reasons to address the issue of disease beyond its personal effects. The global impact of physical illness is profound: In the United States alone, chronic disease costs hundreds of billions of dollars every year. In 2001, the United States spent $300 billion on cardiovascular disease, $100 billion on diabetes, and $117 billion on the costs associated with overweight people and obesity.[2]

As part of the effort to focus on prevention, seemingly disparate lines of research have converged into a new discipline of mind-body medicine that examines the relationship between the mind, the emotions, and the body. Mind-body medicine is based on the premise that mental and emotional processes (the mind) can affect physiological function (the body), and a large body of evidence now supports this connection.[3]

Under the support of a National Institutes of Mental Health grant, physicians and researchers David Spiegel and Sara Stein write, "Once believed to be autonomously functioning mechanisms, the nervous, endocrine, and immune systems are now known to be integrally connected, with exquisitely sensitive communications and interactions."[4]

These and other researchers have shown that what we think and how we feel appear to have powerful effects on the biological functions of our bodies, especially on the immune system. It also shows that there is a complex, dynamic interaction between the mind and the body. Finally, it opens the revolutionary possibility that we can work with our physicians by virtue of our attitudes and our emotions, not just our biological systems.

## A Definition

The scientific investigation of how the brain affects the body's immune cells and how the immune system can be affected by behavior is called *psycho-neuroimmunology*, a term coined in 1964 by Dr. Robert Ader, director of the division of behavioral and psychosocial medicine at New York's University of Rochester. In their landmark study, Ader and his colleagues showed that immune function could be classically conditioned.[5] The science of psychoneuroimmunology (PNI) focuses on the interaction between the mind, the brain, the nervous system, and the immune system. PNI investigates the relationship between psychosocial factors, the central nervous system, the immune system, and disease.[6]

As a science, PNI receives the endorsement of the National Institutes of Health and the support of prominent researchers. Candace Pert, a psychopharmacologist with Maryland-based Peptide Research and a visiting professor with the Center for Molecular and Behavioral Neuroscience at Rutgers University, points out that "separate disciplines make it difficult to make progress. I think we're moving toward a much more interdisciplinary way of looking at things."[7]

David L. Felten, professor of neurobiology and anatomy at the University of Rochester School of Medicine in New York, agrees. "The field of psychoneuroimmunology, as a scientific discipline—and I'm not talking about people who hang crystals from their rear-view mirrors, I'm talking about hard-core research—is showing that the nervous system and the immune system communicate with each other massively, extensively, and continuously," he says.[8]

Though there is still some skepticism about the concepts behind it, PNI researchers are proving that the way people think and feel influences the immune system. Immunologists, physiologists, psychiatrists, psychologists, and neurobiologists "who have explored the murky boundary between mind and body now suspect that certain negative psychological states, brought on by adversity or a chemical imbalance, actually cause the immune system to falter."[9] Some even go so far as to claim that positive attitudes, such as a feeling of control, may in some way "inoculate against disease and act as a valuable supplement to conventional medical care."

Psychoneuroimmunologists focus on the link between the mind, the brain, the nervous system, and the immune system, and though these links are solid, researchers are still not sure whether they *cause* disease or *influence* the development of disease. Because evidence is still being gathered from a host of long-term studies, most researchers warn against overenthusiastic interpretations of the findings. Nonetheless, they view the new field—whether it goes by the name of *psychoneuroimmunology* or simply *behavioral medicine*—as the hottest and most promising area of medical research today.[10]

The evidence for such a link has accelerated remarkably in the past few years. An article in *Time*[11] cited some examples: A ten-year follow-up study at Stanford University showed that women who were ill and received psychotherapy in groups survived nearly twice as long as similar women who didn't. Dr. Dean Ornish of the Preventive Medicine Research Institute in California showed that a mind-body program can reverse even severe coronary artery blockage after only a year, and he says the program may prevent it as well. Other studies have enabled researchers to predict which people in a group will become ill—based on nothing more than psychological profiles.

In yet another example of the growing body of evidence supporting the link between mind and body, the late Norman Cousins, formerly the editor of the *Saturday Review* and a member of the UCLA medical faculty, twice intrigued both the medical community and the public by overcoming usually fatal conditions—one, a massive heart attack, and another, an advanced case of ankylosing spondylitis (a degenerative spinal disease). Cousins followed his physicians' regimen each time, but also infused himself with vast doses of positive emotions and laughter. According to Cousins himself, he was healed not only by the miracle of modern medicine but also by the healing emotions of love, hope, faith, confidence, and a tremendous will to live. Because of his experiences, both with his own illness and with the hundreds of patients he saw, he became an acknowledged authority on the power of emotion. Cousins's belief that emotion plays a profound part in bringing on disease and helping to combat it is not his alone.

## A Brief History

The concept of and controversy surrounding the effect of emotions and stress on health are not new; the relationship between physical and psychosocial well-being has existed throughout history and across cultures.[12] More than 4,000 years ago, Chinese physicians noted that physical illness often followed episodes of frustration. Egyptian physicians of the same period prescribed good cheer and an optimistic attitude as ways to avoid poor health. Half a millennium before the birth of Christ, Hippocrates, considered the father of medicine, cautioned physicians that curing a patient required a knowledge of the "whole of things," of mind as well as body. That philosophy persisted for hundreds of years. In one of the best-known examples, the Greek physician Galen observed during the second century A.D. that melancholic women were much more prone to breast cancer than women who were cheerful.

In 600 A.D. in India, a well-regarded compilation of texts called the *Astangahradaya Sustrasthana* demonstrated a strong relationship between mental state and disease. The texts counseled physicians to "reject" patients who were "violent, afflicted with great grief, or full of fear." Further, it gave a poor prognosis to patients who were afflicted by intensely negative emotions. The texts warned that emotions such as hatred, violence, grief, and ingratitude are stronger than the body's capability for healthy balance, and those patients who could not abandon their negative emotions create new diseases as fast as a physician can heal an old one.

However, the suggested relationship between mental state and disease has not gone unchallenged. In the seventeenth century, the musings of philosopher-scientist René Descartes had a dramatic impact on the "holistic" attitude and philosophy of medicine. Descartes hypothesized that there were two separate substances in the world: matter, which behaved according to physical laws, and spirit, which was dimensionless and immaterial. The body was material, and the mind spiritual. His notion of a fundamental, unbridgeable chasm between the body and the spirit—between the brain and the mind—came to dominate not only medical philosophy but religious philosophy as well.

Research supported Descartes's theory, as it gained momentum throughout the beginning of the twentieth century. Robert Koch, a German country doctor, found that germs cause anthrax in sheep; this became one of the most significant medical discoveries of the time. In crude experiments, he recovered the anthrax germs from dying sheep, injected them into healthy sheep, and then watched those healthy sheep sicken and die of anthrax.

Since anthrax germs caused only anthrax disease, and no other disease, Koch theorized that every disease had a simple, specific cause: germs. The most respected medical authority of the time, Rudolf Virchow, disagreed; he subscribed to the theory that germs undoubtedly play a role in disease, but that many other factors were involved such as environment, heredity, nutrition, psychological state, preexisting health, and stress. However, Koch held stubbornly to his view, and so did most other practitioners of his day.

American physiologist Walter Cannon conducted a series of experiments early in this century that provided physical proof that glands in the body respond to stress. His early experiments demonstrated the relationship between stress and the hypothalamus, pituitary, and adrenal glands, and Cannon established himself as a pioneer of the relationship between the body's response to stress and its physiological symptoms. Several decades later, Austrian-born physician Hans Selye conducted brilliant and sophisticated experiments that gave us what we now know as the "fight-or-flight response" to stress.[13]

It was not until the 1960s that researchers began studying the immune system in earnest. The first time PNI was referred to as a science was in a 1964 paper by G. F. Solomon entitled "Emotions, Immunity, and Disease."[14] The immune defense system proved to be so complex that researchers were overwhelmed with the task of unraveling its parts and functions.

In the next major milestone, Stanford University psychiatrist David Spiegel and psychotherapist Irvin Yalom led support groups in the 1970s for women with advanced stages of breast cancer. The groups used a form of therapy in which they expressed their emotions about their cancer; Spiegel and Yalom found that the women who participated in the group therapy survived twice as long as the women who didn't participate in the therapy. The research attracted substantial attention from the medical community.

Not until the 1980s did immunologists finally start looking at the growing evidence that there might be anatomical links between the brain, the nervous system, and the immune system. This body of evidence split into three areas of research:

- The interaction between the nervous system, the immune system, and the neuroendrocine system
- The psychosocial components that influence immunity and their effects on health and disease
- The influence of immunity on psychological disorders and behavior

It is important to note that data from the last two branches of research are much more difficult to gather and interpret, leading to frequent controversy about research findings.

Today, the broad spectrum of scientists who devote their time to the study of the brain-immune system link concentrates on how emotions work to either enhance or cripple immune response. The most extensive current research is focusing on the effects of stress and depression on immunity.

## The Mind-Body Connection Today

As mentioned earlier in this chapter, the work of psychologist Robert Ader, whose key experiments laid the foundation for the field of mind-body research, gave the following evidence for connections between the mind, the immune system, and the nervous system:[15]

- The central nervous system is linked to both the bone marrow and the thymus (where immune system cells are produced) and to the spleen and lymph nodes, where such cells are stored.

- Scientists have found nerve endings in the tissues of the immune system. The lymphoid organs, such as the spleen, are thoroughly laced with nerve fibers.

- Changes in the brain and spinal cord affect how the immune system responds. That's not all: When researchers trigger an immune response in the body, there are changes in the way the brain and spinal cord function.

- Researchers have discovered that lymphocytes (important immune system cells) respond chemically to hormones and neurotransmitters, and that they can actually produce hormones and neurotransmitters. And receptors for neuromodulators and neurohormones have been found on the T lymphocytes.[16]

- Emotions trigger the release of hormones into the system—adrenaline, noradrenaline, endorphins, glucocorticoids, prolactin, and growth hormones, among others.

- Cells that are actively involved in an immune response produce substances that send signals to the central nervous system.

- The body's immune response can be influenced by stress; stress and other psychosocial factors can make the body more susceptible to infectious diseases (such as the common cold), autoimmune diseases (such as arthritis), or cancer.

- The body's immune response can be "trained," modified by the same kind of classical conditioning used in psychological experiments to train dogs.

- Immune function can be influenced and changed by psychoactive drugs, including alcohol, marijuana, cocaine, heroin, and nicotine.

■ The research into the relationship between the mind and the body has dramatic implications for treatment.

The way that we recognize, define, speak about, and behave in relation to our emotions may be heavily influenced by cognition, culture, history, location, gender, and other individual factors. With that in mind, physicians and surgeons on the cutting edge of technology are coming to realize that emotions as we perceive them play an extremely powerful role in both sickness and health. Dr. Theodore Miller of the renowned cancer institution, Memorial Hospital in New York, urged his fellow cancer surgeons to follow his example and not operate on patients who are convinced they will not survive surgery. In an address to the Society of Surgical Oncology, Miller told the surgeons that these patients usually do die, despite a technically successful operation.[17]

At least part of the power of emotions on health is due to their effect on the immune system. Jonas Salk, developer of the first polio vaccine, concluded years of his own scientific research by saying that "the mind, in addition to medicine, has powers to turn the immune system around." That power is so great, says Salk, that he advocates a major clinical study of the effects of emotions on the body, requiring dozens of years, millions of dollars, and an enormous number of scientists and children. It would be worth the investment, he says, if the study showed us conclusively that children who were positive and in control thrived and stayed healthier than their peers. "The people who do such a study," he concludes, "will be the poets of biology."[18]

As a science, PNI is still considered to be in its infancy, but already a number of medical schools are integrating it into their curricula and a host of federal grants are underwriting increased research. Most important, conferences on immunology now include at least one seminar on the relationship between the brain and the immune system. An increasing number of physicians are acknowledging that how a patient thinks and feels can be a powerful determinant of physical health.

# PNI: The Major Components

## The Brain

Five hundred years before the birth of Christ, the Greeks knew the brain as a three-pound organ inside the head.[19] Hippocrates believed that its role was to cool the blood and secrete mucus, which then flowed down through the nose. Through crude clinical observation over the ensuing years, beliefs about the brain and its function changed. In the Middle Ages, scientists regarded the brain as the seat of the soul. And during our own century, our ability to measure and analyze the electrical activity of the brain has generated major advances in understanding its function.

## What the Brain Is

The brain is a very privileged organ: It has a heart to supply it with blood, lungs to supply it with oxygen, intestines to supply it with nutrients, and kidneys to remove poisons from its environment. The most important part of our nervous system, it is the focal point of organization. For the body to survive, the nervous system, and particularly the brain, must be maintained; all other organs will sacrifice to keep the brain alive and functioning when the entire body is under severe stress.

By weight, 90 percent of the central nervous system is located inside the head in the form of the brain. A long extension of the brain, the spinal cord, descends down the back inside the spinal column. Nerves branch out to the sensory organs—the eyes, ears, and nose—from both the brain and the spinal cord. Nerves also branch out to the muscles, the skin, and all the organs of the body.

The brain itself is made up of nerve cells and nerve fibers. If you looked at a cross-section of the brain, you would see mostly gray matter (containing cells) and white matter (containing fibers surrounded by a fatty insulation called myelin). The fibers and nerves of the spinal cord, as well as those that branch out through the body, are also insulated with myelin; this insulation serves to isolate the nerve fibers so that electrical nerve impulses can't "short out."

Brain functions are modulated by **neuropeptides,** body chemicals that act directly on the nervous system—at least seventy have been identified, including endorphins (which regulate pain relief and happiness), enkephalins (which regulate pain relief), glucocorticoids (which regulate mood, sexual behavior, sleep, and food intake), and adrenaline (which regulates fear).[20] These neuropeptides alter behavior and mood, and they reside in various receptors.

The receptors are proteins with three-dimensional folding patterns that provide a site where cells of all types receive most of their information about what surrounds them. In essence, a signaling molecule (called a "ligand") fits into the receptor site and influences the behavior of the cells. These molecules, or ligands, can be free molecules (like hormones) or can be on the surface of other cells. When the molecules are located on the surface of other cells, the cells must come into actual contact in order for them to communicate.[21] The brain stem is rich with receptors, and certain types of receptors are also found on the cells of the central nervous system and the immune system.

The neurotransmitters are responsible for the direct transfer of signals from one cell to another through the receptors. The neuropeptides set the "tone" by altering how effective the transfer of signals is.

### *What the Brain Does*

Simply stated, the brain masterminds nerve impulses that are carried throughout the body and sends information to various parts of the body. It controls voluntary processes such as the direction, strength, and coordination of muscle movements; the processes involved in smelling, touching, and seeing; and other processes over which you have conscious control. The brain also controls many automatic, vital functions in the body, such as breathing, the rate of the heartbeat, digestion, bowels and bladder, blood pressure, and release of hormones.

Finally, the brain is the cognitive center of the body where ideas are generated, memory is stored, and emotions are experienced. The emotions that so affect the body originate in the brain, then, and this process explains the brain's powerful influence over the body as well as its link to the emotions and the immune system.

We are still learning about how the brain functions. For years, researchers believed that memories exist in the brain as fixed traces, carefully filed and stored. They taught that memory exists in a small seahorse-shaped section of the hippocampus and that other functions are centered in other localized areas of the brain. New research and a group of pioneering experts are now challenging that assumption.

In his book *The Invention of Memory: A New View of the Brain*, physician Israel Rosenfield presents the view that our brain is not "neatly and permanently wired up by our genes. Rather, whatever connections between nerve cells (neurons) we started with are continually reshaped by our experiences. It's a Darwinian struggle up there, and only the fittest connections— the ones that help us survive in our particular environment—get strengthened. Because experiences and contexts differ for each person, so do the connections. And since the demands of our own life vary over time, so do the patterns of connections, as some win and some lose."[22]

The philosophy of these pioneering scientists is "a radical departure from the past: Instead of having fixed memories, we invent what we remember. That is, we recategorize what we've learned, depending on the situation. We're creative magicians: The rabbit we pull out of memory's hat is different from the rabbit that went in—and so is the hat."[23]

According to Rosenfield's theory, we constantly reshape what enters our brain and we constantly assign new meaning to it. Our memory, he says, is inexact and fragmentary. His theory has begun to gain support in the scientific community, and even those who cannot wholeheartedly endorse it still admit that previous, rigid philosophies about the brain may not be entirely correct. Even if the theory is only partly valid, it may help explain how the brain so readily interacts with the emotions it produces and how its effect works on the body. According to Rosenfield, "A mental life cannot be reduced to molecules. Human intelligence is not just knowing more, but reworking, recategorizing, and thus generalizing information in new and surprising ways."[24]

The experience of emotion, then, "has less to do with specific locations in the brain and more to do with the complicated circuitry that interconnects them and the patterns of nerve impulses that travel along them," according to new research. California neuroscientist Floyd Bloom sums it up when he compares the manufacture of emotion to a television set. "There are individual tubes," he points out, "and you can say what they do, but if you take even one tube out, the television doesn't work."[25]

### Emotions Produced by the Brain

The emotions produced by the brain are, in a very real sense, a mixture of feelings and physical responses—and every time the brain manufactures an emotion throughout its loose network of lower brain structures and nerve pathways known as the limbic system, physical responses accompany those emotions. A report published in *U.S. News and World Report* presents a vivid picture of what happens as feelings and physical responses are combined:

> Seeing a shadow flit across your path in a dimly lit parking lot will trigger a complex series of events. First, sensory receptors in the retina of your eye detect the shadow and instantly translate it into chemical signals that race to your brain. Different parts of the limbic system and higher brain centers debate the shadow's importance. What is it? Have we encountered something like this before? Is it dangerous? Meanwhile, signals sent by the hypothalamus to the pituitary gland trigger a flood of hormones alerting various parts of your body to the possibility of danger, and producing the response called "fight or flight": Rapid pulse, rising blood pressure, dilated pupils, and other physiological shifts that prepare you for action. Hormone signals are carried through the blood, a much slower route than nerve pathways. So even after the danger is past— when your brain decides that the shadow is a cat's, not a mugger's—it takes a few minutes for everything to return to normal.[26]

This description tracks what happens with fear, a relatively uncomplicated emotion. According to brain researchers, the pathways of more complicated sensations, such as sadness or joy, are much more difficult to trace, but they are just as responsible for physical effects in the body.

### Chemicals Produced by the Brain

***Endorphins.***    The brain manufactures natural, morphine-like chemicals called endorphins; the word *endorphin* itself is a derivative of the term *endogenous morphines*. Endorphins work as the brain's natural painkiller, sometimes exerting analgesic effects more powerful than those of narcotic drugs; they also produce a sense of calm, happiness, and well-being (responsible for the well-known runner's high). The hot spot for endorphin receptors is the part of the brain known as the amygdala, or "pleasure center."

The role of endorphins is apparently much more complex than was originally thought. According to a report published in *Psychology Today*, endorphins play a role in "crying, laughing, thrills from music, acupuncture, placebos, stress, depression, chili peppers, compulsive gambling, aerobics, trauma, masochism, massage, labor and delivery, appetite, immunity, near-death experiences, and playing with pets."[27]

Scientists have also found that certain foods give people a "sensory hit" and stimulate the release of endorphins. The result is a "feel good all over" experience that causes us to relate pleasure with food. The main food is sugary sweets. Johns Hopkins psychologist Elliott Blass has found that giving a sugar solution to rats under stress calms them in the same way that administering morphine does. But when the rats are given a drug that blocks the release of endorphins, the sugary solution no longer has a calming effect.[28]

Can there be a downside to all this ecstasy? Apparently so. In moderate amounts, endorphins can produce calm, inspire happiness, kill pain, and give us the thrill of anticipation over a warm-from-the-oven slice of spicy apple pie. But when too many endorphins are released by the brain, the effect can be devastating to the immune system.

According to research conducted at UCLA, a flood of endorphins released in response to pain or stress can bind to the natural killer cells, immune system cells that search out and destroy tumor cells. When endorphins bind to the natural killer cells, they falter and become less effective in their role as the body's "surveillance system"; the immune system may not detect and subsequently destroy invaders.

***Peptides.***    Some of the most exciting brain-body research focuses on peptides, the body's natural chemical messengers. Pioneered by neuropharmacologist Candace Pert, peptide research studies the hormones that govern communication between the brain and the body cells. "There's probably a peptide solution to every medical problem," she says.[29] A band of researchers agrees with her—and believes peptide research may even hold the cure for Acquired Immunodeficiency Syndrome (AIDS).

Peptides are intercellular messengers that are widely distributed throughout the nervous system, the gastrointestinal tract, and the pancreas.[30] "We have currently identified sixty to seventy, a number that may change rapidly as research advances, and they act like a sophisticated game of telephone played by the brain, the immune system, and the other organs and systems,"[31] says Joan Goldberg.

## The Immune System

The immune system is a complex system consisting of about a trillion cells called lymphocytes, or white blood cells, and about a hundred million trillion molecules called antibodies. With these innate defenses, the immune system patrols and guards the body against attackers, both from the outside and from within. The most basic requirement of the immune system is that it can distinguish between "nonself" and "self" cells, and that it can then destroy the nonself invaders.[32] "Nonself" cells, or antigens, are unhealthy, dysfunctional, nonintegrated cells and tissues of the body, as well as foreign invading organisms such as bacteria and viruses. "Self" cells are the healthy, functional, integrated cells and tissues of the body. In destroying nonself cells, the immune system eliminates body cells and tissues that have become mutated or changed by disease or environmental factors.

Such action of the immune system is referred to as natural or innate immunity. Acquired immunity occurs when the immune system is exposed to a certain type of nonself cell. The next time an individual encounters the same antigen, the immune system is primed to destroy it. The degree of immunity depends on the kind of antigen, its amount, and how it enters the body. Infants are born with relatively weak immune responses, but they do get natural immunity during the first few months of life from antibodies they receive from their mothers. Children who are nursed receive even more antibodies through breast milk. In addition to acquiring immunity naturally, it is possible to be immunized with a vaccine. Vaccines contain microorganisms that have been altered so they produce an immune response but not full-blown disease.

According to Dr. Steven Locke, the associate director of Psychiatry Consultation Services at Beth Israel Hospital in Boston, the immune system does not operate within a biological vacuum but is sensitive to a number of outside influences. Locke sums up the role of the immune system as "a surveillance mechanism that protects the host from disease-causing microorganisms. It regulates susceptibility to cancers, infectious diseases, allergies, and autoimmune disorders."[33]

A variety of factors influence immunity and the immune system, including genetics, gender, age, and personality traits. When something goes awry in the immune system, infection results; when the entire immune system is compromised, as in AIDS, victims eventually die from overwhelming infections.

## Lymphoid Organs

The organs of the immune system are spread throughout the body.[34] They are generally referred to as lymphoid organs because they are concerned with the growth, development, and deployment of lymphocytes, the key operatives of the immune system. Lymphoid organs include the bone marrow, thymus, lymph nodes, and spleen, as well as the tonsils, appendix, and clumps of lymphoid tissue in the small intestine known as Peyer's patches.

Cells destined to become lymphocytes are produced in the bone marrow cells in the hollow shafts of the long bones. Some of these cells, known as stem cells, migrate to the thymus, a multilobed organ that lies high behind the breastbone. Stem cells that mature in the thymus are called T cells; there, they multiply and mature into cells capable of producing an immune response. Other lymphocytes, which appear to mature either in the bone marrow itself or in lymphoid organs other than the thymus, are called B cells.

Lymph nodes are small bean-shaped structures distributed throughout the body in strings in the neck, armpits, abdomen, and groin, for instance. Each lymph node contains a variety of specialized compartments. Some house T cells; others, B cells. Still others are filled with another type of immunocompetent cell, macrophages, which are discussed in the next section. Lymph nodes also contain webbed areas that enmesh antigens. The lymph node brings together the various components that are needed to produce the body's immune response.

Lymph nodes are linked by a network of lymphatic vessels similar to blood vessels; they carry lymph, a clear fluid that bathes all of the body's tissues and that contains a variety of cells, most of them lymphocytes. Like a system of small creeks and streams that empty into progressively larger rivers, the vessels of the lymphatic network merge into increasingly larger tributaries. At the base of the neck, the large lymphatic ducts empty into the bloodstream.

Lymph and the cells and particles it carries, including antigens (cell-surface glycoproteins that the body recognizes as foreign) that have entered the body, drain out of the body's tissues, seeping through the thin walls of the smallest lymph vessels. As the lymph passes through lymph nodes, antigens are filtered out and more lymphocytes are picked up. The lymphocytes, along with other assorted cells of the immune system, are carried to the bloodstream, which delivers them to tissues throughout the body. The lymphocytes patrol everywhere for foreign antigens, then gradually drift back into the lymphatic system to begin the cycle all over again.

During their travels, circulating lymphocytes may spend several hours in the spleen, an organ in the abdomen that contains a high concentration of lymphocytes. Anyone whose spleen has been damaged by trauma or disease is very susceptible to infection.

# The Immune System in Action

The immune system stockpiles a tremendous arsenal of immunocompetent cells. By storing just a few cells specific for each potential invader, it has room for the entire array. When an antigen appears, these few specifically matched cells are stimulated to multiply into a full-scale army. Later, to prevent this army from proliferating wildly, like a cancer, powerful suppressor mechanisms come into play.

*Lymphocytes* are the white cells that bear the major responsibility for carrying out the activities of the immune system; the immune system contains about a trillion of them. The two major classes of lymphocytes are the B cells and the T cells. The *B cells* secrete antibodies; each specific antibody exactly matches a specific invading antigen, much as a key fits a lock. These antibodies inactivate the antigens, rendering them incapable of causing disease. The body is capable of making antibodies to millions of antigens.

*T cells* do not secrete antibodies, but their help is essential for antibody production. The T cells act as both messengers and destroyers in the fight against pathogens. T cells ravage healthy cells from another person's body, which is why organ transplant recipients have problems with rejection. Some T cells become helper cells that turn on B cells or other T cells; others become suppressor cells that turn these cells off. Scientists believe there are as many as 100 million different varieties of T cells and another 100 million antibodies.

*Natural killer cells* are granular lymphocytes. As their name suggests, they attack and destroy other cells. They are called natural because they go into action without prior stimulation by a specific antigen. Most normal cells are resistant to natural killer cell activity. Most tumor cells, as well as normal cells infected with a virus, however, are susceptible. Thus, the natural killer cell may play a key role in immune surveillance against cancer, hunting down cells that develop abnormal changes.

*Macrophages* and *monocytes* are large cells that act as scavengers, or phagocytes: They can engulf and digest marauding microorganisms and other antigenic particles. Monocytes circulate in the blood, whereas macrophages are seeded through body tissues in a variety of guises.

Macrophages play a crucial role in initiating the immune response by "presenting" antigens to T cells in a special way that allows the T cells to recognize them. In addition, macrophages and monocytes secrete an amazing array of powerful chemical substances called *monokines* that help to direct and regulate the immune response.

*Granulocytes*, like macrophages and monocytes, are phagocytes and thus are capable of enveloping and destroying invaders. They contain granules filled with potent chemicals that enable them to digest microorganisms.

These chemicals also contribute to inflammatory reactions and are responsible for the symptoms of allergy.

Approximately twenty proteins circulate in the blood in inactive form and make up the immune system's complement system. The complement substances are triggered by antibodies that lock onto antigens; the result is often the redness, warmth, and swelling that occur with inflammation. They can also rapidly kill bacteria and other pathogens by puncturing their cell membranes.

## Malfunctions

Fortunately, the immune system usually functions according to plan. Unfortunately, there are factors that can cause breakdown or failure of the immune system. For example, the immune system weakens as we age. With aging, the thymus shrinks; at age twenty it has lost approximately 75 percent of its size and function, and it is virtually gone by age sixty. The result is a significant change in the number and activity of T cells. Aging also upsets the ratio of helper to suppressor cells, resulting in turning off the immune response. Still another effect of aging is the production of antibodies by B cells.

The immune system can also be suppressed by cancer, and it can be damaged by the drugs and radiation therapy used to treat cancer. These treatments kill the rapidly growing cancer cells in the body, but can also destroy normal cells, especially those of the immune system.

The body can also develop a serious overreaction to substances that are usually harmless. In this malfunction of the immune system, there is a severe allergic reaction; the result can be a condition like asthma or anaphylactic shock.

A similar malfunction of the immune system is what researchers have termed *autoimmune disease*. The fine mechanisms of the immune system become unbalanced, and the immune system reacts to normal body tissues as though it were allergic to them. Simply stated, the body attacks itself. Many of these diseases are serious, progressive ones, such as rheumatoid arthritis and systemic lupus erythematosus, a disease in which the immune system mistakes the body's own tissues as the enemy, attacking and destroying them.

Cells of the immune system themselves may undergo malignant transformation, resulting in diseases such as lymphoma or leukemia. Finally, the immune system may be damaged or even destroyed by viral infections (such as AIDS) or congenital diseases that cause abnormalities in the immune system. Such immune system failures are called immunodeficiency diseases. When the immune system breaks down as a result of these diseases, the body is overwhelmed by infections and cancers because it can't destroy invading organisms.

We've known for years that disease can affect the immune system, but a more recent series of studies gives ample evidence that thoughts and emotions can also. Although a number of hormones and neurotransmitters can modulate the immune system, all of these are subservient to the emotions and beliefs of the individual.[35]

## The Brain-Immune System Connection

The brain directs physiological processes in two ways: *neural*, communicating with cells through the nerves that innervate the glands and organs, and *endocrine*, stimulating the production of circulating hormones that then communicate with the cells.[36]

The connection between the brain and central nervous system and the immune system allows the mind to influence either susceptibility or resistance to disease. For example, the thymus gland plays an essential role in the maturation of immune system cells, and researchers have discovered extensive networks of nerve endings laced throughout the thymus gland.[37] Rich supplies of nerves also serve the spleen, bone marrow, and lymph nodes, giving further evidence of a link between the brain and the immune system.

Further, the cells of the immune system seem equipped to respond to chemical signals from the central nervous system. For example, the surface of the lymphocytes has been found to contain receptors for a variety of central nervous system chemical messengers,[38] such as catecholamines, prostaglandins, serotonin, endorphins, sex hormones, thyroid hormone, and growth hormone. National Institute of Mental Health researchers discovered that "certain white blood cells were equipped with the molecular equivalent of antennas tuned specifically to receive messages from the brain."[39] Macrophages and lymphocytes—themselves immune system cells—also produce hormones called *cytokines* that signal the brain in the same way as traditional hormones.[40]

More than three decades ago, Soviet researcher Elena Korneva discovered at the Institute of Experimental Medicine in Leningrad (now St. Petersburg) that she could produce changes in the immune system by selectively damaging different parts of the hypothalamus. Expanding on that theory, French researcher Gerard Renoux showed not only that the brain influences immunity, but also that different sides of the brain exercise different kinds of immunity. Renoux's brain experiments on mice show the profound influence of the brain—and the differing influences as well. When Renoux removed a third of the left side of the mouse's brain, the mouse could no longer respond with vigor to foreign material. When part of the right brain was removed, the number of T cells in the mouse's spleen was decreased.

Because of these receptors on the lymphocytes, physical and psychological stress alter the immune system. Stress has been shown to affect the T cells, B cells, natural killer cells, and lymphocytes. One of the most frequently implicated ways in which stress alters immunity, however, is by suppression of the natural killer cells, which could have important implications on cancer prognosis and the progression of HIV infection.[41]

Stress causes the body to release several powerful neurohormones—including catecholamines, corticosteroids, and endorphins—which bind with the receptors on the lymphocytes and alter immune function. Corticosteroids, in fact, have been found to have such a powerful influence in suppressing the immune system that they are widely used to treat allergic conditions (such as asthma and hay fever) and autoimmune disorders (such as rheumatoid arthritis and rejection of transplanted organs). These corticosteroids and other brain chemicals are unleashed by the hypothalamus, a section of the brain that is a virtual drug factory. The chemicals released by the hypothalamus have the most profound effects on the immune system.

The link between the mind and the immune system has gained a new dimension with the growing evidence that psychosocial factors directly affect immune function. The resulting findings have the potential of influencing a wide range of disorders, including allergies, infections, autoimmune diseases, and even cancer.

PNI research has demonstrated that our psychological, behavioral, and physical processes are closely integrated. Illnesses don't just happen: many are caused by bacteria, viruses, fungi, or other microbes. But what factors determine whether you will fall ill when exposed to these? What determines your immunity?

Part of immunity seems determined by emotions—how you think and feel. What is going on inside your mind, your heart, and your spirit may have tremendous impact on what happens to your body. In a thirty-year study of initially healthy young men, those with the most mature emotions and psychological style—including a sense of humor, an altruistic bent, and so on—were the healthiest thirty years later.[42] After thirty-five years, only 3 percent of those who dealt with the stresses of life in a mature, adaptive way had any chronic illness, as compared with the 38 percent who were either dead or chronically ill in the other group (who coped by using denial, blaming, repression, and intellectualization).

The result of this study supports the case for a new way of practicing medicine. There are several solid principles behind the notion of mind-body medicine. First, mind-body medicine appears to work through complex physiologic systems that are not normally under voluntary control.[43] For example, the production and release of natural opioids (painkillers) can be stimulated by hypnotic suggestion—and can be so powerful that patients can undergo surgery without the use of anesthesia. Biofeedback training can alter blood pressure, heart rate, and other vital signs. Meditation can bring about muscle relaxation, reduced heart rate, and slowed breathing. The physiological conditions that result from these types of mind-body medicine are directly opposite of the physical effects of stress—and work to promote, not impair, health.

The second principle behind mind-body medicine is that the peptides carry not only information about the nervous system and the body's physical functions, but also information about the emotions. That's not all: Information about the emotions is carried throughout the body, potentially impacting every body system.

## The Immune System and Emotion

In reality, it may be too simplistic to say that emotions cause disease. More accurately, emotions are only one important factor in the body's ability to execute resistance mechanisms when it is exposed to causative factors. Normal homeostasis, the optimal balance of hormones, immunity, and nervous system functioning, protects us from the many threats to health we encounter daily. Disrupted emotional responses, and feeling "out of control," lead to disrupted homeostasis. Physiological processes then get out of control. Interestingly, the same part of the midbrain that controls most automatic homeostasis and keeps physiology balanced also controls emotional response, allowing responses to be "enough, but not too much."

There's a physiological reason why emotions can impact health. Different parts of the brain are associated not only with specific emotions, but also with specific hormone patterns. The experience ("release") of certain hormones, then, is associated with different emotional responses, and those hormones affect health.[44] As one example, we know that emotionally induced shifts in hormones can lead to chronic disease, such as high blood pressure. When a person is aggressive and anxious, too much norepinephrine and epinephrine are secreted, even at rest. The arteries thicken, and the excess hormones cause blood vessel muscles to constrict. The gradual rise in blood pressure can then result in hypertension, stroke, or heart failure.[45]

Other studies have borne similar results. It has long been believed, for instance, that as many as 70 percent of all people who go to a gastrointestinal specialist have irritable bowel syndrome, a mixture of pain, diarrhea, constipation, nausea, and sometimes vomiting. Most are women, and most have some kind of an emotional problem. One-fourth of gastroenterology patients have major depression.

One scientific study reported in the *Medical Journal of Australia* tested what would happen when irritable bowel syndrome patients received psychotherapy instead of conventional medical treatment for their condition. The result was that symptoms among the treated patients improved dramatically. After receiving counseling for their emotional upsets, 89 percent of the patients reported less pain as a result; 96 percent had less diarrhea, 90 percent had less constipation, 92 percent were less nauseated, and 81 percent had less vomiting. Researchers who conducted the study concluded that "the symptoms of irritable bowel syndrome were seen as a physical expression of emotions caused by recent loss or ongoing stressful life situations."[46]

Feeling these emotions is only one factor in the subsequent development of disease. Many researchers believe that the inability to express emotions is an even greater cause of disease. Studies have confirmed that the failure to perceive and express emotions can lead to various disease states.[47] Yale surgeon Bernie S. Siegel, well known for his humanistic work with cancer patients, put it this way:

> *Patients must be encouraged to express all their angers, resentments, hatred, and fears. These emotions are signs that we care to the utmost when our lives are threatened. Time after time, research has shown that people who give vent to their negative emotions survive adversity better than those who are emotionally constricted. Among patients with spinal-cord injuries, those who express strong grief and anger make more progress in rehabilitation than those with a more stoical attitude. Mothers who show great distress after giving birth to a deformed infant give the child better care than those who seem to take the misfortune calmly. In a study of people living near Three Mile Island, Dr. Andrew Baum found that those who showed their rage and fear suffered far less from stress and psychological problems than those who took a "rational" approach. Unexpressed feelings depress your immune response.*[48]

In a battery of tests conducted by Leonard Derogatis, it was found that breast cancer patients who showed little emotion were the ones who died early on. The "survivors" were the ones who felt and openly expressed a lot of anger, fear, depression, and guilt.[49] Apparently, the process of suppressing emotion contributed to the tenacity of the disease.

Infectious diseases—such as infectious hepatitis or gonorrhea—are caused by identifiable microorganisms such as bacteria or viruses. But emotions can even determine in part how susceptible we are to these infectious agents, and whether they will actually make us sick.

An excellent example is the herpes simplex virus, which causes fever blisters and cold sores. Most adults harbor this virus in a quiescent state at all times. It often resides around the nostrils and the mouth but remains dormant and does not cause sores. Sometimes, in response to lowered resistance, it flares up, especially when the person is ill with something else (such as the common cold). Many times, it flares up in response to emotional upset. In fact, mental stress is the most common precipitant of herpes skin lesions.

A number of studies have demonstrated the power of emotions in bringing on an attack of herpes virus infection. In one, students who had a high prevalence of cold sores throughout college found that their cold sores occurred less frequently after graduation, when stress levels were lower.[50]

Medical officer Jerome M. Schneck at California's Fort MacArthur recalls a soldier who could accurately predict when his herpes simplex infection would become active. He knew that as soon as he felt hostile emotions, he could anticipate a breakout. He also learned that if he channeled his hostility into something else (such as reading), he was able to prevent the lesions from erupting.[51]

One of the reasons why strong negative emotions may be linked to illness is that negative emotional response, whether it be stress, anger, or sadness, may disrupt the immune system. When you experience strong emotions, your body responds much like it would in the classic "fight-or-flight" response model. Endocrine system activity sends hormones coursing through the bloodstream, which in turn send messages back to the nervous system. As the chemical response gradually builds, your body reaches its physical threshold and ability to deal with the stress of negative emotion; thus, one becomes more susceptible to illness.

Evidence also suggests that emotions send chemical messages to the brain; in response, the brain alters involuntary physiologic responses. The resulting alteration may affect the way the immune system responds to messages from the brain in the presence of disease.[52]

One of the most startling examples of how the mind can alter the immune response was discovered by accident. In 1975, Dr. Ader wanted to condition mice to avoid saccharin. He accomplished this by feeding the mice saccharin while simultaneously injecting a drug that caused upset stomach and that, incidentally, also suppressed the immune system. Associating the saccharin with the stomach pains, the mice soon learned to avoid the sweetener.

Ader then decided to try to reverse the taste aversion to saccharin. This time, Ader gave the same mice saccharin again, but without the drug that caused upset stomach. He was startled to find that the mice who had received the highest amounts of sweeteners during the initial conditioning died when they received saccharin alone. Ader speculated that he had so successfully conditioned the mice that saccharin alone now weakened their immune systems enough to kill them.[53] No previous research had documented a link between the mind and the immune system; until Ader's work, the two were assumed to work independently of each other.

New research indicates that the immune system may be affected by any kind of emotion, negative or positive. In one study, natural killer cells were taken from both depressed and nondepressed people; the natural killer cells were then placed in contact with cancer cells. The natural killer cells from nondepressed people quickly surrounded and destroyed the cancer cells; those from the depressed people did nothing.[54]

Because of findings like these, a number of agencies within the National Institutes of Health (NIH) have called for increased clinical trials to integrate the techniques of mind-body medicine with those of traditional medicine—treatment that relies on drugs and surgery. And as physicians become more comfortable with this knowledge, medicine that addresses both the mind and the body will become a routine component of whole-person clinical care.

## The Role of Religion

Throughout recorded history, most religions have included healing practices; all early human civilizations dealt with physical illness in spiritual or religious terms, including the Mesopotamian, Egyptian, Indian, Chinese, Greek, and Roman civilizations.[55] These healing methods often used supernatural kinds of treatment, such as incantations, prayers, or religious pilgrimages. Until the last several decades, no one considered that the healing associated with spiritual or religious beliefs could actually be tied to natural mechanisms, such as psychosocial and behavioral factors.

More than 850 studies have now been completed showing that spiritual and religious factors have substantial impact on the factors that increase health and immunity. Religion and spirituality help people cope with stress; in one survey, 78 percent of Americans of all ages—and nearly 90 percent of older adults—said religion provided comfort and support.[56] Almost half of the medical patients in another survey indicated that religion was the *most important factor* in enabling them to cope with serious illness; the other half said it helps to a moderate or large degree.[57] Religion and spirituality have also been shown to contribute to positive emotions—such as life satisfaction, happiness, well-being, optimism, and hope—which have been shown to help protect the immune system. People who are involved in religious practice also consistently report stronger social support—a finding that holds true even for those who participate only in private religious practices, such as prayer.[58] Those who attend religious services have a significantly higher number of in-person contacts, nonkin ties, telephone calls, and instrumental support, all of which benefit health. In the last decade, twelve of thirteen studies have demonstrated a significant relationship between greater religious involvement, better physical health, and longer survival.[59]

There are several other reasons why religious and spiritual practice enhance physical health and improve immune function:[60]

- **Health behaviors.** Religious involvement has been associated with a lower incidence of many high-risk behaviors such as cigarette smoking, alcoholism, drug use, risky sexual activity, drinking while driving, and failure to use seat belts. While these certainly explain some of the association between religious activity and health, researchers caution that they should not minimize the importance of religion itself.

- **Health care practices.** Often because of the increased social support, people involved in religious practice are more likely to have their medical illnesses diagnosed sooner, monitored more regularly, and treated more effectively. People who are active in religious faith also tend to be more compliant with medical treatment.

- **Stress buffering.** Spiritual faith and religious involvement tend to produce a more hopeful and optimistic worldview, which helps people cope with both short-term and chronic stress. Religious people tend to turn to their faith for help in dealing with stressful situations (including serious illness and death) instead of to practices that could harm them, such as alcohol, cigarettes, or drugs.

Only a handful of studies have investigated the relationship between religion and immunity; while these are promising, additional research needs to be done to determine actual causes and effects.

## The Emotion-Immunity Connection in Heart Disease, Cancer, and Other Conditions

Research into the impact of emotions on immunity is gradually changing the way we look at disease, and it has prompted even more research by scientists eager to determine the depth of the connection.

### Heart Disease

Solid research shows that psychological factors can be substantial risk factors for both coronary artery disease and myocardial infarction.[61] Psychological risk factors have been classified into three categories, depending on their duration:

- **Acute triggers,** like acute stress or outbursts of anger. Outbursts of anger can cut off oxygen to the heart, resulting in myocardial infarction; acute anger has been shown to double the risk of heart attack. In

advanced stages of cardiovascular disease, angry outbursts can cause
the rupture of arterial plaque, resulting in stroke or heart attack.

- **Factors that last from several weeks to several years,** including
exhaustion and depression.

- **Chronic factors,** including negative personality traits (such as hostility) and low socioeconomic status.

Angina—chest pain that occurs when the heart muscle is temporarily
deprived of oxygen—can be caused by physical exertion, but is also aggravated by emotional stress. "Excessive stress can trigger an angina attack,"
points out James L. Levenson, assistant professor of psychiatry at the Medical College of Virginia. "In some forms of stress the adrenal glands secrete
epinephrine—the hormone associated with the 'fight-or-flight' response.
This, in turn, increases heart rate and blood pressure and hence the workload on the heart. . . . Some patients may be more vulnerable to artery
spasms at these times."

According to comprehensive research, the most common feature of
sudden cardiac death is "marked emotional perturbation," a flood of strong
emotion. The most provocative emotional circumstances that lead to sudden death include the death of, or threat of injury to, a loved one; the early
grief period following any loss; and the threat of personal injury.

Extreme emotional stress in people with otherwise structurally normal
hearts can lead to primary arrhythmias (disturbance in heart rhythm that
causes it to beat unusually fast or slow). In people who have coronary
artery disease, the effects of emotional stress are even more severe and can
result in angina, silent ischemia, or fatal arrhythmias.

In one study of twenty-five people who suffered life-threatening
arrhythmias following acute emotional stress, eleven had no heart disease.
Two follow-up studies showed that people can suffer life-threatening disruptions of the heart rhythm in response to emotional stress, even if they
have no underlying heart disease.

An emotional upheaval can drive up blood pressure; getting extremely
angry can "make your blood boil." According to a report in the *Journal of
Nervous and Mental Disease*, data from forty-eight studies over a ten-year
period show that the primary psychological characteristics of many people
with high blood pressure are anger and hostility, difficulty with interpersonal contacts, and frequent denial and self-repression.[62] The reason is
physiological: Strong emotion causes the body to pump epinephrine (popu-
larly called adrenaline) into the system. Adrenaline has two effects on the
cardiovascular system: It speeds up the heart, and it constricts the blood
vessels. The result is high blood pressure.

## Cancer

Until recently, cancer was not thought to be influenced by thought or emotion. Now, however, researchers are convinced that the immune processes involved in tumor growth may indeed be subject to psychosocial influences.[63]

One of the most solid connections and research directions has been the influence of stress on cancer. Research has focused on two possible relationships: the impact of stress on disease progression and the impact of stress on immunity.[64]

### Stress and Cancer Progression

In a study of women with family histories of cancer, researchers found that these women had lower natural killer cell activity, as did women who were suffering from stress, regardless of their family histories. The findings suggested that stress not only could make the women more susceptible to cancer, but also could impair the ability of the immune system to recover from changes caused by stress.[65]

In a series of studies spanning five years, researchers found an association between stress and the progression of breast cancer and decreased natural killer cell activity.[66] When examining these and other studies, however, caution should be used: The reduced natural killer cell activity caused by stress may indeed impair immunity and contribute to the progression of the cancer—or, on the other hand, the progression of the cancer itself might trigger a cytokine or other hormone that reduces the number of natural killer cells.

Stress can also impact immunity and contribute to cancer progression because of its impact on the neuroendocrine system. We know that stress causes the adrenal glands to produce cortisol—and we know that cortisol suppresses the immune system. Cortisol has also been shown to stimulate the growth of tumors by increasing blood flow to the tumors. Adrenal hormones other than cortisol that are produced in response to stress have also been shown to increase tumor growth.[67]

### Stress and Immunity in Cancer

According to the most widely accepted theory, cancer cells are constantly being formed from normal cells in the body, but according to Jerome Frank, "as long as the individual's natural immune system holds up, these cells are detected and destroyed before they can begin to multiply. When a person's body defenses break down, the cells grow and reproduce and cancer develops. It may be that psychological factors affect the strength of the immune system, and thereby play a part in the occurrence of cancer."[68]

Some studies at the University of Pennsylvania involved injecting cancer cells into animals under much mental stress, then comparing their responses with those of nonstressed animals that were similarly injected. The stressed animals were further divided into two groups: One was truly victimized, the stressor being out of their control, whereas animals in the other group were given warnings that allowed them to abort the stressor. Their ability to reject the cells and remain cancer-free revealed some striking differences in the groups. Those in the stressed group that had control over the stressor immunologically rejected the cancer 63 percent of the time, as compared with only 28 percent in the "victim" group. Animals that were not stressed rejected the cells 60 percent of the time, revealing a trend seen repeatedly in many such studies: It's not the actual stress that is most important, but rather the ability to deal well with stress and an ability to gain a sense of control.

### *Mind-Body Influences on Cancer*

Many studies conducted by researchers throughout the world have shown that cancer-prone persons tend to deny or repress unpleasant emotions, especially anger, hostility, and depression. As one researcher put it, "They seem to be out of touch with their own wants and needs, choosing to effect a permanent pleasant attitude and personality, regardless of the bleakness of their inner lives."[69]

The connection between repressed emotions and the development of cancer was recognized in a research setting as early as two decades ago. Dr. Caroline B. Thomas of Johns Hopkins Medical School did an exhaustive thirty-year study to determine how well psychological factors predicted five different disease states. This was one of the first prospective studies in that it detailed the psychological characteristics of people before they were diagnosed with disease.

Dr. Thomas and her team found that the disease most correlated with psychological traits was cancer. They also determined that three specific characteristics predispose a person to developing cancer: a perceived lack of closeness with one or both parents, responding to stress with a sense of hopelessness, and bottling up emotions or having impaired emotional outlets.

The emergence of specific emotional patterns among many cancer patients led researchers to identify what they call "the cancer personality" (a spin-off from the kind of research that led to identification of the Type A personality). According to researchers, those who have a cancer-prone personality often equate close personal relationships with suffering and rejection—possibly because of negative emotional experiences in childhood—and they conceal their true feelings of isolation behind a mask of cheerful self-confidence.[70]

In commenting on the trademarks of a cancer-prone personality, psychologist Eugene Blumberg noted that "we were impressed by the polite, apologetic, almost painful acquiescence of the patients with rapidly progressing disease, as contrasted with the more expressive and sometimes bizarre personalities of those who responded brilliantly to therapy with remissions and long survival."[71] The patients in Blumberg's study who had the fastest-growing tumors tended to be "consistently serious, overcooperative, over-nice, overanxious, painfully sensitive, passive, apologetic personalities," and had been all their lives. Another specialist in catastrophic illness, Lawrence LeShan, pointed out that "the big thing the majority of cancer victims have in common is that they have lost their major outlet for creative energy. The death of a spouse, retirement, whatever, has closed off their channel of expression, their uniqueness."

Repression of emotions has been linked so closely with cancer proneness that many researchers are now considering it a valid risk factor for cancer. Several long-term studies have stressed the link between cancer and emotions. One of the best-known was conducted on medical students who attended Johns Hopkins University between 1948 and 1964. Students were shown a series of ten Rorschach inkblots and were asked to describe what they saw. Twenty years after the last students were given the inkblot tests, psychologist Pirkko L. Graves and her colleagues rated the responses on an eleven-point scale that pinpointed varying degrees of positive and negative emotions.[72]

Graves and her colleagues had not set out to do a cancer study; initially they had wanted to see what kinds of emotions led to later mental illness. They found that those whose pattern of scores indicated distant, withdrawn approaches to relationships and poorly balanced emotions were more likely to have developed a severe mental disorder by 1984. And, much to their surprise, the researchers found that the same pattern of scores was linked to the later appearance of cancer, particularly cancers of the stomach, pancreas, rectum, large intestine, and lymph nodes such as Hodgkin's disease, leukemia, and multiple myeloma.

Refining the original study, Graves and her colleagues chose 972 medical students from the study and divided them into five groups based on fourteen psychological measures. They then kept track of the students for thirty years. Those who suppressed their emotions were sixteen times more likely to develop cancer than those who expressed their emotions freely and took active measures to relieve their frustrations or anger.

Similar findings emerged from a controversial long-term study conducted in Yugoslavia by University of South Florida psychologist Charles D. Spielberger and his Dutch colleague Henk M. van der Ploeg. Although some believe their study was flawed, it did show that repression and denial of emotions on a regular basis were related to increased risk for both cancer and heart disease.

Some studies show that emotions can be even more powerful as a predictor of cancer than factors such as cigarette smoking.[73] Cigarette smoking is a direct cause of lung cancer. Although the majority of those who develop lung cancer are cigarette smokers, most cigarette smokers do not develop lung cancer. Researchers hoping to find the difference between the smokers who develop cancer and those who don't studied more than 1,000 industrial workers in Glasgow, Scotland, who came to a health clinic with respiratory complaints. Dr. David Kissen and his colleagues tested all of the men psychologically before performing a physical examination and rendering a diagnosis.

He found that those who had cancer when they came to the clinic displayed what he and his colleagues called "a striking inability to express emotions." The inability was significant enough that they were vastly different from the men who did not have cancer.

Researchers who saw the results of Kissen's study were eager to perform a similar test. Two of them, Dr. R. L. Horne of the Shreveport Veterans Administration Hospital and Dr. R. S. Picard of the Washington University School of Medicine, believed that, if Kissen's findings were correct, they could actually predict which patients had cancer based on psychological findings alone. The group headed by Horne and Picard used a variety of studies on lung cancer, including Kissen's, to develop a composite scale of psychological variables. They then began testing patients who came to the hospital complaining of respiratory complaints, and, based on the results of the psychological testing, they made predictions about which patients had lung cancer. They made these predictions without the benefit of any physical examination. The result was that they were able to predict which men had cancer and which had benign lung disease with 73 percent accuracy, a rate researchers regard as "highly significant."

In discussing the results of their study, Horne and Picard maintain that "emotional repression is part of a personality pattern that led to grave difficulties in coping with life's challenges and sorrows. After the loss of a central relationship—with a person or a valued job—those with cancer often reported profound depression, which had predated the cancer by six to eighteen months."

## Diabetes

The link between emotions and diabetes was made as early as the seventeenth century, when British physician Thomas Willis noted that diabetes first appeared in many cases among patients who had experienced significant life stresses. Nearly 200 years later, Claude Bernard, considered the father of modern physiology, found that he could produce diabetes in a normal animal by making a lesion in the area of the hypothalamus. That finding helps explain why there could be a link between stress, anxiety, and diabetes, which may be linked to an upset in the central nervous system.

Recent research shows that there may very well be a "diabetic personality": those most prone to diabetes are characterized by decreased alertness, apathy, and depression. Some researchers also believe that diabetics are more prone to immaturity, passivity, masochism, and perhaps even sexual identity problems. Children with diabetes have a greater tendency for anxiety, aggressiveness, and problems with self-perception. Interpretation of this association needs to be tempered, however, by the fact that some of these behaviors could be affected by erratic blood sugar control.

## Chronic Pain

Research has shown that the pain center of the brain—the anterior cingulate cortex (ACC)—is directly influenced by emotions. As a result, emotional pain can cause literal physical pain. In a study by UCLA scientist Naomi I. Eisenberger published in *Science*, research shows that a rejected lover's broken heart may cause as much distress in the pain center of the brain as an actual physical injury.

In commenting on the study, Bowling Green State University psychologist Jaak Panksepp wrote, "Throughout history, poets have written about the pain of a broken heart. It seems that such poetic insights into the human condition are now supported by neurophysiological findings."

While patients with chronic pain overuse the health care system and drive up health care costs, they rarely get significant relief from their symptoms when given traditional medical treatment. Convincing evidence shows that mind-body medicine is much more effective in the treatment of chronic pain.

In one important study,[74] more than 100 patients with various types of chronic pain symptoms received mind-body treatment. At the end of the first ten weeks, the patients still had pain, but reported less anxiety, depression, and hostility. As treatment continued, the pain began to decrease, and the other symptoms continued to improve as well. By the end of a year, the patients were visiting the clinic 36 percent less often; visits continued to decline during the second year of treatment. The savings from medical care were significant during the first year, and doubled during the second year. The implications? Using mind-body therapies to treat victims of chronic pain could result in improvement for the patients and cost savings for the health care system.

Interest in studies like this one is so high that the National Institutes of Health convened a technology assessment conference to examine the usefulness of combining behavioral approaches with traditional treatments for patients with chronic pain and insomnia. Participants in the conference included experts in behavioral medicine, pain medicine, sleep medicine, psychiatry, nursing, psychology, neurology, behavioral sciences, and neurosciences. They concluded that behavioral medicine approaches should definitely be used in the treatment of both chronic pain and insomnia.

Based on current studies, researchers estimate that as much as 95 percent of all back pain—some of the most stubborn chronic pain—is triggered by the psyche, not by physical abnormalities or by heavy lifting. According to New York psychiatrist Hans Draus, back muscles tense up in response to emotional stress. If the muscles remain tensed too long, they start to hurt. In people whose backs hurt the most, the best predictor of pain is a psychological problem, such as depression.[75] Tense muscles are more prone to injury—so those who are emotionally upset and whose back muscles are tense are more likely to injure their backs with even minor exertion.

## Mind-Body Influence on Other Conditions

Research has solidly shown a mind-body component in a host of other conditions:

### Allergies and Asthma

The process involved in allergy is fairly basic: The white blood cells, part of the body's defense system, mistake a harmless substance (such as wheat or pollen) for an enemy agent. In response, the white cells produce antibodies that latch onto cells in the nose, throat, lungs, stomach, intestines, or skin in readiness for battle. The result is a full-blown allergy attack. The most common antibody produced in allergy is Immunoglobulin E (IgE). Research has shown that stress and emotional strain cause the level of IgE in the blood of animals to increase. In one study, guinea pigs were subjected first to stress and then to a chemical irritant. They showed greater skin sensitivity to the irritant than did a similar group of mice that had not first been stressed. Studies of humans show similar results.

Physiologically, asthma is much the same as allergies. Repeated studies have shown that bronchial asthma is closely tied to emotional factors; feelings of frustration and conflict are often what trigger an attack. Psychiatrist Iris R. Bell concludes that, based on scientific evidence, any period of stress or intense emotion can weaken the immune system so that you react more easily to food or chemicals, which can increase susceptibility to either asthma or allergies.

### Arthritis

A wide variety of studies has focused on the causes of arthritis, and emotional upheaval or stress keeps surfacing as a significant factor in the disease. In one study, researchers found that arthritis sufferers "try overly hard to be nice to other people, to not lean on others for emotional support, and to stow things away down inside, especially anger." Researchers who conducted the study pointed out that those traits antedated the arthritis, not the other way around.

The situation is similar for sufferers of rheumatoid arthritis. Many have a history of long-term tension or emotional upheaval in their lives. In addition, says clinical psychologist Robert Fathman, they are generally full of inner turmoil, likely to be excessively conscientious, fearful of criticism, frequently depressed, and battling a poor self-image. The end result, according to Fathman, is that "these people have so much repressed anger that it 'eats them up.' The anger gets turned against the person herself." Fathman also pointed out that perhaps one reason women are afflicted with rheumatoid arthritis as much as four times more frequently than men is "because of what we do to little girls in our society. We teach them that it's wrong to get angry." Renowned rheumatologist Loring T. Swaim concluded, after years in private practice, that emotional factors are crucial in the development, and perhaps even the causation, of rheumatoid arthritis. Based on results of the studies being done today, a growing number of researchers are agreeing with that assessment.

## Dental Cavities

Emotions have been shown to play a role even in the development of dental cavities. Based on the results of a handful of studies, researchers at the Temple University School of Dentistry say that stressful thoughts and emotions can actually contribute to the mechanisms that cause dental caries. In one test, researchers analyzed the saliva of a group of twelve dental students both before and after a twenty-minute meditation session. The saliva was opaque and contained moderate to high levels of bacteria before the meditation session. After the students had become deeply relaxed, their saliva became watery and translucent, and bacteria levels decreased. "Considering the salivary changes that occur during stress," the researchers noted, "it could be hypothesized that chronic stress would be a causative factor in the development of dental caries." The same factors are apparently at play in gum disease as well.

## Stomach Ulcers

In a series of tests designed to determine the most likely causes of gastric ulcers, gastroenterologists Charles Richardson and Mark Feldman found that ulcer patients had a much higher prevalence of emotional distress than volunteers who did not have ulcers. The physicians and their colleagues at the University of Texas Health Sciences Center at Dallas found that certain emotions, especially hostility, resentment, guilt, and frustration, are associated with increased acid in the stomach, which contributes to ulcers.

Researchers have also discovered that in many cases, stress appears to be less important than is an infection with a bacterium called *H. pylori.*

### Irritable Bowel Syndrome

Emotions are linked to irritable bowel syndrome, a painful combination of cramping, diarrhea, and occasional vomiting. According to Johns Hopkins Medical School Associate Professor of Behavioral Biology William E. Whitehead, the gastrointestinal tract is particularly susceptible to emotional stress and "very readily comes under the influence of external factors and events." He says that irritable bowel syndrome tends to occur among people who overreact to everyday worries; sufferers tend to be both more anxious and more depressed than others. They may have nagging concerns about family problems, work problems, or finances, and studies show that they usually have a number of other stress-related problems, such as headaches or insomnia.

### Pregnancy-Related Problems

Major emotional setbacks in a woman's life during pregnancy can determine the course of the pregnancy and can even result in premature delivery and low birth weight. Psychosocial stress during pregnancy alters the mother's immune system, which has negative effects on the pregnancy and birth—including infection during pregnancy, complications during pregnancy, and less than optimal development of the infant.[76] Researchers who studied more than 200 women at St. Mercy's Hospital in Manchester, England, showed that low birth weight and prematurity were associated with major life events. Stressful events had the greatest impact, the researchers said, when they occurred during the final three months of pregnancy.

### Sexual Dysfunction

Research that gives credence to folklore shows that emotions and emotional stress cause real physiological changes that result in sexual dysfunction. Helen Singer Kaplan, head of the sex therapy and education program at Payne Whitney Clinic of New York Hospital, says, "Depression, stress, and fatigue can damage sexuality profoundly. When a patient is severely depressed, sex is the furthest [sic] thing from his mind. Even moderately depressed patients lose interest in pursuing sexual activity and are very difficult to seduce and arouse." Even people with "normal sexual appetites can psychologically turn themselves off with overwhelming problems," maintains Wanda Sadoughi, director of the sexual dysfunction clinic at Chicago's Cook County Hospital. "By the time some patients come to the clinic, they are having major dysfunctional problems . . . but before all that occurred, the first symptom some of these people had was a loss of desire." Strong emotions and emotional stress affect the central nervous system, causing it to curtail sharply the body's testosterone supply. Testosterone is essential in both men and women for normal sexual desire and performance.

### The Common Cold

Research shows that while negative emotions can give the immune system a beating, even small pleasures can give it a big boost. In a study reported at the annual meeting of the Society for Behavioral Medicine, psychologist Arthur Stone of the State University of New York Medical School tracked 100 men for three months. He found that both stress and pleasure had an effect on the immune system, but here's the real news: Stone and his colleagues found that stress weakened the immune system for one day, whereas pleasurable events enhanced the immune system for three days. "Having a good time on Monday still had a positive effect on the immune system on Wednesday," he reported, "but the negative immune effect from undesirable events on Monday lasts for just that day."

## The Mind and Longevity

Can the way that we think and feel directly impact longevity? One interesting study that looked at the factors that influence longevity was conducted in an area of southern Sweden comprised of one major city, eight smaller towns, and a number of small communities and rural districts.[77] For each person in the study, researchers did the following:

- Conducted a medical examination that included, among other things, taking blood tests, taking blood pressure measurements, obtaining a medical history, and asking questions about smoking habits, alcohol consumption, and diet
- Conducted a psychological assessment that included, among other things, tests for memory, learning retention, reaction time, behavior, and personality rating
- Gathered sociological data that included, among other things, marital status, type of housing, socioeconomic status, satisfaction with professional life, education, social network, feelings of loneliness, and formal/informal social support
- Interviewed each person about quality of life, both during their entire life span and at the time the interviews were conducted

Researchers found that genetics definitely played a role in whether the people in the study reached the age of 100. There were also several medical factors that played a key role; the two most important were body composition and blood pressure. The incidence of severe disease was also low. Most in the study had never smoked. But researchers also identified a number of factors indicating that the mind plays a powerful role in longevity.

According to the study, the centenarians were more responsible, capable, relaxed, easygoing, and emotionally stable, and less prone to anxiety than the population in general. Social characteristics seemed to be especially important. Most had grown up in stable homes; their parents had been extremely long-lived. (While the mean age of death for their fathers was 71.6 years and for their mothers was 74.3 years, the average age for survival from birth at that time in Sweden was only 40 years for men and 44 years for women.) Marriage played an important role; only 2 percent of the centenarians had been divorced, and only 19 percent had never married. Only 9 percent said they often felt lonely. They felt their quality of life—both at present and over their lifetimes—had been good.

Other studies show that the impact of the mind on longevity probably has to do with the relationship between the mind and the immune system. Generally, old age is associated with decline in immunity. The thymus gland stops influencing the growth and development of white blood cells at around the age of sixty. The T cells become less responsive with age and decline in numbers during the three years before death. While the B cells do not decline in number, they lose the ability to function with age. And most studies indicate that the body produces fewer natural killer cells as it ages.[78]

Research has shown that impairment of the immune system is probably not characteristic of aging per se, because a considerable percentage of the elderly maintain robust and healthy immunity. Instead, these changes may be due in part to the fact that the events of old age—such as retirement, loss of an active role in society, and bereavement—are likely to cause a high level of stress, and we know that stress impacts the immune system.[79]

Depression and bereavement, common during old age, have also been shown to impair immunity. Research shows that the more depressed a person is during bereavement, the greater the impairment of the immune system. Thirty-five studies found that depression was related to significant alterations in immunity, including reduced white blood cells and lowered natural killer cell activity—both of which affect the ability to fight off disease. The effect of depression may be partly related to stress (since depression can either *cause* stress or *result from* stress) and partly related to the way depressed people tend to behave: the depressed tend to sleep less, eat a less balanced diet, get less exercise, drink more alcohol, and smoke. The immune effects of depression have been found to be even greater among the elderly or those who are hospitalized.[80]

Other stressful events associated with aging include:

- A reduction in income that often accompanies retirement
- Increased economic stress

- Progressive loneliness (caused by death of a spouse, move or death of friends, and/or being forsaken by children)
- Isolation (caused by institutionalization)
- Poor or declining physical health caused by age-dependent diseases
- Loss of mobility
- Physical disability
- A perception of uselessness

Those who adapt—who learn to cope with these changes—tend to suffer far fewer health effects than those who do not, further indicating that stress instead of aging may be the major culprit in reduced immunity with aging. Those who are unable to adapt suffer impaired immunity as they age; the result is an especially high frequency of autoimmune and infectious diseases.

## Criticisms of the Mind-Body Approach

The field of PNI and the resulting application of mind-body medicine do not lack controversy—and are not without their critics and detractors.

Some who criticize the research accurately point out that just as the immune system itself is extremely complex, so are the studies that attempt to unravel its functioning. According to one work on PNI, the complexity of research includes "biobehavioral involvements, endocrine measure, immune indicators, and health outcomes. When one also takes into account the heterogeneity of study designs, the problem of drawing broadly based conclusions and generalizing results appears overwhelming."[81] Researchers, say the authors, need to be aware of potential limitations, subtle biases, "holes" in the data (areas where few studies have investigated potential relationships), and the temptation to make generalizations—especially when combining the findings of several different studies.

Other general criticisms of PNI and mind-body medicine include:[82]

- The general tendency to isolate mind-body health from sociopolitical, economic, and environmental health—which of necessity disregards factors like poverty, limited access to health care, and risky environmental factors
- The relative neglect of some important areas of health, such as smoking addiction
- The danger that mind-body approaches could supplant advanced drugs and high-tech treatment plans for chronic illness, which makes mind-body medicine a "competing" approach instead of a complementary one

- The cost in terms of training and time commitment to bring practitioners up to speed with mind-body approaches at a time when medical clinics are being forced to cut budgets in the face of managed care cutoffs

## The Challenge for the Twenty-First Century

A unique challenge—and unique opportunity—faces the field of medicine as we continue through the twenty-first century. Consumer confidence in traditional medicine is waning. In an article directed at primary care physicians, the medical director of a family clinic wrote:

> *In spite of impressive advances in immunology, imaging, and therapeutics, many patients are increasingly dissatisfied with their medical care. The side effects and inadequacies of many drugs and procedures have been discussed at length in the lay press, and many Americans have begun to look beyond conventional medicine for health care. Not surprisingly, most people seeking out unconventional therapies are those with chronic diseases. Although the treatment of many acute and infectious illnesses has improved, it has become clearer that the biomedical health care model is not equally effective for all types and stages of illness. Many physicians have noticed that patients experiencing emotional stress often complain of chronic physical symptoms that respond poorly to medications. This phenomenon has led to a growing scientific movement charged with exploring the mind's capacity to affect the body.*[83]

Clearly, there are some limitations in both behavioral and traditional treatments. For example, a person with meningitis needs intravenous antibiotics; a person with appendicitis requires immediate surgery. Behavioral treatment would be inappropriate in situations like these. But for vast numbers of patients who suffer with stress-related complaints, traditional medicine falls short, and behavioral techniques can offer tremendous benefits. And for chronic and degenerative diseases that have not responded well to traditional treatment—including some cancers, AIDS, osteoarthritis, collagen vascular diseases, chronic fatigue, and chronic pain—a combination of traditional and behavioral treatments may provide the answer. Some believe that mind-body therapies are best used in conjunction with appropriate standard medical therapies, and may be most effective for stress-related illnesses.[84] As physicians were instructed in the professional journal *Primary Care*, "Mind-body therapies have been used successfully for many varied medical conditions. . . . The potential uses are vast, but research has not yet unequivocally defined which medical conditions are most improved by mind-body therapies."[85]

When it comes to exploring the mind's capacity to affect the body, we have learned a great deal—but there is still far to go. The body of knowledge we have so far is exciting, full of promise for the prospect of a whole new horizon on how we look at and treat disease—and, most important, burgeoning with possibilities of how we might prevent it. But, to paraphrase Stanford University psychologist David Spiegel, who wrote in the *Journal of the National Cancer Institute*, we have entered the twenty-first century with twentieth-century science and technology and a nineteenth-century understanding of what it tells us about mind-body relationships.

Almost three decades ago, physicians were challenged to embrace a model of health and illness that recognized psychological and social variables as important contributors to health and disease. The ensuing twenty-five years of important scientific work have altered the specific applications, but not the general implications, of that challenge.

## ENDNOTES

1. Joel S. Lazar, "Mind-Body Medicine in Primary Care: Implications of Applications," *Primary Care* 23(1; March 1996): 169.
2. Centers for Disease Control and Prevention, National Center for Chronic Disease Prevention and Health Promotion, Chronic Disease Prevention, Chronic Disease Overview.
3. Delia Rossetto Chiaramonte, "Mind-Body Therapies for Primary Care Physicians," *Primary Care* 24 (4; December 1997): 788.
4. Karl Goodkin and Adriaan P. Vissar, eds. *Psychoneuroimmunology: Stress, Mental Disorders, and Health* (Washington, D.C.: American Psychiatric Press, Inc., 2000), 105.
5. Janice K. Kiecolt-Glaser and Ronald Glaser, "Psychoneuroimmunology: Past, Present, and Future," *Health Psychology* 8(6; 1989): 677–82.
6. Goodkin and Vissar, 1.
7. Franklin Hoke, "Alternative and Conventional Biomedical Research: A Creative Synergy," *The Scientist* 8(5; March 7 ,1994): 1.
8. Hoke.
9. Gina Maranto, "Emotions: How They Affect Your Body," *Discover* (November 1984): 35.
10. From Bob Wechsler, "A New Prescription: Mind over Malady," *Discover* (February 1987): 52–53.
11. Maranto, 11; and Wechsler, 53.
12. Historical data are summarized from "Emotions and the Body," *Executive Health Report* 11 (10; July 1985): 1–4; and Gina Maranto, "The Mind Within the Brain," *Discover* (May 1984): 34–43.
13. Maranto, "Emotions," 36.
14. G. F. Solomon and R. H. Moos, "Emotions, Immunity, and Disease: A Speculative Theoretical Integration," *Arch Gen. Psych.* 11 (1864):657–674.
15. Daniel Goleman and Joel Gurin, eds. *Mind/Body Medicine: How to Use Your Mind for Better Health* (New York: Consumer Reports Books, 1993), 58–59.
16. J. C. Fidelibus, "An Overview of Neuroimmunomodulation and a Possible Correlation with Musculoskeletal System Function," *J. Manipulative Physiol. Ther.* 12 (4; 1989): 289–92.
17. "Emotions and the Body."
18. Maranto, "Emotions," 38.

19. Donald B. Calne, *The Brain* (Bethesda, MD: U.S. Department of Health, Education, and Welfare, Public Health Service, National Institutes of Health, NIH Publication #79-1813), 7–10.
20. G. Miketta, TRIAS, ed., *Netzwerk Mensch*, 1st ed. (Stuttgart: Georg Thieme Verlag, 1991).
21. Phil Evans, Frank Hucklebridge, and Angela Clow, *Mind, Immunity, and Health: The Science of PNI* (London: Free Association Books, 2000), 15.
22. Israel Rosenfeld, *The Invention of Memory: A New View of the Brain* (New York: Basic Books, 1988).
23. Anne H. Rosenfeld, "Brain Attack," *Psychology Today* (May 1988): 68.
24. Israel Rosenfeld, 69.
25. Erica E. Goode, "Accounting for Emotion," *U.S. News and World Report*, June 27, 1988, 53.
26. Erica Goode.
27. Janet L. Hopson, "A Pleasurable Chemistry," *Psychology Today* (July/August 1988): 29.
28. Paul Raeburn, "Eater's High," *American Health* (December 1987): 42.
29. Joan Goldberg, "Peptide Power," *American Health* (June 1990): 35–41.
30. Marvin R. Brown and Laurel A. Fisher, "Brain Peptides and Intercellular Messengers," *Journal of the American Medical Association* 251 (10): 1310–14.
31. Goldberg.
32. John L. Stump, "Threads of Psychoneuroimmunology in Sport," *The Sport Journal* 6 (1; Winter 2003).
33. Signe Hammer, "The Mind as Healer," *Science Digest* (April 1984): 49.
34. National Institute of Allergy and Infectious Diseases, *Understanding the Immune System* (Bethesda, MD: National Institutes of Health, NIH Publication #85-529), 2–10.
35. A. Harrington, "Probing the Secrets of Placebos," *Alternative and Complementary Therapies* (September/October 1995): 299–304.
36. Evans et al.
37. Dossey, 105–6.
38. Stephen S. Hall, "A Molecular Code Links Emotions, Mind, and Health," *Smithsonian* (June 1989).
39. Shannon Brownlee, "The Body at War," *U.S. News and World Report* July 2, 1990, 48–54.
40. Evans et al., 53.
41. Goodkin and Vissar, 13.
42. Arthur J. Barsky, *Worried Sick: Our Troubled Quest for Wellness* (Boston: Little, Brown, and Company, 1988).
43. Eugene Taylor, Ching-Tse Lee, and John Ding-E Young, "Bringing Mind-Body Medicine into the Mainstream," *Hospital Practice* (May 15, 1997): 183.
44. Helen Carter, Christine McKenna, Roderick MacLeod, and Robyn Green, "Health Professionals' Responses to Multiple Sclerosis and Motor Neurone Disease," *Palliative Medicine* 12 (5; 1998): 393.
45. James P. Henry, "The Arousal of Emotions: Hormones, Behavior, and Health," *Advances* 6 (2): 59–62; and James P. Henry, "Neuroendocrine Patterns of Response," in R. Plutchik, ed., *Biological Foundations of Emotions* (New York: Academic Press, 1986), 37–60.
46. William Gottlieb, "Your Emotions and Your Health: A Woman's Guide," *Complete Woman*, 8–10.
47. J. P. Henry and P. M. Stephens, *Stress, Health, and the Social Environment: A Sociobiologic Approach to Medicine* (New York: Springer, 1977).

48. Bernie S. Siegel, *Love, Medicine, and Miracles* (New York: Harper and Row Publishers, Inc., 1986).
49. Siegel.
50. *General Dentistry* (November/December 2003).
51. Reported in Herbert Benson, *The Mind/Body Effect* (New York: Simon and Schuster, 1979).
52. "Emotions Linked to the Immune System," *Better Health* 4:12, 1–2.
53. Joel S. Lazar, "Mind-Body Medicine in Primary Care: Implications and Applications," *Primary Care* 23 (1; March 1996): 169.
54. Stump.
55. H. G. Koenig, M. McCullough, and D. B. Larson, *Handbook of Religion and Health* (New York: Oxford University Press, 2001).
56. Princeton Religion Research Center, 1982, 120.
57. H. G. Koenig, "Religious Beliefs and Practices of Hospitalized Medically Ill Older Adults," *International Journal of Geriatric Psychiatry* 13: 213–24.
58. Harold G. Koenig and Harvey Jay Cohen, *The Link Between Religion and Health: Psychoneuroimmunology and the Faith Factor* (New York: Oxford University Press, 2002).
59. Koenig and Cohen.
60. Ibid.
61. Willem J. Kop, "The Integration of Cardiovascular Behavioral Medicine and Psychoneuroimmunology: New Developments Based on Converging Research Fields," *Brain, Behavior, and Immunity* 17 (2003): 233–7.
62. "Mind/Hypertension Link Certain, Researchers Say," *Brain/Mind Bulletin* (July 1989): 2.
63. Goodkin and Vissar, 109–10.
64. Ibid.,111.
65. D. H. Bovbjerg and H. Valdimarsdottir, "Familiar Cancer, Emotional Distress, and Low Natural Cytotoxic Activity in Healthy Women," *Ann. Oncol* 4 (1993): 745–52.
66. Goodkin and Vissar, 112.
67. Ibid.,115.
68. Jerome D. Frank, "The Medical Power of Faith," *Human Nature* (August 1978): 40–47.
69. Steven Locke and Douglas Colligan, *The Healer Within* (New York: E.P. Dutton, 1986).
70. Frank.
71. Locke and Colligan.
72. Bruce Bower, "The Character of Cancer," *Science News* 131 (1987): 120–1.
73. Joan Borysenko and Myrin Borysenko, "On Psychoneuroimmunology: How the Mind Influences Health and Disease . . . and How to Make the Influence Beneficial," *Executive Health* 19:10, 1983.
74. Chiaramonte.
75. Christie Aschwanden, "A Cure for the Back Blues," *Health* 15 (2; March 2001): 158.
76. M. Coussons-Read, M. Okun, and S. Simms, "The Psychoneuroimmunology of Pregnancy," *Journal of Reproductive and Infant Psychology* 21 ( 2; May 2003): 103–12.
77. S. M. Samuelsson, B. Bauer Alfredson, B. Hagberg, G. Samuelsson, B. Nordbeck, A. Brun, L. Gustafson, and J. Risberg, "The Swedish Centenarian Study: A Multidisciplinary Study of Five Consecutive Cohorts at the Age of 100," *International Journal of Aging and Human Development* 45 (3; 1997): 223–53.

78. Taylor et al.
79. Luisa Guidi, Augusto Tricerri, Daniela Frasca, Marcello Vangeli, Andrea R. Errani, and Carlo Bartoloni, "Psychoneuroimmunology and Aging," *Gerontology* 44 (1998): 250.
80. Guidi et al.
81. Goodkin and Vissar, 10.
82. Henry Dreher, "A Challenge to the Mind-Body Health Movement," *Advances in Mind-Body Medicine* 17 (2; Spring 2001): 147.
83. Chiaramonte, 787.
84. Ibid.,790.
85. Ibid.,791.

CHAPTER 2

# *The Impact of Stress on Health*

*The only difference between a diamond and a lump of coal is
that the diamond had a little more pressure put on it.*

—Anonymous

## Learning Objectives

- Define the health effects and costs of various types of stress.
- Clarify the key elements of job stress.
- Identify the physiological effects of stress on specific body systems.
- Differentiate between healthy and unhealthy stress.
- Understand how to handle stress.

"Is stress good or bad?" For millenia philosophers, spiritual guides, physiologists, and now physicians and health educators have been exploring the remarkable ramifications of that question. No one is free of stress. According to figures from New York's American Institute of Stress published in Time magazine, 90 percent of all American adults experience high stress levels one or two times a week; a fourth of all American adults are subject to crushing levels of stress nearly every day. A survey of American women revealed that 57 percent felt excessively distressed much or most of the time.

## Definitions of Stress

Practitioners gathered at the 1949 Conference on Life and Stress and Heart Disease provided some of the first formal recognition that stress could precipitate chronic disease. Here, stress was given one of its earliest formal definitions: "A force which induces distress or strain upon both the emotional and physical makeup."[1]

Our understanding of stress has come a long way in the last four or five decades. Stress researcher Hans Selye, whose work in the early half of the twentieth century was among the first to identify stress and its effects on the body, defined *stress* as a nonspecific response of the body to any demand. The early pioneers of stress research categorized all stress as negative or bad; today, we understand that stress is anything in the environment that causes us to adapt, and that a "stressful" situation can be either happy (like the birth of a baby) or sad (like the death of a loved one).

We also understand that stress isn't limited to what goes on in our thoughts. We know that stress is "a nonspecific automatic biological response to demands made upon an individual."[2] Scientifically speaking, stress is "any challenge to homeostasis," or the body's internal sense of balance. Stress is a biological and biochemical process that begins in the brain and spreads through the nervous system, causing hormone release and eventually exerting an effect on the immune system. These three systems—the nervous system, the endocrine system, and the immune system—comprise the primary intercommunicating connections designed to maintain *homeostasis*, that is, to maintain all bodily functions in a balanced, controlled way. Disturbance in any one of these three systems will be expressed by responses in the others. Simply stated, the stress response usually starts in two major systems: (1) the nervous system, which reacts almost simultaneously; and (2) the endocrine (or hormone) system, which takes longer to react but persists much longer. Stress sets off a complex domino effect in the body, involving an entire series of body systems and a whole range of powerful hormones.

By itself, situational stress is not inherently either good or bad for health. Much depends on the way one thinks about it, and thus deals with it. We know that stress does not do the same thing to all people. One researcher defined stress as the point at which the organism's ability to perform easily is exceeded by the demands put on it, and stated that the result, psychophysiological strain, can be tempered by a person's coping ability and by moderating factors.[3] For example, recent, fascinating research in New Zealand shows that, depending on how genetics dictate that one handles a neurotransmitter called serotonin, a person may be born with a genetic propensity to be either more stress resilient or stress vulnerable. At the same time, a person's learned styles of coping with stress play a major role in whether those genetics are fully expressed.

A good example of how stressful situations can be altered by perception and outlook was witnessed by Colorado cardiovascular researcher Dr. Robert Eliot while he was traveling in the Middle East.[4] In downtown Riyadh, Saudi Arabia, Eliot saw two Arabs, both driving Mercedes, crash into each other. The two men, uninjured, jumped out of their cars and began hugging and laughing instead of yelling at each other, as Eliot would have expected. Curious about their odd exchange, Eliot asked his interpreter what the two men were saying. The interpreter explained that the two men were thanking Allah for the chance to meet this way.

Plenty of evidence confirms that the way you perceive stress has a lot to do with how stress affects you. American Institute of Stress President Paul J. Rosch likens stress to a ride on a roller coaster. "There are those at the front of the car, hands over head, clapping, who can't wait to get on again," he points out, "and those at the back cringing, wondering how they got into this and how soon it's going to be over." Or, to put it another way, one roller-coaster passenger "has his back stiffened, his knuckles are white, his eyes shut, jaws clenched, just waiting for it to be over. The wide-eyed thrill-seeker relishes every plunge, can't wait to do it again."[5] The roller coaster provides the same stressor, but the passengers have two very different responses. This illustrates that stress is not always "out there" being done to us as much as it is "in here," determined by the ways we have learned to think about the stressor.

## Distress and Eustress

Paul Rosch points out that differences in perception can cause some stress to be good stress (*eustress*) rather than bad stress (*distress*), and he uses symphony conductors as an example. "They work long hours, travel frequently, deal with prima donnas and sensitive artists, yet they live long and productive lives. They've got positive vibes going. They enjoy what they're doing, have pride of accomplishment, the approbation of their peers, and the applause of the audience, all positive stresses."[6] Whether the stress of work is good or bad appears to depend not so much on how busy one is, but on what drives that hard work: love of it, curiousity about it, and satisfaction in it (eustress)—or being driven by fear of failure, anxiously trying to prove oneself (distress). Boredom and understimulation can also be distressful. While distress may cause health problems, eustress may actually improve health.

Eustress promotes productivity and facilitates our efforts; distress leads to a loss of productivity and causes health problems.[7] As one writer describes it, eustress is exhilarating: You're under control but excited, like riding a canoe in a swiftly flowing stream. The opposite happens with distress: Out of control, you feel like a victim in a runaway train.[8] The key to good health, the researchers say, is learning how to turn bad stress (distress) into good stress (eustress).

Stress occurs whenever there is change and whenever we are forced to adapt to that change. Because change occurs nearly constantly, stress just *is*. And just as the body must adapt to changes in temperature, or blood pressure to changes in position (standing up), those who adapt well to psychosocial change (resilience) have much better health outcomes.

Distress has been shown to affect almost all body systems, resulting in cardiovascular disease, neuromuscular disorders (including migraine headache and chronic back pain), respiratory and allergic disorders, immunologic disorders, gastrointestinal disturbances (including peptic ulcer disease, irritable bowel syndrome, nausea, vomiting, and diarrhea), skin diseases, dental problems, and a host of other disorders. Since most diseases are caused by a variety of different factors instead of a single cause, stress probably does not cause illness, but various studies have demonstrated a strong link between distress and the onset of disease. In preventing disease, the best strategy is to eliminate as much distress as you can, and to change your attitude toward the things you can't prevent. This is the process of turning distress toward eustress.

Today, brain research is booming; scientists from a wide range of disciplines have entered the field, and great strides are being made toward finding out exactly how emotions impact health.

## Types of Stress

Basically, there are three types of stress: physical, psychological, and psychosocial.

- **Physical stress** involves stressors in the environment—such as environmental pollution, constant noise, or an inadequate supply of oxygen.

- **Psychological stress** stems from the way we react toward anything that is threatening us, whether the threat is real or imagined.

- **Psychosocial stress** involves stressors from interpersonal relationships and conflicts with people around us. It can also occur when there is isolation as a result of inadequate social interactions.[9]

# The Stress Response

When the body becomes stressed, regardless of the source of the stress, it undergoes what scientists now recognize as the stress response. The stress response is, simply stated, the fight-or-flight response used by primitive people as they faced the various threats in their environment. When facing one of their enemies—a saber-toothed tiger, let's say—their bodies reacted in a very specific way that prepared them to either fight the tiger or run for their lives.

Unfortunately, our bodies still react the same way to threats—real or imagined—even though for today's stressors, either fighting or fleeing is usually inappropriate. As Boston University psychiatrist Peter Knapp pointed out, "When you get a Wall Street broker using the responses a cave man used to fight the elements, you've got a problem."[10]

Each phase of the stress response carried with it benefits for the primitive man or woman who faced physical dangers, and those same benefits have become hazards for the modern man or woman who faces the social stresses of our day. Let's look at a dozen phases of the stress response and examine why yesterday's benefits are today's drawbacks.[11]

1. The **adrenal glands** start pumping out a group of hormones such as cortisol, cortisone, and catecholamines (the body's chemical messengers of stress). In the right amounts, these are critical to life (if the adrenal glands are removed, death follows within a few days). But when secreted in excessive amounts, they can impair the immune system and reduce tissue healing,[12] making it difficult to fight off even a minor cold. Too much cortisone over a prolonged time causes lymph glands to shrivel, bones to become brittle, and blood pressure to rise, and can even cause blood sugars to spike into diabetic ranges.

2. The **thyroid gland** pumps out thyroid hormones, which accelerate metabolism and helped primitive people burn fuel faster to give them energy for fight or flight. It does the same thing to us today, but because we're not engaged in life-or-death battles, it produces a different set of symptoms: insomnia, shaky nerves, heat intolerance, and exhaustion. It contributes to some people losing weight under stress.

3. The **hypothalamus** releases endorphins, powerful natural painkillers that enabled primitive people to fight or flee even when injured. But chronic, relentless stress depletes endorphins and can in turn aggravate migraine headaches, backaches, and even arthritis pain. The hypothalamus, located at the place in the brain that connects thinking to peripheral body processes, also releases the brain's key initiator of the stress response, corticotropin-releasing hormone (CRH). CRH, injected into the midbrain, causes anxiety and upregulates the nervous system to overrespond to stimuli (a cause of several very common medical problems).

4. **Sex hormones** (progesterone in females and testosterone in males) are reduced. That served an important function in primitive times: The decreased libido and fertility came in handy during times of drought, overcrowding, and decreased food supply by giving the community fewer mouths to feed, and it redirected attention from amorous adventures to the threat at hand. Sadly, the same thing happens to you under stress: You may lose your sex drive, become infertile, or suffer from sexual dysfunction (such as premature ejaculation or failure to reach orgasm). Women under acute stress may precipitate a menstrual period early. With unrelenting, chronic stress, they may be more likely to bleed irregularly or not at all (amennorrhea).

5. Coordination of the **digestive tract** shuts down. In primitive people, all blood was diverted to the muscles, rendering them capable of extraordinary feats of power; the mouth went dry, too. The same things

happen today. Eating while under stress can result in stomach bloating, nausea, abdominal discomfort or cramping, and even diarrhea. The dry mouth problems persist, too. Ask any public speaker whose mouth is so dry that he or she can't speak. Dry mouth is such an acute symptom of stress, in fact, that in China it's used as a lie detector test.

6. Release of **sugar** (glucose) into the bloodstream is followed by a boost in insulin to metabolize it, something that provided primitive people with "fuel for the sprint" or a burst of short-lived energy. That same scenario today can cause either high or low blood sugars. Continuously high insulin levels can cause weight gain and lead to elevated blood pressure and lipids (cholesterol).

7. **Cholesterol** is released into the bloodstream, mostly from the liver; it took over where blood sugar left off in supplying sustained energy to the muscles. But today's man or woman under chronic stress doesn't generally need more cholesterol to sustain energy, so the cholesterol is deposited in the blood vessels. The result is well documented by our nation's rate of heart disease fatalities.

8. The **heart** begins racing, a physiological response that pumps more blood to the muscles and lungs, carrying more fuel and oxygen to the muscles, something primitive people needed when under duress. Blood flow to the muscles of the arms and legs increases 300 to 400 percent. The result today is high blood pressure; left unchecked, it can lead to stroke, heart attacks, or kidney problems.

9. Breathing rate increases, providing greater air supply. While usually helpful, the increased demand on the **lungs** can be problematic for people with lung disease, such as asthma.

10. The **blood** thickens and coagulates more readily. Thickening of the blood enabled primitive people to stop bleeding from a wound. When the blood turns thick under stress today, the result can be heart attack, stroke, or embolus (blood clot).

11. The **skin** "crawls," blanches, and sweats. This heightened the sense of touch, provided a cooling mechanism for overheated muscles, and diverted blood away from wounds. Today, it decreases the resistance of skin to electricity (the principle behind most lie detector tests).

12. All **five senses** become acute. In primitive people, pupils dilated to enhance night vision, overall mental performance was sharpened, the senses of hearing and touch were improved, and the entire body was brought to peak function. The same thing happens today, but without the burst of physical energy that brings an end to a sporadic stressful situation, we are more likely to suffer from chronic stress. Thus, the

senses are constantly on red alert, sometimes resulting in pain from stimuli that shouldn't cause such pain, such as a migraine worsening in response to light, sound, or smells.

Prolonged stimulation of the twelve phases of the stress response leads to what Robert S. Eliot calls the *vigilance reaction*.[13] According to Eliot, while the vigilance reaction may have once protected us from external dangers or scarcity, today it wreaks havoc on our bodies. Hypervigilance can cause the nervous system to overrespond to various normal stimuli, leading to such common diseases as irritable bowel syndrome, palpitations, migraine, chronic pain, anxiety disorders, and even medically unexplained neurological symptoms such as dizziness, numbness, or tingling.

## Costs and Outcomes of Stress

Stress is costly. Obviously, no one can put a precise price tag on the various health costs of stress, but figures from a variety of sources give us a fairly good idea of its devastating impact. For example, researchers at the American Institute of Stress estimate that more than 75 percent of all visits to health care providers result from stress-related disorders. The American Academy of Family Physicians estimates that two-thirds of all office visits to family doctors are prompted by stress-related symptoms. Just among the nation's executives, an estimated $10 to $20 billion is lost each year through absence, hospitalization, and early death; much of it as a result of stress.[14] The National Council on Compensation Insurance says that stress-related claims account for almost one-fifth of all occupational disease.[15] Fully one-fourth of all workman's compensation claims are for stress-related injuries, and researchers estimate that 60 to 80 percent of all industrial accidents are related to stress.

Stress-related symptoms and illnesses are costing industry a conservatively estimated $150 billion a year in absenteeism, company medical expenses, and lost productivity. The results of a study at New Mexico State University suggest a strong relationship between stress and absenteeism. Other studies show that stress accounts for more than 20 percent of the costs associated with high job turnover, strikes, work stoppages, absenteeism, and decline in productivity.[16]

Left unchecked, unremitting stress can also shorten your life. In one long-term study that gives a particularly good measure of the effects of stress, researchers studied more than 600 people over twelve years. Investigators tested each study subject at the beginning of the period, asking if they suffered from distress; at the end of the twelve years, they discovered that the existence of distress at the study's outset was a good predictor of who would die during the period of the study. Even when researchers tried to "juggle" the results—by controlling for factors such as smoking, cholesterol levels, obesity, or high blood pressure, or by excluding people with chronic heart disease—the figures remained the same.[17]

A similar study in Sweden followed 752 men for seven years. Researchers found what they expected: The men who were under stress were more likely to die prematurely than those who weren't under stress. But the researchers also found something a little unexpected: The type of stress matters, too. In the Swedish study, certain kinds of stress had more pronounced effects than others. For example, those who felt insecure at work had a 2.4-fold increased risk of dying. Those who had been divorced or separated from their wives or who were in serious financial trouble during the year before the evaluation had triple the risk of dying. And those who had been sued had 7.7 times the risk of dying prematurely than those who had not. Overall, say the researchers, suffering three or more stressful life events more than tripled the risk of dying for the men involved in the study.[18] One might wonder, of course, whether the greater culprit for health risk was the external act of being sued or divorced, or perhaps some personality characteristic that made them more likely to get divorced or sued. For example, men may have been angry, cynical, hostile, or belligerent, characteristics that made them more likely to divorce or be sued.

The good news is that stress doesn't have to knock you out. Research shows that some people manage to be resilient to stress; others exhibit what scientists call "hardiness," an ability to resist the ill effects of stress. Research has also indicated that there are things that help you cope better with stressors. To figure out where you stand, it's important to know the factors that lead to stress, the physiological reactions of the body when under stress, and the way that stress can compromise the immune system and lead to illness.

# Factors Leading to Stress

Feeling stressed arises both from external events and from one's way of thinking about them. During the early 1950s, University of Washington psychiatrist Thomas Holmes noted that tuberculosis had occurred among patients after a cluster of disruptive events, such as a death in the family, a new job, or a marriage. Based partly on that observation and partly on his extensive research, Holmes pronounced that the single common denominator for stress is "significant change in the life pattern of an individual." Holmes emphasized that stress did not cause the tuberculosis—tuberculosis bacteria had to be present—but that stress somehow weakened the body or made it more vulnerable to the disease.[19]

Branching out in his research, Holmes began to search for specific links between disease and what he called *life events*, those things in life that call for the greatest adjustment. He found that the more life events a person was subjected to within a brief period of time, the more likely he or she was to become ill. Holmes developed a social-readjustment rating scale along with his colleague Richard Rahe; commonly known as the Holmes-Rahe scale, it assigns a numerical score to the almost four dozen stressors, or life changes, that increase the risk of disease. Subsequent research by hosts of independent scientists has verified the accuracy of the Holmes-Rahe scale.

## The Holmes-Rahe Scale

The testee scans the list of life changes, pinpoints the ones experienced within the last year, and adds up the numerical scores to get a total. The items in the Holmes-Rahe scale, along with their numerical scores, are:

100 Death of spouse

73 Divorce

65 Marital separation

63 Jail term

63 Death of close family member

53 Personal injury or illness

50 Marriage

47 Fired at work

45 Marital reconciliation

45 Retirement

44 Change in health of family member

40 Pregnancy

39 Sexual difficulties

39 Gain of new family member

39 Business readjustment

38 Change in financial status

37 Death of close friend

36 Change to different line of work

35 Change in number of arguments with spouse

31 Mortgage or loan over $10,000

30 Foreclosure of mortgage or loan

29 Change in responsibilities at work

29 Son or daughter leaving home

29 Trouble with in-laws

28 Outstanding personal achievement

26 Wife begins or quits work

25 Change in living conditions

24 Change in personal habits

23 Trouble with boss

20 Change in work hours or conditions

20 Change in residence

19 Change in recreation

19 Change in number or type of church activities

18 Change in number or type of social activities

17 Mortgage or loan under $10,000

16 Change in sleeping habits

15 Change in number of family get-togethers

15 Change in eating habits

13 Vacation

12 Christmas

11 Minor violations of the law

According to Holmes and Rahe, if you score between 150 and 199 in one year, you have a 37 percent chance of getting sick during the following year. If you score between 200 and 299, your chances of getting sick jump to 51 percent. And if you score over 300, you have a 79 percent chance of getting sick during the following year.

Note that not all the items on the scale are "bad" things. Few of us would consider things like marriage, an outstanding personal achievement, a vacation, or Christmas to be negatives. Also, some items could be either negative or positive. A change in the number of arguments with your spouse, for instance, might mean that you are having fewer arguments and getting along better than ever.

The key word is *change.* Each item on the Holmes-Rahe scale describes something that causes us to change our routine, to adapt. The thing that requires change or adaptation can be positive or negative.

The mind is extremely powerful. Research has shown that merely thinking about one of the stressors on the list can evoke emotions so strong that they can induce the stress response. Isolating one of the items on the list, Holmes said that "a person often catches cold when a mother-in-law comes to visit. Patients mentioned mothers-in-law so often that we came to consider them a common cause of disease in the United States."[20]

## Major Life Events and Cancer

Without an adaptive attitude or perception, major life events can weaken the system enough to bring on serious illness or disease. Yale oncologist and surgeon Bernie S. Siegel attributes some of the cancers of his patients to traumatic loss or crisis in their lives. One study of children with leukemia showed that thirty-one of the thirty-three in the study had experienced a traumatic loss or move within the two years prior to their diagnosis. A separate study at Albert Einstein College of Medicine found that children with cancer had twice as many recent crises as similar, cancer-free children. Even career reversals may play a role, says Siegel: "The defeats of Napoleon Bonaparte, Ulysses S. Grant, William Howard Taft, and Hubert Humphrey have often been implicated in their fatal cancers."[21] This is not to say that stress causes cancer, but it may play a role in one's resistance to the usual causes.

Still another study involved more than 3,000 women who came to the Heidelberg University Gynecological Clinic for breast examination. The women who were not diagnosed with cancer were compared to those who did have cancer as diagnosed through various tests. Researchers determined that three life events had significant relationships to the development of cancer. One was the death of the mother before the woman was sixteen. The second was divorce, separation, or widowhood at any time during the woman's life. And the third was at least one traumatic event during World War II that caused considerable disturbance (researchers noted events like air raids, the death of close relatives, becoming a refugee, transfer of population, encampment, being buried alive, or injury to relatives as among the most disturbing).[22]

A study of 8,000 cancer patients with various types of tumors concluded that "in most of the cases, the cancer appeared during a period of severe and intense life stress often involving loss, separation, and other bereavements."[23] To sort out genetic factors from those attributable to stress, W. H. Green at the University of Rochester studied identical twins, one of whom had developed leukemia, and found that one twin in each pair usually developed leukemia shortly after a major psychological upheaval, while the stress-free twin did not.

## Hassles

Another factor involved in stress is what researchers call *hassles*. The theory is aptly illustrated in an excerpt from a poem by Charles Bukowski:

> . . . *It's not the large things that*
> *send a man to the*
> *madhouse . . . no, it's the*
> *continuing series of*
> *small tragedies*
> *that send a man to the madhouse . . .*

*not the death of his love but a shoelace that snaps*
*with no time left. . . .* [24]

Research into stress shows that it's not always the major events, but sometimes the minor hassles, that can accumulate and cause problems—things like running out of gas on the way to work, having unexpected company drop in, or getting delayed at a busy intersection. Various studies show that hassles are strongly related to episodes of illness, even when there are no major life events to consider.

As an example, psychiatrist and behavioral scientist Ian Wickramasekera points out that men "who experience such important life changes as divorce or the death of a wife may then be exposed to a wave of minor hassles (paying bills, dressing children, cooking, or doing the laundry) as they encounter new responsibilities (moving from father and husband, for example, to father and housekeeper)." Wickramasekera, director of the Eastern Virginia Medical School's Behavioral Medicine Clinic and Stress Disorders Laboratory, adds that a person in this kind of situation often develops back pain, headaches, stomach distress, or chest pain. "Sometimes it is not the mountain in front of you," he says, "but the grain of sand in your shoe that brings you to your knees."[25]

One group of researchers found that hassles have a greater impact on health than do major life change events—and that the influence of major life changes may actually be indirect. Major life changes may influence health because they cause an increased number of minor hassles.[26]

## Attitudes Toward Stress

Your attitudes, perceptions, and the way you look at stressful events in life appear to be even more important than the events themselves, and can help you resist the ill effects of stress. A perfect example of resilience to stress was uncovered by University of Michigan researcher Louis Ferman. He found a "hard-luck victim" who had been laid off three times: first in 1962 when the Studebaker Corporation folded, next in the 1970s by a truck manufacturer that went under, and finally during cutbacks at a Chrysler plant. Ferman said that by all accounts, "He should have been a basket case, but he was one of the best-adjusted fellows I've run into." Asked his secret, the man replied, "I've got a loving wife and go to church every Sunday."[27] The specifics of creating healthy attitudes toward stress will be taken up later in this chapter, the discussion of stress resilience.

## Age-Related Stressors

*Prenatal.*    People are susceptible to different stressors at different stages of their lives. The impact of stress begins before we are even born: A variety of studies have shown that chronic stress during pregnancy contributes to preterm labor.[28] And stress experienced by a pregnant woman has definite physiological effects on her unborn baby. In one study of more than 500 rural women, those who experienced increasing stress levels between the second and third trimester had a significantly higher rate of complications, including neonatal death, neonatal illness, and low birth weight. These findings held true even when the researchers figured in all the standard risk factors.[29] Even nonspecific psychosocial stress can cause problems in the fetus and complications at and immediately following birth. Specifically, one group of researchers found that stress during the pregnancy was associated with "deviant behavior" during the first five days of life. Babies born to stressed mothers cried more, slept less, were more irritable, and did not eat or have bowel movements with normal frequency.[30]

There is some evidence that the neurochemical abnormalities of major stress, depression, or anxiety disorders may influence the fetal brain development in ways that affect personality and behavior long after delivery. For example, during a study of pregnant animals, when the mother-to-be was stressed for a protracted period, the male offspring were much more withdrawn and reserved than those of nonstressed mothers, exhibiting more female-like behavior. Speculation has been raised about whether the depression seen in children of depressed mothers is all genetic or could be influenced by in utero programming of the developing brain by the mother's neurohormones. This raises some very practical dilemmas for the physician and mother when, while pregnant, she may get moderately depressed or have panic disorder. If these problems cannot be controlled without medication, is the risk to the baby greater if the mother goes untreated or takes medication that may or may not be safe during pregnancy? With the more recent data documenting risks to the baby when the mother has mental stress disorders, more physicians are opting to treat with medication when it's really needed. The improved results at and after birth tend to support that decision, and even long-term effects on the baby are beginning to encourage treating the mother's depression or anxiety.

***Children and Adolescents.***   The most tremendous stress an infant faces, of course, is its own birth.[31] Other infant stress is related to the syndrome known as "failure to thrive" (a child simply does not grow, despite the fact that there is no known biological problem). Researchers also believe that, while some amount of stress is healthy for an adult, infants do not benefit from any stress at all.[32] The first year of life is, in some very important ways, critical to the global worldview a person carries. "Is the world a safe and nurturing place, or it is hostile and dangerous? Can I express my needs and feelings safely and will they be honored, or am I likely to get zapped if I do so?" Things as simple as how a cry is responded to can establish longstanding attitudes and expectations in the baby and can later affect the person's ability to express feelings and needs or can influence the person's propensity to look at the world in a hostile, competitive way. Much mental programming occurs in these early years, even if there is no conscious memory of whence it arose. Either abuse or neglect early in life has been shown, both in animals and children, to activate the gene for the brain neuropeptide Corticotropin-Releasing Factor (CRF). The resulting long-term increases in this brain hormone cause significant anxiety and upregulate the nervous system to overrespond to stimuli. This chronically overresponsive nervous system is responsible for much of the increased pain, bowel symptoms, and anxiety experienced by such individuals, even later in life.[33]

School-aged children are understandably stressed by many of the same things that stress preschoolers—divorce of parents, serious illness that requires hospitalization, and witnessing violence. But when school enters the picture, so does a whole new host of stressors. According to researchers, the most common stressors of school-aged children include anxiety about going to school, bullies, changing schools, conflicts with the teacher, forced competitiveness, difficulty with classmates, fads, dares with classmates, failing exams or getting failing grades, failing to make an athletic team, having to give oral reports in front of the class, learning disorders, being unable to complete homework assignments, lack of parental interest in achievements, parental pressure to achieve, dealing with the reputation of older siblings (bad or good), worrying about taking tests, and even special recognition (for making the honor roll, winning a debate match, and so on). A significant amount of stress stems from peer teasing—about, for example, being overweight, being of a different race, wearing glasses, having red hair, or wearing dental braces.[34]

Characteristically, school-aged children react to stress in a number of behavioral ways. They may regress (start wetting the bed or sucking their thumbs, for example), have problems getting along with classmates, lose motivation or concentration, become irritable, or withdraw. These can also be signs of clinical depression in children. But, according to researchers, there is a number of physical signs and symptoms as well: School-aged kids under stress may suffer headaches, stomachaches, poor appetite, and sleeplessness.[35]

Parental reaction to the stress-induced illness can also be important. If illness becomes a safe haven because much nurturing and attention are given, it can become an unconsciously automatic response ("illness behavior") when safety and nurturing are needed. It may be kinder in the long run to make it a not-so-pleasant time, perhaps with bed rest, isolation, and not much that's fun to do—administered with kindness, of course. This is a tricky call, because serious organic disease may heal faster with loving support.

Typical stressors in adolescence include the major transitions of moving from dependent childhood to independent adulthood, yet not being fully equipped for such independence.[36] Parents are wise to understand that this is a time when the need for independence and acceptance is foremost. A teenager knows he or she must become his or her own person, autonomous and "okay." The problem, often, is that a teen lacks the experience to make wise decisions, and parents may undermine the very empowering of their children by offering what they call "constructive criticism" in ways that imply they are not capable or acceptable and that they need to depend on the parent to make the right decision for them.

*Adults.*    College students are generally stressed by academic pressure, course overload, career decisions, self-doubt, changing roles in the family, and the pressures associated with developing intimate relationships. Young and middle-aged adults often suffer from family and career stressors, and often financial problems.

The elderly face the unique stresses associated with adjusting to retirement, failing health, deteriorating sight and hearing, the loss of friends and family members, and the stress of facing their own death.[37] A major source of distress for those who are aging is Western society's notion that one's worth as a person depends on productivity and on looking young. In societies where wisdom and understanding are venerated, elders tend to thrive and to look forward to old age. It is, of course, possible for one to come to that conclusion on his or her own, regardless of the notions of others.

*Miscellaneous Stressors.*    Plenty of miscellaneous stressors can sap energy and contribute to physical illness, regardless of age. These include poor health habits (poor nutrition, poor sleep patterns, or drug abuse.)

## Job Stress and Health

"This job's killing me!" The often-heard complaint contains more than a kernel of truth. The stress connected with certain kinds of jobs can, indeed, hurt your health, and if stress on the job gets too intense, it can kill you. On the other hand, good and satisfying work can greatly enhance health, well beyond not working at all. So what makes the difference?

High-powered executives who cope with the stress of running corporations, humoring clients, balancing budgets, and solving personnel problems are not those most likely in danger. They're under stress, but research indicates that the people most likely to be negatively affected by job stress are the ones who have little control or decision-making power: assembly line workers, factory workers, or computer operators who are constantly scrutinized by supervisors. Another high-risk group is middle management, who are often given tasks from above with which they may disagree, but then with the burden of getting those who they manage to carry the task out— again feeling a lack of control both from above and below. Jobs that seem without meaning and purpose, or without recognition for work well done, can also lead to health problems.

## The Frequency of Job Stress

How many Americans suffer from work-related stress? It's difficult to come up with an exact number, but there are some pretty good estimates. Stress on the job led 34 percent of all American employees to consider quitting their jobs in 1990, as reported in a study conducted by Northwestern National Life Insurance Company. According to the study, 46 percent of American workers find their jobs highly stressful.[38]

A recent Gallup poll conducted for the National Occupational Information Coordinating Committee came up with similar figures. It determined that about half of all Americans say that job stress affects their health, personal relationships, or ability to do their job.[39] Of the employed adults who responded to the poll, a fourth said that job stress had interfered with off-the-job relationships. One in five said that the stress had interfered with their ability to do their job. The same number, 20 percent, said that job stress had affected their physical health. The poll also found that fewer than half of all employed Americans were on the career or job path they had planned. The rest were influenced by family or friends, got their jobs by "chance," or grabbed the only job they could find. Well over half (65 percent) said that, given a chance to start over, they would look more carefully at their career options. Finally, almost a third of the workforce hoped to change jobs within the next three years.[40]

## Job Burnout

A surprising number of people today, particularly in helping professions in larger companies, are experiencing burnout. For example, in a survey of the physicians in the Sacramento (California) Medical Society, 40 percent said they felt some symptoms of depression, and a third were planning to leave their practices within three years.[41] Much of this comes from feeling a loss of personal control and a loss of meaning in the work. This phenomenon often follows excessive demands, expectations of ever-increasing productivity, and management scrutiny. Long work hours combined with lack of recreation and sleep frequently trigger burnout.

The loss of meaning is a major source of burnout, even in healing professions where the primary reason for choosing that work was originally its inherent great meaning and value. Overwork (often driven by "productivity" concerns), loss of sleep, and lack of recreation can drive caregivers to want to just get the basics done so they can leave. An interesting study of this phenomenon involved the measurement of attitudes of medical interns at the beginning and end of their grueling internship year (invariably with excessive workloads and sleep deprivation):

**Table 2.1**    A Survey of Medical Interns[42]

|  | Normal Population | Beginning of Year | 9–12 Months Later |
|---|---|---|---|
| **Profile of Mood States** | | | |
| Anxiety | 13.5 | 10.8 | → 10.4 |
| Depression | 14.1 | 5.1 | → 10.7 |
| Anger/hostility | 9.6 | 3.8 | → 10.5 |
| Fatigue | 10.6 | 4.7 | → 10.4 |
| **Interpersonal Reactivity Index** | | | |
| Empathic concern | 10.6 | 22.0 | → 20.7 |
| Personal distress | 10.9 | 8.8 | → 10.7 |

Note: Numbers indicate percentage of those surveyed.

Note that these young physicians came out of school with significantly better moods, energy, and empathy (and less anger) than the general population, but by the end of a hard job year, many of these benefits had been trained out of them.

Why are we working so hard that we burn out? Back in the 1930s, Americans (and subsequently, increasing numbers in other countries) got hooked on the notion that one's worth as a person is determined by his or her measurable productivity, often in terms of money, competitive status, or hours worked. And each year we are expected to be more productive than the year before. Consider how we calculate one's "worth." Those of old age in the United States may be seen as not of much value, because they are less "productive" in the quantifiable sense. A fascinating paradox is that the incessant demand by employers for measurable productivity actually causes *less* productivity because it leads to stress-related illness and burnout.[43] The current demand from above to generate ever-increasing numbers, measurable productivity that this year must be more than last year's, and that must be better than someone else's, is driving workers and managers toward exhaustion.

The thought that worth equals productivity is driving us toward many of the very common stress-related chronic illnesses described in this book. It is a thought worth challenging. Sometimes a philosophical checkup can be even more valuable than a medical checkup with such illnesses. Is it true that the numbers one generates is the primary determinant of his or her worth and value? In some Asian countries, most people yearn to achieve old age. Why? Because one's worth there is seen in terms of wisdom, character, and the ability to provide vision and hope (rather than simply quantifiable numbers). Such character qualities may require time away from work to reflect on what the good life is really all about, to see the beauty of life, and to nurture relationships.

## The Price We Pay for Job Stress

Estimates are that job stress costs American industry more than $150 billion a year from proven underproductivity absenteeism, illness (resulting in health insurance payouts and workers' compensation claims), employee turnover, and even theft and sabotage. That presents a hefty bill to American companies—estimated by one researcher to be about $1,700 per employee per year for a medium-sized manufacturing firm. It can add up to more than the company's profits.[44]

The costs are due to a number of different factors. Some estimate that 60 percent of all absence from work is caused by stress-related disorders[45] (and that anywhere from 60 to 90 percent of all visits to health care professionals are for stress-related disorders[46]). One study estimates that, in the United Kingdom alone, 100 million working days are lost each year because "people cannot face going to work."[47] And American employers spend some $700 million per year replacing employees below retirement age because of coronary heart disease incapacity.[48]

In an attempt to dull the effects of job stress, many of the nation's workers are turning to drugs and alcohol on the job, and the results are staggering. According to a report in *Time* magazine, "Illegal drugs have become so pervasive in the U.S. workplace that they are used in almost every industry, the daily companions of blue- and white-collar workers alike. Their presence on the job is sapping the energy, honesty, and reliability of the American labor force, even as competition from foreign companies is growing ever tougher."[49]

Job stress-related employee claims are skyrocketing; analysts say they escalated more than 300 percent in a single year in California.[50] During the last decade in that same state, more than half of all worker compensation cases were for disorders that stemmed from stress on the job.[51] A study of workers with back pain in Seattle revealed that job satisfaction was significantly more important than severity of injury in determining whether a worker became disabled (requiring payments) or returned to work.[52] Mental depression has been shown to be the major source of on-the-job loss of productivity,[53] yet curiously, employers (fearful of insurance premium increases) have been the largest barrier to getting full insurance coverage for treating such mental disorders and to changing job characteristics to minimize the risk of depression. (A five-company study in Michigan found the rates of depression in high-demand, low-decision-latitude jobs to be 57 percent, while the rate in low-demand, high-decision-latitude jobs to be 18 percent.)[54] In addition, the same job characteristics associated with more depression are also linked to significantly more coronary events.[55]

To sum it up, says New York Medical College psychiatrist Paul J. Rosch, who heads the American Institute of Stress, "Work stress may be America's number-one health problem."

## Health Effects of Stressful Jobs

Work is the source of a great deal of "ordinary" stress. In one British study, researchers for the National Survey of Health and Development questioned more than 1,400 twenty-six-year-old men. Those who were under stress were asked to pinpoint the source of their stress. Surprisingly, only 8 percent of the men reported stress at home or in some other arena of their personal lives. A staggering 38 percent reported work as the source of severe stress in their lives, and almost half of those said they were physically ill as well.[56]

In still another study, forty-three different occupational groups were assessed for coronary risk. The executives, who seemed to be under all kinds of stress, fared well. It was the blue-collar workers, who are in actuality under the greatest job stress, who had the highest blood pressure, highest cholesterol levels, and highest triglyceride levels. And it wasn't only risk factors. The blue-collar workers had higher rates of cardiovascular mortality as well.[57]

In a series of studies done at Cornell University Medical College, researchers evaluated a total of 260 men who worked at various jobs in New York City. Men who worked in high-stress jobs—those characterized by plenty of pressure but little power to make decisions—were more than three times as likely to have high blood pressure as the men who worked in low-stress jobs.[58] This was further confirmed in a second three-year follow-up study.[59]

Apparently, the boss—and the boss's style—have a lot to do with mediating the effects of a stressful situation on the job. Researchers studied nearly 200 AT&T employees during a tumultuous period; those with supportive bosses suffered only half the illness of those with unsupportive bosses. Those with unsupportive bosses, in fact, suffered two times the illness, obesity, sexual problems, and depression that their colleagues with supportive bosses did.[60]

Studies show that job stress can even continue to affect people after they retire. One Swedish study followed more than 600 men who had retired. The Swedish researchers found that those who had job stress while working had nearly twice the relative mortality risk after retirement. Researchers also found that if job stress during work had been coupled with weak social support, the risk of early death jumped by more than 400 percent.[61]

How could such significant health problems arise from stress? Some of the pathophysiological mechanisms are discussed in a section later in this chapter.

## How Much Work?

Both too little or too much work has ill effects. Unemployment can be devastating to health. One of the most conclusive studies was conducted in Scotland and reported in the *British Heart Journal*.[62] Researchers were puzzled by coronary heart disease rates in the country: Scotland has one of the highest death rates in the world from coronary heart disease, but there is a vast difference from one region to another. They studied men in fifty-six local regions, and they looked at all kinds of factors, ranging from typical socioeconomic factors to amount of annual rainfall and hardness of drinking water. The strongest predictor of coronary heart disease among the men in the study was found to be unemployment.

Reports released by Johns Hopkins University economist M. Harvey Brenner and University of Utah economists Mary Merva and Richard Fowles show that every increase of one percentage point in the unemployment rate results in a 3.1 percent increase in deaths due to a stroke and a 5.6 percent increase in deaths due to heart disease. Brenner also found that unemployment was associated with the same cardiovascular effects in Scotland and Sweden.[63]

On the other hand, excessive work is also a problem. Workaholism is a compulsive disorder, described by one writer as being "as ravaging and insidious as alcoholism or eating disorders."[64] Another called it "the only lifeboat guaranteed to sink." Diane Fassel, author of *Working Ourselves to Death*, calls it "a killer stalking our society."[65] Most important, it can strike anybody; it's not the domain of the high-powered executive. Factory workers can get it, as can housewives (who dedicate sixteen hours a day to being the perfect wife and mother) and children (who are driven to excellence and participate in a host of extracurricular activities at school). Workaholics are stricken with a disease "that affects them not only physically but also emotionally, mentally, and spiritually." Fassel says that characteristic health problems of workaholics include severe headaches, backaches, high blood pressure, and ulcers. An inordinate number have heart attacks or strokes. "Some die," she adds. "Some who survive are scared enough to get help. Others continue working from their hospital beds, until the next attack occurs."[66]

Like men, women fill more than their fair share of high-stress jobs; however, they have less than their fair share of active jobs, often with high demand and low control. Some experts believe that the future scope of women's health may be altered as a result.[67] The type of work and support of coworkers plays a significant role. In the Framingham heart study, women in clerical jobs had twice the coronary disease as homemakers, and this quickly accelerated beyond that if the job atmosphere was hostile and unsupportive.[68] Further, a woman who works outside the home is still usually the person primarily responsible for rearing the children and maintaining the home—doing the laundry, scrubbing the floors, cooking, and essentially having two full-time jobs.

## Job Characteristics

Just as some stress is critical to life, some stress is essential on the job. It's what keeps us motivated, inspired, and productive—as long as it's kept to a healthy level, and a person has some sense of control as to how to deal with it well. In their book *Healthy Work*, authors Robert Karasek of the University of Southern California and Dr. Tores Theorell of Sweden's National Institute for Psychosocial Factors and Health say that the following are characteristics of healthy jobs:

- **Skill discretion.** Your job allows you to make maximum use of your skills and provides the opportunity for you to increase or broaden your skills.

- **Autonomy.** Your job allows you some sense of control. You don't feel as though you are a child being disciplined. You get to participate in long-term planning, and your employer allows flexible hours.

- **Control.** You control the machines at your workplace, not the other way around.

- **Psychological demands.** You have some say over the magnitude of the demands placed on you, and the routine demands you are faced with are mixed with new, unpredictable challenges that help keep the job exciting.

- **Social relations.** You're encouraged to collaborate with your coworkers. There's a sense of teamwork and support.

- **Social rights.** When problems arise, democratic procedures are used to solve them. If you have some kind of a grievance, you know there's an accepted way for you to solve it.

- **Meaningfulness.** Your job has some meaning for you. You know what you're producing, and who it's for. You have ready access to feedback from your customers (the people you work for all day).

- **Integration of family and community life with work.** The people on the job share the responsibilities of running the business, so there's time—and energy—left over for activities other than work.[69]

How do these job characteristics affect health outcomes? Based upon their studies among blue-collar Swedes, researchers Karasek and Theorell summarize quantifiable job effects this way: "For an adult of your age and sex the average life expectancy is thirty more years, but for you, in your psychologically desirable job, it is thirty-seven years. In addition, your job carries with it a 13 percent chance of depression and a 10 percent chance of exhaustion, versus the respective averages 27 percent and 25 [in less desirable jobs] . . . resulting in a life that is seven years longer and twice as free from psychological distress. . . . It is difficult to develop reliable monetary estimates of [job] stress-related losses. . . . But one fact is beyond dispute: the cost is very large."[70]

The authors also note, "While firms must make a profit to survive, it is even more important that the population itself survive, and in a healthy state. New balance sheets will have to be developed." Suppose our business firms were able to see that all their workers are the firm itself, and were committed not only to quantifiable output (economic health), but to the total well being (health) of all in the firm as well? How might we then reshape our work to fit with the proven effects of healthy jobs?

## How Much Stress Is Enough?

Every job is going to include some stress.[71] It might be thunderous noise and wilting heat from the blast furnace of a steel plant, or it might be the inescapable deadlines of reporting for a newspaper. It might be the monotonous repetition of working on an assembly line, or the crushing stress of running a multimillion-dollar corporation. No one would want a job that is totally devoid of stress. Some stress is what makes life (not to mention a job) interesting. But what are the signs that enough is enough, when you've inched over the line toward stress that is debilitating?

Basketball great Bill Russell of the Boston Celtics described the rush that can come from the right level of job stress when he told how the pressures of a pro game begin to percolate: "It usually began when three or four of the ten guys on the floor would heat up," he explained. "The feeling would spread to other guys, and we'd all levitate. . . . The game would be in the white heat of competition, and yet somehow I wouldn't feel competitive. . . . I'd be putting out the maximum effort . . . and yet I never felt the pain. My premonitions would be consistently correct. . . . There have been many times in my career when I felt moved or joyful, but these were moments when I had chills pulsing up and down my spine."[72] It's a level of stress that provides a sense of cohesion, intense satisfaction, great challenge, supreme accomplishment, and personal control.

When there's enough stress to stimulate challenge and satisfaction and control, you'll feel certain emotions and you'll find that your job performance meets certain standards. An optimum level of stress is characterized by high energy, mental alertness, high motivation, calmness under pressure, thorough analysis of problems, improved memory and recall, sharp perception, and an overall optimistic outlook.[73] The signs of too little or too much stress on the job are much the same. Whether absence of job stress has created a monotonous environment devoid of challenge and excitement, or you're in over your head at a job you can't perform to anyone's liking, the signs generally include boredom, apathy, a high accident rate, frequent grievances, absenteeism, a negative outlook toward the employer, widespread fatigue, insomnia, changes in appetite, increased errors, indecisiveness, and increased use of tobacco, drugs, or alcohol.[74]

In summary, keys to healthy work involve creating some sense of personal control, establishing a sense of support, finding intrinsic meaning and purpose in one's work, and hoping to create even better things to come.

## Factors that Influence How We Cope with Stress

Researchers have found that, in addition to the numerous stressors mentioned above, various important factors enable people to cope better with it. For example, genetic susceptibility to distress may be indicated by parents or grandparents who die before the age of sixty-five.[75] The Wisconsin Primate Laboratory, studying mother monkeys for their stress resilience to separation from their family, found that the animals could be bred in stress-resistant and stress-vulnerable strains.[76] One way this happens may relate to the similar genetic inheritance observed for depression and for alcoholism. For example, a person may inherit the tendency to produce much of an enzyme (monoamine oxidase, or MAO) that removes brain neurotransmitters (such as serotonin and dopamine) involved in maintaining control and pleasurable mood. Animals prone to alcoholism by genetics have lower than normal function of these neurotransmitters; treating them with medication that restores serotonin to normal causes a reduction in their voluntary consumption of alcohol.

If these neurotransmitters are removed too rapidly by MAO, a person tends to be shy, "on guard," more antisocial, and more prone to seeing the negatives in life—and, as a result, more distressed. If the MAO is low, on the other hand, the neurotransmitters increase and a person is more likely to be a risk-taker who fails to see dangers.

Factors that increase the ability of children to cope with stress include gender (girls are generally more resilient under stress, though researchers are not sure why), high intelligence, easygoing temperament, a strong internal locus of control, the availability of adults who exhibit warmth and structure, and families with a high socioeconomic status.[77] Attitudes and learned ways of thinking about situations are major factors in the ability to cope with stress. Other factors include a good sense of humor, a well-balanced and nutritious diet, realistic goal setting, plenty of sleep, thorough job preparation, financial security, stability at home, an understanding of stress, and use of relaxation skills.[78] More documented protective factors include high self-esteem, learning to be flexible and innovative in solutions, close personal relationships, having success/mastery experiences, self-discipline (including good control of time), and positive expectancy (hope).

## The Physiological Reactions to Stress

When something sets off the complicated series of physiological responses in the body, the resulting "stress response" involves a series of more than 1,400 known physiochemical reactions. Some of the most common signs and symptoms of stress include headache, backache, insomnia, tightness in the neck and shoulders, indigestion, loss of appetite or excessive eating, and a pounding heartbeat.

The aches and pains we feel in response to stress can be the result of a complex physical reaction. For example, the neurotransmitters serotonin and norepinephrine fall under chronic distress. These same neurotransmitters that are so key to mood and anxiety responses are also important modulators of pain.[79] When they run low in the central nervous system, pain is *upregulated*—that is, a small pain stimulus becomes perceived as a much greater stimulus. Often chronic pain is the result of these neurotransmitter effects of chronic distress. Thus, antidepressant medications or behavioral interventions (such as gaining a sense of control) that raise these central neurotransmitters can be very helpful to reduce chronic pain.[80]

As introduced in Chapter 1, the basics of the physiological reaction to stress were first discovered in 1936 by stress pioneer Hans Selye. Selye called the pattern the general adaptation syndrome.[81] General adaptation syndrome states that there are three inherent stages to the body's reaction to stress. For decades, researchers have studied the syndrome, and Selye's theories have held up to all levels of scientific scrutiny. The general adaptation syndrome is an excellent summary of the physiological changes that follow stress; its major stages are as follows:

1. *Alarm reaction*. In the first stage, the alarm reaction, the body immediately responds to stress; various physiological changes occur that enable the body to combat stress (the fight-or-flight reactions discussed earlier). One of the changes that occurs almost immediately during the alarm reaction is depression of the immune system; normal resistance is lowered, and the victim becomes more susceptible to infection and disease. If the stress is brief, the body's response is limited to that of the alarm reaction. When the stress ends, so does the reaction. The body tends to bounce back and recover quickly.

2. *Resistance*. In stage two, resistance, the body makes physiological changes that enable it to adapt to prolonged stress. The body actually works overtime to bring immune response and resistance up to par. During this second stage, the body's immunocompetence is actually stronger than it normally is, an attempt by the body to keep itself in fighting form. At this stage of increased immune response, a person may get disorders of excess immunity, such as increased allergies or autoimmune diseases (where the immune system attacks the body's own tissues).

3. *Exhaustion*. The body eventually loses the ability to keep up with the demands that stress puts on it and it enters the third stage, exhaustion. Simply stated, the body has its limits. They're different in every person, but when the body reaches its limit, protective immune function breaks down, sometimes with mixtures of too much antibody immunity causing allergies and, at the same time, too little cellular immunity causing susceptibility to infection. This results in some of the diseases of adaptation, the diseases we know as stress-related disorders.[82]

Note that there is significant difference between the acute and chronic stress responses. The immune response in many ways parallels the emotional one. Studies of stress must always take this difference into account. It's much easier to test the effects of short-term, acute stress than to test the effects of chronic stress, which has many more unknown variables.

How quickly a person bounces back from short-term stress depends on that individual's body. How well one withstands long-term stress is an individual thing, too. So is the determination of how long you can go on without breaking down and becoming exhausted. The same factors listed above that allow coping with stress play into how susceptible a person is to developing chronic stress and its illnesses. A particularly important factor is the way we think about the stress. Different modes of thinking produce significantly different responses. For example, the comment, "You're looking good!" could be received by an older person as a compliment, as patronization, or as an implication that the person looks good for such an old person. In each case, the stress response would be very different.

There apparently is even a difference between the way men and women respond to stress. New research shows that though women complain more about the symptoms of stress, such as headaches and backaches, they actually suffer fewer long-term stress-related problems, such as cardiovascular disease. Researchers aren't sure why, but they think the key may lie in female hormones. In one study, women asked to perform stressful tasks registered higher blood pressure and higher heart rates after menopause than before.[83] Other reasons may well involve a woman's greater propensity to express feelings and seek support.

What exactly is the stress response? There is no simple answer, but you can begin to understand some of the profound effects of stress by understanding how it affects major body systems.

## *Stress and the Brain*

The brain is usually the first body system to recognize a stressor. It reacts with split-second timing to instruct the rest of the body how to adjust to the stressor. The latest research shows that the brain continues to stimulate the "stress reaction" for as long as seventy-two hours after a traumatic incident.

The brain is not a good discriminator of stressors. It reacts the same whether the stress is physical (you are almost hit by a car that comes careening around the corner when you step off the curb), emotional (your boss calls you in for another of his "talks"), or even immune-mediated (your body is confronted by a threatening infection). And if the brain over-responds to an emotional stressor, it may well overrespond to a pain or gut stressor, or even an immune stressor, resulting in allergy. What that reaction entails, basically, is the release of a cascade of hormones and brain chemicals that course through the bloodstream, instructing other organs—such as the pituitary, the thyroid, and the adrenals—to release their respective hormones. Just as the brain is the organ that turns on the stress response, it is also the organ that finally turns it off.

Unfortunately, all this hormonal brain activity takes its toll. The latest research reveals that elevated levels of stress hormones kill off significant numbers of vitally important brain cells. According to Stanford University biologist Robert Sapolsky, the stress hormones, the glucocorticoids, trigger the fight-or-flight response that is intended to save us human beings when we are confronted by danger, "but these all-important glucocorticoids also trigger a curious cascading death of the very brain cells that those hormones are meant to protect."[84] This can result, for example, in reduced memory and impaired thinking. University of Kentucky researchers under the direction of Philip Landfield exposed rats to prolonged stress—five days a week for six months. After only three weeks, the rats showed reduced electrical activity in the hippocampus (the crucial memory area of the brain that is most affected by Alzheimer's disease). When examined in autopsies at the end of six months, the rats that were exposed to stress had lost twice as many brain cells—50 percent of all their brain cells—as same-age rats that had been spared the stress.[85]

In separate studies at Stanford University[86] and at the Rockefeller University Laboratory of Neuroendocrinology, researchers found that the stress hormone cortisol makes the cells of the hippocampus smaller. In addition, it results in fewer nerve branches throughout the hippocampus. And the stress does not necessarily need to be prolonged in order to have a significant effect: Excessive cortisol changes the nerve cells and branches of the hippocampus in as brief a time as three weeks.

Sapolsky emphasizes that it's not the stressor that's important, but the perception of it: "The exact same external event can happen to two different people, and, depending on the psychological baggage of the individual experiencing it, the outcome will be different, the disease will be different."[87]

## Stress and the Endocrine System

The function of the endocrine system, with its network of glands, is to secrete hormones. When the body is under stress, two main hormone groups, the catecholamines and the corticosteroids, are galvanized to combat. The catecholamines—adrenaline (or epinephrine) and norepinephrine—can cause the heart to beat faster, the blood vessels to constrict, the muscles to tense up, the respiratory system to work more rapidly, and the blood to thicken and clot in case of injury.

When catecholamine levels are too high, as in chronic stress, the effects can range from minor problems (such as tics and muscle tremors) to more serious, potentially long-range problems, such as diabetes, heart attack, and stroke. In the blood vessels, for example, norepinephrine can cause damage to the vessel lining that allows cholesterol into the wall and can stimulate clotting, both of which can lead to the thickening (plaque) that causes cardiovascular disease. The other major hormone group secreted in response to stress is the group of corticosteroids, including cortisone and cortisol. Too much cortisol can suppress immunity, cause insulin resistance (leading to weight gain and diabetes), increase blood pressure, and cause the previously mentioned progressive nerve loss in the hippocampus.

The changes that occur in the hippocampus as a result of excessive cortisol mimic the loss of cells that results from aging. Studies done at New York University Medical Center point out that aged people are less able to regulate their stress response, and, as a result, levels of cortisol produced during stress don't return to normal for long periods of time. Under these conditions the aged can suffer rapid destruction of brain cells. The New York researchers believe, as a result, that stress can actually play a role in the development and progression of Alzheimer's disease.[88]

Apparently, stress can also interfere with the hormones that influence fertility. Alice Domar, director of the Behavioral Medicine Program for Infertility at the New England Deaconess Hospital, conducted a small study that demonstrated that stress—in this case, from a lack of emotional support—may have an adverse effect on the hormones that influence fertility. Again, Domar warns that her study involved only a small number of patients, and she's hesitant to draw "definitive conclusions," but urges more study of stress and infertility.[89] Clearly, stress can contribute to some infertility; even worrying about not being able to get pregnant can become a self-fulfilling prophecy (worry is picturing the negative happening: for example, being unable to conceive). A common scenario is an "infertile" mother who, when she quits "trying" and adopts a baby, then becomes pregnant. There may be more than just stress involved here, such as the power of pictured expectations: The brain has a way of creating in the body what is being pictured.

Perhaps the most serious complication of chronic high cortisone levels is suppression of the immune system. High cortisol levels can cause shrinkage of the spleen and thymus, which are vital for the production of white blood cells. Known as powerful immunosuppressants, each of the corticosteroids, especially cortisol, "breaks down lymphoid tissues in the thymus and lymph nodes, reduces the level of T helper cells and increases T suppressors, and inhibits the production of natural killer cells. Cortisol also reduces virus-fighting interferon."[90] (Nevertheless, cortisol is not the whole story in stress-induced immunosuppression.)

According to research investigating the link between stress hormones and the immune system, a wide range of diseases is associated with elevated cortisol levels including cancer, hypertension, ulcers, heart attack, diabetes, arthritis, stroke, Parkinson's disease, multiple sclerosis, myasthenia gravis, and a variety of infections. Researchers believe that elevated cortisol levels associated with stress may contribute to psychoses of the aged, depression, "and even perhaps Alzheimer's disease. . . . Elevated cortisol levels are even reported to be a useful predictor of suicide."[91]

## Stress and the Gastrointestinal System

How the gastrointestinal system reacts to the challenges of stress depends in large part on personality traits, say researchers. A study that called on men to solve arithmetic problems and anagrams while under stress showed that some had an increase in gastric acid while others actually had a decrease. The difference, say the researchers, was due to personality traits—in other words, the way people coped with stress.[92] Those who produce too much acid may be at risk for stress-induced ulcers of the stomach or upper small intestine.

One study showed that the important factor seems to be *perceived* stress. More than 4,500 people took part in the National Health and Nutrition Examination Survey Epidemiologic Follow-Up Study. At the beginning of the study, participants did not have peptic ulcer disease; during the thirteen years of the study, researchers followed the participants to see who developed it. Interestingly, during that time, those who perceived themselves as stressed were 1.8 times more likely to develop ulcers than those who did not perceive themselves to be stressed, regardless of how many stressors actually existed.[93]

Other than ulcers, a far more common effect of stress on the gastrointestinal tract is that of "functional bowel disorders," such as irritable bowel syndrome, nonulcer dyspepsia, and esophageal spasm. These are the most common disorders diagnosed in gastroenterology clinics, and they are highly associated with central nervous system disorders (more than 80 percent of patients also have clinical depression or anxiety disorders).[94] This association of depression and anxiety with functional bowel problems makes sense, because their cause really resides not so much in the bowel as in the central and intestinal nervous systems. Abnormalities of the same neurotransmitters involved with stress and depression are the primary culprits in causing the bowel to overrespond to normal bowel stimuli, such as eating food (causing excessive spasm, pain, and bowel movement abnormalities).[95] These same neurotransmitter abnormalities cause the nervous system to overrespond to stress stimuli in an anxiety disorder.

## Stress and the Cardiovascular System

As early as 1628, physician William Harvey maintained that "every affection of the mind that is attended either with pain or pleasure, hope or fear, is the cause of an agitation whose influence extends to the heart."[96] Today, stress is recognized as a major contributor to heart disease. In his book *From Stress to Strength,* cardiologist Robert S. Eliot describes exactly how stress causes coronary artery disease:

- First, stress causes the blood pressure to spike. The increased pressure of the blood pounding through the vessels pummels and weakens the delicate, protective inner lining of the arteries.

- When the lining is damaged, the body starts its first attempt at repair: Fats are deposited in the arteries. The result? Blood vessels are narrowed, blood circulation is slowed, and the likelihood of clotting becomes high.

- The body continues its arsenal of healing: Platelets are mobilized to the damaged arteries. Clots start to form. More fatty material is deposited, and the arteries finally become rigid and inflexible.

That would be bad enough, but when stress continues or recurs, blood pressure spikes again in response to the stress. Now, look at what happens to the arteries already rendered inflexible by earlier stress:

- The inflexible border on the underside of the fatty deposit is distorted and torn by surges in blood pressure.

- The underside of the fatty deposit (the plaque) is filled with tiny blood vessels in an attempt to send nutrients to the damaged artery. When surges in blood pressure cause them to tear, they bleed into the softer surrounding tissues under the plaque. In time, this bleeding dislodges the plaque.

- Once it's dislodged, this rigid, fatty plaque is pushed outward, causing instant obstruction of an already narrowed vessel.

- As the brain recognizes the injury, it instructs the remaining flexible sections of the artery wall to constrict. The result? A sizable length of the artery itself is narrowed.

- Finally, the heart is deprived of oxygen, because oxygenated blood can't circulate through the diseased and narrowed arteries. Heart tissue then dies because of cardiac infarction.[97]

Researchers have noted that in parts of the world where stress is uncommon, so is heart disease.[98] And stress can be life-threatening to a person who already has coronary heart disease: Stress causes the heart to speed up, the blood to circulate more quickly and with greater force, and the blood pressure to escalate. It's a deadly combination to someone whose arteries are already narrowed by disease, as one can imagine from the scenario Eliot describes above. The result is coronary occlusion, damaged heart tissue, and, sometimes, cardiac arrest.[99]

***Mechanisms of Stress: Effects on the Heart.***   Increases in heart rate and blood pressure caused by stress contribute to the increased load on the heart. Stress-induced high blood pressure is even greater among men whose arteries are already clogged by atherosclerosis (characterized by fatty deposits).[100] According to North Carolina A&T researcher Andrew Goliszek:

*The stress of factory noise, for example, has been closely linked to high blood pressure in factory workers exposed to prolonged, daily noise; flood victims experiencing devastating property and financial loss have developed permanent high blood pressure during their recovery periods; and executives in their early thirties, who were chronically angry and hostile but who suppressed their anger and hostility because they couldn't express themselves, developed high blood pressure before they reached their fifties. Even school children are susceptible to high blood pressure when placed in stressful situations.*[101]

Added to this scenario is the problem with some people whom researchers have dubbed "hot reactors," people whose blood pressure seems normal at rest but shoots up to dangerously high levels during stress.[102] Again, this relates to a sensitive nervous system overresponding to stimuli. Eliot estimates that as many as one in five people exhibits undetected daily blood pressure changes that place him or her at high risk for stroke or sudden cardiac death.

"I call those with the most extreme heart and blood pressure responses hot reactors," Eliot maintains. "They burn a dollar's worth of energy for a dime's worth of trouble." And, according to Eliot, they "are pressure cookers without safety valves, literally stewing in their own juices." The worst part of it all, according to Eliot, is that "these people do not suspect that their bodies are paying a high price for overreacting to stress."[103]

What kind of price do hot reactors pay? Eliot has identified ten possible complications of hot reacting: permanent high blood pressure, damaged blood vessel linings, atherosclerosis, accelerated blood clotting, ruptured heart muscle fibers, heart rhythm disturbances, kidney and heart failure, heart attack, stroke, and sudden death.[104]

At the opposite end of the spectrum is the finding that humans who reduce stress enjoy the benefit of lower blood pressure. Research by psychologists at Harvard University followed residents of eight Massachusetts nursing homes for three years. Researchers randomly selected some of the patients in each nursing home and taught each to meditate as a way of reducing stress. At the end of three years, the survival rate among the people who meditated was 100 percent: Not a single one of the patients who meditated had died, and most had significant drops in systolic blood pressure. Among the patients who did not meditate, survival rate was only 62.6 percent.[105]

***Serum Cholesterol.***    Researchers have also shown that stress can elevate levels of serum cholesterol. In one of the first studies showing a link, researchers followed forty accountants who, because of their work, were forced to meet stressful deadlines at specific times of year. The researchers found that the most strenuous work periods coincided with the highest levels of cholesterol, even though the diets and activity levels of the accountants remained unchanged.[106] Friedman, Rosenman, and Carroll reported that, during the period from January 1 to April 15, the cholesterol levels of the accountants rose as much as 100 points over their normal levels.[107]

A number of studies duplicate these findings. One group of researchers measured serum cholesterol levels of medical students a few hours before final examinations and again forty-eight hours later. In all but one student, the serum cholesterol value was an average of 20 percent higher in the stress period before the exam. A similar study showed that the highest cholesterol levels among military pilots in training occurred during examination periods. And studies among college students showed an increase of 11 to 17 percent in cholesterol levels during testing periods.

Almost any kind of stress can cause significantly increased amounts of cholesterol to be released into the bloodstream. A number of studies show that shift work is extremely stressful, particularly for those on the night shift. One study found that night labor was associated with significantly elevated cholesterol levels.[108]

***Spasm in Damaged Blood Vessels.***   Traditional risk factors fail to account for half the cases of clinical coronary artery disease worldwide,[109] yet more than a half million deaths in the United States every year are attributed to arteriosclerosis. Stress delivers a double whammy to people who already have coronary artery disease: Stress causes vessels already choked by plaque to narrow even more, boosting the chance for heart attack. In studies at Harvard Medical School, researchers put subjects under stress to determine the multiplied effect of stress on already damaged arteries. While under stress, the damaged arteries constricted 24 percent more and blood flow declined by 27 percent in the damaged vessels, though it didn't decline in the smooth vessels.[110] This coronary spasm is increased even more if the person has clinical depression (see Chapter 6).

In one study, researchers monitored patients hospitalized in London who were being evaluated for possible coronary bypass surgery. The researchers carefully studied heart function but also measured the levels of stress hormones in the urine and asked patients themselves to record their feelings at various times during the day. The findings showed that the higher the levels of stress hormones in the urine, the more frequent the episodes of silent ischemia.[111]

***Cardiovascular Disease Events.***   Research efforts have shown a strong link between stress and sudden cardiac death. In one study, researchers examined a hundred cases of sudden cardiac death drawn from a coroner's records. The researchers found that almost two-thirds of the victims were under moderate to severe stress on the final day of life, and more than one in five were experiencing acute stress during the last thirty minutes of life. The coroners' reports revealed stressors such as receipt of divorce papers, a fight over a game, an automobile accident, and an attack by dogs as some examples.[112] The sudden deaths were probably due to an irregular heart rhythm caused by catecholamines and increased heart demand as a result of stress.

A growing body of research has shown that, among heart disease patients, mental stress is as dangerous to the heart as physical stress.[113] In a study conducted at the UCLA School of Medicine, subjects were given both mental and physical stress tests; all had been diagnosed as having heart disease. The mental stress caused ischemia in more than half the patients. Researchers found that asking patients to discuss their own shortcomings caused almost the same intensity of heart reactions as did strenuous riding of a stationary bicycle.[114]

While early research on cardiovascular disease centered on diet and exercise, it has taken a dramatic swing toward the examination of stress as a leading factor. Maryland psychologist David Krantz summarizes heart disease as "some interaction of mind, body, and behavior. Your coronary risk probably depends on how your mind interprets situations, how your body reacts, and how often your behavior leads you into stressful situations."[115] This connection between stress and cardiovascular disease will be discussed in more detail in Chapter 3.

## Stress and the Immune System

As research continues into the link between stress and the immune system, as discussed in the psychoneuroimmunology section of Chapter 1, fascinating medical outcomes of that effect continue. For example, research shows that stress can even cause susceptibility to the common "cold." Psychologist Sheldon Cohen and his colleagues at Carnegie Mellon University assessed stress levels for more than 400 healthy adults. A "stress index" was determined, based on symptoms of depression, the number of recent major stressful events, and their assessment of how well they were coping. They were then given nasal drops that contained a small dose of five respiratory disease (common cold) viruses. Those with the highest stress index ran twice the risk of getting a cold and more than five times the risk of becoming infected with a cold virus. The study, says Cohen, "clearly suggests that stress helps produce a susceptibility to colds."[116]

In a similar study done in England, 100 people were asked to keep a diary of things that happened, how they felt about them, and their health. "Uplifts"—experiences that brought pleasure or happiness—were found to decrease significantly in the four days before people developed a cold. Interestingly, the number of "uplifts" seemed more important than the number of hassles, which wasn't as strongly associated with colds. People also reported that they had been feeling more angry, tense, and skeptical during the four days before getting a cold.[117]

Other research also shows that different ways of *coping* with stress seem to modify the impact of stress on immunity. Early research showed that the ability to control and predict stress decreased the physical consequence of that stress; in well-known experiments, laboratory rats that could predict or control a series of shocks were able to avoid the ill effects of stress suffered by the rats that could *not* predict or control the shocks.[118] In the same way, different styles of coping with stress appear to affect the way stress impacts the immune system.[119]

Scientists have come up with a veritable shopping list of conditions caused or aggravated by stress: coronary heart disease, arteriosclerosis, atherosclerosis, high blood pressure, coronary thrombosis, stroke, angina pectoris, respiratory ailments, ulcers, irritable bowel syndrome, ulcerative colitis, gastritis, pancreatitis, diabetes, hyperthyroidism, migraine headache, myasthenia gravis, epileptic attacks, chronic backache, kidney disease, chronic tuberculosis, allergies, rheumatoid arthritis, systemic lupus erythematosus, impotence, infertility, psoriasis, eczema, cold sores, shingles, hives, asthma, Raynaud's disease, multiple sclerosis, cancer, and an entire spectrum of endocrine and autoimmune problems, to name just a few. Physicians caution, however, that "few of these diseases are caused or triggered solely by stress." Other factors must also be considered.[120] While enough bacteria in the right place can cause disease in almost anyone, some people exposed to the usual causes of disease get sick, and some do not. The difference usually resides in that person's "host resistance" to illness. Immunity is part of that resistance. And several mental factors also have proven to be important in host resistance, such as loving support and mature coping styles. (See the chapters on social support and disease-resistant personality such as Chapter 8.) On the other hand, some mental factors undermine resistance, such as hostility, fear, or depression (also discussed in later chapters). Some of these mental factors optimize both immune and mental responses.

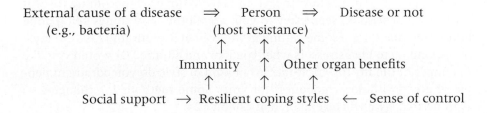

While several factors are involved, findings of continuing research is clear: Stress plays a moderate to major role in a whole Pandora's box of diseases.

## Self-Perceptions of Stress

Obviously, stress can be very detrimental. And, just as obviously, no one can live without some stress. Are we all, then, destined to become victims of stress? Fortunately not.

The researchers who have pinpointed the effects of stress also know that the way a person perceives stress and the way he or she copes with it can keep it from making him or her sick. Attitudes, beliefs, and perceptions can help keep humans well. Ample evidence, cited throughout this book, shows how factors like optimism, faith, hope, and a good explanatory style can help overcome the devastating effects of stress.

Epidemiologist Leonard Sagan remarked that "whether altered conditions are viewed as threatening or challenging, and whether the consequences contribute to personal growth or apathy and despair, is the result of the interaction of two factors: the magnitude and quality of the external stressor and the capacity of the individual to cope."[121]

## How to Protect Yourself from Stress

Since everyone is confronted with stress, are there ways we can protect ourselves from the adverse effects of stress? Absolutely! One of the first ways, says Baylor College of Medicine psychologist Michael Cox, is to face the stress head-on. Recognize it, and get ready to deal with it. "Avoiding and denying that stress exists won't make it go away," he says. "Look at different ways you can change the situation to lessen the stress, make your decision, and face the stress head on. Action is the fastest way to reduce the level of stress."[122] Be prepared for the worst possible scenario, but then leave it behind and work for the best outcome.

Sometimes, for health, a philosophical checkup can be even more useful than a medical one. What is life all about for you? Does life have more to do with proving yourself competitively by generating production numbers, or does it have more to do with discovering and experiencing the sources of joy? Or perhaps learning how to give and receive love? Or becoming wise? If joy or love or wisdom seems key to you, are all the busy things being done enhancing that, or are some getting in the way of it (your joy)? Is your style of responding to life's stressors what you like and admire? Or would you like to temper or modify it somewhat? What kind of style do you admire in people of great wisdom or goodness for you? Some methods for changing to your desired style will be explored in Chapter 24.

Following are some ideas from cardiologist Robert S. Eliot and others as to how you can reduce the effects of stress:

- Develop what Eliot calls a game plan for your personal aspirations, both short-term and long-term ones. Take a personal inventory and reestablish important priorities. You need to balance your talents and goals, similar to the way in which you'd balance your financial portfolio. Work to get things back into balance, and figure out where your long-term goals may be losing out to short-term pressures, Eliot says.

- Do something nice for yourself every day. Take the time to read something you love, soak in a warm bath, take a brisk walk, or call an old friend.

- Commune with nature.

- Develop a system of time management that will help you plan your day without becoming a stressor itself. When you're scheduling your time, remember to leave time for play, time for hobbies and friends, and time for simple relaxation. If you have to, schedule in time for breaks.

- Just as you need to develop a game plan for your personal aspirations, Eliot advises developing a game plan for your career or work. Especially important in today's economy is the ability to adapt, continually assess where you are, look ahead, and anticipate and prepare for change.

- If you commute to work, make sure you plan enough time to arrive without feeling stressed. If you can, turn your commute into something pleasant: ride the bus instead of driving, and take the chance to catch up on some favorite books or magazines. If you have to drive, try out some entertaining tapes or music instead of the usual radio fare.

- Once at work, try the following strategies: Pair up with people you like. Instead of letting the telephone control you, control the telephone; have someone take messages, and block out several periods during the day in which to return calls. Delegate as much work as you can. Do what you can to reduce environmental stresses at work (noise, temperature extremes, and so on). And, at least once a day, concentrate on doing at least one task—no matter how small—that brings you satisfaction.

- Save a little money each month. Take frequent nonbusiness weekends away from home, preferably with your spouse.

- Get married if you're not. Marriage, particularly if carefully nurtured, has been shown to protect against illness.

- Be realistic in your expectations of your children. According to Eliot, it's crucial to accept who they are and let children express their own ideas. Eliot also advocates giving children at least one adult they can look up to and letting them stay closer to home until they have the skills and resources to make it on their own in an increasingly complex world.

- Take a look at your neighborhood. What's going on? Do as much as you can to create a calm, controlled, quiet, comfortable neighborhood and home.

- Pay attention to your physical health. Have regular checkups, and take care of health problems promptly. If you notice unusual symptoms, have a doctor check them out as soon as possible. Above all, believe that you are well.

- Get plenty of sleep. British researchers concluded that flexibility, spontaneity, and originality of thought can be seriously undermined by as little as one sleepless night.

- Eat a balanced diet; avoid tobacco, caffeine, and excess alcohol. During periods of particular stress, go for a small, high-protein meal featuring something like chicken breast, turkey breast, nuts, tuna, or Swiss cheese.

- Get plenty of exercise.

- Stay socially connected. According to Eliot, "Friends are not just nice, they are a necessity." If you have problems, talk them out with a trusted friend; if you're facing something difficult, rehearse it with a friend first. Share your feelings often.

- Develop at least one confidant, someone with whom you can share your deepest thoughts and feelings. And write your thoughts down on a regular basis. Keeping a journal is good, but so is jotting your thoughts on scraps of paper.

- Find and trust in a higher power; develop a sense of spiritual support. Attend your church or synagogue on a regular basis, affiliate with the religious community there, and practice forgiveness on a daily basis. Fill your life with faith; let go of guilt and shame.

- Get a pet! Research has shown that pets reduce stress, lower blood pressure, and provide a type of social support that enhances health.

- Learn to laugh at yourself, and fill your life with humor.

- When things get tough, take a warm bath or shower, or sip a cup of warm herbal tea. And, above all, stay flexible. There may be more ways to cope with any situation than are apparent at first.[123]

## Keys for Handling Job Stress

The same researchers who found that job stress is a killer have also identified a buffer: social support on the job. It might be a boss who treats you with respect. It might be a great feeling of camaraderie with coworkers. It might be regular feedback from customers who appreciate the job you're doing. It might be professional networking with others. Or it might be membership in a labor or professional union. In fact, say researchers Karasek and Theorell, social support on the job "may be one of the most important factors in improving health and well-being in the work environment."[124] As in all other facets of life, the people around us can be the key to good health and long life (see Chapter 9).

In addition to increasing your social support on the job, try the following measures to alleviate job-related stress:

- Take a hard look at the meetings you have to attend. Start by avoiding unnecessary meetings. Could you accomplish the same thing by memo or a few phone calls? When you do find yourself scheduled for a meeting, go in with a clear objective, then stick to the task.

- Set your priorities every morning. Make sure you accomplish at least one thing every day that has high value for you. We all have more items on our "to do" lists than there is time to do them. If one is stuck on the thought, "I have to do it all," frustration results. And usually doing the low-priority items that are right in front of you results in failing on the more subtle high priorities (such as great relationships, for example) for which one needs to consciously block out time. Remember, with "too many things to do," it's really okay not to do it all—and in fact, saying "no" to low-priority items allows you to do your more valued thing. The resultant sense of control over your life is highly health promoting.

- Fridays tend to be "down days," so save the last hour or so on Friday for housekeeping tasks, such as straightening your desk, sorting your mail, returning phone calls, or listing your tasks for Monday. Then save something you really like to do for Monday morning, to get your week started off on a pleasant note.

- Take frequent breaks. You know you need a break when you find yourself daydreaming, you start procrastinating, you have a mental block, or you're feeling tense. Remember that you should take more frequent breaks if you are doing work that requires a lot of concentration. And people who take regular vacations are much less prone to burnout.

- Find meaning and purpose in work.

Rachel Naomi Remen, a physician deeply concerned about the phenomenon of burnout and loss of meaning in the workplace, has found some simple techniques that can be very useful in rediscovering the purpose and meaning you once felt toward your work: She suggests taking ten minutes at the end of the day to journal the answers to the following three questions:[125]

- *"What surprised me today?"*
- *"What moved or touched me today?"*
- *"What inspired me today?"*

Look for the stories. After some time, instead of seeing the answers six or more hours later, you will start to see them as they happen.

Such techniques allow you to recapture the purposes for which you chose your work. For life to be satisfying, your work needs to have intrinsic value—a quality that makes you look forward to going—rather than just the extrinsic rewards. It has been said that happiness consists of meaningful, good work to do and someone to love.

Ultimately, since much of life's stress can only be modified but not eliminated, the real key is turning distress into eustress, the principles of which will be discussed in the chapter on disease resilience and in Chapters 23 and 24.

## ENDNOTES

1. Marc K. Lewen and Harold L. Kennedy, "The Role of Stress in Heart Disease," *Hospital Medicine* (August 1986): 125–38.
2. Ari Kiev, "Managing Stress to Achieve Success," *Executive Health* 24 (1; 1987): 1–4.
3. Dharma Singh Khalsa, "Stress-Related Illness," *Postgraduate Medicine* 78 (6; 1985): 217–21.
4. Susan Jenks, "Further Clues to CAD-Stress Link," *Medical World News* (June 13, 1988): 108.
5. Paul Rosch, "Good Stress: Why You Need It to Stay Young," *Prevention* (April 1986): 29.
6. Ibid.
7. Ruthan Brodsky, "Identifying Stressors Is Necessary to Combat Potential Health Problems," *Occupational Health and Safety* 30–32.
8. Emrika Padus, *Positive Living and Health: The Complete Guide to Brain/Body Healing and Mental Empowerment* (Emmaus, PA: Rodale Press, 1990).
9. Mary F. Asterita, *The Physiology of Stress* (New York: Human Sciences Press, 1985), 4–5.
10. Claudia Wallis, "Stress: Can We Cope?" *Time*, June 6, 1983, 48–54.
11. Peter G. Hanson, *The Joy of Stress* (Kansas City, MO: Andrews, McMeel, and Parker, 1986).
12. Lawrence E. Lamb, "Your Vital Adrenal Steroids (Corticosteroids)," *The Health Letter* 34 (4; 1989): 1–8.
13. Robert S. Eliot, *From Stress to Strength* (New York: Bantam Books, 1994), 24.
14. Kiev, 1–4.
15. Brodsky, 30–32.
16. Ibid.,30–32.
17. P. D. Somervell, B. H. Kaplan, and G. Heiss, "Psychologic Distress as a Predictor of Mortality," *American Journal of Epidemiology* 130 (5; 1989): 1013–23.
18. *British Medical Journal* (October 30, 1993), 1102–5.
19. Hanson.
20. Wallis, 48–54.

21. Bernie S. Siegel, *Love, Medicine, and Miracles* (New York: Harper and Row Publishers, 1986).
22. Horst Scherg and Maria Blohmke, "Associations Between Selected Life Events and Cancer," *Behavioral Medicine* (Fall 1988): 119–24.
23. H. J. F. Baltrush, reported at the Third International Symposium on Detection and Prevention of Cancer.
24. Ibid.
25. Ian Wickramasekera, "Risk Factors Leading to Chronic Stress-Related Symptoms," *Advances* 4 (1; 1987): 21.
26. M. Weinberger, S. L. Heiner, and W. M. Tierney, "In Support of Hassles as a Measure of Stress in Predicting Health Outcomes," *Journal of Behavioral Medicine* 10 (1; 1987): 19–32.
27. Wallis, 48–54.
28. Haim Omer and George S. Everly, Jr., "Psychological Factors in Preterm Labor: Critical Review and Theoretical Synthesis," *Advances* 7 (1; 1990): 11–13, adapted from *American Journal of Psychiatry* 145 (72; 1988): 1507–13.
29. Harold A. Williamson, Jr., Michael LeFevre, and Melvin Hector, Jr., "Association Between Life Stress and Serious Perinatal Complications," *The Journal of Family Practice*, 29 (5; 1989): 489–96.
30. Lynne C. Huffman and Rebecca del Carmen, "Prenatal Stress," in L. Eugene Arnold, ed., *Childhood Stress* (New York: John Wiley and Sons, Inc., 1990), 144–72.
31. Marie L. Lobo, "Stress in Infancy," in Arnold, *Childhood Stress*, 173–92.
32. Lobo, 173–92.
33. Nemeroff.
34. Susan Jones Sears and Joanne Milburn, "School-Age Stress," in Arnold, *Childhood Stress*.
35. Ibid.
36. Robert L. Hendren, "Stress in Adolescence," in Arnold, *Childhood Stress*, 247–66.
37. Age-related stressors summarized from Jerrold S. Greenberg, *Comprehensive Stress Management*, 3rd ed. (Dubuque, IA: Wm. C. Brown Publishers, 1990), 299–393.
38. "Stress in Workplace Is Rising, Survey Says," *Deseret News*, May 8: 1991, 3A.
39. "About Half Suffer from Stress Due to Job, Gallup Poll Says," *Deseret News*, January 11, 1990.
40. Ibid.
41. R. N. Remen, *Int Med News* 1/15/02, p.5.
42. L. M. Belliini, *JAMA* 2002; 287: 3143–46.
43. M. Boles, B. Pelletier, W. Lynch, "The Relationship Between Health Risks and Work Productivity." *J Occup Environ Med.* 2004 Jul; 46(7): 737–45.
44. Walt Schafer, *Stress Management for Wellness* (New York: Holt, Rinehart & Winston, Inc., 1987), 310.
45. Cary L. Cooper and Roy Payne, eds., *Causes, Coping, and Consequences of Stress at Work* (New York: John Wiley & Sons Ltd., 1988), 9.
46. K. Pelletier and R. Lutz, "Healthy People—Healthy Business: A Critical Review of Stress Management in the Workplace," *American Journal of Health Promotion* 2 (3; 1988): 5–12.
47. Cooper and Payne, 10.
48. Ibid.
49. "Battling the Enemy Within," *Time*, March 17, 1986, 52.
50. Ronald B. Goodspeed and Ann G. DeLucia, "Stress Reduction at the Worksite:

An Evaluation of Two Methods," *American Journal of Health Promotion* 4 (5; 1990): 333.

51. "Healthy Lives: A New View of Stress," *University of California Berkeley Wellness Letter* (June 1990): 5.

52. S. J. Bigos, M. C. Battie, D. M. Spengler, L. D. Fisher, W. E. Fordyce, T. Hansson, A. L. Nachemson, J. Zeh, "A Longitudinal, Prospective Study of Industrial Back Injury Reporting." *Clin Orthop.* 1992 Jun; (279): 21–34.

53. B. G. Druss, M. Schlesinger, H. M. Allen Jr., "Depressive Symptoms, Satisfaction with Health Care, and 2-Year Work Outcomes in an Employed Population." *Am J Psychiatry.* 158, no. 5 (May 2001): 731–4.
    Also W. N. Burton, G. Pransky, D. J. Conti, C. Y. Chen, D. W. Edington, "The Association of Medical Conditions and Presenteeism." *J Occup Environ Med.* 46 (Jun 2004): S38–45.
    Also D. A. Adler, J. Irish, T. J. McLaughlin, C. Perissinotto, H. Chang, M. Hood, L. Lapitsky, W. H. Rogers, D. Lerner, "The Work Impact of Dysthymia in a Primary Care Population." *Gen Hosp Psychiatry.* 26, no. 4 (Jul–Aug 2004): 269–76.

54. Robert Karasek and Tores Theorell, *Healthy Work: Stress, Productivity, and Reconstruction of Working Life* (New York: Basic Books, 1990), 176.

55. Ibid.

56. Cooper and Payne; Schafer; Matteson and Ivancevich; and Arthur P. Brief, Randall S. Schuler, and Mary Van Sell, *Managing Job Stress* (Boston: Little, Brown, 1980), 13–14.

57. J. V. Johnson, E. M. Hall, T. Theorell, "Combined Effects of Job Strain and Social Isolation on Cardiovascular Disease Morbidity and Mortality in a Random Sample of the Swedish Male Working Population." *Scand J Work Environ Health.* 15, no. 4 (Aug 1989): 271–9.

58. P. A. Landsbergis, P. L. Schnall, K. Warren, T. G. Pickering, J. E. Schwartz, "Association Between Ambulatory Blood Pressure and Alternative Formulations of Job Strain." *Scand J Work Environ Health.* 20, no. 5 (Oct 1994): 349–63.

59. P. L. Schnall, J. E. Schwartz, P. A. Landsbergis, K. Warren, T. G. Pickering, "A Longitudinal Study of Job Strain and Ambulatory Blood Pressure: Results from a Three-Year Follow-up." *Psychosom Med.* 60, no. 6(Nov 1998): 697–706.

60. "Good Boss, Good Health," *Your Personal Best* (September 1990): 3.

61. Anders Falk, Bertil S. Hanson, Sven-Olof Isacsson, and Per-Olof Ostergren, "Job Strain and Mortality in Elderly Men: Social Network, Support, and Influence as Buffers," *American Journal of Public Health* 82 (8; 1992): 1136–38.

62. I. K. Crombie, M. B. Kenicer, W. C. S. Smith, and H. D. Tunstall-Pedoe, "Unemployment, Socioenvironmental Factors, and Coronary Heart Disease in Scotland," *British Heart Journal,* 61 (2; 1989): 172–7.

63. M. H. Brenner, "Economic Instability, Unemployment Rates, Behavioral Risks, and Mortality Rates in Scotland, 1952–1983." *Int J Health Serv.* 17, no. 3 (1987): 475–87.

64. Bryan E. Robinson, "Are You a Work Addict?" *East/West* (August 1990): 50.

65. Diane Fassel, "Work- and Rushaholics: Spotting a Lethal Disease," *Longevity* (September 1990); 78.

66. Ibid., 78.

67. "Healthy Lives: A New View of Stress," *University of California Berkeley Wellness Letter* (June, 1990); 5.

68. S. G. Haynes, M. Feinleib, "Women, Work and Coronary Heart Disease: Prospective Findings from the Framingham Heart Study." *Am J Public Health.* 70, no. 2 (Feb 1980): 133–41.

69. Karasek and Theorell, Chs. 1–4.

70. Ibid.

71. Cooper and Payne; Schafer; Matteson and Ivancevich; and Brief, Schuler, and Van Sell.
72. "Healthy Lives: A New View of Stress."
73. Rosalind Forbes, *Corporate Stress* (Garden City: Doubleday, 1979), 43.
74. Forbes, 44.
75. Hanson.
76. G. P. Sackett, "Genotype Determines Social Isolation Rearing Effects on Monkeys," *Developmental Psychology* 17 (1981): 313–8.
77. Ann S. Masten, "Stress, Coping, and Children's Health," *Pediatric Annals* 14 (8; 1985): 546.
78. Hanson.
79. Stephen M. Stahl, "Does Depression Hurt?" *J Clin Psychiatry* (2002): 63, 273–4; Also Stephen M. Stahl, "The Psychopharmacology of Painful Physical Symptoms in Depression." *J Clin Psychiatry* (2002): 392–3.
80. H. J. McQuay, et al. "Sysytematic Review of Outpatient Services for Chronic Pain Control." *Health Technological Assessment* 1997;1: i–iv, 1–135; C. Redillas, S. Solomon, "Prophylactic Pharmacological Treatment of Chronic Daily Headache." *Headache* 2000; 40: 83–102; A. G. Lipman, "Analgesic for Neuropathic and Sympathetically Maintained Pain." *Clin Geriatr Med* 1996; 12: 501–15.
81. Andrew G. Goliszek, *Breaking the Stress Habit* (Winston-Salem, North Carolina: Carolina Press, 1987).
82. Ibid.
83. Kelly Costigan, "What Is a Woman's Most Stressful Occupation?" *Complete Woman* (April 1988): 32–33.
84. Jerry Lazar, "New Proof That Stress Ages the Brain," *Longevity* 2 (3; 1988): 25.
85. "Workplace Warning: Stress May Speed Brain Aging," *New Sense Bulletin* 16 (11; 1991): 1.
86. Bruce S. McEwen, "Hormones and the Nervous System," *Advances* 7(1): 1990, 50–54.
87. Ibid.
88. Ibid.
89. "The Stress-Infertility Link," *Longevity* (September: 1993): 26.
90. Michael A. Weiner, *Maximum Immunity* (Boston: Houghton Mifflin Company, 1986).
91. Ibid.
92. G. Holtmann, R. Kriebel, and M. V. Singer, "Mental Stress and Gastric Acid Secretion: Do Personality Traits Influence the Response?" *Editor's Citation Abstract* 35 (8: 1990): 998–1007.
93. R. F. Anda, D. F. Williamson, L. G. Escobedo, P. L. Remington, E. E. Mast, and J. Madans, "Self-Perceived Stress and the Risk of Peptic Ulcer Disease: A Longitudinal Study of U.S. Adults," *Archives of Internal Medicine* 152 (1992): 829–33.
94. Lydiard, et al., *Psychosomatics* 1993; 34: 229–234; also Walker, et al., *Am J Psychiatry* 1990;147:565–72.
95. Gershon. *Aliment Pharmacol Ther.* 1999;13(suppl 2):15-30. Also Humphrey et al., *Aliment Pharmacol Ther.* 1999;13(suppl 2):31-38. 3. Bearcroft et al., *Gut.* 1998; 42 :42–46.
96. Andrew G. Goliszek, *Breaking the Stress Habit* (Winston-Salem, NC: Carolina Press, 1987).
97. Eliot, 30–31.
98. Goliszek.
99. "Stress Can Make You Sick," *Consumer Reports Health Letter* 2(1; 1990): 1, 3.
100. "Can Stress Clog Arteries?" *Consumer Reports on Health* (December 1993): 133.

101. Goliszek.

102. Susan Jenks, "Further Clues to CAD-Stress Link," *Medical World News*, (June 13, 1981): 108.

103. Robert S. Eliot and Dennis L. Breo, "Are You a Hot Reactor? Is It Worth Dying For?" *Executive Health*, 20(10); 1984, 1–4.

104. Eliot, 18.

105. Stephen Brewer, "Anti-Old-Age Stress," *Longevity* (June 1990): 82.

106. Larry A. Tucker, Galen E. Cole, and Glenn M. Friedman, "Stress and Serum Cholesterol: A Study of 7,000 Adult Males," *Health Values*, 2 (3; 1987): 34–39.

107. Eliot, 40.

108. Tucker, Cole, and Friedman, 34–39.

109. John E. Sutherland, "The Link Between Stress and Illness," *Postgraduate Medicine*, 89 (1; 1991): 162.

110. K. A. Fackelmann, "Stress Puts Squeeze on Clogged Vessels," *Science News*, November 16 1991, 309.

111. Marjory Roberts, "Stress and the Silent Heart Attack," *Psychology Today* (August 1987): 7.

112. Peter Riech, "How Much Does Stress Contribute to Cardiovascular Disease?" *Journal of Cardiovascular Medicine* (July: 1983): 825–831.

113. C. Noel Bairey, et al., "Mental Stress as an Acute Trigger of Left Ventricular Dysfunction and Blood Pressure Elevation in Coronary Patients," *American Journal of Cardiology* 66 (1991): 28G.

114. Editors of *Prevention* Magazine.

115. Cited in John Tierney, "Stress, Success, and Samoa," *Hippocrates* (May/June 1987): 84.

116. S. Cohen, D. A. Tyrrell, and A. P. Smith, "Psychological Stress and Susceptibility to the Common Cold," *New England Journal of Medicine* 325 (1991); 606–612.

117. P. D. Evans and N. Edgerton, "Life-Events and Mood as Predictors of the Common Cold," British Journal of Medical Psychology, 64 (1; 1991): 35–44.

118. P. Mormède, R. Dantzer, and B. Michaud, "Influence of Stressor Predictability and Behavioral Control on Lymphocyte Reactivity, Antibody Responses and Neuroendocrine Activation in Rats," *Physiological Behavior*, 43 (1988): 577–583.

119. Robert Dantzer, "Stress and Immunity: What Have We Learned from Psychoneuroimmunology?" *ACTA Physiologica Scandinavia*, 161, supplementum 640 (November 1997).

120. S. I. McMillen, *None of These Diseases*, rev. ed. (Old Tappan, NJ: Fleming H. Revell Company, 1984).

121. Leonard A. Sagan, *The Health of Nations* (New York: Basic Books, 1987).

122. "Learn to Manage the Stress in Your Life," *Healthline* (September 1993).

123. Eliot, 107–144.

124. Karasek and Theorell, 138, (see Figure 4–5 a–b).

125. Remen, 5.

# Part II

# Personality Styles and Health

This portion of the book presents information concerning personality characteristics with consequent effects, and their impact upon health. These health-impacting characteristics or traits can increase the possibility of disease development or affect a disease-resistant personality. The chapters and topics presented in this section are:

**Chapter 3**    *The Disease-Prone Personality*

**Chapter 4**    *Anger, Hostility, and Health*

**Chapter 5**    *Worry, Anxiety, Fear, and Health*

**Chapter 6**    *Depression, Despair, and Health*

**Chapter 7**    *Insomnia and Sleep Deprivation: Health Effects and Treatment*

**Chapter 8**    *The Disease-Resistant Personality*

# The Disease-Prone Personality

*The tragedy of life is what dies inside a man while he lives.*

—Albert Schweitzer

## Learning Objectives

- Define the concept of personality.
- Understand the relationship between personality and disease.
- Explain the existing controversy around disease-prone personalities.
- Identify the "toxic core" of the Type A behavior pattern.
- Explain the traits of the cancer-prone personality.
- Identify personality patterns that have been linked to specific diseases.

Psychologist and clinical professor of community medicine at the University of California Howard S. Friedman wrote, "I have never seen a death certificate marked 'Death due to unhealthy personality.' But maybe pathologists and coroners should be instructed to take into account the latest scientific findings on the role of personality in health."[1]

## Definitions and Foundation

Personality is the whole of your personal characteristics, the group of behavioral and emotional tendencies that distinguish you from everybody else.[2] It is the way your habits, attitudes, and traits combine to make the person that is uniquely you. Because of your personality, you act in a similar and generally consistent way from one day to the next. Personality depends partly on the unique set of genes you inherited from your parents, but it is also shaped powerfully by the family you grow up in, the environment that surrounds you, and the culture and subcultures that influence you.[3]

The theory that personality affects health is, as world-renowned psychologist Hans J. Eysenck put it, a theory "based on centuries of observations made by keen-eyed physicians."[4] The notion that a certain personality type leads to heart disease dates back more than 2,000 years to Hippocrates, and the belief that a certain personality type is associated with cancer goes back several centuries.

One of the first recorded suspicions of a link between personality and disease occurred in the 1940s, when Dr. Franz Alexander treated two women for breast cancer.[5] The two were similar in almost every way, but two years after their mastectomies, one was dying while the other was well. In an effort to explain the differences, Alexander finally turned to personality. The woman who was dying told everyone she was getting well, but underneath her brave facade, she couldn't confront either the disease or its possible outcome. The woman who was well faced her problems head-on. She acknowledged that her situation was tough and then found ways of making adjustments and workable solutions.

Subsequent research on personality and health was pioneered by Yugoslav psychologist Ronald Grossarth-Maticek. Earlier researchers had noted that people with certain illnesses (most commonly heart disease and cancer) had certain personality traits in common, but all of the studies that led to those theories involved people who were already ill. Had the illness itself engendered the personality traits, rather than the other way around?

What science needed was a study involving healthy people—a study that would characterize participants' personality traits, monitor them for a number of years, note which ones got ill, and determine whether there was any correlation between personality traits and the tendency to develop certain diseases.

Grossarth-Maticek took on the challenge. He started by identifying large random samples of subjects. He recorded each person's current physical health, smoking and drinking habits, and other health behaviors. Then he devised several ways to measure personality. At the end, Grossarth-Maticek categorized people into one of six categories: One was prone to develop cancer and one was prone to develop heart disease.[6]

He followed each group closely for at least ten years, some for thirteen years. The results were remarkable. He was able to predict death from cancer with six times greater accuracy than it was possible to predict it based on cigarette smoking.

Among the groups he said were prone to develop cancer (those with inhibited, self-centered expression and a helpless, victimized personality style), almost half did die from cancer, but fewer than one in ten died from heart disease. Among those he predicted to be prone to heart disease (those with a hostile, aggressive personality style and barriers to self-centered expression), more than a third did die of heart disease, but only one in five died from cancer. Among the groups he predicted to be prone to good health, there were relatively few deaths.[7] Though there have been criticisms of and issues with his methodology,[8] to his credit, Grossarth-Maticek's ideas "in the early 1960s agree almost perfectly with the most recent results of American and British research in this field."[9]

Grossarth-Maticek then set out to determine whether the outcome of disease could be affected by changing some personality traits. In one study, he identified people with disease-prone personalities. Then he split that group randomly in half: Half received counseling that included modeling, suggestion, relaxation, visualization, desensitization, and other standard behavioral techniques used to modify personality. The other half received no counseling at all. The group that received counseling had lower death rates from both cancer and heart disease. He later repeated the studies with Eysenck.[10] Together, they found they could reduce by half the death rates from cancer and heart disease with as few as six hours of group therapy.

Grossarth-Maticek's work is the subject of considerable controversy. One report on his work maintains that his claims have "raised eyebrows, skeptical inquiries, and even some charges of scientific fraud."[11] Others charge that his work was riddled with technical and statistical problems that can cast doubt on data.[12] In defense of the work, however, one editor opined,

> *Many great scientific discoveries, of course, have had uncertain and spotty histories. Physicist Niels Bohr won a Nobel Prize for his model of the atom, which turned out to be inaccurate but inspired the research that got it right. Gregor Mendel made serious mistakes in his genetics experiments, but his research led to our modern understanding of human genetics and biology. And despite the criticism, no one, since Grossarth-Maticek began publishing his findings in 1980, has been able to knock down his numbers.[13]*

Even though critical reviews since that time have challenged Grossarth-Maticek's numbers,[14] University of South Florida psychologist Charles Spielberger says that therapies aimed at changing personality traits may have some validity after all. "Even if the benefits of these therapies were reduced by one-half, or two-thirds, one could not reasonably allow the information to be suppressed," Spielberger says. "In the five or ten years needed to replicate these findings, thousands of men and women will die from cancer and heart attacks." As Spielberger points out, preventive psychotherapy isn't going to hurt anyone, and if it helps some, "more power to it."[15]

Regardless of the controversies surrounding Grossarth-Maticek's findings, say the experts, they endow us with hope and encourage further research to pinpoint what influence personality may have on health.

We don't know everything about the link between personality and health, but we do know a great deal about how personality influences health and which personality traits seem particularly connected to certain diseases. A warning is in order, however. With all of our research into the impact of personality on disease, we must carefully avoid blaming any person for his or her illness. Any person can get almost any illness. Personality styles or mental stress do not cause disease so much as they act as a risk factor that, when combined with other risk factors, increases vulnerability.

If you breathe high levels of cigarette smoke or certain other pollutants, there is a good chance that you will develop lung cancer. If you are a woman whose mother and aunts and sisters developed breast cancer, there is a good chance that you will develop breast cancer. In cases like these, your emotional responses may not play a significant role in preventing the cancer. Disease is influenced not only by psychological factors but also by the genes we are born with and the environment in which we live. In fact, most instances of disease are caused by a convergence of factors. As many well-known cases demonstrate, it is a sad fact of life that some people contract cancer and die of it at a young age, regardless of personality or heroic struggle.[16]

Even when people accept blame for an illness, it may be a mistake to assume that they "brought it on" themselves. Such a viewpoint may lead to inhumanity and a lack of compassion for people who need it most.

Why, then, is it important to study the links that we know exist between personality and disease? Because there is a great deal you can do to protect and preserve your own health. It won't work *all* of the time for *all* of the people in *all* circumstances, but a fair share—a majority, in fact—can help themselves stay healthy, and a fair share of those who become ill can help themselves recover.

## Disease and Personality: Exploring the Connection

Most people, whether they know it or not, associate certain personality types with particular illnesses. Workaholics have heart attacks. Worriers get ulcers. People who get too uptight have asthma attacks. In reality, can they be so neatly categorized?

Not yet, but researchers have made tremendous strides in proving that personality does have an impact on health. They have found that the way we look at things, as determined by our personality, may actually contribute to illness (or help keep us well).

A variety of studies dating back more than four decades has exposed the "tip of the iceberg" as far as personality and health connections are concerned. In 1948, a group of medical students at Johns Hopkins University described what they saw in ten Rorschach inkblots. What they saw tells a great deal about their outlook and the substantial differences in their personalities. Some saw the inkblot as a young couple kissing, two people shaking hands, or two dancers; others saw in the same pattern two dogs snarling at each other or two cannibals boiling Macbeth in a kettle.[17]

More than three decades later, psychologist Pirkko L. Graves and her colleagues combined the responses of those medical students with the responses of other groups of students (some of whom had been tested as recently as 1964). Graves rated the students according to an eleven-point scale, then categorized them according to their general personality and personal interaction style.

No one was surprised to learn that the distant, withdrawn students who had a generally "negative" approach to interactions were much more likely to develop a severe mental disorder in the three decades following the first study. What *was* a surprise was that those students were also much more likely to have developed cancer—especially cancers of the stomach, pancreas, rectum, large intestine, and lymph nodes, as well as Hodgkin's disease, leukemia, and multiple myeloma.[18]

Recent analysis looked at the notion that prominent people are more prone to develop Parkinson's disease—and explored the possibility that the traits that lead people to rise to positions of authority might be the same personality traits that increase the risk of Parkinson's disease.[19] In a study that focused on Wilhelm von Humboldt and Adolf Hitler, research showed that those traits—ambition, perfectionism, rigidity, and repressed emotions—appear to boost the risk not only of Parkinson's disease, but also of general infection.

Other research[20] shows that certain personality traits are strongly associated with how people perceive their own health. After studying a large sample of adults aged twenty-five to seventy-four, researchers determined a solid relationship between personality traits and the way people perceive their health. Regardless of whether the people were healthy or ill, several traits were consistently associated with a perception of good health—including openness to experiences, extraversion, and conscientiousness. Similarly, several traits were consistently associated with a perception of poor health, including neuroticism. The association remained significant even after adjusting for factors like age, gender, race, marital status, and education.

## Differing Views on Personality and Disease
### Generic View

Other studies have also shown a link between personality and health. In an analysis of 101 studies conducted between 1945 and 1984, researchers concluded that there are "strong links" between personality and health.[21] While not ready to attach a single personality trait to a single disease, they did conclude that there was a strong connection between certain personality traits and "all diseases except ulcers," the most damaging personality traits being depression, anxiety, anger, and hostility.[22] "Personality may function as diet does: Imbalances can predispose one to all sorts of diseases."[23]

One viewpoint, then, holds that certain personality traits (or, in essence, a certain personality type) cause disease. Researchers who support this point of view believe that there may be a generic "disease-prone personality," but not individual "disease personalities" (such as cancer personality or ulcer personality, for example).

### Disease-Prone Personality View

Other researchers disagree, saying that certain "personalities" or personality traits can be specifically linked to certain diseases. Most prominent in research has been the "coronary-prone personality," the hard-driving and competitive Type A personality who is also hostile, angry, and suspicious. Also prominent in current research is the "cancer-prone personality," characterized by people who demonstrate little emotion, are ambivalent toward self and others, and were not close to their parents.

### Disease Cluster View

A third group of researchers believes that a specific personality may make a person susceptible to a "cluster" of conditions, not just a specific disease. Based on extensive research, Caroline Bedell Thomas and her coworkers at the Johns Hopkins School of Medicine believe that people can be categorized into three broad personality types—alphas, betas, and gammas—which can determine whether they are more prone to become ill or stay healthy.[24]

*Alphas.* Alphas are slow and solid, wary in new situations, gradually adaptable, and undemanding. Only about one-fourth of the alphas became seriously ill in the thirty years of Thomas's study.

*Betas.* Betas are cool and clever, quick to respond to new situations, articulate, and understanding. Only about one-fourth of the betas became seriously ill within thirty years. This group was most prone to be healthiest.

*Gammas.* The group with the greatest health problems were the gammas: either too careful or devil-may-care; often brilliant, but also moody and confused in new situations; and either too demanding or not demanding enough. In one of Thomas's studies, 77 percent of the gammas developed cancer, mental illness, high blood pressure, or heart disease or committed suicide. In another study, half of all the sick students were in the gamma group.

### The Personality Cluster View

A similar viewpoint focuses on personality clusters. Rather than grouping people by personality traits, some researchers have identified what they call clusters or cluster groups—groups that have similar specific personality types. Researchers then identify diseases that seem most closely related to that cluster type. One group of researchers at Georgia State University identified five clusters of illnesses and determined which patterns of personality were strongly associated with each cluster.[25]

## The Controversy

Most researchers now accept the notion of an "immune-prone personality," one whose hardiness enables him or her to tolerate the ravages of stress without becoming ill. There is not such widespread acceptance of the notion that certain personality traits are linked to illness.

Contemporary research on personality and health has been surrounded by controversy for many reasons.[26] First, many physicians are simply not trained to think that way. They want a simple or tangible reason for a disorder so they can "fix it." Second, many physicians still think of the mind and the body as two separate entities that do not affect each other. Third, many physicians (and patients) are skeptical about unusual approaches, including the notion that personality affects health. Finally, the notion that personality affects health is simply not as financially rewarding for a practitioner. Our medical delivery system pays far more for mechanical procedures than for knowledgeable patient teaching and "healing." A surgeon who removes a diseased gallbladder makes hundreds of dollars for an hour's work; not so for a doctor who spends an hour talking to a depressed patient troubled by headaches.

The controversy was fueled a few years ago in response to the report of a study by Barrie R. Cassileth and her colleagues at the University of Pennsylvania. Her research team declared that neither positive attitudes nor feelings of depression or hopelessness had any effect on the survival rates of more than 350 people with advanced cancer. Cassileth's study was printed in the *New England Journal of Medicine*, which prompted pathologist and senior deputy editor of the journal, Marcia Angell, to editorialize, "Our belief in disease as a direct reflection of mental state is largely folklore."[27]

In her editorial, Angell criticized the medical community and the media for giving too much credit to personality and emotions as factors in physical health. "We are told," she wrote, that "type A people are vulnerable to heart attacks, repressed people (especially those who have suffered losses) are at risk of cancer, worry causes peptic ulcers, and so on."[28] Further, Angell said that studies relating personality to health were flawed in their design, analysis, or interpretation and that it was dangerous for patients to believe their emotional attitude can save them from serious illness because it could cause patients to forego necessary medical control in favor of some "method of mind control."[29]

Angell's editorial was incendiary. The journal was flooded with letters from physicians and former cancer patients disputing the editorial's claims. The 60,000-member American Psychological Association issued a statement attacking Angell's piece as "inaccurate and unfortunate."[30] In the years that have followed, the debate has continued.

Shortly after the editorial appeared in the journal, *MD* conducted a poll of its physician readers, asking, "Does emotional state affect disease?"[31] The doctors could hardly have been more unequivocal in their answers: Of the 126 who responded, 124 said yes; only 2 said no. Some of the physicians who responded did not believe that emotions or personality "cause" illness, but almost all conceded that personality has a profound effect on the outcome of an illness.

## Explaining the Differences in People

Regardless of where you stand on the controversy over personality and health, there's one clear fact: We all respond differently to the stresses and problems that confront us in life. Whether it's a bad day or a chronic emotional crisis, some of us sail through valiantly and others of us get sick. Even among those who get sick, there are differences; some suffer from insomnia, others from crippling headaches, and still others from indigestion.

We know that stress can cause physical illness. What we have not known until recently is why it has such a different effect on different people. Researchers think that part of the answer is personality.

The process begins when the brain directs various glands in the body to secrete hormones, which circulate through the bloodstream giving "orders" to various tissues and organs. They may direct the blood vessels to constrict, for example, or instruct the body to metabolize sugar. Once the specific task has been completed, a feedback system signals the brain, and the hormone subsides. Everyone has the same network, the same sets of hormonal switches and cycles. They control how we respond in all kinds of situations, including stressful ones.

If everyone has the same physiological makeup, why do we react so differently? Personality may play a key role—as do diet, accidents, early childhood experiences, and our genetic makeup. These factors create what researchers call weak links, which determine where stress is apt to strike a given person.[32] Psychoanalyst Herbert J. Freudenberger points out that these weak links, part of our personality, are for the most part "learned and reinforced behaviors."[33] It explains why one person under stress gets a backache while another gets an ulcer. In essence, it's another explanation of how personality can affect health.

Regardless of the illness involved, researchers reporting their findings in the *British Journal of Medical Psychology* pointed out perhaps one of the most telling traits of a disease-prone personality. Researchers at the University of Helsinki studied almost 200 people with various diseases and found an amazing difference: Unlike their normal counterparts, those with disease-prone personalities felt more emotionally stable when they were ill. More than anything else, that finding may help us distinguish those who, as Friedman wrote, may suffer "death due to unhealthy personality."[34]

## Type A Personality: The Coronary Artery Disease–Prone Personality

One of the most active areas in health psychology seeks to identify and explain the relationships between personality and heart disease. At every stage of heart disease, state of mind appears to play a role.[35] If recent research is any indication, personality and behavior may play a major role in heart disease. The results of one recent study conducted in India, in fact, determined that coronary-prone behavior patterns *significantly* increase the risk of coronary heart disease.[36]

In a summary of research printed in *Psychology Today*, a writer editorialized,

> *By treating the heart as an unfeeling pump, surgeons have been able to create pacemakers and work their way up to the ultimate in high-tech medicine: the artificial heart. But even as Barney Clark and other courageous patients were testing the electronic pumps, scientists were using chemistry, psychology, and hard data to discover that trouble in the heart may come in part from sickness of the soul.*[37]

That sickness of the soul has evolved over the past three decades from a notion called the "Type A personality" to a broader-based concept that some call the "Type A behavior pattern." Two bits of good news have emerged from the most recent research: First, because the behavior pattern consists of a set of habits, it can be changed. Second, some of the more desirable parts of the Type A behavior pattern (such as increased productivity) apparently do not contribute to heart disease; one can safely retain some of those positive characteristics and change the harmful parts.

Personality traits that increase your risk for coronary artery disease are not inherent flaws. They are patterns of behavior that have been shown through scientific research to boost the chances of developing (or intensifying) heart disease. For ease of discussion throughout this chapter, we will

refer to this collection of personality traits by the name most researchers
have used: the Type A personality.

## Definitions of the Type A Personality

Cardiologist Ray Rosenman, who with colleague Meyer Friedman originated the theory of Type A personality three decades ago, says that Type A
behavior "refers to the behaviors of an individual who reacts to the environment with characteristic gestures, facial expressions, fast pace of activities, and the perception of daily events and stresses as challenges, all leading
to an aggressive, time-urgent, impatient, and more hostile style of living."[38]

Rosenman and Friedman have defined the Type A personality as "an
action-emotion complex that can be observed in any person who is aggressively involved in a chronic, incessant struggle to achieve more and more in
less and less time, and if required to do so, against the opposing efforts of
other things or other persons."[39]

That struggle against time and other people, Friedman contends, is
what causes physical damage. As one researcher put it, Type A personalities
"are not only more hostile, competitive, and impatient" but are also guided
by the central view that they "are indeed responsible for everything, control
everything, and are not only the captains of their own ship but the crew
and cargo as well."[40]

## Foundations of the "Coronary Personality"

The link between emotions and the heart has been recognized for thousands of years and is referred to in the most ancient medical records. Physicians recording their thoughts in the oldest surviving medical "textbooks,"
the Egyptian papyri, stated that, in examining a patient's limbs, they were
examining the heart, "because all his limbs possess its vessels, that is: the
heart speaks out of the vessels of every limb." Medical historians believe
from this passage that the Egyptians were keenly aware of the influence of
emotions on the heart.[41]

### Hippocrates and Others

Early written history is replete with examples of the mind's influence over
the heart; even the Bible speaks of people who were struck dead after some
great emotional upheaval. More than 2,000 years ago, the ancient physician
Hippocrates opined that "this is the great error of our day in the treatment
of the human body, that physicians separate the soul from the body."[42]

In 1628, William Harvey, recognized as a founder of modern physiology
and medicine, published a landmark book in which he provided the first
documented description of the human circulation. After accurately describ-

ing the pathway of the blood through the heart and lungs and via the arteries to the tissues of the body, Harvey echoed the sentiments of the Egyptian physicians in linking the heart to the mind. He wrote, "Every affection of the mind that is attended with either pain or pleasure, hope or fear, is the cause of an agitation whose influence extends to the heart."[43]

A little more than 200 years later, physicians gave even more credence to the effect of the mind on the heart. Researchers of the day noted that soldiers in the American Civil War had something in common with those in Europe's Crimean War: Both had a particular type of heart murmur and certain types of irregular heart rhythms.[44]

The first description of the Type A personality, though it was not given that name, occurred at the turn of the twentieth century by Sir William Osler, an American physician who became professor of medicine at Oxford University. He attributed heart disease to "the high pressure at which men live and the habit of working the machine to its maximum capacity."[45] Other researchers followed; in the 1930s, the Menningers noted that coronary artery disease patients often exhibited a "strongly aggressive personality." A decade later, one psychosomatic medicine pioneer described a "coronary personality," whose pattern consisted of the hard-driving, goal-directed behavior he often saw among coronary heart disease patients.[46]

### Friedman and Rosenman's Research

The most significant and far-reaching work on coronary personality came in the mid-1950s from cardiologists Meyer Friedman and Ray Rosenman. It began as somewhat of an accident: An upholsterer who came to their office to repair some furniture pointed out that the fabric was worn only on the very edge of the couches and chairs. It was a sign, he mused, that the patients were literally "on edge." Armed with evidence that their patients were perched on the edge of their seats, Friedman and Rosenman launched the landmark series of studies that led to identification of the Type A behavior pattern,[47] a pattern they initially dubbed "the hurry sickness."

Why the name "Type A?" This time the advice came from a scientist, not an upholsterer. Friedman and Rosenman began applying for federal funding to conduct their studies, requesting funds to research a "coronary-prone personality." Their repeated requests were denied, apparently because the scientists who were reviewing the funding applications did not believe that personality could increase the risk of heart disease. Finally, a scientist at the National Institutes of Health advised the pair to come up with a more generic name for their research project. Friedman and Rosenman came up with the harmless label "Type A behavior"; they called the opposite personality simply "Type B." With the new name, funding was approved.[48]

Friedman and Rosenman made two bold proclamations:

1. There are literal biochemical reasons why behavior can increase the risk for coronary heart disease.

2. Certain behavior patterns can be used as a tool for predicting who will get heart disease—not just as a detail to be confirmed at a postmortem exam.

In 1960 the two began what was to become the definitive study on Type A behavior pattern: the Western Collaborative Group Study. Working out of San Francisco's Mt. Zion Hospital, they studied 3,154 men, aged thirty-nine to fifty-nine years, who did not show any signs of existing coronary heart disease. The men were tested at the beginning of the study and classified as either Type A or Type B, and any traditional risk factors (such as cigarette smoking or obesity) were recorded.

The men were then observed carefully for eight and a half years. Researchers noted which of the men showed any manifestations of coronary heart disease—angina pectoris (chest pain resulting from arteriosclerosis), "silent" heart attack (changes in the electrocardiogram without physical symptoms), a heart attack requiring hospitalization, or death due to coronary artery disease.[49]

Those who had been classified as Type A at the beginning of the study were more than twice as likely to get heart disease as those who had been classified as Type B. The Type A's developed more angina, had more silent heart attacks, suffered more overt heart attacks, and fell victim to more coronary deaths. They even had more second heart attacks if they survived an initial one.[50]

The Western Collaborative Group Study succeeded in establishing Type A behavior as an independent risk factor for heart disease.[51] Type A behavior was added to the list of heart disease risks, and was accepted as such for nearly two decades. In 1981, in fact, the National Heart, Lung, and Blood Institute concluded that Type A behavior was an independent risk factor of cardiovascular disease.

### The MRFIT Study

Confusion resulted from a second larger study that cast doubt on the relationship between Type A personality and coronary heart disease. The National Heart, Lung, and Blood Institute figured that if people reduced their risk factors, their chances of developing heart disease would also be reduced. Their decade-long study was called the Multiple Risk Factor Intervention Trial (MRFIT). At a cost of more than $100 million, researchers studied more than 12,000 men who did not yet have signs of heart disease but who did have specific factors that placed them at high risk for a heart attack. The risk factors included high blood pressure, high cholesterol levels, and a cigarette smoking habit. Each man was also classified as Type A or Type B; to make sure that classifications were accurate, Rosenman himself made the final determination of status.

The men enrolled in the study were then put in programs to reduce their heart attack risk. Medical treatment reduced blood pressure, diet and medication brought down cholesterol levels, and men stopped smoking. Researchers found no relationship between Type A behavior and any kind of coronary heart disease event. Of ten subsequent studies conducted during the late 1970s and early 1980s, eight also failed to confirm the Type A hypothesis.[52]

## *"Second-Generation" Studies*

More study results surfaced in 1988: Those in the Western Collaborative Group Study who had suffered heart attacks during the eight and a half years of the study were followed for a total of twenty-two years. The researchers learned that if the men survived the first twenty-four hours after a heart attack, the Type A men actually had a significantly better long-term survival rate. In fact, they died at only about half the rate of the Type B's who had heart attacks.

Advocates of the theory began what pioneer researcher Redford Williams calls the second generation of Type A research. They learned that Type A is more of a risk factor for those under age fifty years and that it varies as a risk factor depending on the level of cholesterol in the blood.

In the meantime, a growing number of scientists were investigating the relation between personality and heart disease. Researchers found that some components of Type A behavior were relatively harmless, while others formed what researchers called the "toxic core" of the personality type. With that discovery, both sides of the controversy have been placated. Some components of Type A behavior (the good ones) can indeed increase the chances of survival after a heart attack. But other components of Type A behavior (the bad ones—the toxic core) can significantly increase the risk of suffering a heart attack in the first place.

Recent research shows that depression may also play a factor—but the exact *way* it acts as a risk factor for heart disease is not what scientists originally thought. In a study[53] involving 100 healthy young adults—half of whom were clinically depressed—researchers found that depression caused weight gain. (Interestingly, there was no evidence that the weight gain caused the depression.) The accumulation of adipose tissue caused the release of chemicals that in turn activated an inflammatory response that caused coronary heart disease.

In other recent research,[54] various personality traits have been shown to exert greater impact at different stages of cardiovascular disease. According to the research, hostility appears to have the most significant impact in the early stages of the disease. During the transition from stable to unstable disease, the most significant factors appear to be depression and exhaustion (common in Type A behavior pattern). During acute episodes, the most significant factors seem to be mental stress and anger.

### What "Causes" Type A Personality?

Many factors influence each of us: Genetics determine the color of our eyes, and the way our parents treat each other can influence the way we act in relationships. Some researchers believe that environmental factors are the sole cause of Type A personality; others cite data in an attempt to prove that we inherit Type A behavior as surely as we inherit the color of our hair. In actuality, scientifically interpreted research exists to support both sides.

***Environmental Factors.***    Ray Rosenman, one of the two cardiologists who originated the Type A theory, stands firmly on the environmental side; he maintains that there is little evidence of a genetic component for Type A behavior, although some genetic influence may exist for traits such as drive, competitiveness, compulsiveness, dominance, sociability, and impulsiveness.[55] The greatest influence, according to Rosenman, is adult modeling and conditioning, which he says explains why children tend to behave the same way within family units. It's not the gene pool; it's the way the parents act.[56]

Partly as a result of that modeling, Rosenman says, Type A behavior pattern is more common among children who have parents with higher educational level and higher occupational status, and children who live in urban rather than rural areas. It is more common among boys than girls. It is also more common among children whose mothers work fulltime outside the home.

In a series of studies conducted by Dr. Karen Matthews and her colleagues at the University of Pittsburgh, parents of Type A children were more likely to make critical remarks and were more apt to encourage their children to try harder, even when the children were already doing very well on a specific task. Even discipline seems to play a role. Type B children tend to have parents who explain the reasons behind discipline. Type A children, on the other hand, tend to have parents who use more physical and restrictive disciplinary techniques.[57]

When the University of Pittsburgh researchers zeroed in on family environments, they found that hostile and angry children—those most prone to be Type A—tended to come from families that were "less supportive, less open with their feelings, less positively involved with their children, and more likely to use physical and restrictive techniques in disciplining their children."[58]

***Genetics.***   Just as much evidence indicates that genetics could determine personality, scientists have learned over the past few years that numerous personality traits, even social attitudes and political beliefs, are at least half determined by genetics. According to Duke University's Redford Williams, the traits applicable to Type A personality "have all been found to show strong, clear-cut genetic influences."[59]

Researchers who have attempted to determine the role of genetics in personality formation have generally used twins as study subjects. One such study involved more than 100 pairs of twins living in the Philadelphia area. After studying a number of traits as well as a variety of physical characteristics, it was concluded that some of the physical characteristics, the Type A behavior pattern, and some of the traits that accompany the Type A personality were determined by genetics.[60]

What exactly is inherited? Part of the answer seems to be related to the same neurochemical inheritance that characterizes depression and anxiety (deficient serotonin neurotransmitter function in the brain). The more toxic Type A characteristics are more common in families with inherited vulnerability to these anxiety and depression disorders, and treatment with medication (or exercise) that corrects the serotonin neurotransmitter deficiency reduces Type A behavior.

## Characteristics of the Coronary-Prone Personality

Type A is not so much a specific personality style as it is a set of behaviors. Those behaviors are related to exaggerated neuroendocrine responses that then produce the characteristic behaviors (such as time urgency, hostility, and anger).[61]

Friedman, who originated the concept, says that there are five basic characteristics of the Type A personality. One is free-floating hostility, part of the toxic core that will be discussed in greater detail later. The other four characteristics are insecurity of status, hyperaggressiveness, sense of time urgency, and the drive to self-destruction.

### Behaviors That Are Probably Harmless

Type A's never slow down; they eat, walk, and talk quickly. Type A's are extremely time conscious: they hate to be late, and they hate to be kept waiting. Standing in line is extremely annoying to a Type A personality. In research, Type A personalities have expressed the notion that success comes from doing things quickly. They feel guilty when they are relaxing. In fact, they can't even relax when they are supposed to relax. Even on vacation, they feel a pressing need to be in motion, to be doing something they believe to be useful, instead of just "lying around."[62]

Typical Type A personalities almost always try two or three things simultaneously. A Type A executive, for example, eats a sandwich at his desk while talking on the phone to a colleague and filling out a monthly sales report. Another Type A washes dishes while she watches a television program and talks on the phone to a friend.

Type A personalities are extremely competitive and tend to "keep score" of even insignificant and trivial situations. Almost everyone is competitive when it comes to professional sports or a highly sought-after promotion, but a Type A personality acts that way even in a game of checkers with a child. Extreme Type A's compete when there's nothing to compete for and no one to compete against. They simply have to be the fastest, the smartest, the brightest, and the best.

A key characteristic of Type A behavior pattern is aggression and an aggressive style of speech. Other Type A characteristics include an insatiable drive for success, high ambition, impatience, insecurity, and a constant drive to control others and the environment. Type A personalities tend to set unrealistic goals, and they tend to use other people to achieve their goals. Many are selfish, easily bored, compulsive, and unobservant. Many Type A personalities live dangerously, and with time and fatigue, they may develop a tendency toward self-destructive behavior.

### Insecurity of Status

Occasionally, people who exhibit Type A behavior are truly caught in a position that demands superhuman efforts; much more frequently, however, their careers or family demands are no different than those of others. According to Friedman, Type A's struggle ceaselessly and senselessly to accomplish more and to involve themselves in more, not because demands are being placed on them but because they are placing the demands on themselves. Friedman theorizes that the typical Type A struggles because of a hidden lack of self-esteem and a need to prove him or herself.

Friedman, who has studied a number of famed Type A personalities, found that most of them—including the presidents of huge corporations, bank executives, distinguished military officials, presidents of universities, film stars, and even presidents of the United States—had hidden insecurities. To make up for those insecurities, to soothe their fears about themselves, they dived in with both feet, working furiously to immerse themselves in important and prestigious activities.

## Hyperaggressiveness

Ordinary aggression denotes a desire to compete and win, a wish to achieve. *Hyperaggression*—excessive aggression—is different: It is marked by a ruthless, driving desire to prevail and to dominate at all costs, totally disregarding the feelings or fundamental rights of others. In some cases, it even involves an attempt to destroy the self-esteem of others, an emotional drive that aims to strip others of their security.

Type A's at risk play games not for the enjoyment or the leisure, but to win. They are not merely satisfied with winning, either; they must prove all other players to be worthless and stupid. Someone once said that an aggressive Type A personality couldn't even play a game of Scrabble with a group of children without soundly defeating all of them.

## Sense of Time Urgency

The sense of time urgency manifest in Type A personalities comes from the desire to accomplish too much in too short a time. The Type A is forever setting unrealistic deadlines, vowing to accomplish too much or an unrealistic number of things, and constantly volunteering to take on even more tasks in the face of near-total exhaustion. The Type A personality copes with the incredible pressure of hurry sickness by speeding up all activities and trying to think of or do more than one thing at a time.

Type A personalities walk faster, talk faster, drive faster, eat faster, read faster, and move faster than their more easygoing counterparts. They will do almost anything to avoid waiting in a line, even a short line at a restaurant, a bank, or a ticket counter. They become hostile and irritated if they have to wait for five minutes at the dentist's office; they bristle with anger if a business associate does not arrive for their lunch appointment at precisely the prearranged time.

When they can no longer speed up, Type A personalities often cram their waking hours with accelerated thoughts, plans, and activities. Still not convinced that they are making the most of their time, they try to think about or do two or more things at a time. Such "polyphasic" activity, involving mental time-sharing (the flitting back and forth between subjects), has been shown to induce distress.[63]

## The Drive to Self-Destruction

Many Type A's, even the good-natured, optimistic ones, seem to harbor an unconscious drive to self-destruct. Friedman uses the example of a powerful head of an international corporation who failed to file income tax returns year after year, was finally caught, pleaded no contest, and was forced to resign from his position. His excuse was that he had no time to fill out the forms. Those who worked with him, however, suspected that the stress and strain of the position caused the executive to do something that would give him a release. Another example is President Richard Nixon. Henry Kissinger, who served in Nixon's cabinet and became one of his closest advisors, commented, "It was hard to avoid the impression that Nixon, who thrived on crisis, also craved disasters."

Friedman began to interview heart attack victims during recovery and convalescence. He was startled to learn that more than half had expected the heart attack before it ever occurred—and that they had, in fact, yearned for it. For some, it was the chance to finally be released from the cycle of stress and pressure; for others, it was a chance to at last lay quietly in a hospital bed and concentrate on only one thing: getting better.

### The "Toxic Core" of Type A Behavior

The hurry-sickness attributes of a Type A personality are probably the best known, but they are also the least detrimental to health. The second-generation studies found some behavior elements far more dangerous than others. The set of traits that creates major health risks for the Type A personality—called the "toxic core"—consists instead of hostility, anger, cynicism, suspiciousness, and excessive self-involvement.

*Free-Floating Hostility.*    Free-floating hostility is a permanent, deep-seated anger that hovers quietly until some trivial incident causes it to rupture to the surface in a burst of hostility; it is the tendency to experience anger, irritability, and resentment in response to even common events and to react with antagonism and disagreeableness.[64] Detailed research shows that there may actually be two separate components to free-floating hostility:[65]

- *Expressive hostility*, characterized by frequent expressions of anger and annoyance, the tendency to argue in a loud voice, and the potential for physical aggression when provoked.

- *Neurotic hostility*, characterized by chronic anger, low trust, and hostility that is not openly expressed; by itself, neurotic hostility has not been shown to increase the risk of heart disease, but in combination with expressive hostility it is a potent factor in heart disease.

Researchers Margaret Chesney, Nanette Frautschi, and Ray H. Rosenman believe that Type A persons often have an "enhanced potential for hostility."[66] This potential can be created by either genetic or learned factors. Because the enhanced potential is chronic, or ever present, even minor irritations or upsets can trigger a hostile rage. Type A's who have free-floating hostility react with seething anger and dwell on the objects of their despising. They become irritated and explosive and find it difficult not to become physically abusive. Sometimes the anger that accompanies free-floating hostility is displaced: A woman who gets angry and hostile in a traffic jam may lash out at a child in the back seat, for example.

Important and still-controversial studies have made a startling conclusion about the hostility factor: Apparently you can have many of the characteristics typically associated with the Type A personality—such as competitive drive, an aggressive personality, and impatience—without running the risks of a heart attack, as long as you are not hostile.

Renowned experts, such as Duke University's Redford Williams, point to hostility as one of the most crucial elements in heart disease. "We have strong evidence that hostility alone damages the heart," Williams emphasizes. In one study, hostility was shown to increase the risk of heart disease by a staggering seven times. "The kind of person at risk is someone who generally feels that other people are not to be trusted," Williams adds, "that they'll lie and cheat if they can get away with it."[67]

In a report published in *Psychology Today*, the kind of personality Williams describes as being at highest risk is "deeply suspicious. They feel that they must remain constantly on guard against others, whom they believe are dishonest, antisocial, and immoral." The Duke University team of researchers claims that this kind of hostility predicts not only blockages in the coronary arteries, as measured by X-ray studies of patients suffering chest pains,[68] but also death from heart disease and other causes.[69]

Psychologist Timothy Smith of the University of Utah reported to the 2004 Society of Behavioral Medicine meeting that couples with no history of heart disease developed the early signs of disease if they were hostile and domineering in their interactions—even those over things as basic as household chores, in-laws, money, and children. Smith's research showed that those who were hostile began developing calcium deposits in their coronary arteries—an early sign of arterial damage. The more hostile and strained their relationship, Smith says, "the more severe this silent atherosclerosis tended to be."[70]

Part of the reason why hostile Type A personalities run a greater risk of heart disease is that they more frequently trigger the cascade of potentially damaging hormones that are released as part of the fight-or-flight response. As Williams puts it, "Trusting hearts may live longer because for them the biologic cost of situations that anger or irritate is lower."[71]

Another reason hostility may be correlated so strongly with heart disease is that people who are hostile tend to drive others away, and social support, social networking, and social integration have been repeatedly proven to be strong protectors of health.

In summing up the importance of hostility as a toxic component of Type A personality, Williams says that the coronary-prone hostile personality has three parts: cynical mistrust of other people's motives, frequent feelings of anger, and aggressive expression of hostility toward others without regard for their feelings.[72]

*Anger.*    Another part of the toxic core of the Type A behavior pattern is anger, defined by researchers as "an emotional state incorporating feelings ranging from irritation and aggravation to rage and fury."[73] (Anger is often confused with hostility, which is an habitual way of evaluating people or events in a negative, cynical, paranoid way.) Researchers believe that the powerful combination of hostility and unexpressed anger carries the greatest risk of heart disease.

The particular combination is deadly, say researchers, and it appears to have a much greater impact on health than any single factor. "It isn't the impatience, the ambition, or the work drive," says Redford Williams, explaining the health risk of Type A personality. "It's the anger: it sends your blood pressure skyrocketing. It provokes the body to create unhealthy chemicals. For hostile people, anger is poison."[74]

The greatest risks, researchers believe, are from hostility paired with unexpressed anger, or "anger-in," a specific way of reacting to the people or situations that make a person angry. People who harbor unexpressed anger are not able to express their angry feelings, even when those feelings are appropriate or justified.

There is some disagreement among researchers about the dangers of suppressing anger. In the Western Collaborative Group Study, the men most likely to have a heart attack were the ones who became angry and "blew up" more than once a week. Another study conducted at the University of Michigan School of Public Health measured the way that "cool reflection," suppression of anger, and expression of anger affected blood pressure, and determined that the healthiest approach was "cool reflection": acknowledging the anger but not expressing it with verbal or physical hostility.

It appears that just the presence of ongoing anger may be more important than how it is expressed; thus, cognitive therapy approaches that simply allow the anger to dissolve so it no longer needs to be expressed may be valuable.

*Cynicism.*    Cynicism, anger, and hostility are closely related emotions: As Redford Williams describes it, cynical mistrust of others is the driving force behind hostility. It almost starts a chain reaction, he explains:

*Expecting that others will mistreat us, we are on the lookout for their bad behavior, and we can usually find it. This generates the frequent anger to which the hostile person is prone, and that anger, combined with a lack of empathy for others—a natural consequence of the poor opinion we hold of others in general—leads us to express our hostility overtly, in the form of aggressive acts towards others.*[75]

When cynicism is paired with hostility, the effects can be devastating to health. In one experiment, Duke University Medical Center researchers asked a group of college students (some of whom were hostile and some of whom were not) to solve a difficult series of scrambled word puzzles. Physiological responses, such as blood pressure, were measured during the experiment.

At the end of the first part of the experiment, researchers found that there was no difference between the two groups as they were doing the puzzles. Then they added another factor designed to separate students who were also cynical: Researchers stood over the students while they were doing the puzzles and made snide remarks like "Stop mumbling; I can't understand what you are saying" and "Remember, you're getting paid to do this."

Once the element of harassment was added, the students who were cynical showed sharp differences in physiological responses. They had higher blood pressure, higher blood flow, and more anger while they were doing the puzzles and being harassed, and their blood pressure remained high for fifteen minutes after they did the puzzle. Researchers attribute the changes in the cynical students to the fact that hostile people "view other people's actions and motives very cynically. They thought the researchers were 'out to get them,' felt threatened, and reacted, while low hostiles did not perceive the researchers' actions as a personal attack."[76]

***Suspiciousness.***   Suspiciousness is a trait closely allied to cynicism. In a study at Duke University's Center for the Study of Aging and Human Development, researchers noted that "people who are suspicious are constantly on guard, and there's evidence to suggest that this may raise levels of potentially harmful stress-induced hormones in the blood."[77] In the same study, those who scored high on a test of suspiciousness were significantly more likely to become ill and die during the fifteen years the study was conducted. The greater risk for illness and death due to suspiciousness held up even after researchers took into account other risk factors, such as age, sex, physician rating of functional health, smoking, cholesterol, and alcohol intake.[78]

In a separate study, Friedman and Rosenman studied 1,990 middle-aged men who had not yet developed coronary heart disease. Each man was given the Minnesota Multiphasic Personality Inventory as well as a questionnaire that evaluated sixteen personality factors. The study subjects were then monitored for five years to determine which ones became ill or died. Those most likely to develop coronary heart disease were the suspicious ones.[79]

***Excessive Self-Involvement.***   One of the most interesting theories about Type A behavior and the potential link to heart disease points to a personality trait that researchers think is a killer: excessive self-involvement. A person whose language is excessively peppered with references to I, me, mine, and other self-references seems to be at the greatest risk of all for coronary heart disease.

A trio of researchers working under the auspices of the National Heart, Lung, and Blood Institute and the California Affiliate of the American Heart Association studied first a group of students and, later, 13,000 middle-aged men whom they had determined to be Type A personalities. Two findings were significant: First, blood pressures increased when people made self-references; and second, those with Type A personalities made twice as many references to themselves as did those with Type B personalities. Those who developed coronary heart disease (especially those who died from it) were those who tended to be excessively self-involved.

Self-involvement seems to be such an important factor because people who are self-involved tend to be "hot reactors"; they have extreme cardiovascular reactions when subjected to stress, including precipitous increases in blood pressure and health-harming chemical changes.[80] The excessive self-involvement may be what actually causes the hostility and anger that have been so strongly linked to Type A heart disease. The facts are that self-involvement may be related to, and often accompanied by, other dangerous Type A traits such as hostility.

***Workaholics.***   The characteristics of the Type A personality lead many to confuse Type A with "workaholism," but a workaholic isn't necessarily a Type A. Yale researcher Marilyn Machlowitz, who wrote a dissertation on workaholics, defines them as people "whose desire to work hard and long is intrinsic, and whose work habits almost always exceed the prescriptions of the job and the expectations of those with whom or for whom they work."81 Machlowitz further defines the workaholic as "that blur of a person rushing by with an overflowing briefcase, dictating into a tape recorder, checking the time, and munching on a sandwich."[82]

There are some important distinctions between Type A behavior and workaholics. Type A's tend to have a hard-driving, competitive approach to work because they crave the recognition and approval of others; most workaholics do it because they truly love to work. Type A's play with the same feverish pitch they bring to the office; a workaholic simply prefers work over play and, given the choice, will work instead of play. Type A's are driven and unhappy; many workaholics are satisfied, happy people who genuinely enjoy what they are doing. The difference lies in the motivation behind the hard-working busyness: one person driven by fear of failure and the need to prove oneself worthy, the other by love of work and a sense of mission.

The real difference between workaholics and Type A personalities seems to lie with hostility. The workaholic seldom is hostile. The Type A is almost always hostile. While Type A personalities are hostile and often unhappy, most workaholics, says Machlowitz, are happy.

When does workaholism become a health problem? According to Robert Rosen, director of the Institute on Organizational Health at the Washington Business Group on Health, an inflexible addiction to work is what is unhealthy: "If you're avoiding something or if the need for manipulation and power becomes the overriding fuel for the commitment to work, you're placing yourself at risk of affecting your health."[83] Researchers point out that most health problems occur when workaholics are mixed with nonworkaholics, either at home or in the office. And then, ironically, it's the nonworkaholic who usually pays the price in terms of health risks.

## Effects of Coronary-Prone Behavior on the Body

Coronary-prone behavior causes health problems because it literally wreaks havoc on the body. In his book *Super Immunity*, psychologist Paul Pearsall gives a vivid description:

> *The supersystem sizzles with neurochemical changes, we roast in our hormonal stew, and, as if by some universal wisdom, the body can be stopped in its tracks by adopting an "enough is enough" strategy. We overload, our heads start pounding for attention, our hearts get attacked for our lack of intimacy, and our vessels cause the doctor's mercury gauge to warn us that things are getting too high. Even our bowels can get irritated with us and show their displeasure in their own unique language. Somewhere in our bodies, through our overuse and abuse of our supersystems, something is burning out.[84]*

Type A behavior is essentially an exaggerated stress response, and the body begins pumping out hormones needed to fight or flee. It's the classic fight-or-flight reaction we all have in response to stress, whether mental or physical. The hostile Type A personality lives in a chronic state of what Redford Williams calls vigilant observation.[85] The body is on constant alert. It never relaxes. The result is increases in circulation, blood cholesterol level, blood triglyceride levels, and blood sugar level.

The physical effects of the Type A behavior pattern begin in the hypothalamus, a complex portion of the brain that lies at its base, directly over the pituitary gland. The hypothalamus sends out signals to various parts of the body in response to emotion. The anger and hostility that are chronically experienced by a Type A personality are processed by the hypothalamus as it would process an intense physical struggle. As a result, the system is bathed with excessive catecholamines, epinephrine (adrenaline), testosterone, estrogen, thyroxine, and insulin.

The stress associated with Type A behavior causes these effects:

- An increase in adrenaline-like hormones (norepinephrine) that cause microvascular drainage in blood vessel walls, allowing cholesterol in the blood to seep into the wall and eventually creating atherosclerotic plaques.[86]

- An increase in coronary artery spasm further narrows the vessels supplying oxygen to the heart muscle.

- An increase in blood pressure increases the heart's workload and oxygen requirement. Type A behavior typically results in an increase in norepinephrine, which constricts the blood vessels, resulting in high blood pressure.[87] Several studies have found that high blood pressure is much more common among people with unexpressed anger, especially among those with an "anger-in" style of coping, a very specific Type A trait.[88]

- Blood platelets become more "sticky," part of the process that leads to atherosclerosis and clotting to complete the obstruction of the narrowed arteries. This is a definite risk factor for coronary heart disease.[89]

- All of the above phenomena lead to oxygen imbalance in the heart, resulting in myocardial infarction (heart attack).

A number of studies—including the Framingham Heart Study, the Belgian-French Collaborative Study, and the Japanese-American Study—place the heart disease risk of the Type A personality at more than twice the risk in the population at large.

Unfortunately, the anger and hostility and struggle are chronic, so the body is always pumped full of excess hormones. Even during supposedly "low-voltage" periods of the day, Type A's expose their bodies to "high-voltage" chemicals that can damage and even eventually destroy it. Some of the most profound effects of chronic overload of stress hormones are increased levels of cholesterol and fat, blood platelet changes, alterations in the heart and arteries, excess insulin secretion, magnesium deficiency, and defective immune system function.

## The Emotional Effects of Type A Behavior

Significant links exist between Type A hostility (with its attendant insecurity) and the neurochemical changes that cause depression, which has also now been shown to be a significant coronary risk factor. Many of the same neuroendocrine problems described above for Type A are also features of depression. Overt mental depression occurs more frequently in Type A people,[90] and hostility improves with antidepressant medication.[91]

We know that marriage quality can have a significant effect on heart disease risk. Research published in the *Journal of Applied Social Psychology* shows that Type A's fail to display the sensitivity and understanding that a long-term relationship requires. Psychologist Don Byrne of the State University of New York at Albany says that this not only limits the Type A's chances of tying the marriage knot, but also greatly increases the likelihood of divorce. Cynicism, for example, has been shown to be highly predictive of marital difficulties.

Type A personalities have also been shown to have a weaker network of social support than more easygoing Type B's. Psychiatrist Karen A. Matthews of the University of Pittsburgh points out that some of the "abrasive" interpersonal traits of the Type A personality (such as hostility) may interfere with social relationships, leading to increased social isolation.[92]

Researchers at Duke University Medical Center say that "Type A's with low levels of social support had more severe coronary artery disease than Type A's with high levels of social support. . . . These results are consistent with the hypothesis that social support moderates the long-term health consequences of the Type A behavior pattern."[93] An example of this was a study of 10,000 Israeli men at high coronary risk. Those with loving support from their wives had half the angina incidence of those who lacked such support.[94]

### *Type A Behavior and Heart Disease Risk*

The Type A who seems most at risk is the minimally educated and trained assembly line worker who has the least amount of control over his environment.[95] Close behind is the demanding person who has been placed in a position for which he is not competent or the middle manager given much responsibility but little control. The factors of social support, lack of control, and other situational elements all affect the Type A personality. While various research results may show different rates of risk, they all show one thing: A Type A personality (or coronary-prone personality) definitely increases the risk of heart disease.

Hostile Type A personality increases the risk of heart disease as much as or more than the "standard" risk factors of cigarette smoking, high serum cholesterol, and high blood pressure and is synergistic with them. If Type A coexists with another risk factor, the risk of developing coronary heart disease is four times greater. If Type A personality exists alongside two additional risk factors, the risk of developing coronary heart disease is eight times greater.[96]

The risk from Type A may be even more important at younger ages. In the age bracket of thirty-nine to forty-nine years, Type A men are 6.5 times more likely to have a heart attack.[97]

## Impact on Men, Women, and Children

Women can pay an even greater price for Type A behavior than men do. The prestigious Framingham Heart Study showed that a Type A woman runs four times the risk of heart disease as compared with her Type B sister.[98] Other studies portray the gap as even wider: Statistics from the Western Collaborative Group Study show that Type A women are three times as likely as Type B women to develop angina.[99] Friedman found that Type A women are seven times more likely than Type B's to develop heart disease.[100]

The hallmarks of Type A personality in men are time urgency, relentless drive for achievement, free-floating hostility, and inability to relax. Women have many of the same traits, but they often can't express their hostility as directly.[101] The result is an increasing feeling of isolation and alienation that may be an even more dangerous manifestation for women than busyness or anger.

Children can also exhibit Type A personality and can pay the price in terms of susceptibility to heart disease. The process of coronary heart disease begins early in childhood. "Although present research does not show a direct link between coronary-prone behavior in children and coronary heart disease in adults, there is evidence that children assessed as Type A exhibit behavior patterns similar to those of adults assessed as Type A."[102]

The attitude can also be carried into adulthood. Established research shows that roughly half of all children remain in the personality category they exhibit during childhood.[103] New research reported in *Science News* indicates that "the Type A pattern of aggression and competitiveness shows up early in life and can persist, perhaps putting the individual at risk of heart disease as an adult."[104]

Type A personality manifests itself among children much as it does among adults. Almost all Type A children score high on hostility and anger; many are suspicious.[105] Most have higher achievement test scores and classroom grades, independent of IQ test scores, most likely because of their competitive nature.[106] Type A children also tend to be more outgoing, talkative, and physically active; more aggressive in their interactions with others; and more likely to experience a greater number of aversive significant life events than are Type B children.[107]

## Psychosocial Coronary Risk in Women

According to study results, factors that create significant risk for coronary death in women include being divorced and disempowered,[108] feeling socially isolated,[109] and being depressed.[110] Sudden death in women, presumably from heart rhythm abnormalities, has also been linked to bereavement and to being childless. Interestingly, behavior nearly opposite of the angry, hard-driving Type A man was more predictive of cardiac mortality in women: suppressed (but real) anger, slowness, and low level of arousal (as is seen in depression).

## The Role of Type A Personality in Other Illnesses

The role of Type A personality in heart disease has been acknowledged and widely known for decades, but the health-harming aspects of Type A personality aren't limited to heart disease. In one study reported in the *British Journal of Medical Psychology*, researchers got a glimpse of how broad the impact of Type A personality may be on health. The Type A subjects had not only more coronary heart disease but also significantly more peptic ulcers, asthma, rheumatoid arthritis, and thyroid problems. Conditions that seem particularly related to the presence of Type A personality include ulcers, headache, cancer, genital herpes, and vision problems.

The reported number of diseases per person was dramatically higher among Type A's, even though the Type A subjects in the study were markedly younger than the others. Globally, the Type A's had much more illness. Study leaders concluded that Type A behavior is a general disease-prone condition.[111]

One broad-range study showed that people with Type A personality ran a significantly higher risk of having accidents, dying from accidents, and dying from violence.[112] In another study that involved a group of more than 2,000 men who had survived the Western Collaborative Group Study follow-up period, those who had the fewest Type A characteristics had the best health twenty-two years later.[113]

Type A behavior does increase the risk of developing certain diseases, but there may be a silver lining to the Type A cloud: Internist Brian Miller believes that Type A personality can actually become an asset when a person is fighting disease. "Interestingly," he points out, "I see patients with very driven personalities get better faster than other patients. Apparently, these patients feel there is more to live for."[114] The key appears to be transforming the hostility and cynicism while preserving some of the assertive, active-living characteristics.

The findings about personality and heart disease risk bear other implications for treatment as well. Dr. Dean Ornish, president of the Preventive Medicine Research Institute and well-known for his approaches to heart disease treatment, recommends an approach that includes stringent dietary changes, regular exercise, and stress management. Behavioral approaches such as yoga, meditation, and group sharing have helped reduce hostility and stress—and have been shown to reduce stress hormones, relax the blood vessels, and promote a sense of well-being. "Diet and exercise alone are like a two-legged stool," says Redford Williams. "It's more stable with the third leg, stress management."[115]

In one trial of Ornish's approach, those who included behavioral approaches in their treatment showed 91 percent reduction of angina within the first few weeks to months of the study, saving the expense and trauma of bypass surgery or angioplasty. In another study, Mutual of Omaha used Ornish's program on 194 heart patients and saved $30,000 per patient over the next three years. Based on that success, the federal government is studying the possibility of applying the treatment plan for Medicare patients.[116]

## Type D Personality

Another behavior pattern—the "Type D personality,"[117] characterized by the tendency to experience negative emotions and the inability to express feelings in social situations—has also been linked to heart disease.

A large body of scientists found that certain negative emotions, such as anger,[118] anxiety,[119] depression,[120] worry,[121] and hopelessness,[122] all increased the risk of coronary artery disease. Heart bypass patients who are depressed at the time of their surgery are more than twice as likely to die during the next five years when compared to people whose conditions are the same but who are not depressed.[123] Other factors, including social isolation, have also been shown to impact the heart—and the emotional stress of being alone causes heart attack survivors to die at twice the rate of those who live with others. "They're heartbroken in more ways than one," says Dr. Herbert Benson, president of Boston's Mind/Body Medical Institute.[124]

Apparently the constellation of negative emotions has a much greater impact on the development of heart disease when it is combined with what is referred to as "social inhibition," or the inability to easily make contact with others, talk to strangers, express opinions to others, make "small talk" (even with close acquaintances), carry on an easy conversation, impact others, take charge in group situations, or feel at ease in a group. Researchers have labeled the combination of negative emotions and social inhibition Type D Scale–16 (DS16). Those who score high on both social inhibition and negative feelings are said to have a "distressed" personality (thus the name Type D). Scientists found that the presence of *either* negative emotions or social inhibition without the other did not necessarily increase the risk of heart disease, but that the combination can be deadly.[125]

The problem isn't the *occasional* experiencing of these negative emotions, but the tendency to experience these negative emotions across time and a variety of situations[126] and the tendency to suppress negative emotions.[127] Researchers have also found that people diagnosed with affective disorder are also significantly more likely to develop both fatal and nonfatal coronary artery disease.[128]

Long-range research conducted over a period of ten years involving almost 300 men and women between the ages of thirty and eighty found that Type D personality:[129]

- increases the risk of cardiac death, especially among patients with established coronary heart disease.[130]
- causes increased risk of subsequent heart attack among myocardial infarction patients.
- increases the risk of death by four times among coronary artery disease patients.

Research also shows that close relationships help to ease the emotions related to Type D personality.[131] In one study reported in September 2004 by psychologist Timothy Smith of the University of Utah, simply looking at a picture of someone you love helps reduce the stress response, reducing heart rate and blood pressure. Massachusetts cardiologist Harvey Zarren found that when he rode in an ambulance with heart patients, he asked the patient to describe what he or she loved most in life. The patients' abnormal heart rhythms stabilized and high blood pressure fell to normal. Unlike his colleagues, Zarren never had a patient progress to cardiac arrest while in the ambulance.

## The Controversy

The notion of coronary-prone personality is a controversial one, possibly because behavior is much more difficult to pinpoint as a risk factor than are other, more specific risk factors that can be measured in a laboratory (such as high blood pressure or elevated cholesterol). "Behavior comes from the soft, fuzzy science of psychology, rather than from the hard, precise, biomedical sciences," psychologist Ethel Roskies points out, a fact that may make it difficult for medical researchers to accept the coronary-prone personality. Medical personnel may have even more difficulty with the concept, she adds, "if behavioral modification, rather than conventional medical and surgical techniques, is seen as the treatment of choice for this new type of risk factor."[132]

Still another reason for controversy, says Roskies, is the "personal involvement of most health professionals and scientists with Type A behavior." The competitive selection process itself guarantees that a large majority of professional health care workers are more likely to be Type A, and may thus feel threatened when behavioral issues are brought up. "When we speak of diabetes mellitus or smoking, we are speaking of other people, 'them,' 'out there'; but when we talk about Type A, in contrast, we are talking about ourselves."[133]

Researchers themselves have different concepts of exactly what a Type A personality is, they use different criteria to assess what they believe to be Type A personalities, they rely on people to judge themselves as Type A (a judgment that isn't always accurate), and many researchers have problems judging Type A behavior in anyone except male executives.[134] Self-assessment tests for qualities like hostility are notoriously unreliable because of a well-demonstrated self-delusion. It is, after all, not very socially acceptable to try to prove oneself hostile.[135]

Still, a growing body of evidence links Type A behavior or at least some components of it to the development of heart disease, the likelihood of suffering recurrent heart attacks, and death from heart disease. Important data also link some of the components of Type A behavior with other illnesses as well and with the increased likelihood of premature death.

## Type C Personality: The Cancer-Prone Personality

One of the most controversial notions being explored by medical researchers is that of a cancer-prone personality, a set of traits that predisposes a person to cancer. The exact effect of personality on cancer is difficult to assess: People can be exposed unwittingly to carcinogens that may play a role, and there can also be a vast difference in a number of factors between the time of prognosis and the time of diagnosis. Nonetheless, an increasing number of physicians believes that the trends definitely point to a link between personality and cancer and that these notions give a new and pressing direction to medical research.[136]

The notion of a cancer-prone personality isn't new. The second-century physician Galen noted that "melancholic" women had a greater tendency toward breast cancer than their more "sanguine" counterparts. Medical writers in the eighteenth century described in detail the personality traits and experiences shared by cancer patients. And eminent British physician Sir James Paget noted in 1870, "The cases are so frequent in which deep anxiety, deferred hope, and disappointment are quickly followed by the growth or increase of cancer that we can hardly doubt that mental depression is a weighty addition to the other influences that favor the development of the cancerous constitution."[137]

Researchers became keenly interested in the possibility of a cancer-prone personality during the 1950s, when psychologist Eugene Blumberg began noticing a "trademark" personality among cancer patients in a Long Beach veterans' hospital. He wrote, "We were impressed by the polite, apologetic, almost painful acquiescence of the patients with rapidly progressing disease as contrasted with the more expressive and sometimes bizarre personalities of those who responded brilliantly to therapy with remissions and long survival."[138]

To figure out whether there was any connection, Blumberg administered psychological tests to the cancer patients. The tests measured whether they could release pent-up emotions, how anxious they were, and whether they were depressed. Then he matched test results with patients at intervals and checked to see how rapidly their disease was progressing.

He found that the patients with the fastest-growing tumors were the ones who were "consistently serious, overcooperative, overly nice, overly anxious, painfully sensitive, passive, and apologetic."[139] And they had been that way all their lives. The patients with the slow-growing tumors, on the other hand, were the ones who had developed a way of coping with life's stresses.

At about the same time, physicians at San Francisco's Malignant Melanoma Clinic were becoming interested in the same questions. They had noticed a "disturbing pattern" in the personalities of patients with melanoma (a particularly virulent form of skin cancer). The patients were "nice"—too nice. In fact, they were passive about everything, including their cancer. Could it be a coincidence? The doctors didn't think it was, so they asked University of California School of Medicine psychologist Lydia Temoshok to talk to the patients and determine whether a personality pattern emerged.

After talking in detail to 150 of the clinic's melanoma patients, Temoshok declared that there was a distinct pattern. The cancer patients were indeed very, very nice. They never seemed to express any negative emotion—not fear, or sadness, or anger, or denial, or any of the other emotions common to a patient struggling with a terminal disease. The patients couldn't express negative emotion, assert themselves, acknowledge or attend to physical pain, or admit their own needs. In fact, say the researchers, these patients "were the rock of stability for their families. Even in the face of cancer, they maintained this composure. When one of them was diagnosed, she might say, 'I'm doing fine. But I'm really worried about my husband. He takes things so hard,'" explained Temoshok.[140] These cancer patients, in the face of a painful, devastating, and almost certainly terminal disease, seemed always happy, always in control.

The result of Temoshok's research was what she called the Type C personality—essentially the complete opposite of the hard-driving Type A.

Type C's are overwhelmed by emotions they have not been able to express or resolve. Temoshok found that the Type C was at high risk for cancer:

- The Type C melanoma patients had thicker, more aggressive tumors, both signs of a bleaker prognosis.

- Temoshok was able to predict survival based on the way the patients initially reacted when they heard their diagnosis: Those most likely to die were women who reacted with stoicism and men who reacted with helplessness and hopelessness.

- Melanoma patients were significantly more likely than either healthy people or people with heart disease to repress their emotions (a Type C strategy).

- The melanoma patients who were more able to openly express their emotions also had more lymphocytes (immune cells that are key in fighting cancer) around their tumors. The patients who repressed their emotions had fewer lymphocytes at tumor sites.

- Temoshok found significant associations between every single negative emotional state and recurrence of the disease or death several years later. Temoshok believes that the data show "powerful evidence" that people who died of cancer suffered a collapse of their usual Type C coping style and were then overwhelmed by emotions they couldn't express or resolve.[141]

To test the validity of her theory, Temoshok videotaped detailed interviews with each of the 150 melanoma patients she had originally talked to in the clinic. She then invited a group of her colleagues to look at the videotapes and to help her categorize the patients by what they judged to be each one's personality type: Type A, Type B (relaxed and easygoing), or Type C (passive, overly compliant, and unable to express negative emotions—what Temoshok called "a fragile accommodation to the world"). Temoshok followed the patients' progress for the next year and a half. Most of the Type C's were concentrated in what doctors called the relapser's group, the patients whose conditions worsened or who died.

Based on similar cancer-personality studies that had been conducted during the previous thirty years and a continuation of her own research, Temoshok concluded that behavior and personality may not cause cancer, but certain personality traits affect how an individual copes with stress and may very well affect the outcome of the disease. Other research confirms that rather than *causing* cancer, the identified personality and behavior traits correlate more closely to how aggressively the disease progresses.[142] Temoshok even went so far as to say that people with a Type C personality are likely to have "a worse outcome than might be expected on medical grounds."[143] In discussing the Type C personality, Temoshok points out that it is not actually a personality, but a "behavior pattern." At its origins, she says, is a defense mechanism that is useful in moderation but that later gets out of control.

The findings of the melanoma study and of various follow-up studies have convinced Temoshok of two things. First, she says, changing Type C behavior can both improve the health of people who are already sick and actually help prevent cancer among healthy ones. Some of the most important skills, she says, are developing an awareness of needs, reframing ideas about feelings (feelings aren't bad, but blocking feelings is), learning how to express emotion, taking charge, getting social support, working through hopelessness, and cultivating a fighting spirit.[144]

Second, Temoshok learned that "people did not bring cancer on themselves. No one can be blamed for mind-body factors in cancer, because no one intentionally develops the cancer-prone behavior pattern. . . . When brought about with compassion and self-care, awareness of Type C behavior offers the person opportunities for growth and empowerment, not self-blame."[145]

## LeShan's Analysis

One of the researchers most prominent in the study of a cancer personality is psychologist Lawrence LeShan, who began his research at about the same time Blumberg was puzzling over his "nice" cancer patients in the veterans' hospital.

LeShan interviewed 250 patients who had been hospitalized for cancer, and compared their response to those of patients who had been hospitalized for other diseases. LeShan was fascinated by a striking similarity in the life history of the cancer patients, with three specific "life events" common to the cancer patients:

- Cancer patients described a "bleak" childhood; they had a tense, hostile relationship with one or both parents, and they felt lonely and isolated. They began to feel that a satisfying, "safe" relationship with another person was not possible.

- As young adults, they finally found something to which they were able to make a strong emotional commitment—another person, a cause, a job, or something else. The emotional investment was strong, and that object of emotional investment became the centerpiece of their lives.

- Something happened to take away the object of emotional investment: The spouse died, they were fired from their job, or a beloved child took up with unsavory companions and forsook the family. There was nothing to replace the great void, and six to eight months later these people were diagnosed with cancer.[146]

## Other Research

Another psychologist who noticed a striking similarity in the histories of cancer patients was Claus Bahnson, then at Jefferson Medical College in Philadelphia. In interviewing cancer patients, he, too, found that they had very similar backgrounds; most pronounced was a cold, strict, aloof relationship with their parents. Scottish researcher David Kissen, who has spent the bulk of his career studying the personality traits of lung cancer victims, has also noted the common thread among this particular group— the loss of someone close during childhood and the apparent lack of emotional involvement over the loss.

## Expression of Emotion

The hallmark of the cancer personality, according to Temoshok, is the "non-expression of emotion."[147] Kissen says that whatever emotions they feel are kept bottled up inside. Many have unresolved tension, usually concerning a parent or other family member, but they refuse to express or resolve it.[148] Even when they are experiencing tremendous despair, it is characteristically "bottled up"; while cancer patients are often described by other people as kind, sweet, and benign, this sweetness is "really a mask they wear to conceal their feelings of anger, hurt, and hostility."[149]

In a study by psychologists at the University of Oslo in Norway, researchers examined how personality and culture influenced the likelihood of developing breast cancer. Women whose personalities were characterized by repression, self-blaming defense mechanisms, and the inability to feel or express anger were significantly more likely to develop breast cancer.[150]

## Stress and Cancer

While stress may play a role, researchers believe that stress alone is probably not the cause of cancer. As one put it, "The stress of life changes alone does not induce the development of cancer. There must also be an underlying personality structure that handles such life changes in an unhealthy way. Feelings of loneliness and hopelessness, of being helpless or trapped, often characterize people who develop this dread disease."[151]

Most other researchers agree; based on an analysis of cancer personality studies, one commented that cancer patients are more commonly lonely, angry, rigid, self-sacrificing, repressed, depressed, and hopeless.[152] Others say that cancer patients characteristically react to stress, loss, or change with a feeling of helplessness, hopelessness, or an overwhelming inability to cope. Still others say that repressed anger and negative emotions in general contribute to the progression of cancer.

## Depression: A Factor?

Until recently, researchers believed that the personality trait of depression had a strong link to the development of cancer, but ensuing research shows that depression apparently is not a factor in the development of cancer.

According to research conducted by National Institute on Aging psychologist Alan Zonderman and published in the *Journal of the American Medical Association*, depressed people have no greater risk of developing cancer than the general population.[153] Zonderman and his colleagues studied a group of more than 6,000 people, 1,000 of whom showed signs of depression (such as crying spells, insomnia, loss of appetite, and poor concentration). They followed the medical histories of all 6,000 people for the next ten years. At the end of ten years, 11 percent of the depressed people had developed cancer, but so had 10 percent of the nondepressed ones. The number in each group who had died from cancer during the ten-year period was exactly the same: 4 percent.[154]

Earlier studies that did show a link between depression and cancer were probably flawed for a variety of reasons (too small a sample group, failure to control for other factors, and so on). In concluding his study, Zonderman stated that "we found that depressive systems didn't predict who was going to get cancer or who was going to die from cancer ten years later."[155]

## Other Factors

People who develop cancer tend to be what researchers call loners, people who feel lonely and who face the world with bland, unemotional exteriors. To test that notion, psychologists Pirkko Graves and John Shaffer, along with their colleagues at the Johns Hopkins University School of Medicine, analyzed psychological data collected over almost two decades on nearly 1,000 male medical students at the school.[156] They used personality traits to divide the men into five groups. Then they scrutinized the students' medical records, which had been collected each year over a period of almost forty years.

Graves and Shaffer found that the people most likely to develop cancer were the people who were lonely and unemotional. They developed cancer sixteen times more often than members of the healthiest group. The ones least likely to develop cancer were members of what Graves and Shaffer called the acting-out emotional group—people who were anxious, easily upset, and depression-prone but who expressed their feelings freely. Fewer than 1 percent of the people in the acting-out emotional group developed cancer during the forty years of follow-up.[157]

In one study of breast cancer patients, researchers saw that those who were not lonely seemed to have the best prognosis. Among the breast cancer patients, women with numerous close friends were less likely to die than those who had few or no close friends.[158]

Helplessness and hopelessness have also been strongly associated with cancer, and they appear to influence not only who develops cancer but also who is able to survive it. "It is well-known, if quietly admitted, that the best medicine may be to no avail when given to someone who has already given up the struggle for life," stated one researcher. "Even if there is no strong relationship between the origins of cancer and some personality type, the evidence does suggest that the way in which a person responds to the threat may have a lot to do with surviving the physical insult of cancer."[159]

In fifteen years of following breast cancer patients, researchers found that the ones who survive the longest with no recurrence of disease are also the ones who reacted to their cancer diagnosis in one of two ways: Either they denied that there was anything seriously wrong with them, or they rallied with a "fighting spirit"—a determination to do everything possible to beat the cancer. Fighting spirit also involved a positive expectation and a feeling that they could control their lives, regardless of the cancer. Seven years after appropriate treatment, the survival of the deniers and the fighters was about the same (about 80 percent), but then the protection provided by denial faded. At twelve years, 80 percent of those with "fighting spirit" were still alive, as compared with only 50 percent of those who used denial to cope. Those who succumbed most easily were the ones who kept a stiff upper lip (the stoics, as Greer called them) and the ones who collapsed in a hopeless, helpless, all-is-lost response; only 20 percent of the helpless-hopeless survived at five years.[160] Other studies have confirmed that a strong will to live prolongs survival of breast cancer patients, as does better coping ability in dealing with problems.[161]

With all the research findings that are emerging, most agree that there does seem to be a particular cancer-prone personality—if not one that actually causes cancer, then at least one that contributes to its development, spread, and mortality. But there may still be cautions regarding cancer personality research and theory. In the first place, says one researcher, there is a danger in delving into the personalities of people already diagnosed with cancer: To become a person with cancer is to cease to be a "normal" person, and a cancer victim may look back and interpret everything that happened in life in light of the cancer.[162] Second, asking a cancer patient to recount details from the past makes a researcher reliant on the person's memory.

There's also the natural tendency for recent events to eclipse earlier ones. It's difficult for anyone to look back at a time in life and weigh the particular stresses or events that may have occurred. These weaknesses are precisely why researchers lean more heavily on studies that test an entire population before cancer is ever diagnosed.[163]

That considered, it can likely be helpful to integrate mind-body techniques into cancer treatment and prevention programs. To begin, it has been demonstrated that mind-body techniques help strengthen the immune system, which may mobilize the body to fight the cancer itself. When combined with good nutrition and exercise, particularly helpful practices may include relaxation techniques (such as meditation, guided imagery, and progressive muscle relaxation) and strong social support (supporting and helping others as well as seeking others who can support you).[164]

Mind-body techniques have been shown to help in cancer treatment; even if they have not resulted in a cure, they have improved the quality of life for cancer patients. At Boston's Dana-Farber Cancer Institute, an ancient Chinese movement and meditation technique—qigong—has been used to reduce pain and anxiety among cancer patients. Tens of thousands of cancer patients are now using mind-body techniques to help them cope with pain, depression, and anxiety and to help them sleep better; these techniques include yoga, talk therapy, visualization, tai chi, music therapy, relaxation techniques, and prayers, among others.

Of the nation's twenty-six major cancer centers, fourteen now offer complementary medicine programs that include mind-body techniques, bringing together oncologists and alternative practitioners. The Society for Integrative Oncology, founded by Dr. Barrie Cassileth, chief of integrative medicine at New York's Sloan-Kettering Cancer Center, held its first international conference in late 2004.

Lorenzo Cohen, head of integrative medicine at Houston's M.D. Anderson Cancer Center, says that mind-body techniques will soon become as much a part of standard cancer care as chemotherapy or radiation. "In the not-so-distant future," he says, "oncologists will send patients to learn tai chi or yoga the way cardiac specialists now send patients to stress-management courses after they've had a heart attack."[165]

## The Rheumatoid Arthritis–Prone Personality

Of all the forms of arthritis, rheumatoid arthritis is the most crippling and most devastating. As an autoimmune disease, it is characterized by the immune system turning against the body and attacking the collagen in the joints' connective tissue. Because it isn't associated with wear and tear, rheumatoid arthritis attacks people of all ages, including children.

The disease has long been considered to have a powerful psychological component. Some researchers are so convinced of the arthritis-personality connection that they have described rheumatoid arthritis as the "expression of a personality conflict."[166]

## Identical Twin Study

Study of the link between personality and rheumatoid arthritis began in earnest in the early 1960s, when a team of researchers from the University of Rochester studied eight pairs of identical twins—one of whom had rheumatoid arthritis while the other did not. Because only one twin in each set had the disease, researchers knew that genetics was not a factor.

Researchers interviewed each of the twins—all women—in great detail to determine not only personality traits but also life events that may have led to the diagnosis of rheumatoid arthritis. They found some strikingly similar patterns among the women afflicted with arthritis. In each pair of twins, the one with arthritis seemed to put herself under a great deal of stress; in fact, these women actually seemed to *seek out* stress. The disease seemed to manifest itself only after each woman had decided to dedicate her energies to a particularly stressful or distasteful situation.[167] For example, one woman took a job she really didn't want so she could impress her in-laws. Another gave up personal pursuits to spend her life caring for her psychotic stepfather.

Other striking similarities emerged. The healthy twins felt free to express criticism and to argue but described their marriages as happy ones. The arthritic twins spoke ill of their husbands and apparently put up with considerable abuse in their marriages, yet they never argued with their husbands.[168] In summing up that peculiar dichotomy, one researcher remarked that people with rheumatoid arthritis "will endure stressful situations longer than their siblings. The arthritic patients' inability to express anger may make some situations more stressful to them than these same situations would be to other people."[169]

The healthy women described themselves as people who liked people. They said they were easy to get acquainted with, were active, were constantly busy, were productive workers, and enjoyed life in general. The self-image of the arthritic twins was just the opposite. They described themselves as moody and easily upset. They claimed they were nervous, tense, worried, depressed, and high-strung. While the healthy sisters enjoyed life, the arthritic ones said that they were struggling.

The results of the identical twin study are consistent with what other researchers have found. One researcher who examined more than 5,000 rheumatoid arthritis patients found "that in a high percentage of cases the patients suffered from worry, work pressures, marital disharmony, and concerns about relatives immediately prior to the onset of disease."[170] Others characterize rheumatoid arthritis patients as people who appear to be calm, composed, and optimistic and who rarely, if ever, express anger. Some believe these patients don't even feel anger. On the rare occasions when these patients express anger or rage, they feel overcome with remorse and guilt and feel a strong need to punish themselves. Research has established that people with rheumatoid arthritis are more likely to suffer from emotional disturbance and that they tend to suffer from perfectionism, chronic anxiety, depression, hostility, and introversion.[171]

## The Solomon and Moos Study

Stanford University School of Medicine psychiatrist George Solomon and his colleague Rudolf Moos asked to examine each patient who came into the San Francisco General Hospital emergency room complaining of a tender, inflamed, or "hot" joint. Emergency room personnel administered laboratory tests to each patient—a simple blood test indicates the presence of an antibody in the blood. While patients were waiting for the results of the test, Solomon and Moos asked them to participate in a psychodrama.

Solomon and Moos knew that rheumatoid arthritis patients were characteristically unassertive and inhibited. So they constructed a psychodrama that would put that trait to its most severe test: They asked patients to return an item (an iron for women, a shaver for men) to someone playing a hostile department store clerk. The role required great assertiveness, and the researchers watched carefully as each suspected—but yet undiagnosed—patient play-acted.

Based on how each patient interacted with the "hostile clerk," Solomon made his own diagnosis, predicting which patients would eventually be proven to have rheumatoid arthritis and which would not. He was able to predict with 100 percent accuracy exactly which patients had rheumatoid arthritis simply by watching how they asserted themselves in an unpleasant situation.

Following their initial experiment, Moos compiled everything he could find on the link between personality and arthritis and he became familiar with the case studies of more than 5,000 people with rheumatoid arthritis. Based on his exhaustive studies, he concluded that there was a distinct psychology involved in the rheumatoid arthritis process.[172]

## The Immune System Factor

Since rheumatoid arthritis is an immune disorder, researchers have looked at how the personality affects the immune system among arthritis sufferers.[173]

In both animals and humans, emotional distress has significant effects on both immune dysfunction and the inflammatory response characteristic of arthritis.[174] Rheumatoid arthritis patients have been shown to have an imbalance in the white blood cells (lymphocytes) that regulate much of the immune response. In their blood and joint fluid, rheumatoid patients have a disturbed "immunoregulatory ratio" of helper T lymphocytes (which enhance the immune response) to suppressor T lymphocytes (which decrease the response).[175]

Other neurochemicals that modulate immune function and inflammation are endorphins, the body's natural painkillers.[176] These are well-known to be affected by mental state; for example, happy excitement turns them on, depression turns them off. Less well-known is the fact that endorphins are deficient in both the blood and the brain in many arthritis patients.[177] Endorphins not only reduce pain perception in the brain but also block the release in tissues of inflammation-producing neurochemicals, such as Substance P and prostaglandins. Substance P has also been thought to be a mechanism by which the nervous system might be involved in rheumatoid arthritis.[178]

Two of the traits common to arthritis victims, chronic anxiety and repressed hostility, have been shown in repeated studies to compromise the immune system. In one study, researchers carefully studied thirty-three women who suffered from rheumatoid arthritis. They looked at the number of daily "hassles" each went through, the major challenges they faced, and the amount of psychological distress each one had. They then measured the immune function of each woman. As expected, the researchers found major effects on the immune system, and those effects were stronger among the women who suffered greater psychological distress, major challenges, and minor hassles.[179]

Based on several decades of research into the connection between personality and rheumatoid arthritis, one researcher constructed what he believes to be an accurate picture of the arthritis patient's personality.[180] He maintains that rheumatoid arthritics are likely to be dependent and feel inadequate, but they deny their dependency by overcompensating with an outward facade of independence, self-assurance, and self-control. They are aware of strong, unexpressed feelings of anger, but they are severely blocked in their ability to express anger or other emotions. They tend to court others' favor, but they avoid closeness in interpersonal relationships. They tend to become overactive—a way of dealing defensively with their tensions—and they overreact to even the slightest criticism or rejection. The single most powerful precipitating factor in rheumatoid arthritis "was the loss of, or separation from, important key figures upon whom these patients depended for support."[181]

# The Ulcer-Prone Personality

Physicians have long acknowledged that the physiology behind gastric ulcer is simple: The ulcer sufferer secretes too much gastric acid. That acid eats away at the lining of the stomach, causing erosion; in severe cases, the ulcer becomes perforated, eating a hole through the wall of the stomach. Most ulcers are caused by infection with a bacterium (*Helicobacter pylori*) that interacts with the acid. Whether mental stress in a susceptible person increases the likelihood of persistent *Helicobacter* infection, as it does with other infections, has not yet been studied.

Use of tobacco, alcohol, caffeine (especially coffee), and aspirin have all ✓ been shown to increase gastric acid production. Cigarette smoking is a double-edged sword, since it also delays healing. Certain emotions can also increase acid; the most powerful seem to be frustration, hostility, and resentment. Some people even experience an increase in gastric acid when they see, smell, taste, or chew food—or even think about it.

Anti-inflammatory medications like aspirin (which are more commonly used by stressed patients) can compound the problem by breaking down the mucus barrier that protects the stomach and intestinal lining from the acid.

## Pioneering Research

Recent research has indicated the presence of an "ulcer personality." Much like the cancer personality or arthritis personality, the ulcer personality may actually cause ulcers, or it may figure in determining how severe ulcers become.

One of the first recorded observations of the emotional link to ulcers occurred in the mid-nineteenth century:[182] Dr. William Beaumont had a patient whose abdominal wall had an opening clear into his stomach. That opening afforded the perfect window through which to view the rate of stomach secretion—and Beaumont noticed that the secretion of stomach juices changed when the man became emotionally stressed.

Pioneering research on the ulcer-personality link has been conducted by Dr. Charles Richardson and Dr. Mark Feldman, professors of internal medicine at the University of Texas Health Science Center in Dallas.[183] They found that ulcer patients seem to have the same number of stressful situations as people who don't have ulcers, but they perceive the situations as being far more negative than do other people. When faced with a job change or relocation, for example, ulcer patients perceived disaster and upset instead of adventure or a positive change. In addition, ulcer patients seemed much more likely than others to be neurotic—preoccupied with their own aches and pain and too concerned about their bodily functions. They expected the worst, and felt threatened by a wide variety of situations, even situations that did not pose much of a real risk.

### Characteristic Traits

The ulcer personality is characterized by excessive dependency on others and a tendency to rely on other people in ways that are not healthy. Even though such persons are very dependent, they enjoy far less social support than most healthy people do. Many ulcer patients express the feeling that they have few friends or relatives on whom they could depend in times of crisis. They tend to suffer from excessive worry, annoyance, and fear of common situations or circumstances. And, unfortunately, ulcer patients seem to have more times of crisis than others, possibly because the ulcer personality is also marked by deep pessimism or the tendency to always expect the worst. Finally, ulcer patients who have been given psychological tests show a fairly consistent quality: While other people are able to bend with stress, an ulcer patient tends to break. This tendency leads to higher rates of emotional distress, anxiety, and depression among those with ulcers. The situation is aggravated by doing other things to damage the lining of the stomach, such as drinking too much coffee or alcohol.

But researchers are quick to point out the bright side of ulcer personality research: With help and determination, ulcer patients can learn to change the way they look at things, and with a change in personality traits, the tendency toward ulcers can diminish considerably.

## An Asthma-Prone Personality?

Research shows that several factors may be at work in the personality traits of an asthmatic. Initially, many asthma episodes are caused by bronchial infection or an allergic reaction; air passages narrow, the victim can't get enough air, and that feeling is profoundly distressful. Any attending emotional reaction just makes the asthma worse. Asthma is usually maintained by an inflammatory process in the airways that may have some of the same underlying mechanisms involving the central nervous system as those for rheumatoid arthritis. It is not uncommon to see the airway disease of anxious or depressed asthmatics improve significantly when those mental conditions are treated appropriately.

It is now believed that some people later develop an almost Pavlovian response to whatever triggers their asthma. Simply thinking, "I feel a cold coming on; it's going to cause an asthma attack," or, "The pollen count is going to be high today," can be enough to trigger a full-fledged asthma attack without an actual physical insult.

There's also a vicious cycle among asthmatics, especially childhood asthmatics, that is very difficult to break. An asthma episode tends to engender sympathy, attention, and compassion, and to keep the child home from school. If that's what asthmatic persons need in their life—more sympathy, attention, and compassion—attacks may become more frequent. Although the biology of the attack is very real, it is precipitated by emotional need.

A few traits seem more common among those with asthma. Many are anxious and feel powerless. Even though they are angry and hostile, they feel weak and out of control of their lives. Finally, many feel ready to strike out at those around them.

## Reducing Your Risks

Is it possible to overcome a disease-prone personality? Some researchers think it is. In an address before the National Institute for the Clinical Application of Behavioral Medicine, Henry Dreher suggested the following ideas for change:[184]

- Develop an awareness of your own needs. You can start on a small scale—maybe you need a few minutes alone when you get home from work before you plunge into family life, for example.

- Discover what Dreher calls an "inner guide"—essentially, an awareness of your innermost thoughts and feelings. If you're used to suppressing emotion or ignoring your needs, it can take some real concentration.

- Reframe your ideas about your feelings. If you're troubled by the thought that you are angry toward an abusive parent, stop feeling guilty for your anger. Find appropriate ways to express your anger, work through it, and then build on what is left, even eventually forgiving your abuser.

- Learn the skills of emotional expression. Everyone occasionally feels angry, hostile, disappointed, depressed, or resentful. The key is to acknowledge your emotion, express it appropriately, and then move on.

- Take charge of your medical care; find a physician who will take the time to talk to you, who will explore options, and who will answer questions. Find out all you can, and make your own decisions.

- Get as much social support as you can. A broad network of family and friends is ideal, but you should cultivate at least a few close friends in whom you can confide.

- Work through your feelings of hopelessness. Getting information is the first step; next, figure out what your challenges might be, then work out a game plan for each. As soon as you realize that you have viable options, you'll find that you feel in charge instead of hopeless.

- Cultivate a fighting spirit; be willing to face challenges head-on and to fight to the finish.

To stress components that are more positive and productive, Dr. Meyer Friedman uses the following drills to help people change the negative components of a Type A personality into the health-protective characteristics of an effective Type B:

- Smile at yourself in the mirror for a minute or two.

- Don't interfere with someone who is doing a job more slowly than you would do the same job.

- Eliminate two phrases from your vocabulary at work: "How much?" and "How many?"

- Take regular breaks from work; try daydreaming, meditating, or even playing with your pet.

Other effective practices to modify Type A behaviors can include the following.

***Practice Mindfulness.***    Do one thing at a time, being completely present with full attention. Give yourself with caring creativity to whatever is chosen to be done in the present moment.[185]

- While waiting in lines, practice the enjoyment that comes with socializing or doing relaxation exercises.

- Smile at the competitive antics of yourself or others.

- Drive around the block when you try to beat someone out in traffic.

- Read books that have nothing to do with your vocation.

- Take restful breaks during the day, perhaps using relaxation exercises.

- Eat slowly and mindfully.

- Ask, "What did I do well today, and what's worth remembering?"

- Practice conditioning a relaxation response after exercise and other arousal.[186]

In making the transition, it's more important to envision what you want (valued Type B traits) than to try not to be hostile. (The brain doesn't do well with "not" commands, because it needs to picture clearly the desired outcome before change can occur.) As you try to envision the effective Type B traits, work toward these habits:

- *Have less time urgency:* Give more attention to the central task at hand. Be less eager to move on to something else. Be on time, but without frenzy or rage. Be patient. Contemplate, especially beauty and metaphor. Tend to see the whole more than the parts. Value and enjoy the things you've already done (or you're doing now) as much as the things you will do in the future.

- *Relinquish control:* Delegate. Be tolerant of, or even enjoy, differences. Inspire creative involvement with others.

- *Value yourself:* Appreciate yourself for what you are as much as for what you do. Accept and value yourself as you are. Understand that self-identity is far more than numbers. Feel valued and of worth, regardless of your achievements. Work hard, but don't let failure collapse your self-esteem. Learn to love growth and the process of getting better through mistakes. Compete with yourself, not with others.

- *Get rid of free-floating hostility:* Don't find fault with others to bolster your own ego. Accept with equanimity the trivial errors of subordinates. Enjoy empowering and lifting others. Don't feel tense or induce tension in others. Be self-confident enough to be objective, to see through another's eyes. Be capable of both feeling and expressing affection; enjoy intimate relationships.

The behavior change methods that develop these characteristics are beginning to be proven some of medicine's most valuable preventive approaches!

## ENDNOTES

1. Howard S. Friedman, *The Self-Healing Personality* (New York: Henry Holt and Company, 1991), 1.
2. Clive Wood, "Type-Casting: Is Disease Linked with Personality?" *Nursing Times,* 84, no. 48: 26.
3. Friedman, *The Self-Healing Personality,* 22.
4. Hans J. Eysenck, "Personality, Stress, and Cancer: Prediction and Prophylaxis," *British Journal of Medical Psychology* 61, p. 1, 57–75.
5. Friedman, *The Self-Healing Personality,* 57.
6. S. Yousfi, G. Matthews, M. Amelang, and C. Schmidt-Rathjens, "Personality and Disease: Correlations of Multiple Trait Scores with Various Illnesses," *Journal of Health Psychology* 9, no. 5: 627–47.
7. R. Grossarth-Maticek, D. T. Kanazir, P. Schmidt, and H. Vetter, "Psychosomatic Factors in the Process of Carcinogenesis: Theoretical Models and Empirical Results," *Psychotherapy and Psychosomatics* 38 (1982): 284–302; and R. Grossarth-Maticek, D. T. Kanazir, P. Schmidt, and H. Vetter, "Psychosomatic Factors in the Process of Carcinogenesis: Preliminary Results in the Yugoslavian Prospective Study," *Psychotherapy and Psychosomatics* 40 (1983): 191–210.
8. S. Yousfi et al., "Personality and Disease."
9. Eysenck, "Personality," 30.
10. Ibid.
11. Joshua Fischman, "Fighting Cancer and Heart Disease: The Character of Controversy," *Psychology Today* (December 1988): 27.
12. S. Yousfi et al., "Personality and Disease."
13. Fischman, "Fighting Cancer."
14. "Nineteen Critical Commentaries," *Psychological Inquiry: An International Journal of Peer Commentary and Review* 2, no. 3.
15. Fischman, "Fighting Cancer."

16. Friedman, "The Self-Healing Personality," 94–96.
17. Bruce Bower, "The Character of Cancer," *Science News* 131 (1987): 120.
18. Bower, "The Character of Cancer."
19. R. Horowski, L. Horowski, S. M. Caine, and D. B. Caine, "From Wilhelm von Hunboldt to Hitler: Are Prominent People More Prone to Parkinson's Disease?" *SBU Therapeutics* 6, no. 4: 205–14.
20. R. Goodwin and G. Engstrom, "Personality and the Perception of Health in the General Population," *Psychol Med* 32, no. 2: 325–32.
21. Judy Berlfein, "An Ill Nature," *Psychology Today*, n.d., 16.
22. Ibid.
23. Ibid.
24. Joann Rodgers, "Longevity Predictors: The Personality Link," *Omni*, February 1989, 25.
25. Douglas J. Stanwyck and Carol A. Anson, "Is Personality Related to Illness? Cluster Profiles of Aggregated Data," *Advances* 3, no. 2: 4–15.
26. Friedman, "The Self-Healing Personality,"15.
27. Marcia Angell, "Disease as a Reflection of the Psyche," *New England Journal of Medicine* 312, (1985): 1570–72.
28. Angell, "Disease as a Reflection."
29. Ibid.
30. Ibid.
31. June Zimmerman, "Does Emotional State Affect Disease?" *MD*, April 1986, 30, 41.
32. Joel Davis, "Anxiety Aches," *Self*, January 1985, 100.
33. Steven Locke and Douglas Colligan, *The Healer Within: The New Medicine of Mind and Body* (New York: E. P. Dutton, 1986), 140.
34. L. Kelti Kangas-Jarvinen, "'Psychosomatic Personality': A Personality Constellation or an Illness-Related Reaction?" *British Journal of Medical Psychology* 62, no. 4: 325–31.
35. Anne Underwood, "For a Happy Heart," *Newsweek*, September 27, 2004, 54.
36. S. P. Zodpay and S. G. Raut, "Coronary Prone Behaviour Pattern and Risk of Coronary Heart Disease: A Case Study," *Indian J Med Sci* 52, no. 8: 348–51.
37. T. George Harris, "Heart and Soul," *Psychology Today*, n.d.
38. Ray Rosenman, "Do You Have Type 'A' Behavior?" *Health and Fitness '87 Supplement* S12–S13.
39. Ethel Roskies, *Stress Management for the Healthy Type A* (New York: Guilford Press, 1987), 8.
40. Paul Pearsall, *Super Immunity*.
41. Redford Williams, *The Trusting Heart: Great News About Type A Behavior* (New York: New York Times Books, Division of Random House, 1989), 17.
42. Rosenman, "Do You Have a Type 'A' Behavior?" S12.
43. Williams, *The Trusting Heart*, 19.
44. Rosenman, "Do You Have a Type 'A' Behavior?" S12.
45. Williams, *The Trusting Heart*, 19.
46. Roskies, *Stress Management*, 6.
47. Roskies, *Stress Management*, 8.
48. Williams, *The Trusting Heart*, 22.
49. Ibid., 24–25.
50. Ibid., 25–26.
51. Ibid., 27.
52. Ibid., 37.

53. G. E. Miller, K. E. Freedland, R. M. Carney, C. A. Stetler, and W. A. Banks, "Pathways Linking Depression, Adiposity, and Inflammatory Markers in Healthy Young Adults," *Brain, Behavior, and Immunity* 17, no. 4: 276–85.

54. Willem J. Kop, "The Integration of Cardiovascular Behavioral Medicine and Psychoneuroimmunology: New Developments Based on Converging Research Fields," *Brain, Behavior, and Immunity* 17 (2003): 233–37.

55. Ray H. Rosenman and Margaret A. Chesney, "Stress, Type A Behavior, and Coronary Disease," *Common Psychiatric and Somatic Conditions*, 547–65.

56. Rosenman and Chesney, "Stress."

57. Williams, *The Trusting Heart,* 120.

58. Ibid.

59. Ibid., 122.

60. J. C. Meininger, L. L. Hayman, P. M. Coates, and P. Gallagher, "Genetics or Environment? Type A Behavior and Cardiovascular Risk Factors in Twin Children," *Nursing Research* 37, no. 5: 341–46.

61. Melvin J. Steinhart, *Emotional Aspects of Coronary Artery Disease* (Kalamazoo, Mich.: Upjohn Company, 1984).

62. Steinhart, *Emotional Aspects.*

63. Jon Kabat-Zinn, *Full Catastrophe Living* (Boston: Delacorte Press, 1990).

64. Gary Felsten, "Five-Factor Analysis of Buss-Durkee Hostility Inventory, Neurotic Hostility and Expressive Hostility Factors: Implications for Health Psychology," *Journal of Personality Assessment* 67, no. 1: 179.

65. B. J. Bushman, H. M. Cooper, and K. M. Lemke, "Meta-Analysis of Factor Analyses: An Illustration Using the Buss-Durkee Hostility Inventory," *Personality and Social Psychology Bulletin* 17: 344–49.

66. Ibid.

67. Ibid.

68. R. B. Williams, T. L. Haney, et al., "Type A Behavior, Hostility, and Coronary Atherosclerosis," *Psychosomatic Medicine* 42 (1980): 539–49.

69. R. B. Shekelle, M. Gale, A. Ostfeld, and D. Paul, "Hostility, Risk of Coronary Artery Disease and Mortality," *Psychosomatic Medicine* 45 (1983): 109–14; and J. C. Barefoot, W. G. Dahlstrom, and R. B. Williams, "Hostility, CHD Incidence, and Total Mortality: A 25-Year Follow-Up Study of 255 Physicians," *Psychosomatic Medicine* 45 (1983): 59–63.

70. Underwood, "For a Happy Heart," 55.

71. Chris Raymond, "Distrust, Rage May Be 'Toxic Core' That Puts 'Type A' Person at Risk," *Journal of the American Medical Association* 261, no. 16: 813.

72. Kristina Orth-Gomer and Anna-Lena Unden, "Type A Behavior, Social Support, and Coronary Risk: Interaction and Significance for Mortality in Cardiac Patients," *Psychosomatic Medicine* 52 (1990): 59–72.

73. Roskies, *Stress Management,* 17.

74. Earl Ubell, "The Deadly Emotions," *Parade,* February 11, 1990, 46.

75. Redford Williams, "The Trusting Heart," *New Age Journal,* May/June 1989, 26.

76. Joshua Fischman, "Type A Situations," *Psychology Today,* August 1988, 22.

77. John C. Barefoot, Ilene C. Siegler, John B. Nowlin, Bercedis L. Peterson, Thomas L. Haney, and Redford B. Williams, "Suspiciousness, Health, and Mortality: A Follow-Up Study of 500 Older Adults," *Psychosomatic Medicine* 49 (1987): 450–57.

78. Barefoot et al., "Suspiciousness."

79. Donald E. Girard, Ransom J. Arthur, and James B. Reuler, "Psychosocial Events and Subsequent Illness—A Review," *Western Journal of Medicine* 142, no. 3: 358–63.

80. William H. Hendrix and Richard L. Hughes, "Relationship of Trait, Type A Behavior, and Physical Fitness Variables to Cardiovascular Reactivity and Coronary Heart Disease Risk Potential," *American Journal of Health Promotion* 11, no. 4: 264–71.

81. Tom Ferguson, "Contented Workaholics," *Medical Self-Care,* summer 1981, 20–24.

82. Ferguson, "Contented Workaholics."

83. Sharon Faelton, David Diamond, and the editors of *Prevention* magazine, *Take Control of Your Life* (Emmaus, Pa.: Rodale Press, 1988).

84. Pearsall, *Super Immunity.*

85. Williams, *The Trusting Heart,* 26.

86. Eileen M. Mikat, Jorge V. Bartolome, Jay M. Weiss, Saul M. Schanberg, Cynthia M. Kuhn, and Redford B. Williams, "Chronic Norepinephrine Infusion Accelerates Atherosclerotic Lesion Development in Sand Rats Maintained on a High-Cholesterol Diet," *Psychosomatic Medicine* 53 (1991): 211.

87. Robert S. Eliot, *Behavior and Cardiovascular Disease* (Kalamazoo, Mich.: Upjohn Company, 1989).

88. Neil Schneiderman, Margaret Chesney, and David S. Krantz, "Biobehavioral Aspects of Cardiovascular Disease: Progress and Prospects," *Health Psychology* 8, no. 6: 649–76.

89. Eliot, *Behavior.*

90. S. J. Schleifler et al., "The Nature and Course of Depression Following Myocardial Infarction," *Archives of Internal Medicine* 149 (1989): 1785–89.

91. P. Berzanyi, E. Galateo, and L. Valzeli, "Fluoxetine Activity on Muricidal Aggression Induced in Rats by P-Chlorophenylalanine," *Aggressive Behavior* 9 (1983): 333–338.

92. Denis J. Lynch and Kay Schaffer, "Type A and Social Support," *Behavioral Medicine* (summer 1989): 72.

93. *Psychosomatic Medicine* 4 (1987).

94. J. H. Medalie and U. Goldburt, "Angina Pectoris Among 10,000 [Israeli] Men: Psychosocial and Other Risk Factors," *American Journal of Medicine* 60 (1976): 910–21.

95. Steinhart *Emotional Aspects.*

96. Angell, "Disease as a Reflection."

97. R. M. Suinn, "The Cardiac Stress Management Program for Type A Patients," *Cardiac Rehabilitation* 5 (1975): 13–15.

98. S. Haynes et al., *American Journal of Epidemiology* 3 (1980): 3758.

99. Roskies, *Stress Management,* 14.

100. Meyer Friedman and Diane Ulmer, *Treating Type A Behavior and Your Heart* (New York: Knopf, 1984), 83–102.

101. Michael Castleman, "Are You a Type-A Woman?" *Medical Self-Care,* n.d., 30–33.

102. Tandy J. McClung, "A Profile of Low, Moderate, and High Type A Female Children," paper presented at the tenth anniversary meeting of the Society of Behavioral Medicine, April 1, 1989.

103. Kathy A. Fackelmann, "Child's Aggression May Foretell Heart Risk," *Science News,* July 1, 1989, 15.

104. Fackelmann, "Child's Agression."

105. Carl E. Thoresen, Jean R. Eagleston, Kathleen Kirmil-Gray, and Sue Wiedenfeld, "Examining Anger in Low and High Type A Children and Adolescents," paper presented at the tenth anniversary meeting of the Society of Behavioral Medicine, March 31, 1989.

106. Karen A. Matthews, Catherine J. Stoney, Charles J. Rakaczky, and Wesley Jamison, "Family Characteristics and School Achievements of Type A Children," *Health Psychology* 5, no. 5: 453–67.

107. David M. Murray, Karen A. Matthews, Susan M. Blake, Ronald J. Prineas, and Richard R. Gillum, "Type A Behavior in Children: Demographic, Behavioral, and Physiological Correlates," *Health Psychology* 5, no. 2: 159–69.

108. L. H. Powell, L. A. Shaker, et al., "Psychosocial Predictors of Mortality in 83 Women with Premature Myocardial Infarction," *Psychosomatic Medicine* 55, (1993): 426–33.

109. L. F. Berkman, V. Vaccarino, and T. Seeman, "Gender Differences in Cardiovascular Morbidity and Mortality: The Contribution of Social Networks and Support," *Annals of Behavioral Medicine* 15 (1993): 112–18.

110. Margaret A. Chesney, "Social Isolation, Depression, and Heart Disease: Research on Women Broadens the Agenda," *Psychosomatic Medicine* 55, (1993): 434–35.

111. B. Rime, C. G. Ucros, Y. Bestgen, and M. Jeanjean, "Type A Behavior Pattern: Specific Coronary Risk Factor or General Disease-Prone Condition?" *British Journal of Medical Psychology* 62, no. 3: 229–40.

112. J. Suls and G. S. Sanders, "Type A Behavior as a General Risk Factor for Physical Disorder," *Journal of Behavioral Medicine*, 11, no. 30: 201–26.

113. Shoham-Yakubovich, "How Your Personality Affects Your Health," *Good Housekeeping*, June: 1983.

114. Williams, "The Trusting Heart," 74.

115. Underwood, "For a Happy Heart," 55.

116. Ibid., 56.

117. Johann Denollet, "Personality and Coronary Heart Disease: The Type-D Scale-16 (DS16)," *Annals of Behavioral Medicine* 20, no. 3: 209–15.

118. M. A. Mittleman, M. Maclure, J. B. Sherwood et al., "Triggering of Acute Myocardial Infarction Onset by Episodes of Anger," *Circulation* 92 (1995): 1720–25; and I. Kawachi, D. Sparrow, A. Spiro III, P. Vokonas, and S. T. Weiss, "A Prospective Study of Anger and Coronary Heart Disease: The Normative Aging Study," *Circulation* 94 (1996): 2090–95.

119. D. K. Moser and K. Dracup, "Is Anxiety Early after Myocardial Infarction Associated with Subsequent Ischemic and Arrhythmic Events?" *Psychosomatic Medicine* 58 (1996): 395–401; and I. Kawachi, D. Sparrow, P. Vokonas, and S. T. Weiss, "Symptoms of Anxiety and Risk of Coronary Heart Disease: The Normative Aging Study," *Circulation* 90, (1994): 2225–29.

120. J. C. Barefoot and M. Schroll, "Symptoms of Depression, Acute Myocardial Infarction, and Total Mortality in a Community Sample," *Circulation* 93 (1996): 1976–80.

121. L. D. Kubzansky, I. Kawachi, A. Spiro III, et al., "Is Worrying Bad for Your Heart? A Prospective Study of Worry and Coronary Heart Disease in the Normative Aging Study," *Circulation* 95 (1997): 818–24.

122. S. A. Everson, D. E. Goldberg, G. A. Kaplan, et al., "Hopelessness and Risk of Mortality and Incidence of Myocardial Infarction and Cancer," *Psychosomatic Medicine* 58 (1996): 113–21.

123. Underwood, "For a Happy Heart."

124. Ibid.

125. Johann Denollet, Nathalie Stroobant, Hans Rombouts, Thierry C. Gillebert, and Dirk L. Brutsaert, "Personality as Independent Predictor of Long-Term Mortality in Patients with Coronary Heart Disease," *Lancet* 347 (1996): 8999, 417–21; and J. W. Pennebaker and H. C. Traue, "Inhibition and Psychosomatic

Processes," in H. C. Traue and J. W. Pennebaker, eds., *Emotion, Inhibition, and Health* (Seattle, Wash: Hogrefe & Huber, 1993), 146–63.

126. D. Watson and L. A. Clark, "Negative Affectivity: The Disposition to Experience Adverse Emotional States," *Psychological Bulletin* 96 (1984): 465–90.

127. Denollet et al., "Personality as Independent Predictor," 417–21.

128. J. M. Murphy, R. R. Monson, D. C. Olivier, A. M. Sobol, and A. H. Leighton, "Affective Disorders and Mortality: A General Population Study," *Archives of General Psychiatry* 44 (1987): 473–80; and R. M. Carney, M. W. Rich, K. E. Freedland et al., "Major Depressive Disorder Predicts Cardiac Events in Patients with Coronary Artery Disease," *Psychosomatic Medicine* 50 (1988): 627–33.

129. J. Denollet and D. L. Brutsaert, "Personality, Disease Severity, and the Risk of Long-Term Cardiac Events in Patients with a Decreased Ejection Fraction After Myocardial Infarction," *Circulation* 97 (1998): 167–73.

130. Denollet et al., "Personality as Independent Predictors."

131. *Newsweek*, September 27, 2004.

132. Roskies, *Stress Management*, 5.

133. Ibid., 56.

134. Paul Bennett and Douglas Carroll, "The Assessment of Type A Behavior: A Critique," *Psychology and Health* 3 (1989): 183–94.

135. Friedman and Ulmer, *Treating Type A Behavior*, 62.

136. William H. Redd, "Cancer and Emotions: Is There a Connection?" *Executive Health Report* 26, no. 3: 1, 4–6.

137. Locke and Colligan, *The Healer Within*.

138. Ibid.

139. Ibid.

140. Ibid.

141. Lydia Temoshok and Henry Dreher, *The Type C Connection: The Behavioral Links to Cancer and Your Health* (New York: Random House, 1992).

142. Yousfi et al., 627–47.

143. Locke and Colligan, *The Healer Within*, 133–34.

144. Henry Dreher, "The Type C Connection: A Powerful New Tool in the Fight Against Cancer," in *Proceedings of the Fourth National Conference on the Psychology of Health, Immunity, and Disease*, published by the National Institute for the Clinical Application of Behavioral Medicine.

145. Temoshok and Dreher, *The Type C Connection*.

146. Locke and Colligan, *The Healer Within*, 134.

147. Ibid.

148. Barbara A. Schindler, "Stress, Affective Disorders, and Immune Function," *Medical Clinics of North America* 585–97.

149. Michael A. Weiner, *Maximum Immunity* (Boston: Houghton-Mifflin Company, 1986).

150. K. H. Liste, "Breast Cancer, Personality and the Feminine Role," *Patient Educ. Couns.* 36, no. 1:33-45.

151. Eleanor Smith, "Fighting Cancerous Feelings," *Psychology Today*, May 1988, 22.

152. Schindler, "Stress."

153. Alan Zonderman, "Depression Not Linked to Cancer," *Executive Health Report* 26, no. 3: 5.

154. "Is There a Cancer Personality?" *Johns Hopkins Medical Letter* 2, no. 1: 1.

155. Zonderman, "Depression."

156. Smith, "Fighting Cancerous Feelings," 22–23.

157. Ibid.
158. Alice Domar, "Advice for Asking," *Newsweek,* September 27, 2004, 60.
159. Phillip L. Rice, *Stress and Health* (Monterey, Cal.: Brooks/Cole Publishing Company, 1987), 103–4.
160. S. Greer et al., "Psychological Response to Breast Cancer and Fifteen-Year Outcome," *Lancet* 1: (1990): 49–50; and Greer, Morrison, and Pettingale, *Journal of Psychosomatic Research* 19: 147–53.
161. A. D. Wiseman, *Cancer—The Behavioral Dimensions,* 331.
162. Locke and Colligan, *The Healer Within.*
163. Peg Tyre, "Combination Therapy," *Newsweek,* September 27, 66–67.
164. Domar, "Advice for Asking."
165. Tyre, "Combination Therapy," 67.
166. Barbara Powell, *Good Relationships Are Good Medicine* (Emmaus, Pa.: Rodale Press).
167. Locke and Colligan, *The Healer Within,* 107.
168. Powell, *Good Relationships.*
169. Ibid.
170. Ibid.
171. Friedman, *The Self-Healing Personality,* 85.
172. Locke and Colligan, *The Healer Within,* 108.
173. G. F. Solomon and A. A. Amkraut, "Psychoneuroendocrinological Effects on the Immune System," *Annual Review of Microbiology* 35 (1981): 155–84; G. F. Solomon, N. Kay, and J. E. Morley, "Endorphins: A Link Between Personality, Stress, Emotions, Immunity, and Substance P," in N. P. Plotnikoff, R. E. Faith, A. J. Murgo, and R. A. Good, eds., *Enkephalins and Endorphins, Stress and the Immune System* (New York: Plenum Press, 1986), 129–44; and C. D. Anderson, J. M. Soyva, and L. J. Vaughn, "A Test of Delayed Recovery Following Stressful Stimulation in Four Psychosomatic Disorders," *Journal of Psychosomatic Research* 26 (1982): 571–80.
174. E. M. Sternberg, G. P. Chrousis, R. L. Wilder, and P. W. Gold, "The Stress Response and the Regulation of Inflammatory Disease," *Annals of Internal Medicine* 117, no. 10: 854–66.
175. E. M. Veys, P. Hermanns, G. Verbruggen, J. Schindler, and G. Goldstein, "Evaluation of T Cell Subsets with Monoclonal Antibodies in Synovial Fluid in Rheumatoid Arthritis," *Journal of Rheumatology* 9, no. 6: 821–26.
176. R. A. Good, N. P. Plotnikoff, R. E. Faith, A. J. Murgo, and R. A. Good, Enkephalins and Endorphins, *Stress and the Immune System* (New York: Plenum Press, 1986), v–vi; and Solomon et al., "Endomorphs," 129–44.
177. C. Denko, "Serum Beta Endorphins in Rheumatic Disorders," *Journal of Rheumatology* 9, no. 6: 827–33.
178. J. D. Levine, D. H. Collier, A. L. Basbaum, M. A. Moskowitz, and C. A. Helms, "Hypothesis: The Nervous System May Contribute to the Pathophysiology of Rheumatoid Arthritis," *Journal of Rheumatology* 12 (1985): 406–22.
179. Friedman, *The Self-Healing Personality.*
180. Weiner, *Maximum Immunity.*
181. Ibid.
182. Friedman, *The Self-Healing Personality,* 89; A. R. Rimon, "A Psychosomatic Approach to Rheumatoid Arthritis: A Clinical Study of 100 Patients," *Acta Rheumatologica Scandinavica,* suppl. 13 (1969): 1–154; R. Rimon and L. Riika-Liisa, "Life Stress and Rheumatoid Arthritis: A 15-Year Follow-Up Study," *Psychotherapy and Psychosomatics* 43:38–43; T. W. Smith, J. R. Peck, and

J. R. Ward, "Helplessness and Depression in Rheumatoid Arthritis," *Health Psychology* 9, no. 4: 377–89; A. O' Leary, S. Shoor, K. Lorig, and H. R. Holman, "A Cognitive-Behavioral Treatment for Rheumatoid Arthritis," *Health Psychology* 7 (1988): 527–44; K. Lorig, *Arthritis and Rheumatism* 28 (1985): 680–85; S. Crown, J. Crown, and A. Fleming, "Aspects of the Psychology and Epidemiology of Rheumatoid Disease," *Psychological Medicine* 5 (1975): 291–99; Gringas, *Journal of International Medical Research 4,* (suppl. 2): 41; M. Scott, *Practitioner* 202 (1969): 802; I. Oreskes et al., *Annals of Rheumatic Disease* 27 (1968): 60; and G. G. Haydn, *Annals of Rheumatic Disease* 33 (1974): 274.

183. "Is There an Ulcer Personality?" *Wellness Newsletter,* July 1987, 2; and Sharon Faelten, David Diamond, and the editors of *Prevention* magazine, "Take Control of Your Life: A Complete Guide to Stress Relief," *Prevention* (Emmaus, Pa.: Rodale Press, 1988), 206–7.

184. Dreher, "The Type C Connection."

185. Hal Straus, *Men's Health,* June 1992, 72.

186. See the discussion of the characteristics of coronary-protected individuals in Friedman and Ulmer, *Treating Type A Behavior,* chap. 3.

# CHAPTER 4

# Anger, Hostility, and Health

*Of the seven deadly sins, anger is possibly the most fun. To lick your wounds, to smack your lips over grievances long past, to roll over your tongue the prospect of bitter confrontations still to come, to savor to the last toothsome morsel both the pain you are given and the pain you are giving back—in many ways it is a feast fit for a king. The chief drawback is that what you are wolfing down is yourself. The skeleton at the feast is you.*

—Frederick Buechner

## Learning Objectives

- Explore the difference between anger and hostility, and the significance of each.
- Define the physiological reactions and health effects that accompany anger and hostility.
- Describe effective techniques for managing and even transforming anger and hostility.

Anger has assumed a whole new importance, particularly when it comes to heart disease. What used to be blamed on "the hurry disease," as researchers called it, has now been more accurately identified. You can be a heart-healthy Type A as long as, among other things, you're not chronically angry. The impact of anger on health doesn't stop there. The exploding rage you feel when you get really angry brings with it actual physical changes in your body; the health consequences of anger certainly can include high blood pressure and other coronary problems, but the consequences are much more widespread than that. For example, surging hormones and chemicals affect many organs and systems other than the heart. When you are chronically angry, as Buechner so graphically stated, "what you are wolfing down is yourself. The skeleton at the feast is you."[1]

"Anger kills," says famed Duke University researcher Redford Williams. "We're speaking here not about the anger that drives people to shoot, stab, or otherwise wreak havoc on their fellow humans. We mean instead the everyday sort of anger, annoyance, and irritation that courses through the minds and bodies of many perfectly normal people."[2]

## The Definitions of Anger and Hostility

The terms *anger* and *hostility* are often used interchangeably, but they are not the same.[3] Anger is a transient emotional response that depends on the way one chooses to think about events, usually triggered by perceived provocation or mistreatment. Hostility, on the other hand, is a habitual attitude that may not even require much provocation and is usually associated with cynicism and resentment.[4] Hostile people experience a lot of anger.

What, exactly, is anger? First of all, everyone experiences it. Just watch two toddlers fighting over a favorite set of blocks, a teenager challenging an unreasonable curfew, or an executive whose car gets rear-ended on the way to an important business presentation.

Anger is a temporary emotion. It combines physiological arousal with emotional arousal. It can range in severity all the way from intense rage to "cool" anger that doesn't really involve arousal at all (and might more accurately be described as an attitude, such as resentment).[5] People express anger in all sorts of ways, such as hurling verbal insults, using profanity, slamming doors, or smashing a fist into the nearest available object. Anger can, in fact, often be considered a secondary emotion, that is, a way of expressing blame or communicating discomfort with a more primary emotion such as frustration. When this secondary aspect is realized, one can decide to choose a more healthy way of communicating.

The words we use to describe our anger strongly hint at the turmoil that is going on inside our bodies when we're angry. Social psychologist and anger expert Carol Tavris pointed out some of the most common descriptors:[6]

- His pent-up anger welled up inside him.
- He was bursting with anger.
- I blew my stack.
- She flipped her lid.
- He hit the ceiling.
- Our blood "boils," our muscles tense up, our stomach feels like it's tied up in knots, and our cheeks feel like they're burning up.

The more angry we become, the stronger and more powerful we feel—and the more pressed to "strike out."[7]

The terms *anger* and *hostility* are often used to describe a set of negative emotions, but they differ in duration and intensity. Anger has been defined as a *temporary* emotion that may or may not be accompanied by outward

expressions (physical or verbal). Hostility, on the other hand, is not a tem- ✓
porary emotion, but rather an *attitude*. It is anger that is expressed in aggressive behavior motivated by animosity and hatefulness. "Chronic anger" is
usually hostility. Ongoing hostility is usually associated with a cynical and
suspicious worldview, and sometimes with clinical depression.

"Anger is generally considered to be a simpler concept than hostility or
aggression," explain researchers Margaret A. Chesney and Ray H. Rosenman.
"The concept of anger usually refers to an emotional state that consists of
feelings that vary in intensity, from mild irritation or annoyance to fury and
rage. Although hostility usually involves angry feelings, it has the connota-
tion of a complex set of attitudes that motivate aggressive behaviors
directed toward destroying objects or injuring other people."[8]

Hostility comes from the Latin word *hostis,* which means "enemy." For
the hostile, enemies seem to abound. They are everywhere: at the office, in
the elevator, in the grocery store checkout line, on the freeway, in the
house on the corner. And, because of the health-damaging effects of hostility, hostile people become their own enemy.

Hostility is an ongoing accumulation of anger and irritation. As psychologist Robert Ornstein and physician David Sobel put it, hostility is "a permanent resident kind of anger that shows itself with ever greater frequency
in response to increasingly trivial happenings."[9] Tavris says that "into each
life come real problems that people should be angry about. But hostile personality types get equally angry about cold soup and racial injustice. They're
walking around in a state of wrath."[10] And, the researchers warn, hostility
may go undetected for a long time. One reason for slow detection is that
hostile people deny it[11] and often try to hide it (most actually don't really
want to be hostile). If asked if they are often hostile, they might angrily
reply, "Of course not! What do you take me for, anyway?"

Pioneering researchers like Redford Williams now suspect that the
notorious Type A personality may not play the major role once believed in
heart disease. Instead, a handful of traits—particularly hostility—may be
the actual culprits. According to Williams, about 20 percent of the general ✓
population has a level of hostility high enough to be dangerous to health.[12]
He describes hostility as having three components:

- *Attitude*. Hostile people are generally cynical toward others.
- *Emotion*. Hostile people express frequent anger, especially over petty
  incidents or issues.
- *Behavior*. Hostile people display threatening or aggressive behavior.

Hostility is more than a simple emotion or an isolated angry outburst in
a moment of frustration. And for some reason, hostility rarely stands alone;
it is often intertwined with cynicism, suspiciousness, and self-centeredness.[13]

Researchers have found that the most health-harming kind is free-floating hostility, an attitude characterized by being angry, or on the verge of anger, most of the time, with or without cause. At the best, hostile people are grouchy; at the worst, they are constantly consumed by hatred. Occasional hostility is not the problem; the problem is the constant, slow-burning anger and the willingness to see almost everyone as the enemy.[14]

## Manifestations of Anger and Hostility

Anger has as many different causes as there are situations and people in them. A common one is the frustration of physical or psychological restraint—being held back from something we intensely want or want to do.[15] Others include being forced to do something against our will, being taken advantage of, being insulted or ridiculed, or having plans defeated. Sometimes other primary emotions (such as distress, sorrow, or fear) can lead to anger.

Besides individual differences in the way we feel and express anger, there are also some important cultural differences. In a number of Latin and Arab cultures, the free expression of anger is heartily endorsed; two who are angry with each other may fight because they figure that a strong third party (such as a neighbor or family member) will intervene before things go too far. The Utku Eskimos fall at the opposite end of the spectrum: They ostracize anyone who loses his or her temper, regardless of the reason. Tavris tells of an anthropologist who was shunned for several months by the Utkus when she became angry with some Caucasian fishermen who broke an Eskimo canoe.[16]

Between these two extremes are all kinds of middle ground. The Japanese don't display anger as their traditional Western counterparts do; instead of lashing out verbally, the Japanese assume a neutral expression and a polite demeanor when angry. The Mbuti gatherer-hunters of northeast Zaire take it a step farther; when angry, they laugh. Some individual disputes have become "full-scale tribal laugh fests."[17] These differences illustrate how anger is a chosen, expressive (secondary) emotion.

Hostility, however, shows up with many associated features. Noted Harvard psychiatrist James Gill has compiled a list of such traits. A hostile person, says Gill, notices with irritation the perceived faults of others, has an intense need to win at games or sports, and gets extremely angry (with self and others) at losing. He or she turns most conversations into a debate and argues tenaciously until winning the point. He or she also is extremely demanding and critical, not only of others but also of self, and is extremely sensitive to any kind of criticism or uncomplimentary remark. Even when smiling, the hostile person appears tight and tense, as though ready to quarrel on a second's notice.[18] The key in relating them to hostility, says Gill, is consistency: These aren't occasional attitudes, but habitual and characteristic ways of reacting.

Still another definition of hostility might be obtained from the psychological tests that researchers use to pinpoint it. One of the most standard—and most reliable—is the Hostility Scale, administered as part of the Minnesota Multiphasic Personality Inventory (MMPI). This scale, called the HO scale or the Cooke Medley Hostility Scale,[19] has been most used to study the health effects of hostility. Other shorter scales have also been developed and correlated with heart disease.[20] University of Utah researcher Dr. Timothy Smith used what Redford Williams calls a time-honored way of isolating personality traits from the MMPI test. He administered the test, along with a wide array of other tests, to a large group. Then he studied how the other tests related to the scores on the hostility test. Based on his results, he concluded that the traits most related to hostility were suspiciousness, resentment, frequent anger, and a cynical mistrust of other people.[21]

Cynicism refers to the generally negative view that hostile people have toward humankind; they tend to depict others as selfish, deceptive, and unworthy. They tend to have the same kind of attitude toward the world in general, even when their sense of mistrust is not directed at anyone specifically. Redford Williams claims that those with cynical hostility and cynical mistrust are at the greatest health risk of all.[22]

Hostile people tend to have an attitude of paranoia, attributing hostility to others. They often believe that other people are intentionally out to get them, purposely trying to hurt them. If you wonder if you have too much hostility, examine how you tend to project such attributes onto others.

Timothy Smith also noted that people who tested most hostile were less hardy or resilient, experienced more frequent and severe hassles every day, and derived little satisfaction from their daily social contacts.[23] This inability to thoroughly enjoy life sounds very much like depression, and, in fact, clinical depression often takes the form of cynical hostility, particularly in men. Similar to anxious depressive disorders, hostile people often have a nervous system constantly on guard for impending danger. And the health effects, particularly cardiovascular effects, are very similar between cynical hostility and depression.[24]

It's also possible, says Williams, to get a good mental picture of hostility by looking at its opposite, the trusting heart. According to Williams,

> *[The] trusting heart believes in the basic goodness of humankind, that most people will be fair and kind in relationships with others. Having such beliefs, the trusting heart is slow to anger. Not seeking out evil in others, not expecting the worst of them, the trusting heart expects mainly good from others and, more often then not, finds it. As a result, the trusting heart spends little time feeling resentful, irritable, and angry. From this it follows that the trusting heart*

*treats others well, with consideration and kindness; the trusting heart almost never wishes or visits harm upon others.*[25]

It's like the Law of the Boomerang: What you throw out is what you get back, and you see what you are looking for and expect. The process becomes a self-fulfilling prophecy—if you expect others to be hostile, your automatic behavior prompts their hostility. On the other hand, if you expect them to be kind, your demeanor toward them is more likely to trigger their kindness. This principle is also sometimes called the Law of Expectations.

It is valuable in this discussion to come to know your learned and habitual attitudes by simply asking yourself how you view most people in the world around you: with cynicism, or with trust? Is the world to you more hostile or more kind?

## The Significance of Anger and Hostility

Back when people needed the fight-or-flight response to defend themselves against aggressors, they needed anger. It was important to survival. That surge of energy helped early people defend themselves. Anger enabled them to fight with vigor and great strength.

Our culture evolved much more rapidly than our bodies. We are now a society and a civilization that is expected to deal calmly and rationally with each other. We don't need to fight saber-toothed tigers; our battles are waged in boardrooms and bedrooms. We no longer need the fight-or-flight response as much, but our bodies still respond that way. We call it stress. We seldom need the physical energy of anger, either, but we still get angry. Instead of being a benefit, most regard it as a liability.

In rare cases, anger may play a valuable role in self-defense or in the physical defense of a loved one. Any other time, an angry assault is considered today a violation of both legal and moral ethics, and while the victim may suffer physical harm, the aggressor almost always gets in trouble.[26]

According to researchers, anger rarely exists in isolation. When researchers at the University of Tennessee studied eighty-seven middle-aged women to determine their anger levels, they found that the women who were angry also tended to be pessimistic, lack social support, be overweight, sleep poorly, and lead sedentary lives. The angriest women were also more likely to have existing health problems and to feel they could do nothing to control their problems.[27] Many of these associated features can be driven by the same neurochemistry characteristic of clinical depression abnormalities. This abnormal neurochemistry is also true of "rage attacks." Such rage can also be part of bipolar ("manic-depressive") disorders.

If what current research indicates is true, hostility may have a powerful influence over not only the central nervous system but the body's arsenal of hormones as well. As such, it may play a significant role not only in health and illness but also in premature death. Hostility has such an impact on health, in fact, that the University of Maryland's Theodore M. Dembroski claims it's easy to spot an intensive-care patient in the making: "He's the fellow who mutters and curses to himself if the line at the video store is too long; the one who leans on his horn if you hesitate even a millisecond when the light turns green. He's the hostile man, the one who gets angry over everyday frustrations and expresses those feelings in rude, antagonistic ways."[28]

## Causes of Hostility

Where does hostility come from? How do hostile children get created? What in our makeup may predispose us toward a hostile attitude? Researchers aren't sure, but they're beginning to get clues by studying the lives and backgrounds of people who are hostile. Genetics plays a predisposing role, but learning, particularly early in life, may be even more important and in fact may activate the genetic vulnerability. In one study conducted by University of Kansas researchers Christine Vavak and Kent Houston, 134 college students were given the Cook-Medley Hostility Scale.[29] They were then asked to complete detailed questionnaires about their self-esteem, their health behaviors, their parents' child-rearing practices, and other background factors.

The students who were most hostile seemed to have had an "oppositional orientation" toward people that was developed during childhood. They came from homes where both parents were strict and coercive, used frequent physical punishment or hostile control, and frequently communicated dissatisfaction with the child. Those who scored high on the hostility scale described parents who were less warm and accepting, less likely to have treated the child as an equal, and less likely to have encouraged independent thinking.[30] Those who were the most hostile (as determined by test scores) were also those who had the lowest self-esteem, and those who felt the least amount of acceptance from others. Similarly, another study of the development of hostility in people with coronary disease found it to be related to learned beliefs and attitudes about one's self and others. People who didn't learn self-esteem growing up had a subsequent buildup of negative psychosocial interactions and had poor self-concepts. This poor self-concept was described as hostile in nature and reflects a mistrust of others and a deep sense of isolation.[31]

Finally, the results of at least one sophisticated study indicate that hostility may be more learned than inherited. Researchers came to that conclusion by studying identical twins who had been separated at birth and raised in different families.[32] Researchers learned that hostility often arises from a worldview of a victim, not uncommonly from having experienced the world as a hostile, unaccepting place as a child.

Psychologist Michael J. Strube has seen a pattern of hostility in children as young as age three. One of the main culprits, he says, is "parents urging them to excel, while presenting them with ill-defined goals and little, or ambiguous, feedback."[33]

# The Need to Express Anger

Research has shown that, to be healthy, people need to express or transform anger in a managed, wise way. It is a mandate to confront the things that are making us angry and to work through the anger. According to University of Arizona psychologist Roger J. Daldrup, there are two classic ways of expressing anger in an unhealthy way: misdirecting it or suppressing it completely.[34]

## Unhealthy Expression of Anger

Misdirected anger, Daldrup says, "is the classic kicking the cat because you're angry at your spouse maneuver. Though people who misdirect their anger seem to be expressing it, they are just burying the real problem and creating more problems along the way."[35]

Originally, many recommended that the healthiest response was to give people the opportunity to act out their aggression, with the philosophy that the ensuing "cathartic" effect would ease the emotions and result in dissipated anger and aggression.[36] In one study, people were given unusually harsh (though bogus) feedback about an essay they had written in an attempt to anger them. These angry people were then given the chance to slam a punching bag for two minutes. The theory of researchers was simple: Letting the angry people punch it out for two minutes would reduce their anger and make them less likely to be aggressive later. In fact, the opposite proved true: In a simple contest afterward, those who had punched the punching bag were far more aggressive toward their opponents than angered people who did not pound on a punching bag. The results of the study showed that acting on anger leads to even greater aggression.[37]

At the same time, however, research done by Redford Williams showed that men who openly expressed their anger at the age of twenty-five were more likely to be dead by age fifty than those who did not "get it out" when angry.[38] According to Williams,

> People who "express" their anger are more, rather than less, likely to be more aggressive later and be more, rather than less, likely to have a higher death rate when followed up 25 years later. The simplistic advice, "when angry, let it out," is unlikely, therefore, to be of much help. Far more important is to learn how to evaluate your anger and then to manage it.[39]

The other classic response, complete suppression of anger, doesn't work either, because, says Daldrup, it creates what he calls "the keyboard effect." Once a person starts repressing one emotion, he begins repressing them all, something he likens to pressing down the soft pedal on the piano: "That pedal will soften all the notes on a piano, just as dulling one emotion will dull them all. Sadly, people become used to that feeling of dullness, but the anger is still there, destroying your relationships, sabotaging creativity, or interfering with your sex life."[40] Using denial and repression of emotions as a coping strategy, in the long run, has adverse health effects. So is it best to vigorously express anger or to suppress it? As we will see later, there may be another alternative. This was shown, for example, in a classic forty-year study by George Valliant and colleagues at Harvard, where, compared to more adaptive, mature coping styles, chronically using repression and denial to cope were associated with ten times more chronic illness in middle age.[41]

There are many other unhealthy ways of expressing anger, according to Tavris. Some of the most common ones are miscommunicating, emotional distancing, escalating of the conflict, endlessly rehearsing grievances, assuming a hostile disposition, acquiring angry habits, making a bad situation worse, losing self-esteem, and losing the respect of others.[42]

So if both vigorous expression and suppression of anger are harmful to health, what is one to do? What is needed, researchers agree, is the ability to confront the source of anger and express feelings without getting overwhelmed by the anger. As Carol Tavris put it, "The purpose of anger is to make a grievance known, and if the grievance is not confronted, it will not matter whether the anger is kept in, let out, or wrapped in red ribbons and dropped in the Erie Canal."[43]

According to Daldrup, anger becomes frightening (to you and to others) only when it is repressed for a long time and is then expressed with the "force to turn silverware into metal filings."[44] "If you were discharging anger as it came up for you," he says, "there wouldn't be any extra energy attached to it. You'd be able to say 'I disagree with you' or 'I don't like what you are saying' in a straightforward manner without any extra energy attached to it." Instead of doing that, says Daldrup, most people store up— or "stuff"—their anger. "Stuffing is the only way you'll have enough energy for an explosion."[45] So one needs to level about where they are coming from, but not necessarily in a hostile way.

Preliminary research has shown that bottling up anger can lead to many health consequences, among them heart disease, cancer, rheumatoid arthritis, hives, acne, psoriasis, peptic ulcer, epilepsy, migraine, Raynaud's disease, and high blood pressure.[46] And several researchers agree that expressing anger benefits health as long as the expression itself is healthy. The classic idea about expressing anger in screaming and pounding hysteria doesn't stand up under experimental scrutiny, says Tavris. Instead of helping, this kind of reaction "makes you angrier, solidifies an angry attitude, and establishes a hostile habit. If you keep quiet about momentary irritations and distract yourself with pleasant activity until your fury simmers down, chances are that you will feel better, and feel better faster, than if you let yourself go in a shouting match."[47] In her book *Anger: The Misunderstood Emotion*, Tavris adds, "Ventilating is cathartic only when it restores our sense of control, reducing both the rush of adrenaline that accompanies an unfamiliar and threatening situation and the belief that you are helpless and powerless."[48]

The way you deal with anger will have considerable impact on your health, say the researchers. If you get momentarily irritated at something, one approach might be to distract yourself—to concentrate on more pleasant thoughts. But if you start feeling chronic or continual anger at someone or something, more aggressive action is needed to confront your feelings and work through the anger. "If you're angry at something that is trivial but still infuriating, you can choose to distract yourself," says Tavris, "but if you're continuously angry at someone, you have a problem. You need to look at that problem and work on solving it."[49]

## Healthy Expression of Anger

One of the keys to the healthy expression of anger is to face the situation early, before it has a chance to accumulate and fester. Dr. Lenore Walker, one of the nation's top experts on domestic violence, points out that "you can either talk yourself into getting angrier, or you can talk yourself out of it. You have a choice. When you learn to recognize anger and work through it early on, it tends to go instead of grow."[50]

Remember that anger is usually not a primary emotion, but more commonly is a chosen way of expressing blame for other feelings, such as frustration. We often think the only alternatives when angry are to either vent it with rage or stuff it. But there is another important alternative. Outside provocations are not really the cause of the anger. Rather, the cause is rooted in the way we choose to think about the provocation, and thus respond to it. Changing the way one thinks about the provocation can completely dissipate the anger, resulting in no need to either express or stuff it. The anger simply dissipates.

For example, a man who had a heart attack was asked by his physician about the circumstances preceding chest pain.[51] "It's my boss," he replied. "Every time he comes in the office, he chews us out and puts us down. Everyone hates the guy, and every time he came around, I got chest pain, until finally I had my heart attack. We couldn't say anything to him, because the last guy who got angry with him lost his job!" However, on quiet reflection as to why his boss used such tactics, the employee said, "It's because he is so insecure. He has to put everybody down to make himself look more important and correct."

"I wonder if maybe he's hurting inside," replied his physician, "and just doesn't yet know a better way to get *real* sense of worth. That must be a painful way to live."

After long discussion, the heart attack patient softened and said, "Maybe you're right. Maybe the guy acts like a turkey because he just doesn't know a better way to deal with his own problems."

"What do you think would happen if, instead of feeding his insecurity with your own anger and subtle putdowns, you chose instead to help heal the insecurity that drives his dumb behavior?"

"I don't think I could do that. I really hate this guy," was the patient's response. But eventually he agreed to try and feel his boss' insecure discomfort for just a few hours, and attempt to ease that underlying cause instead of just condemning the behavior that came from it. Before long, this enterprise turned into a day, then a week. Coming back, he said, "This is amazing to me. My anger is just gone. It's hard for me to believe, but I actually feel sorry for him, even a little compassion. I've been trying to find some things about him that make him feel valued. That was hard to do at first, but it's easier now. And for what it's worth, he's not putting me down as much any more. And I don't really feel tense around him any more, even when he pulls his old tricks."

This employee had discovered a great secret about dealing with anger:

1. The boss was not the real cause of his anger; instead, his anger was caused by his own rigidly judgmental thinking about the boss.

2. Coming (with some difficulty) to think differently about his boss, in more understanding ways, dissipated the anger.

3. The key principles here are those of self-assertion: *Speak the truth in kindness.* That is, level honestly about your own point of view, but do it in a way that honors and lifts the other person, rather than putting him or her down, either overtly or within yourself. Such proper expression of anger becomes liberating and empowering for both you and the others involved. The goal of expressing anger in healthy ways, then, is to face it directly, wisely transform it, and thus get rid of it.

## How the Body Reacts: The Health Effects of Anger and Hostility

According to one researcher, "Medical research shows that no matter how many times you work out at the gym or how careful you are to eat correctly, you're putting yourself at risk if you don't manage your anger effectively."[52]And the most recent research shows that the effects of anger are diverse and widespread.

To understand the broad consequences of anger, consider the wide range of physiological reactions that go with it:[53] changes in muscle tension, scowling, grinding of teeth, glaring, clenching of fists, flushing (redness of the face), goosebumps, chills and shudders, prickly sensations, numbness, choking, twitching, sweating, losing self-control, or feeling hot or cold. Common medical problems associated with chronic anger and hostility include fatigue, pain in the neck or jaw, ringing in the ears, excessive sweating, redness, hives, acne, itching, severe headache, migraine headache, belching, hiccuping, peptic ulcers, chronic indigestion, diarrhea, constipation, intestinal cramping, loss of appetite (without accompanying weight loss), and frequent colds.[54] Even more serious problems, such as heart attacks and strokes, will be discussed below.

Psychologist G. Stanley Hall wanted to get a clear picture of how people feel when they are angry, so he gave several thousand people questionnaires that helped examine their responses to anger. The responses were remarkably similar among the 2,184 people who completed the questionnaires. Anger, they said, produced "cardiac sensations, headaches, nosebleed, mottling of the face, dizziness, tears, snarls, or a complete inability to vocalize."[55] Those reactions are probably due in part to the immediate physical changes that accompany anger, much like those described for stress or the classic fight-or-flight response. The heart and respiration speeds up, blood pressure rises, the digestive process slows down, and the muscles tense up, all in readiness for action.

The chronic repression of anger, then, has physical effects very similar to those of chronic stress. According to Carnegie-Mellon historian Peter Stearns, author of *Anger: The Struggle for Emotional Control in America's History*, chronic anger "is an insidious thing, because we aren't even aware that we are repressing. We think we are free to express anger, but we're not as free as we might believe."[56]

The results of repressed, chronic, or prolonged anger can be devastating. Such chronic anger usually involves either inherent hostility or the unwillingness to let go of the misery of blaming what someone has done to hurt us. Psychologist Ted Grossbart points out that one of the two most "common human agonies that provide the underlying fuel for skin diseases" is anger.[57] In his research, Grossbart has traced a number of disfiguring skin disorders and rashes—among them eczema, hives, warts, and genital herpes—to anger. When patients are helped to work out their anger, Grossbart says, the skin disorders improve dramatically.

Anger also apparently predisposes its victims to the common cold. Some of the most comprehensive research connecting the two has been con-

ducted at Cornell Medical School and at the Great Lakes Naval Medical
Research Unit. Researchers exposed a group of men of similar medical status to the cold virus. Only the ones who were depressed, angry, and frustrated got sick; the rest stayed healthy. Even more important, say the
researchers who conducted the studies, was the powerful effect of simply
recalling episodes of anger. While simply talking about anger, the
researchers say, the patients were more likely to develop nasal congestion,
mucoid discharge, and even asthma attacks.[58]

The effect of anger on susceptibility to colds may be because of its effect
on immunity, particularly on S-IgA, the antibody in the saliva that helps to
protect against the common cold. In one study, volunteers watched videos
and looked at pictures designed to make them angry. Researchers found
that the anger resulted in a significant reduction in S-IgA for as long as five
hours after the emotion of anger was experienced—therefore reducing the
volunteers' ability to resist the common cold virus.[59]

Anger has been shown to be a major cause of migraine headaches. In
detailed research, a large percentage of migraine sufferers have been those
who are unable to express anger verbally. Mismanaged anger, anger that is
either suppressed or misdirected, has also been shown to be a major factor
in bulimia and anorexia.[60]

It is believed that unexpressed anger can affect the heart as well.
Lynda H. Powell, psychologist at Rush-Presbyterian-St. Luke's Medical Center in Chicago, found that women who survived one heart attack but who
kept a lid on their anger and had a pattern of reacting slowly to outside
events were the ones most likely to suffer fatal heart problems. In commenting on the study, University of California psychologist Margaret A.
Chesney said that it challenges traditional thinking: For men, expressing
anger and hostility can lead to heart problems. Apparently, the opposite can
be true for women: Repressing anger and hostility leads to heart disease.[61]

Hostility highly correlates with worsening medical symptoms. A Danish
random sample of 3,426 men and 3,699 women (aged forty or fifty years)
showed that high symptom load was predicted by cynical hostility as measured by the eight-item Cynical Distrust Scale. Those high in hostility had
over twice as many distressing physical symptoms.

Changes in hostility over one's life also play a role in other risk factors
for health outcomes. Hostility tends to peak in late adolescence and reach a
nadir in middle age, then tends to stabilize into old age.[62] However, a long-
term study following the course of hostility from college to middle age
showed that those whose hostility increases over those years had double
the risk of obesity, inadequate social support, and depression (all health risk
factors) as well as reduced life achievements.[63] The same study showed that
higher hostility in the late teen years predicted unhealthy behaviors and

worse health appraisals thirty years later. This suggests the need for those more angry and hostile in early life to actively pursue strategies to change those patterns. This can be done using some of the suggestions at the end of this chapter and in the last two chapters.

Researchers who have zeroed in on hostility have learned that the emotions related to it have very specific physical effects on the body, effects far more pronounced than those associated with other emotions.[64] The effects of hostility are so devastating because hostility does two things to the body:

1. Hostility causes the constant, unending release of stress hormones, especially norepinephrine, which, when continuous, cause significant pathological changes in a variety of ways.

2. Hostility weakens the branch of the nervous system designed to calm the body down after an emergency.

To understand why hostility is so harmful to health, it's important to understand what happens in both these scenarios.

## Hostility, Hormones, and Neurotransmitters

In essence, chronic hostility causes two kinds of chronic stress reactions: (1) the fight-or-flight response (the body prepares to confront or flee from an enemy), and (2) vigilant observation (the body stays constantly "on guard" in case it should be threatened). Hostility causes both reactions simultaneously— a "double whammy" for the body to deal with continuously.

While stress or a perceived danger may cause occasional or short-term reactions of this kind in the body, hostility is a constant, chronic condition. A hostile person goes throughout the entire day in this condition. (Many hostile people don't even get relief at night while sleeping; researchers have shown that stress hormones are secreted throughout the night and eliminated in the urine around the clock.)

To begin with, hostility causes the body to release Corticotropin- $\checkmark$ Releasing Hormone (CRH), which mobilizes the whole sequence of stress hormones. CRH instructs the pituitary gland and the adrenal glands to secrete stress hormones like cortisol and catecholamines (such as norepinephrine). The result is a classic stress response: Blood pressure increases, the heart beats harder and faster, insulin resistance occurs, the liver releases stored sugar, cholesterol rises, and clotting increases. As you might imagine, all of these are significant coronary risk factors, particularly if operating chronically.

Those reactions in themselves wouldn't be so bad if they happened only occasionally, and if there were a physical way for the body to overcome the reaction. With hostility, neither is the case. And there's a possibly lethal reaction connected with hostility as well: The constant on-off of stress hormones that accompanies hostility can trigger both heart rhythm abnormalities (and cardiac arrest) and also coronary artery spasm, resulting in a heart attack.[65] This spasm, and the increased clotting, are due not only to hormones like norepinephrine but also to the effects of hostility and its associated depression of neurotransmitters such as serotonin.

In the central nervous system, serotonin relieves stress and calms anger (and falls when control is lost). Genetic deficiency in brain serotonin function can set a person up to be more depressed or hostile. But serotonin is also stored in platelets, the little blood entities that initiate clotting. When brain serotonin falls (as with chronic anger or feeling out of control), a tissue receptor (serotonin type 2) becomes more sensitive, and the result is more clotting[66] and blood vessel spasm, and ultimately more heart attacks and strokes. A heart attack is caused by the occurrence of three things: Artery narrowing (plaque), artery spasm, and then a clot to finish off the occlusion. As you can see, all three are rapidly accelerated with hostility or chronic depression.

Let's take a look at the effects of hostility on some principal stress hormones that can have definite hazardous effects, mostly on the circulatory system.

### Epinephrine and Norepinephine (Catecholamines)

Epinephrine, sometimes called adrenaline, constricts the blood vessels, especially the minute ones in the extremities. At the same time, it causes the heart to work harder and stimulates the heart muscle. As a result, the heart pumps rapidly in high-pressure spurts, driving blood pressure dangerously high.

Sometimes called noradrenaline, norepinephrine also causes the blood vessels to constrict; it is generally released when blood pressure is too low. In addition, persistently high norepinephrine disturbs the platelets and the red blood cells, and damages the endothelium (the lining of the heart and blood vessels), leading to the influx of lipids into the wall and creating a place for platelets to adhere, causing clotting to occur. In carotid artery ultrasound studies, hostile people get more rapid plaque formation, and thus artery narrowing.[67] This is particularly true in those with hypertension.[68] And, interestingly, meditative stress reduction that lowers these catecholamines reverses the artery thickening.[69]

Studies have shown that people who are hostile (people traditionally labeled Type A) release much more epinephrine and norepinephrine into their systems, and they release much more norepinephrine if confronted with a challenge. In an early study by Friedman and Rosenman (the researchers who pioneered the Type A theory), a group of men were seated at a table.[70] In the middle was an expensive bottle of French wine. Each man was given a pile of puzzle pieces and told that whoever solved the puzzle first would win the bottle of wine.

The men eagerly began trying to put together the puzzle. Soon, loud rock music began to blare out of concealed speakers in the room. The men worked for several minutes, the music blasting, until researchers told them to stop. (No one completed his puzzle, because some of the pieces had not been provided.)

Researchers had drawn blood samples from the men at the beginning of the experiment, and they drew samples again after they told the men to stop working on the puzzle. All the men in the study had similar levels of epinephrine and norepinephrine before they started competing for the bottle of wine, but the Type A men—the hostile ones—had much higher levels of norepinephrine after trying to win the contest.[71] Similar effects are seen in runners "who have to win." The extreme competitiveness counters the benefits of the exercise, compared to those who exercise for the fun and value of it.

In a similar experiment, New York City researcher David Glass asked firemen and policemen to volunteer for a study in which they played Pong, a computer game. Each man had the same opponent: a man who was introduced as a fireman or policeman but who was in reality a colleague of Dr. Glass and an expert Pong player. The expert won every game. But it didn't stop there: As he played, he disparaged the opponents—for their lack of skill and their clumsiness—and even impugned their manhood. As in the first experiment, blood samples were taken before the game began and again after it was finished. The Type A men who were most hostile had significantly higher levels of epinephrine in their blood than did the calmer, more easygoing men.[72]

## Cortisol

A corticosteroid, cortisol is the most potent hormone released by the body in an effort to defend itself. Cortisol inhibits the breakdown of epinephrine and norepinephrine, in essence making it very difficult for the body to calm down after a perceived emergency or threat. To make matters worse, it increases the body's responsiveness to epinephrine and norepinephrine, rendering those hormones more potent. Second, cortisol releases chemicals that further damage the endothelium (the cells lining the heart and blood vessels). Finally, in addition to damaging the vessels, cortisol causes an increase in the level of fats, insulin, and sugar in the blood, all known contributors to heart disease. Both cortisol and catecholamines cause insulin resistance, leading to a state called "the metabolic syndrome" that puts people at high cardiovascular risk. With insulin resistance, the insulin level rises to compensate, and high insulin can also raise both cholesterol and blood pressure.

## *Prolactin*

Prolactin has a dual effect on the cardiovascular system: It releases calcium into the bloodstream, and it makes the blood vessels more vulnerable to the effects of epinephrine and norepinephrine. In addition, prolactin has some role in regulating blood pressure. Prolactin rises in response to a fall in the central neurotransmitter dopamine, which often runs low in depressed, cynical people. The lack of dopamine is one reason why such people have difficulty experiencing joy.

In addition to the specific effects of each individual stress hormone released in response to hostility, the hormones working together have several effects:

1. The hormones working together further increase the risk of acute cardiac events.[73]

2. The fluctuation of the hormones released during hostility can trigger spasms of the coronary arteries, resulting in a heart attack.

3. The group of hostility hormones (especially epinephrine, norepinephrine, and cortisol) contribute to premature development of arteriosclerosis.

4. The combination of hormones secreted during hostility interferes with the body's natural messengers that reduce blood pressure. Under normal conditions, tiny "thermostats" (called "baroreceptors") in the walls of the blood vessels send messages to the brain to restore blood pressure to normal. Stress and hostility hormones inactivate these baroreceptors, leaving them unable to signal a reduction in blood pressure. As a result, blood pressure stays elevated and can be driven even higher by epinephrine; in addition, the heart rate is less variable (a significant predictor of cardiac events).[74]

5. The hormones compromise the immune system, making the individual less resistant to disease. According to researchers at the University of Texas Cancer Center, norepinephrine and other stress hormones block the ability of macrophages (scavenger cells that provide resistance against disease) to kill tumor cells.

6. Hormones released in response to hostility interfere with the body's DNA repair system. As a result, the body loses its first line of defense against a number of diseases, including cancer.

7. The hostility hormones block the entry of sugar into brain cells. If this condition persists long enough, brain cells are deprived of sugar for an extended time and may malfunction.

All of this combines to end up in well-demonstrated adverse effects on health outcomes of many types.[75]

## Anger: The Cancer Connection

Studies on the effects of stress on cancer vary between different kinds of cancer. Some conducted as early as the 1950s show a link between anger and ✓ some cancers. Most often implicated is chronic anger with an inability to appropriately express that anger. Researchers who were interested in exploring the link between anger and cancer studied the life patterns of approximately 400 cancer patients during the 1950s. There was a common thread among them: Many seemed unable to express anger or hostility in defense of themselves. The same patients were able to get angry in the defense of others, or even in the defense of a cause, but not in defense of themselves. A more recent Michigan study that prospectively followed nearly 700 people for seventeen years found a similar pattern: Suppressed persistent anger was associated with not only more cancer deaths but also mortality from all causes.[76]

Other studies of cancer patients, especially women with breast cancer, indicate that the style of expressing anger (or the ability to express it at all) seems to have considerable impact on the development and spread of cancer. In one study, researchers interviewed a group of women with breast disease; some had benign breast disease and others were later diagnosed with breast cancer. Before the diagnoses were made, interviewers made notes on the anger style of each woman. The women who were later diagnosed as having breast cancer had an entirely different anger style than those who had benign breast disease. The cancer victims were much more likely to suppress their anger and then finally explode with anger when they could no longer hold it in. Many didn't express anger at all, and those who did let it go all at once. It is important to know that prospective studies of this kind (first measuring anger, then following over time for the development of subsequent effects) are far more reliable than retrospective studies (looking back with recall) making such comparisons.

In a retrospective study, Marjorie Brooks, an assistant professor at Jefferson Medical College, surveyed 1,100 women who did not have breast cancer and compared the results of the surveys to those of fifteen women with benign tumors and fifteen women with malignancies. The results made a strong case against anger. Both the women with benign tumors and the women with malignant tumors had experienced much more anger during the previous year than had the 1,100 women who had no breast disease. More of the women with malignancies were frequently angry when compared to the women with tumors that were benign. And when compared to the women in normal health, more of those with benign tumors had felt angrier during the previous year.

There was also a big difference in the way the women expressed anger. Women in normal health tended to get angry and then forget about it. They

were able to confront the situation that made them angry, work quickly
through their angry feelings, and move on without anger. The women who
had benign breast disease tended to get angry and stay angry. Interestingly,
the women with malignant tumors got angry, but either they didn't express
it or they apologized for it, even when they were in the right.

A number of other studies have linked suppression of anger with cancer. In Lydia Temoshok's study of malignant melanoma patients, those who
suppressed anger had fewer lymphocytes at their tumor sites. When
Temoshok and her colleagues taught some of the patients ways to express
their anger, tumor growth in those patients stopped.

The ability to express anger may even affect survival rates among cancer patients. In one prospective study, researchers found that patients who
were able to express negative emotions—anger, hostility, guilt, depression,
and aggression—survived longer than the patients who said they had fewer
negative emotions.[77]

## An Angry/Hostile Heart, an Ill Heart

As you might suspect from the mechanisms above, perhaps one of the most
devastating effects of anger is on the heart and the circulatory system.
Among all emotional factors, hostility (and its associated depression) is an
important determinant of cardiovascular disease.[78] According to research
data published in the *New England Journal of Medicine*, mismanaged anger is
perhaps the principal factor in predicting cardiovascular disease.[79] According
to Redford Williams, not all the aspects of a Type A personality are harmful
to the heart, but one of the aspects that is definitely a risk is anger.[80] There is
still some controversy over the notion of Type A personality as it relates to
heart disease risk. It's not the busy-ness of Type A that is toxic to the cardiovascular system, but the cynical hostility. According to the researchers, all
Type A's are not at increased risk of coronary heart disease—only those who
are hostile. The most toxic mix is hostility, anger, cynicism, antagonism, and
mistrust.[81] Heart-harming hostility is characterized by anger-proneness,
resentment, suspicion, and the tendency to view photographs of strangers
as unfriendly or dangerous.[82] It is also hallmarked by explosive and vigorous
vocal mannerisms, competitiveness, impatience, and irritability.

As an example of his concept, Williams points out the person who is
stuck in a long line of traffic when he needs to get to an appointment on
time. "Anyone will be stressed if he really has to keep an appointment,"
Dr. Williams explains. The person who is at risk, though,

> *may not even have a real deadline or an important appointment to keep, and
> still becomes angry and hostile in a short period of time. And he'll immediately*

*think that the whole thing is someone's fault—that the police are incompetent because they aren't directing traffic properly, for instance. He'll get annoyed at the motorists in the other lane, because he thinks they're staring at him. His breathing will become deeper and faster. He may start honking the horn. The anger and resentment just keep building up. He may even try to drive up on the shoulder to get around the other cars.[83]*

It's that kind of person, Williams says, who is at risk of a heart attack or other major illness.

The emotion of anger itself can have a direct effect on angina (chest pain) and heart attack. In fact, a study released by the American Heart Association says that people who can't keep their tempers under control and who tend to explode in anger during arguments double their risk of heart attack, especially during the two hours following an episode of intense anger.[84] That risk jumps to triple the risk of heart attack among those who have lower educational levels.[85] The study, conducted by Dr. Murray Mittleman of Harvard University Medical School, involved more than 1,500 men and women. Research published in the May 2000 edition of *Circulation* found that people who are highly prone to anger are nearly three times more likely to have a heart attack, and even those who have moderate anger have a significant risk of illness and death from coronary heart disease.[86]

In one study, University of Michigan research scientist Mara Julius studied 696 married and single adults for twelve years. As one part of her study, she gave every subject a questionnaire to determine whether he or she was angry and, if so, how the anger was expressed. Of the questionnaire respondents, the ones with the highest blood pressure were those who suppressed anger, expressed anger but then felt guilty, or never protested an unjustified attack. Even more fascinating was Julius's findings on death from high blood pressure: A person with high blood pressure who suppresses anger is five times more likely to die than is a high blood pressure victim without suppressed anger.[87] However, persistent blood pressure effects of anger seem highly dependent on whether the person continues to ruminate on the perceived offense.[88] The article describing this observation is subtitled, "At Least Don't Ruminate on It!" This is important overall advice about anger. Refuse to hang on to it, and it will be far less likely to hang on to you.

Suppressed anger may be a particularly lethal factor. New research shows that heart disease rates are significantly higher among both men and women who are unable to express their anger appropriately. One study, which followed 2,500 men for a period of nine years, found that men who suppress their anger are 75 percent more likely to develop heart disease than men who let their anger out or who talk about their anger.[89] In a separate study, researchers at the University of Pittsburgh School of Medicine found that middle-aged women who suppress their anger have a much higher rate of heart disease, especially when suppressed anger is combined with hostility and anxiety.

Hostility has a more potent adverse cardiovascular effect than anger alone, and is a leading factor in heart disease risk. Researchers studied more than 400 patients at Duke Medical Center to determine coronary artery health and personality traits. More than 80 percent of the men who were classified as Type A and who also measured high in hostility had seriously diseased coronary arteries; only half of the other men did. For women, the risk was even more significant: 50 percent of the hostile Type A women had seriously diseased arteries, while only 12 percent of the others did.[90]

Anger might affect the heart muscle itself, partly due to the diseased arteries supplying inadequate oxygen to the muscle. A study by researchers at Stanford University and the University of California, San Francisco, evaluated eighteen people with known coronary disease and nine healthy people. For each, researchers studied the pumping ability of the heart under a variety of conditions; in particular, they measured the percentage of blood that was squeezed out of the left ventricle with each contraction, a measure known as the ejection fraction. Among subjects with heart disease, anger caused a 5 percent drop in the ejection fraction, decreasing the heart's pumping capacity.[91]

Other tests proved that anger causes abnormalities in the wall of the heart similar to those that accompany intense exercise and more intense than those caused by a mental challenge, such as arithmetic.[92] In one study, heart disease patients who merely *recalled* an event that made them angry experienced a decrease in the amount of blood pumped out by the left ventricle.[93] Research shows that patients with this kind of compromise are almost three times more likely to suffer a cardiac event.[94]

Williams performed a study linking hostility to high blood cholesterol, a leading risk factor in heart disease, and his results showed that hostile teenagers are as likely as adults to have high cholesterol. "People with high hostility at nineteen tend to have high cholesterol levels at forty," Williams said in summing up the study, which was presented to the American Heart Association.[95] For the study, Williams and his colleague, Dr. Ilene C. Siegler, studied 830 subjects who took personality tests at the University of North Carolina. They followed the men and women for twenty years. Those who scored high on a hostility scale while in college tended, twenty years later, to have high levels of total cholesterol in their blood but low levels of HDL cholesterol (the beneficial kind).

In addition to elevations in cholesterol and blood pressure, hostility also seems correlated to other coronary risk factors as well. For example, elevated blood homocysteine, which is highly correlated to heart attack risk, is also significantly elevated in hostile people. Interestingly, in a Greek study, there was somewhat of a linear relationship between the degree of hostility and the blood level of homocysteine. Specifically, a 10-unit increase in the hostility scale was associated with a rise in homocysteine levels.[96]

A very high predictor of cardiovascular events is the metabolic syndrome, characterized by insulin resistance that then contributes to weight gain, high lipids, and elevated blood pressure. The development of the metabolic syndrome is much higher in cynically hostile people, and this seems to be an important mediator of the cardiac disease seen in hostility.[97]

Several large-scale and long-term studies have linked hostility to coronary artery disease. In one, again spearheaded by Williams and his colleagues, more than 2,280 Duke University Medical Center patients were studied for signs of Type A behavior and for the trait of hostility. The patients had been referred to the medical center for coronary angiography, a diagnostic procedure for determining the extent of coronary artery obstruction. Researchers found that they could predict which patients would be found to have coronary artery disease by pinpointing which ones were hostile, and that hostility served better than Type A as a predictor.[98]

In a similar study as part of his work at Duke University, Williams selected 400 patients admitted to the medical center for coronary arteriography (a study to determine blockage of coronary arteries).[99] Cardiologists let Williams test patients before their arteriogram; each patient was interviewed and given the MMPI. Based on interviews and psychological test scores, Williams determined which of the patients were hostile; then, cardiologists performed the arteriograms.

Williams was fascinated by his findings. In previous studies, Type A personality had always been a predictor of heart disease. It still was, but Williams found that hostility was an even more accurate and powerful predictor. In his study, 70 percent of the patients who were hostile had at least one major blockage of a coronary artery (as compared to 48 percent who were not hostile). Type A people were 1.3 times more likely to have a blockage than non–Type A's, but hostile people were 1.5 times more likely to have blockages than the nonhostile people were.[100] Overall, hostility seemed to be the most influential factor. According to Williams, "Not only did people with higher [hostility] counts have more severe arteriosclerosis, but the [hostility] scores were also associated with arteriosclerosis even more strongly than were Type A scores."[101]

What, then, are the long-term outcomes of hostility? Several prospective studies are convincing. More than 3,000 healthy men between ages of forty-five and fifty-five years were studied for more than eight years in the San Francisco area; all the men were free of apparent coronary artery disease when the study began, and researchers watched them carefully over the years for signs of disease. When the study began, researchers taped interviews with each man and used the interviews to rate each person's potential for hostility. The hostile patients developed heart disease at a much higher rate than those who did not show signs of hostility. Furthermore, the men who reported getting quite angry at least once a week and expressing it outwardly were much more likely to develop heart disease than the hostile men who did not feel or express anger as often.[102]

In still another study of more than 1,800 factory workers in Illinois, study subjects were carefully followed for more than twenty years. Researchers found that the factory workers who were high in hostility had 1.5 times more heart disease than those who weren't and that hostility was significantly associated with death from all causes over the twenty-year period.[103] Interestingly, there was also an increased rate of cancer among the men with high hostility scores.[104] In a smaller but still convincing study, more than 255 young physicians were tested for personality traits and then followed for twenty-five years. The death rate from heart disease and from all causes in general was six times greater for the physicians who measured high in hostility.[105]

Several follow-up studies involving middle-aged men who had taken the MMPI twenty-five years earlier showed that the effect of hostility on both coronary disease and mortality was much stronger among younger men than among the middle-aged ones. For younger hostile men, the risk of disease was four to six times greater; for hostile middle-aged men, the risk dropped to 1.5 times. As a result, researchers now theorize that early hostility may most accurately predict premature health problems. As Williams pointed out, "Once middle age is reached, the surviving men with hostility traits may represent a group of biologically hardy survivors."[106] Perhaps a more useful explanation is that people can learn to be less hostile with passing years, now proven to reduce the health risk previously present.[107] Even elderly people can learn to reduce hostility, with significant improvement in their health outcomes. In a study at the Ochsner Heart and Vascular Institute in New Orleans, elderly persons with hostility symptoms had greater weight ($p = 0.02$); four times higher anxiety and depression scores ($p < 0.0001$); two times higher scores for multiple, unexplained medical symptoms ($p < 0.0001$); and 17 percent lower scores for quality of life ($p < 0.001$) compared with elderly persons without hostility symptoms. ($P$ values of less than 0.05 are scientifically convincing as being significant.) Importantly, in these elderly patients, marked reduction in hostility and improvements in other risk factors occurred following interventions to reduce the hostility and stress reactions.[108] In people who have had heart attacks, both young and old, such interventions can also significantly reduce second attacks and coronary mortality (sometimes by more than 50 percent, even more than some medication interventions).[109] Such interventions will be discussed in Chapters 23 and 24.

Learning to respond with less anger may be particularly important for those with a strong family history of heart attacks and strokes. The risk of inheriting cardiovascular disease, once thought to be primarily due to inheriting traditional risk factors such as high cholesterol, has now been shown by Mark Ketterer and his colleagues to be far more related to inheriting the tendency (both neurochemical and learned) to be hostile or depressed.[110] This means that these mental issues more powerfully mediate the inheritance of heart disease than do other medical factors. Ketterer also has shown that one's assessment of his or her own hostility is not nearly as reliable as that of a spouse or close friend, and that, in fact, "denial scores" (spouse/friend assessments minus self-assessments) are even stronger predictors of coronary disease severity and mortality.[111] You need to listen to and trust the opinion of those close to you (even more than your own opinion) as to whether you may be a bit too angry and hostile.

## Hostility and Mortality

A number of researchers who have attempted to pinpoint the health effects of hostility have found that it contributes to premature death from many causes, including cancer. In one study, students in law school were given a battery of psychological tests intended to measure hostility. In a twenty-five-year follow-up, researchers found that only 4 percent of the nonhostile lawyers died from any cause, but 20 percent of the hostile attorneys died during the same period.[112]

Duke psychologist John Barefoot agrees that hostile or cynical attitudes can lead to premature death. Barefoot and his colleagues followed 500 middle-aged participants for fifteen years. All had similar health and lifestyle patterns. Those who scored high on hostility tests had more than six times the death rate of those with low scores. When the researchers followed up on death records at the end of the study, about one-fifth of the participants had died; the survivors were generally the ones with low hostility and less suspiciousness.[113]

The same group followed 968 people who started out with coronary disease, and found that over fifteen years hostility predicted a 33 percent higher mortality rate compared to that of the less hostile.[114]

### The Psychological Effects of Anger

The reactions to anger aren't limited to the body. A host of studies shows that anger is linked to an array of psychological symptoms and behaviors, too. In one, reported in the *American Journal of Health Promotion*, anger was assessed in middle-aged women. Those who were angry generally got inadequate sleep and too little exercise and used a greater than average number of over-the-counter drugs. The angry women in the study also showed lower optimism and a greater number of (and more severe) daily hassles, had less social support, and had lost an important relationship during the previous year.[115] Such anger is frequently associated with clinical depression (particularly bipolar depression), and this seems particularly true for men. Similarly, some people with similar neurochemical abnormalities to clinical depression struggle with rage attacks, even with minimal provocation. This can be related to excessive neuron firing in these disorders, and may at times need medical treatment.

## Which Hurts More: Expressing or Suppressing?

There has been disagreement in the scientific community about which is more dangerous to health: expressing anger or suppressing it. That controversy has been sparked by recent research that shows that anger, regardless of how or whether it is expressed, is detrimental to health. According to Williams, "There is something wrong with being angry: whether you keep it to yourself or let it show; if you have a lot of anger day in and day out, you have a significant increase in risk of premature mortality."[116]

In one study, blood pressure screening was done at the offices of the Massachusetts Division of Employment Security among people who had previously been working but who had involuntarily lost their jobs.[117] Researchers posted an announcement in the hall saying that free blood pressure screening would be performed; volunteers were weighed and asked to be seated for five minutes before blood pressure was taken. While the volunteers waited, they filled out brief questionnaires that sought information on health history and demographics. Questions also determined the style of anger of each respondent.

Three blood pressure readings were taken for each volunteer, and researchers adjusted their data according to age, social class, and obesity. When survey data were controlled for these factors, researchers found a surprisingly consistent result: There was a significant relationship between suppressed anger and systolic blood pressure. The more anger was suppressed, the higher was the blood pressure.

According to studies, suppressed anger is especially dangerous for ✓ women—and for more reasons than the increased cancer noted above. Researchers at the University of Michigan conducted an eighteen-year study of 700 people. They found that women who suppress their anger are three times likelier to die early of any cause than are those who express it. Men, they found, were at higher risk from suppressed anger only if they already had high blood pressure or chronic bronchitis. (Deaths from chronic bronchitis can occur from anger-induced airway spasm.) In commenting on the study, Estelle Ramey, professor emerita of physiology at Georgetown University Medical School, said that women suffer more "when they hold their anger in because they don't have a choice. A man can decide to keep his temper because it's the gentlemanly thing to do. But a woman may have to suppress her anger because she'll trigger male violence if she lets go."[118]

And what about the people who sometimes express anger, and sometimes repress it? Now research has found that people who have it both ways—who both express and suppress anger—are most prone of all to coronary heart disease.[119] Fortunately, there is a third alternative that doesn't require either angry expression or suppression. The third alternative goes after the actual cause of the angry feelings: the thinking that causes the anger. We tend to believe that the provoking situation causes the anger. But, in reality, situations do not themselves make us angry; our chosen thinking about them does. That is, we make ourselves angry about situations by the thinking we choose. It goes like this:

$$\text{Situation} \rightarrow \text{Chosen (or learned) thinking} \rightarrow \text{Feelings}$$

Notice that feelings (such as anger) do not arise directly from the situation, but are created by the thinking. Let's illustrate this concept. Suppose a teenager has been rebelling against his parents, provoking them with putdowns and refusing to listen to anything they have to say. The parents get angry, even furious. They react by attempting to take control of him. But it's not working, and their frustration leads to even more anger.

Then, in a moment of quiet reflection and seeking for deeper wisdom, they realize their son is trying to become independent, one of the jobs of the teenage years. He's just not doing it well, because he's thinking, "Independence is doing the opposite of what you're told," not realizing that real and rational independence is doing whatever gets the best consequences, whether he was told to do it or not. Wise rationality for the teen would likely include building bridges with those around him, particularly those from whom he could use some support. On the parents' side, once they realize the difficult nature of their son's struggle to understand independence, and that mature independence is also what they want for him, feelings soften. In quiet moments of wisdom, they begin to feel compassion for him instead of anger. Wanting to empower and lift their child instead of retaliate with their own putdowns, they start searching for ways to gently do that empowering. And suddenly, out of new compassion, the anger is gone. A new, wiser way of thinking, more in line with their values about what great parents do for their children, has created feelings very different from anger.

If the feelings are destructive (making you miserable, hurting relationships, and causing loss of control), the thinking that causes those destructive feelings is usually somewhat irrational or in violation of one's deeper wisdom. This principle is the basis of some of the most effective psychotherapy methods, such as cognitive therapy or rational behavioral therapy.

What is the third alternative for dealing with anger, then? Come to think about the situation in new ways that are more rational and more in line with your deeper wisdom and values. Then the anger tends to dissipate and no longer needs to either be expressed or suppressed.

What does all this boil down to? Anger can compromise health and shave years off life. Williams sums up the situation this way: "Trusting hearts may live longer. For them the biological 'cost' of situations that anger or irritate is lower. . . . So that's what they mean when they say that nice guys finish last. It's because most of the angry, hostile, nasty ones aren't in the race anymore!"[120]

## What To Do if Anger Is a Problem

Does all the above mean you can never feel anger? No. Yale oncologist and surgeon Bernie Siegel tells us, "Anger has its place, so long as it is freely and safely expressed rather than held inside where it can have a destructive effect and lead to resentment and hatred."

So how can you get a handle on anger? Try these suggestions:

- Next time you start feeling angry, or when you encounter a situation that you know causes anger, distract yourself. Meditate, listen to a favorite concerto through a pair of headphones, or close your eyes and imagine something you really love (like that border of yellow tulips that breaks through the sodden ground at the edge of your road every spring). Often in this relaxed, meditative state, new, more rational ways of thinking about the situation will appear.

- It sounds trite, but it works: When you feel like you're really going to explode, take two or three very deep breaths and count to ten, slowly. Just taking a pause will help you get your perspective so you can express your feelings in a more appropriate way.

- One of the best ways to get a handle on anger is to practice forgiveness. If you need some ideas on how to start forgiving others, see the suggestions in Chapter 14.

- Social connectedness goes a long way toward getting rid of anger. Do what you can to get connected: Find a confidant, get a pet, cuddle.

- Finally, when you start to feel angry, step back. Take a critical look at your negative thoughts. Think about your thinking, and discover wiser, larger, more rational ways to view the situation. Reason with yourself. Then laugh![121]

If ongoing hostility is the problem, in addition to the above suggestions, try some of Diane Ulmer's recommended drills:[122]

- Practice smiling at others and complimenting them.
- Practice giving yourself permission to stay calm when things don't go the way you want.
- Practice laughing at yourself.
- Play fun games.
- Stop using obscenities.
- Look for opportunities to say, "Maybe I'm wrong."
- Volunteer to help people who are less fortunate than you are.
- Learn more about the spiritual practices and teachings of your chosen religion.
- And, something mentioned by several researchers, including Williams: Pretend that today is your last day.[123]

If ongoing anger seems to be caused by blaming someone or circumstances for hurting you, realize that holding on to that blame is not hurting them, but will only eat you alive. The Hindus would say you are giving away your energy, even your spirit, to the one (or circumstances) you are blaming. They might advise, "Call your energy (your spirit) back! Don't give it away any longer." Give up the false notion that they are now controlling you to be so angry. Only your own thoughts are doing that. So let go of the blame, and be the way you want to be regardless of what someone else has done. Take back control of your experience of life. This is the power and value of forgiveness, no matter how grievous the fault. Forgiveness is not giving an undeserved gift to the perpetrator. It is about taking back control of your life and health.

Ellen Goodman, a writer for the *Washington Post*, summed up the sentiment eloquently in a piece about New Year's resolutions. In calling for the resolution to be a civil, social creature, she wrote,

*This may be a peak period for the battle against the spread of a waistline and creeping cholesterol. But it is also within our willpower to fight the spread of urban rudeness and creeping hostility. Civility doesn't stop nuclear holocaust and doesn't put a roof over the head of the homeless. But it makes a difference in the shape of a community, as surely as lifting weights can make a difference in the shape of a human torso.*[124]

## ENDNOTES

1. Source unknown.
2. Redford Williams and Virginia Williams, *Anger Kills* (New York: Random House/Times Books, 1993), xiii.

3.  T. W. Smith, "Hostility and Health: Current Status of a Psychometric Hypothesis," *Health Psychology* 11 (1992): 139–50.

4.  B. E. Hogan and W. Linden, "Anger Responses Styles and Blood Pressure: At Least Don't Ruminate about It!" *Ann Behav Med* 27 (2004): 38–49.

5.  Carol Tavris, "On the Wisdom of Counting to Ten," in P. Shaver, ed., *Review of Personality and Social Psychology*, vol. 5 (Sage, 1984), 170–91.

6.  Tavris, "On the Wisdom of Counting to Ten," 173–74.

7.  Karen Judson, "Anger: The Shapes of Wrath," *BH & L* (February 1988): 57–58.

8.  Margaret A. Chesney and Ray H. Rosenman, *Anger and Hostility in Cardiovascular and Behavioral Disorders* (Washington, D.C.: Hemisphere Publishing Corporation, 1985).

9.  Robert Ornstein and David Sobel, *The Healing Brain* (New York: Simon & Schuster, 1987), 181.

10. M. W. Ketterer, J. Denollet, A. D. Goldberg, P. A. McCullough, S. John, A. J. Farha, V. Clark, S. Keteyian, J. Chapp, B. Thayer, and S. Deveshwar. "Men Deny and Women Cry, but Who Dies? Do the Wages of 'Denial' Include Early Ischemic Coronary Heart Disease?" *J Psychosom Res.* 56, no. 1: 119–23.

11. Ibid.

12. Ibid.

13. Redford Williams, *The Trusting Heart: Great News about Type A Behavior* (New York: Times Books, Random House, 1989).

14. Paul Bagne, "Rude Awakening," *Men's Health*, October 1990, 34–35.

15. Izard, *Human Emotions*, 329–30.

16. Tavris, "On the Wisdom of Counting to Ten," 175–76.

17. Sharon Faelten, David Diamond, and the editors of Prevention Magazine, *Take Control of Your Life: A Complete Guide to Stress Relief* (Emmaus, Pa.: Rodale Press, 1988), 84.

18. Carl E. Thoresen, "The Hostility Habit: A Serious Health Problem?" *Healthline*, April 1984, 5.

19. W. Cook and D. Medley, "Proposed Hostility and Pharasaic Virtue Scales for the MMPI." *J Appl Psychol* 38 (1954): 414–18.

20. M. W. Ketterer, J. Huffman, M. A. Lumley, S. Wassef, L. Gray, L. Kenyon, P. Kraft, J. Brymer, K. Rhoads, W. R. Lovallo, and A. D. Goldberg, "Prospective Study of a Self-Report Type A Scale and Risk of Coronary Heart Disease: Test of the MMPI-2 Type A Scale." *Circulation.* no. 6, 100: 686–7; and K.W. Ketterer, "The Ketterer Stress Symptom Frequency Checklist: Anger and the Severity of Coronary Artery Disease," *Henry Ford Hosp Med J.* 38, no. 4: 207–12.

21. Ibid.

22. Williams, *The Trusting Heart*, 71.

23. Ibid., 66.

24. A. Rozanski, J. A. Blumenthal, and J. Kaplan, "Impact of Psychological Factors on the Pathogenesis of Cardiovascular Disease and Implications for Therapy." *Circulation* 99 (1999): 2192–2217; and W. Jiang, R. R. K. Krishnan, C. M. O'Connor, "Depression and Heart Disease: Evidence of a Link and Its Therapeutic Implications." *CNS Drugs* 16 (2002): 11–127.

25. Tavris, "On the Wisdom of Counting to Ten," 173–74.

26. Izard, *Human Emotions*, 333–34.

27. "How Anger Affects Your Health," *Wellness Letter*, January 1992, 5.

28. Diane K. Ulmer, "Helping the Coronary Patient Reduce Hostility and Hurry Sickness: A Structured Behavioral Group Approach," *The Psychology of Health,*

*Immunity, and Disease,* vol. A, 587; in Proceedings of the Sixth International Conference of the National Institute for the Clinical Application of Behavioral Medicine.

29. J. C. Barefoot, K. A. Dodge, B. L. Peterson, W. G. Dahlstrom, and R. B. Williams, "The Cook-Medley Hostility Scale: Item Content and Ability to Predict Survival," *Psychosomatic Medicine* 51 (1989): 46–57.

30. Brent K. Houston and Christine R. Vavak, "Cynical Hostility: Developmental Factors, Psychosocial Correlates, and Health Behaviors," *Health Psychology* 10, no. 1: 9–17.

31. C. D. Sofhauser, "Psychosocial Antecedents of Hostility in Persons with Coronary Heart Disease," *J Holist Nurs.* 21, no. 3: 280–300.

32. D. Carmelli, R. H. Rosenman, and G. E. Swan, "The Cook and Medley HO Scale: A Heritability Analysis in Adult Male Twins," *Psychosomatic Medicine* 50, no. 2: 165–74.

33. George Valliant, et al., *New England Journal of Medicine* 1978; also M. Seligman and C. Peterson, *Learned Optimism* 1990.

34. Roger Daldrup, "How a Good Dose of Anger Therapy Can Restore Peace of Mind," *Your Personal Best*, April 1989, 8.

35. To come.

36. B. J. Burshman, R. F. Baumeister, and A. D. Stack, "Catharsis, Aggression, and Persuasive Influence: Self-Fulfilling or Self-Defeating Prophesies?" *Journal of Perspectives in Social Psychology* 76 (1999): 367–76.

37. Redford B. Williams, "Conferences with Patients and Doctors: A 69-Year-Old Man with Anger and Angina," *Journal of the American Medical Association* 282 (August 25, 1999) 8.

38. J. C. Barefoot, K. A. Dodge, B. L. Peterson, W. G. Dahlstrom, and R. B. Williams, "The Cook-Medley Hostility Scale: Item Content and Ability to Predict Survival," *Psychosomatic Medicine* 51 (1989): 46–57.

39. Williams, "Conferences with Patients and Doctors," 8.

40. Daldrup, "How a Good Dose of Anger Therapy," 8.

41. George Valliant, et al., *New England Journal of Medicine* 1978; and M. Seligman and C. Peterson, *Learned Optimism* 1990.

42. Tavris, "On the Wisdom of Counting to Ten," 170–91.

43. Ibid., 170–91.

44. Daldrup, "How a Good Dose of Anger Therapy," 8.

45. Ibid., 8.

46. Izard, *Human Emotions,* 351.

47. Tavris, "On the Wisdom of Counting to Ten," 170–91.

48. Carol Tavris, *Anger: The Misunderstood Emotion* (New York: Touchstone, 1982).

49. Tavris, *Anger.*

50. To come.

51. To come.

52. Hendrie Weisinger, "Mad? How to Work Out Your Anger," *Shape*, January 1988, 86–93.

53. Tavris, *Anger.*

54. Elizabeth Weiss, "How Anger Affects Our Bodies," *New Woman*, December 1984, 98–103.

55. Tavris, *Anger.*

56. Karen Judson, "Anger: The Shapes of Wrath," *BH & L* (February 1988): 57–58.

57. Steven Locke and Douglas Colligan, *The Healer Within: The New Medicine of Mind and Body* (New York: E. P. Dutton, 1986), 183.

58. Weiss, "How Anger Affects Our Bodies," 98–103.

59.  Glen Rein, Mike Atkinson, and Rollin McCraty, "The Physiological and Psychological Effects of Compassion and Anger, Part 1 of 2," *Journal of Advancement in Medicine* 8, no. 2: 87–105.

60.  Tavris, *Anger*, 170–91.

61.  Bruce Bower, "Women Take Un-Type A Behaviors to Heart," *Science News* 144: 244.

62.  I. C. Siegler, "Hostility and Risk: Demographic and Lifestyle Variables," in A. W. Siegman and T. W. Smith, eds., *Anger, Hostility and the Heart* (Hillsdale, NJ: Lawrence Erlbaum, 1994) 199–214.

63.  I. C. Siegler, P. T. Costa, B. H. Brummet, et al., "Pattern of Change in Hostility from College to Midlife in the UNC Alumni Heart Study Predict High Risk Status," *Psychosomatic Medicine* 65 (2003): 738–45.

64.  J. L. Marx, "Coronary Artery Spasms and Heart Disease," *Science* 208 (4448): 1127–30; and E. Braunwald, "Coronary Artery Spasm," *Journal of the American Medical Association* no. 17: 1957–59.

65.  Marx, "Coronary Artery Spasms," 1127–30; and Braunwald, "Coronary Artery Spasm," 1957–59.

66.  F. Laghrissi-Thade, *Biol Psychiatry* 42 (1997): 290–95.

67.  D. E. Polk, *Psychosomatic Med* 63 (2001): 107.

68.  M.E. Bleil, *Psychosomatic Med* 63 (2001): 184.

69.  A. Castillo-Richmond, *Stroke* 31, no. 3: 568–73.

70.  To come.

71.  Judson, "Anger: The Shapes of Wrath," 57–58.

72.  Williams, *The Trusting Heart*, 83–84.

73.  Daldrup, "How a Good Dose of Anger Therapy," 8.

74.  R. Virtaaanen, A. Jula, J. K. Salminen, et al., "Anxiety and Hostility Are Associated with Baroreflex Sensitivity," *Psychosomatic Medicine* 65 (2003): 751–56.

75.  T. Q. Miller, T. W. Smith, et al., "A Meta-Analytic Review of Research on Hostility and Physical Health," *Psychol. Bull.* 119 (1996): 322–48.

76.  E. Harburg, N. Kaciroti, L. Gleiberman, and M. A. Schork, "Expressive/Suppresive Anger Coping Responses, Gender, and Types of Mortality Followup," *Psychosom. Med* 65 (2003): 588–97.

77.  James W. Pennebaker and Harald C. Traue, "Inhibition and Psychosomatic Processes," in Harald C. Traue and James W. Pennebaker, eds., *Emotion Inhibition and Health* (Seattle, Wash.: Hogrefe & Huber Publishers, 1993), 152–53.

78.  M. W. Ketterer, G. Mahr, and A. D. Goldberg, "Psychological Factors Affecting a Medical Condition: Ischemic Coronary Heart Disease," *J Psychosom Res.* 48, nos. 4–5: 357–67.

79.  Ornstein and Sobel, *The Healing Brain*, 181.

80.  To come.

81.  R. B. Williams, Jr., T. L. Haney, K. L. Lee, Y-H. Kong, J. A. Blumenthal, and R. E. Whalen, "Type A Behavior, Hostility, and Coronary Atherosclerosis," *Psychosomatic Medicine* 42, no. 6.

82.  John Droubay Hardy and Timothy W. Smith, "Cynical Hostility and Vulnerability to Disease: Social Support, Life Stress, and Physiological Response to Conflict," *Health Psychology* 7, no. 5: 448.

83.  "The A Is for Anger," *Men's Health*, July 1989, 10.

84.  Williams, "Conferences with Patients and Doctors," 8.

85.  M. A. Mittleman, M. Maclure, M. Nachnani, J. B. Sherwood, and J. E. Muller, "Educational Attainment, Anger, and the Risk of Triggering Myocardial Infarction Onset," *Archives of Internal Medicine* 157 (1997): 769–75.

86. Janice E. Williams, *Circulation*, May 2000.

87. "Depression, Anger, and the Heart," *Harvard Health Letter*, February 1993, 7.

88. Hogan and Linden, "Anger Responses Styles and Blood Pressure," 38–49.

89. *Journal of Epidemiology and Community Health*, 1998.

90. Looke, et al., *The Healer Within*, 183.

91. Matthews, *Psychosomatic Medicine*.

92. A. Rozanski, C. N. Bairey, D. S. Krantz, et al., "Mental Stress and the Induction of Silent Myocardial Ischemia in Patients with Coronary Artery Disease," *New England Journal of Medicine* 318 (1988): 1005–12.

93. G. Ironson, C. B. Taylor, M. Boltwood, et al., "Effects of Anger on Left Ventricular Ejection Fraction in Coronary Artery Disease," *American Journal of Cardiology* 70: 281–85.

94. W. Jiang, M. Babyak, D. S. Krantz, et al., "Mental Stress-Induced Myocardial Ischemia and Cardiac Events," *Journal of the American Medical Association* 275 (1996): 1651–56.

95. Ilene C. Siegler, Bercedis L. Peterson, John C. Barefoot, and Redford B. Williams, "Hostility during Late Adolescence Predicts Coronary Risk Factors at Mid-Life," *American Journal of Epidemiology* 136, no. 2: 146–52.

96. D. B. Panagiotakos, C. Pitsavos, C. Chrysohoou, E. Tsetsekou, C. Papageorgiou, G. Christodoulou, and C. Stefanadis, "Increased Plasma Homocysteine Concentrations in Healthy People with Hostile Behavior: The ATTICA Study." *Med Sci Monit.* 10, no. 8: CR457–62. Epub 2004 Jul 23.

97. T. L. Nelson, R. F. Palmer, and N. L. Pedersen, "The Metabolic Syndrome Mediates the Relationship between Cynical Hostility and Cardiovascular Disease," *Exp Aging Res.* 30, no. 2: 163–77.

98. Redford B. Williams, Jr., "Hostility, Anger, and Heart Disease," *Drug Therapy*, August 1986, 43.

99. To come.

100. Ketterer, et al., *The Healing Brain*, 181.

101. Ornstein, et al., *The Healing Brain*, 181.

102. Carl E. Thoresen, "The Hostility Habit: A Serious Health Problem?" *Healthline*, April 1984, 5.

103. Thoresen, "The Hostility Habit," 5.

104. Williams and Williams, *Anger Kills*, 36.

105. J. C. Barefoot, W. G. Dahlstrom, and R. B. Williams, "Hostility, CHD Incidence and Total Mortality," *Psychosomatic Medicine* 45 (1983): 59–63.

106. Williams, "Hostility, Anger, and Heart Disease," 43.

107. Siegler, et al., "Pattern of Change," 738–45.

108. C. V. Lavie and R. V. Milani, "Impact of Aging on Hostility in Coronary Patients and Effects of Cardiac Rehabilitation and Exercise Training in Elderly Persons," *Am J Geriatr Cardiol.* 13, no. 3: 125–30.

109. M. Friedman, *Am Heart J* 112 (1986): 653–65; and J. A. Blumenthal, et al., *Arch Int Med* 157 (1997): 2213–23.

110. M. W. Ketterer, J. Denollet, J. Chapp, S. Keteyian, A. J. Farha, V. Clark, M. Hudson, A. Hakim, A. Greenbaum, J. Schairer, and J. J. Cao, "Familial Transmissability of Early Age at Initial Diagnosis in Coronary Heart Disease (CHD): Males Only, and Mediated by Psychosocial/Emotional Distress?" *J Behav Med.* 27, no. 1: 1–10.

111. M. W. Ketterer, J. Denollet, J. Chapp, B. Thayer, S. Keteyian, V. Clark, S. John, A. J. Farha, and S. Deveshwar, "Men Deny and Women Cry, but Who Dies? Do the Wages of 'Denial' Include Early Ischemic Coronary Heart Disease?" *J Psychosomat Res* 27 (2004): 1–10.

112.   Kathy A. Fackelmann, "Hostility Boosts Risk of Heart Trouble," *Science News* 135 (1989): 60.

113.   J. C. Barefoot, B. L. Peterson, W. G. Dahlstrom, et al., "Patterns of Hostility and Implications for Health," *Health Psychology* 10 (1991): 18–24.

114.   S. H. Boyle, R. B. Williams, D. B. Mark, B.H. Brummett, I. C. Siegler, M. J. Helms, and J. C. Barefoot, "Hostility as a Predictor of Survival in Patients with Coronary Artery Disease," *Psychosom Med.* 66, no. 5: 629–32.

115.   Sandra P. Thomas and Madge M. Donnellan, "Correlates of Anger Symptoms in Women in Middle Adulthood," *American Journal of Health Promotion* 5 no. 4: 267–72.

116.   Williams, "Conferences with Patients and Doctors," 8.

117.   Joel E. Dimsdale, Chester Pierce, David Schoenfeld, Anne Brown, Randall Zusman, and Robert Graham, "Suppressed Anger and Blood Pressure: The Effects of Race, Sex, Social Class, Obesity, and Age," *Psychosomatic Medicine* 48, no. 6: 430–35.

118.   "Women Who Suppress Anger Die Sooner," *American Health*, July–August 1991.

119.   James W. Pennebaker and Harald C. Traue, "Inhibition and Psychosomatic Processes," in Harald C. Traue and James W. Pennebaker, eds., *Emotion Inhibition and Health* (Seattle, Wash.: Hogrefe & Huber Publishers, 1993), 152–53.

120.   Redford Williams, cited in "The A Is for Anger," 11.

121.   Bernie Siegel, *Peace, Love and Healing: Bodymind Communication and the Path to Self-Healing* (New York: Harper & Row, 1989), 28.

122.   Ulmer, "Helping the Coronary Patient," 592; and M. Friedman and D. Ulmer, *Treating Type A Behavior and Your Heart* (New York: Fawcett, 1984).

123.   Williams, *Anger Kills.*

124.   Ellen Goodman, "Thoughts for a New Year," *Reader's Digest*, January 1989, 118.

# CHAPTER 5

# Worry, Anxiety, Fear, and Health

*I have had many troubles in my life,*
*but the worst of them never came.*

—James A. Garfield

## Learning Objectives

- Define worry.
- Understand generalized anxiety disorder, panic disorder, and other common anxiety disorders.
- Define somaticizing.
- Discuss the effects of worry and anxiety on the body.
- Discuss the health consequences of fear.

Worriers slide into the seat of an airplane, snap the seatbelt closed, and worry that the plane might crash. They worry that a fussy toddler might have contracted chickenpox. They worry that their term paper wasn't good enough or that they'll be fired because they called in sick one too many times.

Worry is something most Americans are familiar with. According to statistics from a variety of studies, only about a third classify themselves as nonworriers, people who worry less than an hour and a half each day. More than half classify themselves as moderate worriers, people who worry between 10 and 50 percent of the day and may or may not be troubled by worrying. The rest are chronic worriers, people who worry more than eight hours a day.[1]

Andrew Matthews of Louisiana State University says that worry might be a form of increased vigilance against threats, a form of problem solving, or a way to rehearse potentially unpleasant events. If you use it to prepare for and deal with a bad situation, it can be beneficial. If it becomes excessive, it can harm health.[2]

# Definitions of Worry

According to clinical psychologist Thomas Pruzinsky of the University of Virginia,

> *[Worry is] a state in which we dwell on something so much it causes us to become apprehensive. It differs from the far stronger emotion we call fear, which causes physical changes such as a racing pulse and fast breathing in our bodies. Worry is the thinking part of anxiety.*[3]

Worry is a preoccupation with potential dangers or pain in the future. And, says Pruzinsky, most people who report to a doctor that they are worried say they worry anywhere from 80 to 95 percent of the day.[4]

Worrying reflects our attempts to cope mentally with our concerns and fears. It's not always bad; worry might be useful if it helps us become more vigilant in the face of real danger, or helps us take steps that will keep something negative from happening. Worry becomes harmful when there's no way to keep our worries from becoming reality or when worrying becomes so pervasive that we are immobilized by it.[5] More often than not, what we are worrying about never happens, but the worry makes us feel like we are living the catastrophe anyway. Worry may be appropriate in a situation where there are real wolves growling at the door, but frequently we create imaginary wolves—and our body then reacts as if they were actually there.

Sometimes worry feels like we are pouring energy into preventing the anticipated catastrophe, but, in fact, the worry may help make the catastrophe more likely to happen. This observation is based on what might be called "The Law of Expectations." For example, if you have to give a talk and you are worrying a lot about it, the energy you spend worrying seems like you are doing something to prepare. In fact, however, your worry is causing you to visualize failure, create unconscious images of being unprepared, or visualize making a fool of yourself. Anytime you visualize failure, it tends to become a self-fulfilling prophecy—the image you "practiced" will come up when it's time for you to speak and will generate behaviors (such as the worried-about forgetting, stammering, or being seen as incompetent) that are more likely to lead to failure. Worrying is like visualizing negative performance, versus visualizing positive performance. Highly successful athletes, performers, or speakers often use positive visualization, the process of generating practiced successful images, in order to perform well during actual performance. Worrying is like practicing failure; it is like living with the failure, even though it may never happen.

Surveys show that the most common sources of worry for Americans are family and relationships, job or school, health, and finances. According to Jennifer L. Abel, associate director of the Stress and Anxiety Disorders Institute at Pennsylvania State University, most people worry about 5 percent of the time. Chronic worriers, on the other hand, spend an average of about 50 percent of their time worrying. And some, says Abel, worry 100 percent of the time.[6]

Of those chronic worriers, most worry elaborately. In one study demonstrating this point, psychologists compared twenty-four chronic worriers with twenty-four people who say they don't worry. The psychologists then gave both groups a scenario: What if you got bad grades? The nonworriers fashioned simple responses: They might get into trouble with their parents, or might feel embarrassed for a few days. The chronic worriers, however, were characterized by responses that progressed quickly from bad grades to the more catastrophic possibilities of loss of control, mental illness, pain, deterioration, and even death and hell.[7]

## Generalized Anxiety Disorder

Some people have what is called *generalized anxiety disorder,* a problem disabling enough to require medication.[8] Generalized anxiety disorder is characterized by:[9]

- excessive worry about many things (as opposed to a specific situational problem).
- worry that is present more than half the time for many months (by definition, more than six months).
- significant body tension and several physical symptoms.

The physical symptoms associated with generalized anxiety disorder are similar to those that are part of panic disorder (see Table 5.1 on page 177), but are often more prolonged and less dramatic. Generalized anxiety is often also accompanied by symptoms of depression and its associated physical illnesses (see Chapter 6). For example, fatigue, which is often seen with depression, is even more predictive of anxiety and its commonly associated sleeplessness.[10] Other physical symptoms often seen with depression, but even *more* predictive of anxiety, include musculoskeletal and back pain, chest pain, heart palpitations, dizziness, numbness or tingling, and trouble swallowing.[11] Of people with major depression, 70 percent also have clinical anxiety problems. Generalized anxiety results in much physical and occupational disability and in high levels of medical care and costs.[12]

According to the National Institute of Mental Health, the anxiety disorders that stem from worry and social anxiety are the United States' most commonly reported mental health problems.[13] And what starts in the mind as worry can have a profound effect on the body.

## Panic Disorder

A classic example of mind-body interaction is created when a person experiences spontaneous, usually unprovoked anxiety attacks coupled with several dramatic physical phenomena. The diagnosis requires that at least four of the symptoms listed in Table 5.1 (page 177) occur simultaneously during these usually brief but frightening attacks. Just as the attacks often come on for no clear reason, they also stop spontaneously after five to thirty minutes. If you or someone you know has one of the symptoms in the list, determine whether any of the other listed symptoms also occur during these discrete attacks. If so, it is very likely a panic attack. As noted, these often occur without provocation, often as a spontaneous neurochemical event. Sometimes the feeling of anxiety itself is absent, since it is only one of the potential symptoms.

The problem is that panic disorder, which is very effectively treatable, often goes undiagnosed and thus untreated for prolonged periods of time. If it remains untreated, phobias often develop, usually out of an irrational fear of returning to the place or situation where the first attacks occurred. These phobias can become very disabling, sometimes making a person very fearful to return to work, to drive, or to even leave home.

The medical effects of panic disorder can also be very significant. The physical symptoms of panic disorder can be dramatic and very bothersome, often leading to many tests (usually all with normal results) and multiple medical visits. Some studies suggest that as many as one-sixth of patients seen in a general medical office are having some form of panic attacks that are causing the physical symptoms they come to have evaluated. The symptoms are not imagined, but rather are related to abnormal nervous system function, usually involving many of the same neurotransmitter abnormalities that cause clinical depression.

## Other Common Anxiety Disorders

Probably the most common anxiety disorder of all frequently goes undetected, often because its very nature causes its victims to hide the fear. Social anxiety disorder is characterized by a sometimes overwhelming, inappropriate fear or embarrassment when under scrutiny by others, or even with the attention of an unfamiliar person in a conversation.[14] Flushing, losing focus, and feeling that others are detecting the embarrassment all create more anxiety, sometimes leading the victim to avoid almost all unfamiliar social contact.

Another impressive form of anxiety is obsessive-compulsive disorder, which is characterized by recurrent stressful thoughts (often lacking sense) that are excessively difficult to dismiss. These obsessive thoughts are accompanied by compulsive, repetitive behaviors that are perceived by most others as very excessive, such as some of the following:[15]

- overcleaning
- multiple checking (such as repeatedly checking to see if the front door is locked)
- saving things (without the ability to discard) to the point of severe clutter
- self-inflicted physical trauma, such as picking the skin
- eating disorders, such as anorexia

These compulsive behaviors are often an attempt to take control, because the victim feels out of control. The part of the brain that maintains bodily and emotional control (the limbic system) is not functioning correctly in anxiety disorders, and the subsequent feeling of things being out of control elicits controlling behaviors. Controlling behaviors are, for example, a symptom of serotonin deficiency in that part of the brain (and often improve greatly with techniques that improve that serotonin function.)

One other anxiety disorder worth mentioning is posttraumatic stress disorder, which is usually triggered by a very traumatic event; the event is characterized by flashbacks and nightmares that cause the victim to mentally re-experience the trauma repeatedly.[16] One often avoids circumstances that remind him or her of the trauma.

All of these "disorders" involve abnormally exaggerated responses of the central nervous system to stimuli; the symptoms listed in Table 5.1 (page 177), if occurring individually or particularly in combination, are highly likely to have some associated anxiety. For example, in a study done in two general medicine clinics at the University of Utah, if patients had a combination of dizziness and numbness or tingling, 93 percent had an associated anxiety disorder.[17] If these disorders interfere with life, they commonly require medical treatment as well as behavioral reconditioning of the nervous system to respond with more control. All anxiety disorder patients also had higher-than-normal physical problems.

## Somaticizing

Somaticizing is the body's way of turning mental stress, usually anxiety, into physical manifestations. People afflicted with the phenomenon of somaticizing, those whom some experts have come to call the *worried well*,

**Table 5.1**    Physical Symptoms of Panic Disorder

**Cardiopulmonary**

Shortness of breath

Palpitations (heart pounding, racing, or skipping)

Chest pain or pressure

**Ear, Nose, and Throat**

Dizziness

Choking

**Gastrointestinal**

Abdominal distress (indigestion, nausea, or diarrhea)

**Neurological**

Numbness and tingling

Weakness

**Autonomic Nervous System**

Sweats

Hot flashes or chills

Tremors or shakes

Source: R. Spitzer et al., *Diagnostic and Statistical Manual IV,* American Psychiatric Association.

are usually anxious or worried. *Worried well* is clearly a misnomer, because such a person is far from well, but the term implies no clear-cut organ damage to explain the person's physical symptoms. In a classic study of primary care patients, Kurt Kroenke and his colleagues studied patients coming into a primary care clinic, following the evaluation of the most common symptoms seen (many of which are classic anxiety disorder symptoms). After three years of tests and follow-up, an average of only 17 percent ever received a clear-cut organic diagnosis! The rest (83 percent) went organically "unexplained."[18] It is this very common group of patients that is highly likely to have some of the nervous system dysregulation associated with anxiety and depressive disorders.

The person's biological abnormality lies within the regulation mechanism of the central nervous system. The same neurochemical abnormalities and dysregulation that causes anxiety and depression disorders can at times show up physically without many emotional components. Also, if a person is unwilling to face emotional difficulties, they may subconsciously "somatize" them, or convert them into physical complaints.[19] As many as two-thirds of all patient visits to the doctor may be made by these worried well, and because some physicians don't recognize the mental basis of the physical complaints, these patients are often sent from one physician to another without being helped.[20] Hosts of studies compiled over the past three decades have shown that addressing the central nervous system issues that underlie somatized physical problems can cut health care costs by an estimated 5 to 80 percent per year.[21]

Psychologist Nicholas Cummings, who founded the Hawaii-based Biodyne Institute, says that "some patients spend as much as $28,000 a year in a fruitless attempt to isolate a physical cause for what is basically an emotional problem. . . . On some days these patients saw four different physicians." Cummings says the emotional problems of anxiety and worry have to be addressed if there is to be an improvement in the patient's condition, and says he never disputes the reality of patients' difficulties: "I can say with all honesty: 'I know you hurt. But as long as you're here, tell us a bit more about you.'" Cummings adds that addressing the emotional problems often helps when other treatments have failed.[22]

## Effects on the Body

Physician Marty Rossman explains that worry "creates negative images about some future event like a deadline or a test. The down side is that chronic worry can overwork and wear down the immune system, leading to chronic stress, a state that has been associated with numerous ailments, from headaches to heart disease."[23]

When people somatize an emotion like worry into a physical complaint, they literally feel something physically. But worry can actually cause physical changes that can compromise many body systems, and physical illness can result. The brain has considerable capacity to create bodily responses in line with practiced, visualized expectations. This is the physical expression of the Law of Expectations mentioned above for worried behaviors. This is well proven by the placebo effect: when a person expects to do well with a particular treatment, the brain has a way of eliciting that expected effect, clear down to cellular levels at times. Medical studies repeatedly find that it's far more effective to give a placebo than to do nothing; that's the reason why good scientific studies of a medical treatment regimen require that treatment be compared to a *placebo control* (a group of people who are given a placebo).

Worry is literally practicing the visualization of the imagined catastrophe, and the brain has the capacity to elicit physical and behavioral responses that fit with that visualization, thus often creating some of the very problems about which you worry. While we attempt to separate the behavioral or emotional responses from the physical ones, the brain does not differentiate these two so neatly—it tends to elicit an oversensitive physical response at the same time it sends out an oversensitive emotional or behavioral response.

## The Association of Anxiety with Common Medical Illnesses

Who gets sick the most? A study of all patients coming in for physical illness at two general medicine clinics at the University of Utah revealed that 47 percent had an identifiable anxiety disorder (42 percent also had diagnosable depression, and more than half of all patients coming in had some kind of anxiety or depressive disorder).[24] Linn et al., found similar numbers in clinics at UCLA. Yet these disorders are present in fewer than 15 percent of the general population. That means that more than half of general medical patients are coming from the 15 percent of the population that is anxious or depressed! In addition, often what drives a person to see a physician is not the physical symptom itself as much as anxiety about what that symptom means. Once reassured that it is not serious, the problem may be quite tolerable.

High utilizers of medical care are particularly likely to have anxiety and depression disorders.[25] *Anxiety disorder* includes the entities described above (such as panic disorder, generalized anxiety disorder, obsessive-compulsive disorder, posttraumatic stress disorder, or social anxiety disorder). Any of these anxiety disorders commonly includes, in addition to the symptoms in Table 5.1, other physical symptoms, such as pain,[26] or allergic problems[27] such as hives. In addition, many very common medical disorders have a high relationship to anxiety.

For example, a person with migraine headaches has four times the normal rate of depression but *thirteen times* more panic attacks than the general population.[28] When carefully evaluated, of people coming to an emergency room or cardiology clinic with chest pain, 40 percent are having panic attacks,[29] and another 25 percent have other kinds of diagnosable anxiety disorders.[30] Treatment of noncardiac chest pain with antidepressant medications (and perhaps stress-reduction techniques) that increase serotonin in the nervous system, *even in the absence of depression or anxiety disorders*, reduces the chest pain by as much as 80 percent.[31] This suggests that the same neurochemical (namely, serotonin) abnormalities seen with anxiety are important in the chest pain.

Of people with irritable bowel syndrome (the most common disorder seen in gastroenterology clinics), 40 percent are having panic attacks, and 80 to 90 percent are having some form of anxiety or depression disorder.[32] Anxiety is similarly highly associated with dyspepsia, one of the most common upper intestinal symptoms.[33] And treatment of the anxiety, either with medication[34] or stress-reduction techniques,[35] can be very helpful for irritable bowel problems. In fact, antidepressant medications used for anxiety disorders have long been some of the most effective ways to treat these intestinal disorders, even in the absence of depression.[36] Roughly 40 percent of people with esophageal spasm[37] and half of those with heart palpitations[38] are having panic attacks[39] (and the diagnosis is often missed until much later).

Similar very high associations of panic, generalized anxiety, and depression disorders are present with common muscle pain problems such as fibromyalgia[40] or myofascial pain syndrome. For example, chronic back pain (the fourth most common symptom in primary care clinics) is highly associated with anxiety disorders, and when present, the anxiety precedes the back pain 95 percent of the time.[41] This is not to say that the pain is imagined, but rather that the pain system is overresponsive, just as the stress response system (or bowel system) is overresponsive in these disorders.

The reason for these striking associations lays in the fact that migraines, irritable bowel syndrome, fibromyalgia, depression, and anxiety disorders all have similar underlying neurochemical abnormalities in the brain, such as deficient functions of the neurotransmitters serotonin, norepinephrine, GABA, and dopamine.[42] Serotonin and GABA in the brain tend to quiet down the response to a stimulus or stressor. These substances act in the parts of the brain called the limbic system and the hypothalamus, which maintain control of many body systems, preventing those systems from having too little or too great a response. If serotonin function (and that of other quieting neurotransmitters such as GABA) is low, many systems overreact to a stimulus: too much bowel response to food (irritable bowel), too much immune response (multiple allergies or chemical hypersensitivity), too much pain response to a pain signal (headache and fibromyalgia), and too much stress response to a stressor (anxiety disorders). Anxious people tend to diffusely have too much spasm of smooth muscles—those that contract the intestines, bladder, airways, and blood vessels in response to a stimulus. All of these organs can thus become disordered in a very real way in people with anxiety.

These same "overresponsive" disorders are also characterized by too high a level of neurochemicals (such as Substance P or glutamate) that magnify responses to an unpleasant stimulus (like pain). Depressed and anxious people thus tend to have too much pain. This pain is not imagined, but is overprocessed and magnified in the nervous system. Normally when a pain signal from peripheral tissue arrives in the brain, the brain sends back a signal to inhibit and control the pain signal. That downward inhibitory tract is driven by the neurotransmitters serotonin, norepinephrine, and dopamine, all of which run low in the central nervous system of abnormally depressed and anxious people. (When central nervous system norepinephrine runs low, it tends to be too high in the periphery, causing some of the damage noted in previous chapters—see Chapter 2.) So the downward inhibitory tract does not work well in anxiety disorders, and the result is overresponsiveness to many stimuli, creating unnecessarily painful symptoms.

Correcting these nervous system chemical abnormalities, both with medications and with other treatments that do not involve drugs, can dramatically improve all these very common "dysregulation" problems. The medications used for these problems are usually antidepressants, so named because they were first used to treat depression. But they often work well for these hypersensitivity disorders even when the symptom of depression is absent. Such medications are not simply symptom-relieving pills, but rather they tend to normalize regulation and neurotransmission in the nervous system. Treatments other than medication involve attention to good sleep and exercise and particularly stress-reduction approaches, all of which can improve these same neurotransmitters (see Chapters 23 and 24).

## Worry and the Circulatory System

Worry has been shown to have effects on the heart and circulatory system as a whole. Researchers interested in the effects of worry tested 125 patients for a year following their heart attacks. A real distinction developed between the ones who worried about their condition and the ones who didn't: Those who worried were significantly more likely to have arrhythmias (abnormal heart rhythms that can lead to sudden, fatal heart attacks).[43] In fact, cardiologist Robert Eliot catalogues examples of people who have been literally "scared to death." A sudden surge of stress hormones like catecholamines can cause immediate heart muscle damage (necrosis) and abrupt arrythmias that cause sudden death. This was, for example, documented in sudden deaths in the Caribbean after its victims were frightened by a voodoo curse.[44]

Worry has been related to high blood pressure in a number of studies. Some of the most convincing ones involved animals in the laboratory. In one, researchers confined monkeys in a cage in which they had to press a bar once every twenty seconds for twelve hours a day to avoid electrical shocks. After a few months, the monkeys developed high blood pressure. Researchers removed the bar from the cage and stopped delivering electrical shocks. What happened then was the real surprise: The monkeys' blood pressure skyrocketed!

Apparently, the monkeys worried constantly about not being able to avoid the shocks, even though none was delivered. Examinations of the monkeys showed that the arteries to the skin, kidneys, intestines, and muscles were tightly contracted, causing tremendous increases in blood pressure.[45]

A similar thing happened when researchers placed mice in a room with a cat that was confined in a cage. The cat was never let out of the cage, and was never allowed or enabled to chase the mice. Within six to twelve months, the mice all developed high blood pressure. They apparently were worried about the cat, and their constant worrying caused high blood pressure.[46]

## Worry and Asthma

In primary care medical clinics, two-thirds of those with asthma have an anxiety or depression disorder.[47] From scientific tests, we know that the emotion of worry causes the body to produce the chemical acetylcholine, which causes the airways to contract. When enough acetylcholine is secreted, the effect on the lungs is asthma. The muscles around the bronchioles constrict so tightly that air can no longer flow freely through them. Another important mechanism for anxiety triggering asthma involves the serotonin system, which can also trigger smooth muscle spasm in the airways. Central serotonin function runs low in people with anxiety disorders. When central nervous system serotonin function is low, a serotonin receptor called $5HT_2$ upregulates—that is, becomes more sensitive. When stimulated, this hypersensitive receptor causes smooth muscle spasm, as seen not only in asthma but also in blood vessels,[48] bowel,[49] and bladder[50] (causing such common medical problems as irritable bowel or bladder problems and headaches).[51]

Obviously, then, anxiety can have a significant impact on victims of asthma. In one study, researchers simply told a group of asthmatics that they were being exposed to pollens and other aggravating agents. Then the researchers stood back and watched what happened. More than half of the asthmatics developed a full-blown asthma attack, even though no pollens or other irritants were actually present. Worry that it would happen triggered the attack.[52]

In a similar study, children with asthma were observed to determine the effect of various emotions on their illness. Most saw their parents as overbearing or rejecting, and these children constantly worried that they might not measure up or be accepted. To test a theory, researchers sent the parents on a paid vacation. They left the children with trained observers and watched what happened in the parents' absence. Half of the children improved dramatically without any other treatment. They stopped worrying, and their blood levels of acetylcholine diminished.[53]

One study of asthma patients found that stress-reduction techniques (relaxation and visualization coupled with thinking differently about the stressor) were as effective as airway dilator (relaxant) medication in preventing asthma attacks.

## The Effects of Uncertainty

One specific kind of worry, uncertainty, has been shown to create a particularly devastating kind of stress. Uncertainty is not knowing. It's being confronted with a complex situation that the person can't figure out. It's confusion over what is meant by a person or situation. It's a situation that is not predictable and, therefore, a situation in which the individual can't determine how to act. If it gets confusing enough or unpredictable enough, it can cause feelings of futility or helplessness and can lead to considerable distress.[54]

Studies involving uncertainty prove the point. One researcher studied a group of 100 patients in a Veterans Administration hospital. Each had rated an upcoming event—treatment, surgery, or the like—as being extremely stressful. When the researcher probed into each patient's situation, however, he found an amazing thing: The patients were not really stressed over the event itself. They were stressed because of uncertainty. They did not have enough information about the event. They didn't feel they knew exactly what was going to happen to them. They didn't really understand the outcome. It was the uncertainty, not the event itself, that caused all the upset.[55] Now, several well-controlled studies of providing information before surgery, detailing what to expect and what to do about it, have been shown to significantly improve surgical outcomes such as complications, time spent in the hospital, and costs. Similarly, for women delivering babies, a woman at the bedside who conveys support and knowledge about what to expect greatly improves obstetrical outcomes[56] (see Chapter 23).

Uncertainty keeps a person in a constant state of semiarousal, putting a heavy burden on the body's ability to adapt to stress. It's the same reason that predictable pain is so much less stressful: You are capable of learning when it is safe to "lower your guard" and relax. Not knowing when a pain or a shock is coming means having to stay on guard—tensed and stressed—all the time.

A series of studies demonstrates the effect of uncertainty. A report by the British Health Service monitored the prevalence of peptic ulcers during World War II, when England was being bombed frequently by enemy troops.[57] People living in the center of London, where the bombings were regular and predictable, suffered a 50 percent increase in the rate of gastric ulcers. In contrast, the increase in ulcer rate among residents on the outskirts of the city, where the bombings were extremely unpredictable, was six times greater than among the residents of London's central district.

In an experiment in New Jersey, two psychologists divided a group of laboratory rats into two groups.[58] Rats in the first group were given electrical shocks at random and without warning. Rats in the second group were also given electrical shocks, but were warned of the impending shock shortly before each one was delivered. The rats that were given unpredictable shocks developed gastric complications at a significantly greater rate than the rats whose shocks were predictable.

It works likewise with people. A psychologist in New York interviewed college students and kept track of their health histories during the year.[59] He noted not only when the students reported being sick but also the circumstances that preceded and surrounded the episodes of illness. He found that they reported being sick most often following events in their lives that were undesirable. Furthermore, most of the sickness followed events that were not only undesirable but also left the students uncertain about how much control they had.

Other studies show that undesirable life events and uncertainty are a deadly combination. Undesirable life events alone don't usually result in illness, nor do uncontrollable life events about which we are uncertain. But when the two are paired up—when events are both undesirable and unpredictable—there is a "significant impact" on health that usually results in illness.[60]

All of this suggests the value of learning the ways that highly resilient people view uncertainty. The approach is based on hope and on enjoying challenge. Much of future life is uncertain. Trying too hard to control it, particularly when its details are uncontrollable, will be fraught with frustration, and then anxiety. Studies of resilient people show that they enjoy a new challenge and fully expect to creatively solve problems as they arrive.[61] The process of uncertainty for them involves an opportunity to learn, to create, and to once again rise to the occasion. This is turning distress into eustress (see Chapter 2), and the result is better health.[62]

## The Health Consequences of Fear

When worry escalates, the result is fear. Everyone has experienced fear. A swimmer of only moderate skill might be afraid of swift waters; a child might be afraid of the dark. A hiker will probably experience fear on hearing the distinctive warning of a rattlesnake; a jogger might feel fear when confronted with the bared fangs of a Doberman pinscher. According to Norman Cousins, "Fear and panic create negative expectations." Then, he says, "One tends to move in the direction of one's expectations."[63] Fear causes the heart to race, the head to spin, the palms to sweat, the knees to buckle, and breathing to become labored. The level of arousal that results is similar to the effects of stress, and the human body can't withstand it indefinitely.

Fear causes the body to secrete epinephrine, or adrenaline, a hormone also secreted in response to stress. Fear floods the system with epinephrine. Its most powerful effect is on the heart: Both the rate and strength of contractions increase. Blood pressure soars. The body is stimulated to release other hormones, which act on various other organs and systems. In essence, the body is put on alert. If the fear is intense enough, all systems can fatally overload.

Medical history is replete with examples of people who were literally frightened to death.[64] Take, for instance, Pearl Pizzamiglio. Fifteen minutes after she started the 11 P.M. shift at the In-Town Motor Hotel in Chevy Chase, Maryland, Michael Stewart walked in with another man. Stewart handed her a paper bag with a note that said, "Don't say a word. Put all the money in this bag and no one will get hurt." Pizzamiglio put $160 in the paper bag, the men fled, and she called the police. Two hours later, Pearl Pizzamiglio, aged sixty, free of any history of heart problems, was dead of heart failure. Stewart was arrested and charged with murder; the jury decided that, indeed, a simple paper bag and a piece of paper could be considered instruments of death. Stewart had, literally, scared Pizzamiglio to death.

In another incident, Barbara Reyes was spending her Memorial Day weekend floating on a raft on Georgia's peaceful Lake Lanier. The calm of the peaceful, warm afternoon was shattered when a man riding a motorized jet ski roared within a foot of the forty-year-old Reyes. In a panic, Reyes paddled to shore, collapsed, and died. Randolph Simpson, the Gwinnett County coroner who examined Reyes, said, "There's no question she was literally scared to death." The man who roared by on the jet ski was arrested and charged with involuntary manslaughter.

One forty-five-year-old man died of fright as he stepped to a podium to give a speech. An elderly man sitting on his lawn collapsed and died when a car jumped the curb and appeared to be headed straight for him. Panamanian dictator Omar Torrijos reportedly amused himself by killing a prisoner with an unloaded gun; the sound of the blanks firing was enough to scare the man to death. And in the year 840, Bavarian Emperor Louis died of fright when he saw a solar eclipse.

The physical effects of fear are the same whether the fear is perfectly understandable or illogical. A surge of catecholamines occurs. When dogs are injected with catecholamines, the hormones released in response to fear, they die. Autopsies reveal certain characteristic lesions on the surface of the heart, presumably an effect of the catecholamines. The same lesions are visible under microscopic examination on the hearts of 80 percent of all victims of sudden cardiac death. While much of the evidence on being scared to death is anecdotal, some is very scientific. Consider, for example, the monitoring of Air Force test pilots. Eliot studied scientific documentation from five separate incidents. In each, Air Force test pilots lost control of their aircraft and were not able to eject. "Their electrocardiograms were being monitored from the ground," Eliot points out. "These people died before they hit the ground, and they died of fright."[65]

One of the most dramatic examples was provided by Bernard Lown, a renowned Harvard cardiologist who witnessed an incredible incident involving a middle-aged woman who had been hospitalized with tricuspid stenosis, a non-life-threatening narrowing of a heart valve. As they were making their rounds one morning, doctors entered this woman's room. Her physician turned to Lown and the other doctors who were gathered around her bedside and announced, "This woman has TS." The doctors then left the room. The woman for some reason decided that TS meant "terminal situation." She began to hyperventilate and sweat profusely, and her pulse shot up to 150. Upon learning of her fear, her doctor tried to explain and calm her, but in vain. She died later the same day of heart failure.[66]

Strongest of all fears are phobias, fears that are irrational and inappropriate. A phobia is an intense fear of an object or situation that would not frighten most people. Victims of phobia become almost immobilized, rearranging their entire life to avoid the feared object or place. One of the most common phobias is agoraphobia, or fear of going out into open spaces (stores, restaurants, theaters—anywhere outside a "safe" place, like home). Other phobias include fear of being trapped in a cramped space, fear of speaking in public, fear of dogs, fear of eating in public, fear of heights, and fear of blood. An estimated 13 million Americans have a phobia of some kind.[67] Many phobias begin first with the unprovoked attacks of panic disorder (a spontaneous neurochemical event). Others can arise from a terrifying traumatic experience.

When a phobic encounters the feared object or situation, the result is a panic attack or phobia attack, and the effect on the body is the same as the well-known fight-or-flight response. In this case, the emphasis is on flight.

And, again, fear enters the picture. The most severe physical reactions occur before an encounter with the dreaded object or situation. The mere anticipation of what might happen is enough to cause pain and disability on its own. Hormones surge into the bloodstream, and the body is intensely stressed. It can't endure the state of arousal for long. If the fear is prolonged or intense, the body can literally short-circuit or gradually become devastated by the physical effects of stress.

# What to Do About Worry and Anxiety

If you're a worrier, can you stop? Researchers suggest the following techniques:[68]

- **Learn to solve problems.** According to Dr. Timothy A. Brown, associate director of the Center for Stress and Anxiety Disorders at the State University of New York, most worriers jump from one topic to another without reaching any solutions. To reduce uncertainty, contemplate exactly what you would do if the worst possible scenario occurred— have a plan. Then go to work to create an outcome that is not the worst.

- **Work on improving your thoughts.** Pennsylvania State University's Jennifer L. Abel says that doesn't mean seeing the world through rose-colored glasses. Worriers, she points out, see the world through cracked glasses: "Our goal is to give people clear glasses, so they see things more accurately." Anxiety comes not so much from stressing situations as it does from the way one practices thinking about those situations. More mature, rational thinking about the same situation creates far less anxiety.

- **Use visualization and deep breathing** to get you through the worry. Visualizing yourself wisely dealing well with the concern greatly reduces anxiety.

- **Let go of catastrophizing.** Remember the Law of Expectations: Picturing the catastrophe (worry) is like practicing failure. Practice visualizing success instead. Imagine how a wise, capable person might handle this situation.

- **Focus on what's going on right now.** Stay completely in the present moment. According to Abel, worry is almost always future-oriented, "so if we can focus on what we're doing right now—the sentence we're reading, the voice of the person speaking—rather than thinking about what someone might say next, we're better off." Dr. Jon Kabat-Zinn has proven significantly improved health outcomes from the highly successful stress-reduction program he created at the University of Massachusetts. His program is built primarily around the principle of learning how to stay in the present moment (called *mindfulness*).[69] Methods for learning this are described in detail in his book *Full Catastrophe Living*, and also in the works of Thich Nhat Hanh.[70] The Harvard Mind Body Clinic also focuses on learning this technique to elicit the relaxation response.[71] Achieving central nervous system quieting from mindfulness involves practicing meditative methods: It begins with focusing on the breath or a mantra-like sound or word, and learning to be able to choose where to give your attention (disregarding distractions). And feeling the power of giving attention wherever you choose increases the personal sense of control.

■ It seems odd, but it works: Dr. Michael Vasey, assistant professor of psychology at Ohio State University, has joined a number of other researchers in advising people to **set aside a worry period,** a specific period of time every day (researchers suggest thirty minutes). During that entire period, focus completely on your worry and try to think of solutions to your problems. According to Vasey, "If you practice focusing on worries and thinking of solutions for 30 minutes each day for several weeks, your anxiety starts to taper off. You'll get better at generalizing solutions or realize it's not worth worrying about." Unload the worries: Write down first steps to the solutions, and tomorrow's to-do list, well before going to bed.

■ Be sure to get enough sleep (seven to eight hours for most people).

■ Keep in mind that many anxiety disorders, such as panic disorder, generalized anxiety disorder, obsessive compulsive disorder, or posttraumatic stress disorder, particularly if depression is also present, may need a course of medication (usually "antidepressants") to help correct the underlying biochemical abnormalities.

The longer anxiety and worry go without some kind of intervention, the more difficult they are to reverse. Anxiety is very treatable, particularly if treated *early,* and doing so not only improves symptoms but also helps to prevent its many medical problems.

## ENDNOTES

1. Sharon Faelten, David Diamond, and the editors of *Prevention, Take Control of Your Life: A Complete Guide to Stress Relief* (Emmaus, Pa.: Rodale Press, 1988).
2. "Worrying Well," *Berkeley Wellness Letter* (June 1993).
3. Amy H. Berger, "Are You a Chronic Worrier?" *Complete Woman,* October 1987, 58.
4. Berger, "Are You a Chronic Worrier?"
5. Faelten, Diamond, and the editors of *Prevention, Take Control of Your Life.*
6. Cathy Perlmutter, "Conquer Chronic Worry," *Prevention,* November 1993, 75.
7. "Worrying Well."
8. Susan Ince, "People Who Worry Too Much," *Weight Watchers Women's Health and Fitness News,* 1990, 3.
9. R. Spitzer et al., *Diagnostic and Statistical Manual IV* (Washington, D.C.: American Psychiatric Association, 1998).
10. N. L. Smith, Citation award paper presented to the American Psychosomatic Society annual meeting, *Psychosomatics* abstracts 1996.
11. J. Shavers, *The Identification of Depression and Anxiety in a Medical Outpatient Setting and Their Correlation to Presenting Physical Complaints,* Ph.D. diss., University of Utah, 1996.

12. P. P. Roy-Byrne, "Generalized Anxiety and Mixed Anxiety-Depression: Association with Disability and Health Care Utilization," *Journal of Clinical Psychiatry* 57, suppl. 7: 86–91.
13. Berger, "Are You a Chronic Worrier?" 58.
14. Spitzer et al., *Diagnostic and Statistical Manual IV.*
15. Ibid.
16. Ibid.
17. Smith, American Psychosomatic Society.
18. K. Kroenke et al., *American J of Medicine* 86 (1989): 266.
19. Winifred Gallagher, "Treating the Worried Well," *American Health*, January–February 1988, 36.
20. Carol Turkington, "Help for the Worried Well," *Psychology Today*, August 1987.
21. Turkington, "Help for the Worried Well."
22. Ibid.
23. Will Stapp, "Imagine Yourself Well," *Medical Self-Care*, January/February 1988, 27–30.
24. Smith, American Psychosomatic Society; and Shavers, *The Identification of Depression and Anxiety.*
25. W. Katon, M. Von Korff, E. Lin, et al., "Distressed High Utilizers of Medical Care," *General Hospital Psychiatry* 12 (1990): 355–62.
26. S. F. Dworkin, M. Von Korff, and L. LeResche, "Multiple Pains and Psychiatric Disturbance: An Epidemiological Investigation," *Archives of General Psychiatry* 47 (1990): 239–44.
27. A. I. Terr, "Environmental Illness: A Clinical Review of 50 Cases," *Archives of Internal Medicine*, 146 (1986): 145–49.
28. N. Breslau and G. C. Davis, "Migraine, Physical Health, and Psychiatric Disorder: A Prospective Epidemiological Study in Young Adults," *Journal of Psychiatric Research* (1993) 27: 211–21.
29. H. Arnesen, O. Ekeberg, T. Husebye, and S. Friis, "Panic Disorder in Chest Pain Patients Referred for Cardiological Outpatient Investigation," *J Intern Med* 245, no. 5: 497–507.
30. W. Katon, M. L. Hall, J. Russo, et al., "Chest Pain: Relationship of Psychiatric Illness to Coronary Arteriographic Results," Also see R. Mayou, *Br. Heart J* 72 (1994): 548–53; *Am J Cardiol* 63(1989): 1399, and *Am J Med* 84 (1988): 1–9.
31. I. Varia, *Am Heart Jl* 140 (2000): 367–72.
32. R. B. Lydiard, M. D. Fossey, W. Marsh, and J. C. Ballenger, "Prevalence of Psychiatric Disorders in Patients with Irritable Bowel Syndrome," *Psychosomatics* 34 (1993): 229–34; and E. A. Walker, P. P. Roy-Byrne, and W. J. Katon, "Irritable Bowel Syndrome and Psychiatric Illness," *Am J Psychiatry* 147 (1990): 565–72.
33. G. Magni, F. diMario, G. Bernasconi, et al., "DSM-III Diagnoses Associated with Dyspepsia of Unknown Cause," *Am J Psychiatry* 144 (1987): 1222–23.
34. P. Poitras, M. Riberdy Poitras, V. Plourde, M. Boivin, and P. Verrier, "Evolution of Visceral Sensitivity in Patients with Irritable Bowel Syndrome," *Dig Dis Sci* 4, no. 4: 914–20; R. E. Clouse, 1991 and 1987; and J. E. Richter, 1986.
35. T. N. Wise, *Psychosomatics* 23 (1982): 465–9; also Poitras, "Evolution of Visceral Sensitivity," 914–20.
36. D. A. Drossman, "Review Article: An Integrated Approach to the Irritable Bowel Syndrome," *Aliment Pharmacol Ther* 13, suppl. 2: 3–14.
37. R. E. Clouse and P. J. Lustman, "Psychiatric Illness and Contraction Abnormalities of the Esophagus," *New England Journal of Medicine* 309 (1983): 1337–42.

38. A. J. Barsky, P. D. Cleary, R. R. Coeytaux, and J. N. Ruskin, "Psychiatric Disorders in Medical Outpatients Complaining of Palpitations," *Journal of General Internal Medicine* 9 (1994): 306–13.

39. Katon et al., "Chest Pain," 1–9. (Of chest pain patients with normal coronary angiograms, 43 percent had panic disorder and 36 percent had major depression.) Similar results were found by B. Beitman, V. Mukerji, J. W. Lamberti, et al., "Panic Disorder in Patients with Chest Pain and Angiographically Normal Coronary Arteries," *American Journal of Cardiology* 63 (1989): 1399–403.

40. D. L. Goldenberg, "Psychological Symptoms and Psychiatric Diagnosis in Patients with Fibromyalgia," *Journal of Rheumatology* 16, suppl. 19: 127–30; and T. A. Ahles, M. B. Yunus, and A. T. Masi, "Is Chronic Pain a Variant of Depressive Disease? The Case of Primary Fibromyalgia Syndrome," *Pain* 29 (1987): 105–11.

41. P. B. Polatin, *Spine* 18 (1993): 66–71.

42. I. J. Russell, H. Vaeroy, M. Javors, and F. Nyberg, "Cerebrospinal Fluid Biogenic Amine Metabolites in Fibromyalgia Syndrome and Rheumatoid Arthritis," *Arthritis Rheum* 35 (1992): 550–56.

43. "Heart Attack: Can You Worry Yourself to Death?" *Medical Abstracts Newsletter*, November 1988, 3.

44. Robert S. Eliot, *Is It Worth Dying For?*

45. J. P. Henry, J. P. Meehan, and P. M. Stephens, "The Use of Psychosocial Stimuli To Induce Prolonged Systolic Hypertension in Mice," *Psychosomatic Medicine*; R. P. Forsyth, "Blood Pressure Responses to Long-Term Avoidance Schedules in the Restrained Rhesus Monkey," *Psychosomatic Medicine* 31 (1969): 300; and R. P. Forsyth, "Regional Blood Flow Changes During 72-Hour Avoidance Schedules in the Monkey," *Science* 173 (1971): 546.

46. Henry et al., "The Use of Psychosocial Stimuli."

47. Shavers, *The Identification of Depression and Anxiety*.

48. P. M. Vanhoutte, "Serotonin, Hypertension and Vascular Disease," *Neth J Med* 38, nos. 1–2: 35–42; and A. E. Doyle, "Serotonin Antagonists and Vascular Protection," *Cardiovasc Drugs Ther* 4, suppl. 1: 13–8.

49. G. Engel, D. Hoyer, H. O. Kalkman, and M. B. Wick, "Identification of 5HT2-Receptors on Longitudinal Muscle of the Guinea Pig Ileum," *J Recept Res* 4, nos. 1–6: 113–26.

50. M. L. Cohen, "Canine, but Not Rat Bladder Contracts to Serotonin via Activation of 5HT2 Receptors," *J Urol* 143, no. 5: 1037–40.

51. A. Srikiatkhachorn and M. Anthony, "Serotonin Receptor Adaptation in Patients with Analgesic-Induced Headache," *Cephalalgia* 16, no. 6: 419–22; and P. J. Goadsby and J. W. Lance, "Physiopathology of Migraine," *Rev Prat* 40, no. 5: 389–93.

52. T. J. Luparello et al., "The Interaction of Psychologic Stimuli and Pharmacologic Agents in Airway Reactivity in Asthmatic Subjects," *Psychosomatic Medicine* 5 (1970): 500.

53. K. Purcell et al., "Effect on Asthma in Children of Experimental Separation from the Family," *Psychosomatic Medicine* 31 (1969): 144.

54. Phillip L. Rice, *Stress and Health: Principles and Practice for Coping with Wellness* (Monterey, Calif.: Brooks/Cole Publishing, 1987), 80–81.

55. Rice, *Stress and Health*, 80–81.

56. J. Kennell, et al., "Continuous Emotional Support During Labor in a U.S. Hospital: A Randomized Controlled Trial," *Journal of the American Medical Association* 265 (1991): 2197–201.

57.  Rice, *Stress and Health*, 80–81.

58.  Ibid.

59.  Ibid.

60.  Ibid.

61.  Suzanne Ouellette Kobasa, "How Much Stress Can You Survive?" *American Health*, September 1984, 67.

62.  Aaron Antonovsky, *Unraveling the Mystery of Health: How People Manage Stress and Stay Well* (San Francisco: Jossey-Bass, 1987), 36–37.

63.  Norman Cousins, *The Healing Heart* (New York: W. W. Norton, 1983).

64.  Examples are from Edward Dolnick, "Scared to Death," *Hippocrates*, March–April 1989, 106–8.

65.  Dolnick, "Scared to Death," 106–8.

66.  Ibid., 106–8

67.  Faelten, Diamond, and the editors of *Prevention, Take Control of Your Life*, 97.

68.  Perlmutter, "Conquer Chronic Worry," 76–80.

69.  Jon Kabat-Zinn, *Full Catastrophe Living* (New York: Delacorte Press, 1990).

70.  Thich Nhat Hanh, *The Miracle of Mindfulness: A Manual of Meditation* (Boston: Beacon Press, 1976).

71.  H. Benson and E. Stuart, *The Wellness Book* (New York: Carol Publishing Group, 1993).

# CHAPTER 6

# Depression, Despair, and Health

*One who expects completely to escape low moods is asking the impossible. Like the weather, life is essentially variable, and a healthy person believes in the validity of his high hours even when he is having a low one.*

—Harry Emerson Fosdick

## Learning Objectives

- Identify the meaning and prevalence of depression.
- Explain the neurobiology of depression as it affects physical problems.
- Describe the effects of depression on body systems and health outcomes.
- Identify ways to treat and deal with depression.

Life is a series of natural ups and downs. Everyone who lives feels intermittent sadness and grief. While those intermittent sad moods can be depressing, they don't really constitute depression.

## A Definition

The word *depression* has several meanings:

1. As a normal human affect, it's caused by the disruption of normal life balance, loss, conflict, or trauma.

2. Depression can be a symptom of a physical illness, or a medication side effect.

3. Clinical depression is also a biological syndrome based on neurochemical abnormalities; that's the definition used throughout most of this chapter.

4. Finally, depression can be a combination of all three. And any of these can follow a crisis.

Depression as an illness is not a normal reaction, but can occur even without a clear reason. It is much more than an occasional sad mood. Usually in depression, the pleasure centers in the brain don't work well, and the punishment centers are on overdrive, so even good things feel bad. This phenomenon causes the "perception error" of depression, where everything seems negative.

Sometimes depression involves quitting or just plain giving up. A person who is depressed feels that the present conditions and the future possibilities are intolerable. A more severely depressed person may even "go on strike" from life, doing less and less, losing interest in people, abandoning hobbies, and giving up at work, because nothing feels pleasurable or good.[1]

One reason why depression is difficult to define is its elusiveness. Steven Paul, chief of clinical neuroscience at the National Institute of Mental Health, says that depression is "like a fever, in that it's often an unspecific response to an internal or external insult. Like fever, it has a number of origins and treatments."[2]

Frederick Goodwin, the scientific director of the National Institute of Mental Health, says that depression is the richest, most striking example in psychiatry, and possibly in all of medicine, of the relationship between the mind and the body.[3] Another dramatic example of that connection is panic disorder (discussed in Chapter 5), which usually is highly associated with depression. Rather than being a single illness or condition, many experts believe it is a group of mood disorders that strike with varying intensity. No one yet has all the answers, but one thing is certain: Depression, together with its neurochemical cousin, anxiety, has some profound effects on who gets sick and, in particular, who comes to see the physician. Many of the neurochemical abnormalities, and thus medical illness connections, are similar between depression and the anxiety disorders discussed in Chapter 5.

Have you ever wondered if you have clinical depression? Answer the following questions from the Patient Health Questionnaire (PHQ9) (Table 6.1).[4]

The PHQ9 is drawn from the Prime MD Today questionnaire, which was carefully validated against detailed diagnostic interviews in large numbers of primary care medical patients.[5] The PHQ9 was found to be very reliable for making the diagnosis of clinical depression. If five or more of the answers are present more than half the days, or nearly every day, that by definition is "major depression." Three or four such positive answers would be considered "minor depression," which has the same medical implications as major depression, particularly if the low-grade depression has gone on for a long time. Minor depression present for more than two years is called "chronic dysthymia."

Other important types of depression include bipolar mood disorders, in which the mood fluctuates up and down more precipitously. The "ups" can

**Table 6.1**     Patient Health Questionnaire (PHQ9)

**Over the past two weeks, how often have you been bothered by any of the following problems?**

| | Not at All | Several Days | More than Half the Days | Nearly Every Day |
|---|---|---|---|---|
| ■ Little interest or pleasure in doing things | ✓ | | | |
| ■ Feeling down, depressed, or hopeless | ✓ | | | |
| ■ Trouble falling or staying asleep, or sleeping too much | | ✓ | | |
| ■ Feeling tired or having little energy | | ✓ | | |
| ■ Poor appetite or overeating | ✓ | | | |
| ■ Feeling bad about yourself, or that you are a failure or have let yourself or your family down | | ✓ | | |
| ■ Trouble concentrating on things, such as reading or watching television | ✓ | ✓ | | |
| ■ Moving or speaking so slowly that other people could have noticed, or the opposite—being so fidgety or restless that you have been moving around a lot more than usual | ✓ | | | |
| ■ Thoughts that you would be better off dead, or of hurting yourself in some way | ✓ | | | |

be too excited, happy, or impulsive in a risky way, or, instead of happy, may be agitated, irritable, and angry. Much of the chronic anger discussed in Chapter 4 can result from the neurochemistry of depression. You will notice in the PHQ9 several symptoms of dysregulated (too much or too little) basic "vegetative" functions such as appetite, sleep, or movement. When sleep and appetite are too much, a person may have "atypical depression," which is more likely to be bipolar.

## Prevalence and Manifestations

If you survey the U.S. population at any given time, about 7 percent of all women and 3 percent of all men have major depression; probably another 4 to 5 percent have minor depression, and 8 percent have major anxiety disorders. The percentages go even higher in winter. During their lifetime, nearly one-fourth of all women suffer clinical depression.[6] The percentage of teenagers with diagnosed clinical depression has increased more than fivefold over the past forty years.[7] Teenage depression is more likely to be bipolar, an important realization because bipolar problems need to be treated differently than major depression.

Medically, depression is a huge problem. Approximately one-fourth of all primary care medical patients come from the 15 percent of the population with major depression and anxiety disorders. That climbs to almost half of all patients if you include minor depression and anxiety disorders (like chronic dysthymia). Almost half of the top users of medical care are those with major depression.[8] Only about one-third of the depressed are recognized and treated, and that drops to fewer than one-fourth of those with anxiety.[9] This lack of accurate diagnosis arises largely because depression and anxiety cause so many medical symptoms, and often because patients don't want to recognize a "mental" component to their medical illness. (Clinical depression and anxiety are combined here because they so often overlap and because they appear to be caused by some of the same neurochemical abnormalities.) About 70 percent of depressed people also have a diagnosable anxiety disorder and nearly a third have generalized anxiety disorder,[10] that is, nearly continuous background anxiousness. In essence, huge numbers of people whose underlying mental problems go untreated repeatedly return complaining of medical problems. Treating the depression has proven to greatly reduce not only suffering and disability but also medical illness and costs as well (see Chapter 23).

People in all walks of life and of all ages suffer from depression. Depression occurs among the young—and when it does, it greatly increases the likelihood of physical illness and leads to tobacco and alcohol dependence, and drug abuse during adulthood.[11] Depression seems particularly rampant among downtrodden persons and women. According to Martin E. P. Seligman, "Women are twice as likely to suffer depression as men are, because, on the average, they think about problems in ways that amplify depression. . . . Women tend to contemplate their depression, mulling it over and over, trying to analyze it and determine its source."[12] That may lead to blaming others erroneously for the depressed feelings. Studies show that depression is prevalent among people with poor social support and a dearth of supportive relationships.[13] Sometimes the biological depression makes such relationships much more difficult. Spouses will comment, "I'm damned if I do and damned if I don't. Anything I do will be seen as negative" (even giving a compliment). And then the disturbed relationship may be blamed for exacerbating the depression. Well-known people have also struggled with the "black dog of depression"—Abraham Lincoln, Ernest Hemingway, Winston Churchill, Sylvia Plath, Thomas Eagleton, and even biblical figures, including Saul, and Nebuchadnezzar.[14]

Depression can lead to suicide. Some experts estimate that as many as 15 percent of those with untreated depression eventually resort to self-destruction.[15] The problem may be even more pronounced among the adolescent victims of depression, particularly those who are bipolar. Elliot S.

Gershon, chief of the clinical psychogenetics branch of the National Institute of Mental Health, states,

> *The chilling fact is that we may be on the verge of an epidemic-like increase of mania, depression, and suicide. The trend is rising almost exponentially and shows no signs of letting up. I would go so far as to say this is going to be the public health problem of the 1990s and beyond if the trend continues.*[16]

According to several studies of the elderly, depression is often associated with illness, disability, isolation, bereavement, and poverty.[17] And according to a study of more than 11,000 people published in the *Journal of the American Medical Association,* people with depression had worse physical, social, and role functioning, and were in worse physical health. They suffered even more bodily pain than did people with a chronic medical disease such as arthritis, back problems, gastrointestinal disease, or diabetes.[18] Depressed people have five times the normal disability rates.[19] If you compare the most common chronic medical diseases, only severe heart or pulmonary failure comes close to depression in causing disability. Overall, costs of depression in the United States in 1990 were estimated at $53 billion per year, and only about 10 percent of that was outpatient treatment costs.[20] When workplace costs were added, the figure was $77.4 billion. By 2000 the overall cost had remained relatively stable, despite the fact that depression treatment rates increased by 50 percent during that ten-year period. The increased treatment costs were countered by a fall in the workplace costs when treated workers became more productive.[21] (These figures don't include the costs of treating medical illness caused by undetected depression.)

People with depression have two and a half times more physical illnesses, and four times the normal mortality rate[22] (63 percent of that mortality due to cardiovascular conditions). Additionally, medical patients often feel they are depressed because of the impact of their medical illness, but interestingly, when the depression itself is treated, the physical problems often greatly improve.

## Causes of Depression

Most researchers today think that certain brain circuits are fragile and that this renders some people vulnerable to depression. That fragility is determined primarily by the deficient function of the neurotransmitter chemicals, such as serotonin, norepinephrine, and dopamine, that enable brain signals to be transmitted from one cell to the next. That deficiency of brain neurochemical function can often be genetic, and it may explain why depression sometimes runs in families. The familial tendency is real. One early but well-known study of the Amish in Pennsylvania showed that all twenty-six suicides between 1880 and 1980 were members of only four extended families.[23]

In commenting on the studies and the tendency of depression to run in families, John Mann, director of the laboratory of psychopharmacology at Cornell Medical College, explains, "Serotonin levels are under some genetic control to begin with, and this suicidal tendency appears to be an inherited biochemical trait."[24] To separate the genetic causes from depressed behavior learned from families, studies of identical twins adopted to different families have shown a very clear inheritance pattern, even among those raised by very upbeat families. Nevertheless, the cause is not entirely predetermined by genes, though heredity is an important factor in creating vulnerability to stress.

This interaction between stress and genetics was nicely demonstrated in a lengthy follow-up study in New Zealand. Genes for the "serotonin transporter" that removes serotonin from the connections between nerve cells (neural synapses) were found. Two types of gene alleles (short and long) were identified. Then the effect of stressful events on people with different inherited combinations of these genes was determined. If a person had two short alleles (one from each parent), they were much more vulnerable to stress causing clinical depression than if long alleles were inherited. If two long alleles were inherited, a person was much more stress resilient, with little depression developing despite much situational stress; the protection presumably created better serotonin function. This study seems to show that rather than arguing over whether depression is inherited or learned by experience, both interact with each other in a very real way. These same serotonin transporter genetics predict suicidality,[25] and can affect other mental illnesses as well.[26]

Older theories (which have been criticized) say that depression primarily occurs as a result of a severe adverse life event or a series of less serious difficulties that gradually erode self-esteem. One scientist who believes that theory is Dr. George W. Brown of the Department of Social Policy and Social Science at the University of London's Royal Holloway and Bedford New College. Brown compiled the results of ten different studies. They show, he says, that 88 percent of depressed women had experienced some recent severe life event or a "major difficulty" in their lives.[27]

Later, Brown studied that group of results, paying more attention to the details of the adverse life events suffered by the women. He reported a fifteenfold difference in the predicted risk of depression between women who had the worst assortment of life events and those who reported no adverse life events at all during the period in which the study took place.[28] Again, these stressful events could be interacting with genetic vulnerability.

New understanding of the neurochemistry of depression and anxiety recognizes an important role for corticotropin-releasing hormone (CRH), the neuropeptide that activates the adrenal gland in response to stress. Long-lasting CRH and norepinephrine abnormalities can clearly be triggered by early-life traumatic events, which turn on the gene for CRH. The activated brain CRH then causes the nervous system to be excessively sensitive to stimuli and, in essence, to remain on guard for danger, even after the trauma is long gone.[29] The previously activated gene, cranking out CRH, has a hard time turning back off, even though there is no more trauma. If interventions to quiet things down are not used, the sensitized nervous system then overreacts to pain, stress, and other stimuli, sometimes indefinitely. We debate, "Is the depression caused by nature (genetics) or nurture (learned)?" but here we have a case of the nurture turning on the nature.

So which is the cause of depression, inherited neurochemistry or repeated negative experiences that cause both abnormal neurochemistry and a depressed habit pattern? Episodes of depression coming out of the blue, for no reason, certainly make a case for a neurochemical cause. Nevertheless, some further fascinating experiments in mental conditioning again suggest it may be both. Most people have heard of the classical mental conditioning experiments with Pavlov's dogs. Measurements of digestive processes (saliva, enzymes, etc.) were made when the dogs ate food. Then each time they ate, a bell was rung. Before long, the brain became conditioned to expect food when the bell rang, and in a classic mind-body way, ringing the bell with no food elicited the digestive response (a mental expectation carried to cellular levels). Similarly, under unrelenting stress they cannot control, people and animals show depletion of brain serotonin activity. If the pattern is repeated several times in association with a certain place or situation, long after the stressor is gone, subsequent exposure to the same place or situation will cause a drop in serotonin function and a rise in CRH. Serotonin suppression becomes a conditioned response. (Once again, the body has an immense capacity to produce physiological responses that the brain "expects," including the depressive and physical effects of neurochemical changes.) In the case of learned, conditioned neurochemical changes likely to cause depression, the effect can combine with genetic predisposition to sustain even the biological depression. There is some evidence that repeated depressive episodes can even condition the enzymes that allow genes to express themselves physically to respond so as to lay down "hardwired" neurological circuits that automatically create a depressed or hypersensitive response that is more resistant to treatment, the so-called kindling phenomenon.[30] Sometimes this phenomenon is called *neuroplasticity,* a conditioned hardwiring of neurons to overrespond to stimuli. The practical implications of this kindling over time is that these depression and anxiety (and pain) disorders need to be treated as early as possible, to avoid their becoming hard-wired and thus more difficult to reverse.

This same kindling phenomenon shows up with increases in another neurotransmitter that contributes to depression, *Substance P.* Substance P is a pain-promoting transmitter that is high in depression and chronic stress and accounts for some of the excess pain and oversensitivity to stimuli seen in depression. Repeated pain conditions a nervous system to produce increasingly more Substance P chronically, resulting in more chronic pain. Since both depression and chronic pain conditions have similar neurochemical abnormalities, one would then expect them to strongly overlap, as they do. Some ask whether the pain causes the depression or the depression causes the chronic pain, but the fact is that both are caused by similar neurochemical abnormalities in the central nervous system.

More recently, new concepts are developing that suggest some depression could be the result of immune and inflammatory system activation.[31] These observers even speculate that lingering viruses (such as cytomegalovirus) play a role in creating clinical depression,[32] much like the depressed and achy feelings one has with a flu illness. This becomes confusing in the chicken-and-egg sense; does the inflammatory activation trigger depression, or does depression trigger the inflammatory and immune activation (or do they both trigger each other)?[33]

One theory about the cause of depression, then, combines a variety of perspectives. As reported in *Psychology Today* and proposed by psychiatrists Hagop Akiskal of the University of Tennessee and William McKinney, Jr., of the University of Wisconsin:

> *Assume, first, that a person is genetically susceptible to depression, meaning that certain circuits in the brain areas particularly concerned with pleasure and rewarding experiences are chemically fragile and somewhat easily upset. Give that person some early traumatic experiences and undermine confidence and self-esteem, such as the loss of or separation from a parent at a critical stage of development. Add the kind of psychological stress later in life that echoes the early loss and places unusual demands on the already vulnerable reward system. (Events are particularly likely to affect people with few social supports—family, friends or lovers.) The brain's response to this is felt as a diminished ability to experience emotion, including pleasure. Paradoxically, this lack of emotion, this emptiness, is deeply felt and incredibly painful. At the same time, activity decreases, as do sociability and the opportunity for pleasure and rewards: One tries less, gets less and feels worse.[34]*

One other important consideration in the onset of depression is poor nutrition. Amino acids such as tryptophan that converts to serotonin in the brain, or tyrosine that converts to norepinephrine, are essential and also require certain vitamins (such as $B_6$ and $B_{12}$) that make up the neurochemicals. Deficiencies of these nutrients can also lead to a "chemical" depression.[35] (See Chapter 22 on nutrition.) Patients who have responded well to antidepressants, and are then deprived of these nutrients, relapse back into depression while still taking the medication.[36] Such medications need these building blocks to work, and people who lack the nutrients may develop depression that responds to their replacement.

## Characteristics of Depression

Depression has been called the common cold of mental illness,[37] and, like the common cold, it can have a variety of symptoms that reflect the entire spectrum of severity. In some cases of depression, the few symptoms are quite mild; in others, a host of symptoms are quite severe. Medical symptoms that cannot be clearly attributed to organic disease are especially likely to be due to the neurobiology of depression and anxiety disorders (Table 6.2).[38]

These symptoms are not imagined; rather, they arise from a very real physiological dysregulation that occurs when the midbrain (particularly the mesolimbic system) no longer effectively controls those operations, as happens in persons with depression or anxiety disorders. Normal function gets out of balance as do mood and arousal, when the part of the mesolimbic brain that exerts control is not working properly. Again, some chemical neurotransmitters that largely govern function of that part of the brain are serotonin, norepinephrine, and dopamine, the same chemicals that are deficient in persons who suffer depression or anxiety.

The mesolimbic system harbors both the pleasure and punishment centers. When the pleasure center is stimulated electrically, a great euphoria is felt. Animals can become addicted to self-stimulating the pleasure center, even to the point of starving to death while they continue the stimulation. The same effect can be obtained by injecting dopamine (and sometimes serotonin); the release of these is the normal way that the pleasure centers are stimulated when pleasurable thoughts occur. When either is deficient, you can't feel pleasure, even in situations that are normally very pleasura-

**Table 6.2**    Prevalence of Major Depression and Anxiety Disorders in Medical Patients with Organically Unexplained Symptoms

| Symptoms | Unexplained (%) | Depression (%) | Anxiety (%) |
|---|---|---|---|
| Headache | 48 | 53 | 44 |
| Chest pain | 36 | 66 | 66 |
| Back pain | 30 | 53 | 40 |
| Joint pain | 26 | 58 | 48 |
| Shortness of breath | 25 | 64 | 44 |
| "Stomach" problems | 46 | 46 | 40 |

ble. This anhedonia, the inability to experience pleasure, is the hallmark of a neurobiological depression.

On the other hand, if the punishment center in the midbrain is stimulated, a feeling of great dysphoria (unpleasantness, fear, and loss of control) occurs. When the punishment center in an animal is stimulated, the animal cowers, looks everywhere for danger, and, if the stimulus persists long enough, simply gives up. Because these centers are operated by a different set of neurotransmitters, they continue to work well during depression.

What happens, then, for a depressed person? A normally pleasant event feels punishing rather than pleasurable, creating the perception error that makes everything, even good things, look grim. For example, someone gives a compliment, but instead of feeling good, as was intended, a depressed recipient might even feel bad about it and say to herself, "Why did they feel they had to say that? Do I look needy or something? What do they really want out of me, anyway?" Thus a positive is converted to a negative, and usually people around them don't understand what's going on. It's a vicious cycle, because the distress that results compounds the neurochemical problem, which then intensifies the situational distress. The neurochemical imbalance negatively distorts thought, and the stressful thoughts exacerbate the neurochemical imbalance.

Simply stated, then, the illness called depression reflects a disturbance of mood that occurs when the pleasure centers of the brain are not working (or when the punishment centers are working overtime). This illness called depression can be much more, however, and occasionally depressed mood itself can be absent, since it is only one component of the syndrome. In depression, the other automatic "vegetative" functions of the middle brain— appetite, sex drive, sleep, metabolism, energy regulation, modulation of hormone, and immune function—are also dysregulated.[39] The stress response itself is dysregulated, causing either too much of a response to a stimulus (anxiety disorder) or too little of a response ("psychomotor retardation").

This mental state can color the way a person feels and thinks until it affects virtually all the activities that are normally considered a part of daily life. The classic mood associated with depression is a combination of helplessness and hopelessness. Often, there is a disturbance in sleep patterns: A person may sleep much more than normal, may sleep at unusual times, may not be able to fall asleep, or may fall asleep easily but then awaken, unable to fall back to sleep. Partly because of these sleep problems and partly as a result of the depression itself, the person may feel fatigued and lacking energy all the time. Insomnia itself can trigger depression.

Many times, victims of depression also have eating problems. Some overeat, but many lose their appetite and suffer some weight loss. In many cases, depression leads to complete loss in the pleasure of eating. Many who are depressed sharply increase their alcohol consumption, particularly those who also suffer from anxiety. A variety of physical complaints can accompany depression. Most depressed people experience a number of vague physical pains and complaints; some become frantically obsessed with their health and convinced that they are suffering from serious physical diseases. Many lose interest in sex, finding no pleasure in it; others suffer from sexual dysfunction (such as loss of arousal or orgasm).

Many who are depressed struggle with feelings of personal worthlessness; others have vague, usually unjustified guilt feelings. A classic sign is indifference to things that normally held importance in a person's life—family, friends, hobbies, leisure activities, and/or work. Lacking hope, some think about suicide. It may even be possible to predict who is at a higher risk of suicide by measuring some of the neurochemical abnormalities associated with depression.[40] Some of the more meaningful parts of life are lost, along with the ability to savor the things that normally brought great enjoyment—a stroll along a shady street on a Sunday afternoon, a baby's smile, the companionship of good friends.

Researcher Richard Sword has identified what he calls a depression-prone personality, a person who is more likely than others to become depressed. According to Sword, a depression-prone person is ambitious, conscientious, responsible, and hard working; has a high standard of personal honesty and integrity; and sets high standards for others, but even higher standards for him or herself. This person is generally pleasant and seems to be happy, even when inwardly sad. On the other hand, once milder depression develops, anger, irritability, and controlling behavior can increase. Summarizing, National Institute of Mental Health psychiatrist Phillip Gold says that a person with "melancholic depression" has low self-esteem, a sense of hopelessness, intense anxiety about the future, a loss of sleep and appetite, and decreased sexual desire.[41]

In its earlier and most minor forms, inherited neurochemical depression, with its sense of punishment and negative expectations, can tend to put a person more on guard, looking for danger or possible exploitation and disregard by others. This may be manifested as shyness, a feeling of being unaccepted and the need to prove oneself, or hostile cynicism (particularly in men).

## Depression and Premenstrual Syndrome

Women with premenstrual syndrome (PMS) much more often have a history of treated depression than normal healthy women—31 percent, as compared with 6 percent of normal controls, 9 percent of women with heavy menstrual bleeding, and 22 percent of women with significant menstrual cramps.[42] Estrogen has an antidepressant effect on several brain neurotransmitters, and a drop in estrogen in the late cycle appears to be associated with a drop in brain serotonin (and endorphin) function in women who are genetically vulnerable to depression. These women are also more vulnerable to postpartum depression, when estrogen levels fall at delivery, and are probably more susceptible to depression at menopause.

If PMS sufferers are followed long enough, the symptoms may begin to extend back through the entire cycle, worsening at ovulation or before the period. For many, PMS appears to be an early, mild form of depression unmasked by normal hormone changes affecting a vulnerable brain neurotransmitter system. If the PMS is more severe, many of the physical symptoms associated with depression (such as migraine, muscle aches, or bowel symptoms) can appear before the menstrual period, then disappear afterward. Many women find significant relief from PMS with some of the same treatments used for depression—medications that improve serotonin function, exercise, a high-carbohydrate and low-protein diet, stress management and relaxation techniques, and avoidance of stimulants (such as caffeine).

Many women with either PMS or depression crave sweets as the symptoms worsen, which is the brain's attempt to boost serotonin levels. In fact, craving sweets is often a signal that serotonin function is deficient. Why? Serotonin is manufactured in the brain from tryptophan, an amino acid in the diet. To get into the brain, tryptophan has to cross the blood-brain barrier, which protects the brain from potentially dangerous substances in the bloodstream. To do that, it has to compete with the other amino acids in dietary proteins. If there are too many other amino acids, tryptophan has trouble getting into the brain and serotonin production falls. The solution? Eating carbohydrates (either sugars or starches) suppresses competing amino acids and makes it easier for tryptophan to enter the brain. (Starches are better than sugars, because an excessive rebound in adrenaline often occurs in anxiously depressed people as the sugar level falls a few hours after eating; starches reduce that rebound effect.) Some physicians use the disappearance of carbohydrate craving as a signal that the dose of antidepressant medication is adequate.

## Seasonal Affective Disorder

Some people are at increased risk for depression in the winter. Experiments at the National Institute of Mental Health have concluded that the ability to deal with stress—and thus to avoid depression—can be significantly influenced by the amount of sunlight received each day. Data from the studies indicate that some people seem better able to cope with stress, change, and challenge during the spring, summer, and early autumn months. As winter approaches and the days grow shorter and darker, many persons become lethargic, anxious, and depressed.[43] Some of the mechanisms of this seem similar to those causing winter hibernation in animals.

Investigators at the National Institute of Mental Health noticed that during the winter, when there is less light, some people tend to slow down, gain weight, sleep more, and feel depressed. A few even develop more serious problems than just a mild case of the blues. Some become incapacitated. Some even become suicidal.

Believing that light played a role, investigators exposed persons predisposed to suffer from winter depression to strong artificial, broad-spectrum light for at least five hours a day. For those exposed to light, symptoms of depression and distress were significantly reduced or even completely eliminated.[44] The therapeutic light is broad-spectrum white light; yellow incandescent bulbs do not work. Since those early studies, the daily regimen has been much simplified and has produced nearly the same benefits. The usual regimen today is exposure to bright lights for 30–60 minutes in the early morning.

Researchers who have studied the phenomenon of light have noticed that its effects seem to be influenced by geography. The propensity toward depression is more pronounced in northern climates such as the Scandinavian countries and Canada, where sunlight is limited. By contrast, in sunny areas of the world, as on the Mediterranean coast, people are much less likely to suffer from depression. This winter effect is not uncommon: The seasonal depression effect is seen in nearly 10 percent of the population in New Hampshire and 6 percent in New York, but in only 2 percent of those who live in Florida.[45]

What is the effect of the sunlight? While we're not completely sure, we have been able to glean information by studying animals that hibernate in winter. The seasonal behavior changes in animals—migration and hibernation—seem to be related to a light-sensitive area of the brain, the pineal gland. As days grow shorter, less light is transmitted through the eyes to the brain's pineal gland. In response, the pineal gland releases more of the hormone melatonin, which, among other things, suppresses reproduction and heightens survival adjustments.[46] Melatonin, secreted in response to darkness, is also involved in day-night biorhythms of such things as hormone secretion and sleep cycles. Taken orally, melatonin induces fatigue and sleepiness (like that of hibernating animals). Injected, melatonin induces depression (possibly by interfering with serotonin function) and may therefore be the culprit in the darkness-aggravated depression and sluggishness seen in what researchers have now dubbed seasonal affective disorder (SAD). Symptoms can include pain that is worse in the winter (as with some chronic muscle pain conditions, like fibromyalgia), and even the increased prevalence of infections seen during the winter. Anecdotes indicate that light therapy may be effective to help the increased winter pain, though that has not been rigorously studied. Immune function becomes somewhat dysregulated during the winter in victims of SAD, and it improves with light treatment.[47] Scientists working on the projects say, "The sunlight influence seems to be mediated via the retina, in the eye. It is by looking at the light, not just being generally exposed to it, that one obtains the beneficial results."[48] If a person has a clear-cut winter pattern to their depression, light can sometimes be even more effective than antidepressants, or a useful adjunct to those medicines. It's important to remember that SAD could be bipolar depression, and require different treatment than typical depression.

## The Physiological Changes of Depression

Depression obviously has a profound influence on the mind and the emotions, but many studies continue to find that depression has an equally profound influence on the body as well. Researchers have learned that during depression, the body undergoes hormonal and chemical changes similar to those of chronic stress (see Chapter 2). This occurs, says National Institute of Mental Health psychiatrist Phillip Gold, because in depressed people, the mechanisms that normally regulate the stress response fail. "Although depressed people often seem to think and react slowly," he says, "they are actually in a highly aroused state, focusing obsessively on their own sense of inadequacy. This state of mind parallels the heightened sense of awareness and focus that plays a positive role in a short-term response to stress, but in depression that intense awareness and focus is turned inward, with psychologically crippling results."[49] This hyperactivity of the brain in depression is demonstrated on functional MRI scans of the brain, and likely contributes to the anxiety seen with depression. The response to the excessive activity in the bodily parts of the brain is often accompanied by a shutting down of the prefrontal parts that are involved with thinking and decision making.

Normally, when we are challenged, the brain hypothalamus releases corticotropin-releasing hormone (the CRH mentioned in the genetics discussion, above). CRH causes the pituitary gland, which is located near the brain, to stimulate the adrenal gland, which is located near the kidney, to increase its production of cortisol, a compound that, along with adrenaline, heightens the alerting and protecting systems in the body. When stress passes, or as we adapt effectively to longer term stresses, hormone production diminishes, returning again to normal levels.

However, researchers have shown that in certain people subject to serious chronic depression, this endocrine system, once activated, does not seem able to turn itself off. CRH and cortisol levels remain elevated.[50] In a test of adrenal function, the suppression of hormone activity that should occur after the administration of a compound called dexamethasone fails to occur.[51] Consequently, when depressed, it may take an unduly extended period of time for the individual to recover from the impact of stress; or, in some instances, he may not recover at all without medical intervention.[52]

As serotonin function in the brain falls, in parallel the endorphin levels drop and pain-promoting Substance P rises.[53] Endorphins are the brain's own chemicals, designed to relieve pain and help us feel good.[54] (Morphine works to relieve pain largely by stimulating the natural endorphin receptors in the brain.) Depression is a state of endorphin deficiency. Other conditions characterized by low endorphin (and sometimes serotonin) levels include chronic pain disorders, migraine, premenstrual syndrome, and some arthritis. This fall in endorphins and rise in Substance P may partly explain why so many people with depression—approximately 60 percent—have recurrent, multiple pain problems. People with more than one pain complaint are six to eight times more likely to have clinical depression than others, and treatment of the depression often solves the pain problem if it has not become too chronic.[55]

Other important mechanisms of this increased pain seen with depression primarily involve defectiveness of the downward inhibitory tract from the brain down the spinal cord to the sites where pain signals arrive from the body periphery (see Chapter 5 for more information). That inhibitory tract is manned by the same neurotransmitters that are deficient in depression: serotonin, norepinephrine, and dopamine. The result of the deficiencies of these chemicals in depression results in a host of very common hypersensitivity disorders: irritable bowel syndrome, migraine and tension headaches, neurological symptoms (such as dizziness and tingling), and muscle pain disorders like fibromyalgia. If a person has one of these, he or she is likely to have several others, including depression and anxiety disorders.

One painful condition that deserves attention is fibromyalgia, a common problem characterized by chronic widespread muscle pain that causes multiple painful or tender points at sites of muscle insertion, fatigue, and sleep disturbance. The pain is often exacerbated by mental stress; for many, it's also worse in wintertime. Since the pattern of fibromyalgia is so similar to that of depression, some experts have wondered if the same neurochemical link causes both. For example, Dr. Jon Russell at the University of Texas in San Antonio and others have shown that people with fibromyalgia have three times the normal Substance P (which magnifies pain) in the cerebral spinal fluid and low serotonin function that inhibits pain, as also do those with depression.[56] Chronic pain conditions such as fibromyalgia would then be expected to have higher than usual prevalence of depression, and they do. Seventy-one percent of fibromyalgia patients have major depression, and they also have a strong family history of depression.[57] Antidepressants,[58] anticonvulsant medication,[59] stress management,[60] and relaxation techniques,[61] with particular attention to improving deep sleep,[62] are helpful in treatment of fibromyalgia. Also helpful are exercise, a strong physician-patient relationship, and a positive expectation about treatment. Sometimes nutritional supplements that increase nervous system serotonin (such as tryptophan or 5 hydroxytryptophan–5http), or dopamine (D-L phenylalanine), or stabilize sensitive nerve membranes (omega–3 fatty acids) may help.[63] Fibromyalgia can be very successfully treated early on, but if left untreated, over time, kindling occurs, and the excess pain becomes much more difficult to reverse. Excess Substance P and abnormal serotonin function are also seen in other common pain conditions associated with depression and fibromyalgia, such as migraine and irritable bowel syndrome.

Thus, high rates of underlying depression and panic disorder are also often present in persons who have other, more specific medical problems that combine pain with the smooth muscle spasm discussed in Chapter 5. Examples include irritable bowel syndrome ("spastic colon") patients (23 percent have major depression, and more have milder forms), esophageal motility disorder patients (40 percent are depressed, and 38 percent have panic disorder), patients with migraines (4.2 times normal depression rates), and patients with chest pain but normal coronary arteriograms (who have nine times more depression and seven times more panic disorder than normal).

There are a number of medical conditions that can mimic depression—so closely, in fact, that a physician may miss the underlying medical condition altogether. According to Gregory Manov and William Guy of the Department of Psychiatry at Vanderbilt School of Medicine and the Tennessee Neuropsychiatric Institute in Nashville, at least seven major categories of medical disease can charade as depression.[64] But when depressed patients are evaluated for these mimicking medical diseases, they are seldom present. The following can appear—even with careful scrutiny—to be depression:

- A number of **disorders of the central nervous system.** Tumors of the brain—especially slow-growing ones that affect the left hemisphere in general or the frontal or temporal lobes—often cause depressive symptoms. So do multiple sclerosis (especially in its early stages), brain injuries, cerebrovascular accidents (strokes), and chronic bleeding in the brain. Depression is also often the earliest symptom of a developing irreversible dementia, such as Alzheimer's disease, Huntington's chorea, Jakob-Creutzfeldt disease, and Wilson's disease.

- Some **endocrine disorders.** These include both hypothyroidism and slowly developing hyperthyroidism and other disorders of the thyroid gland. Severe depressive symptoms are also characteristic of Addison's disease and Cushing's syndrome (both diseases of the adrenal gland).

- Chronic and debilitating **disorders of the gastrointestinal tract.** Some gastrointestinal diseases do not result in localized gastric symptoms; at times, depression is the only symptom. A classic case is cancer of the pancreas; patients may feel no local pain from the cancer, but almost all suffer from serious depression, making it difficult for a physician to find the real illness. Depression very frequently occurs with Crohn's disease (regional enteritis), ulcerative colitis, and amyloidosis, and may be the only symptom in the early stages of these diseases.

- Chronic systemic illnesses, particularly those involving **infection or inflammation.** Lupus erythematosus is one of the most classic. Chronic infections and infectious diseases (by releasing immune chemicals called interleukins), too, may have direct effects on brain chemistry, leading to serious depression, Such lingering diseases include malaria, tuberculosis, syphilis, viral encephalitis, and meningoencephalitis. Any time an immune response to infections occurs, depressive symptoms are possible. This can cause confusion, because depression itself makes a person more prone to infections.

- **Simple nutritional deficiencies.** Most commonly at fault are vitamin deficiencies, such as niacin, folate acid, and vitamin $B_{12}$. Simple electrolyte imbalances such as low potassium or magnesium can cause all the classic symptoms of depression, too, most often in persons who take diuretics (water pills) and those who eat a strict low-sodium diet.[65]

## Depression and Longevity

Depression can increase mortality in some obvious ways. As mentioned, severe depression can lead to suicide. Depression, even in milder stages, however, also contributes to a higher risk of getting medical diseases that can be lethal. A University of Michigan study involving 6,000 people showed that elderly patients with symptoms of depression were 34 percent more likely to develop a new medical disease than those without depression were.[66]

Depression can also worsen the plight of people who already have a medical problem. Research shows that, when sick people become depressed, they tend to become sicker, need more medication, and spend more days in the hospital. Worst of all, it can actually reduce survival.[67] Mortality rates are four times the normal rate in depressed persons, not so much from suicide as from increased medical illness (63 percent of it cardiovascular disease). The severity and mortality of almost any disease are substantially worse if the patient is also depressed. This is particularly proven for stroke, coronary artery disease, myocardial infarction, heart rhythm disturbances, sudden death, rheumatoid arthritis, certain cancers, multiple sclerosis, Parkinson's disease, epilepsy, kidney disease, psoriasis, acne, and diabetes.[68]

Depression also shortens life in nursing homes. One group of researchers studied 454 patients that were newly admitted to eight nursing homes in the Baltimore area. Depression at the time of admission raised the risk of death within a year by 59 percent, regardless of physical health. Why? Researchers think several factors may be at work, including poor nutrition, inadequate rest, or impaired immune function among depressed persons.[69]

Just how depression shortens the survival time of patients who are already ill is not exactly known, although we do have some important clues. One came from a study of children who died from asthma attacks; twelve who died were compared with twelve who survived their attacks. According to researchers, "Family and personal characteristics of those who died suggested that depression may have played a role."[70] Depression can also worsen the loving, supportive relationships shown to prolong life.

Seven of the children who died—but only two of the ones who survived—came from families marked by marital discord, lack of emotional support, alcoholism, and drug abuse. And eight of the children who died— as compared with three who survived—had talked about death or suicide within a month of the fatal attack.

Researchers who conducted the study and analyzed its results wanted to find out why depression may have contributed to the asthma deaths, so they probed more deeply into the chemistry of depression. According to investigator Bruce Miller, director of the pediatric psychophysiological treatment unit at the National Jewish Center for Immunology and Respiratory Medicine in Denver, depression creates a chemical imbalance in the body that boosts the parasympathetic nervous system. It also upregulates the serotonin 2 ($5HT_2$) receptor discussed for asthma in Chapter 5. The result can be deadly for an asthmatic: The parasympathetic nervous system closes the airways.[71] The increased smooth muscle spasm in the airways is much like the increased spasm of the coronary arteries and bowel seen in depression, in which the abnormal $5HT_2$ receptor plays a role also.[72]

When followed prospectively, depressed people have fairly consistently showed greater mortality risk. In one such study, researchers followed up on 1,593 men and women who had been hospitalized for depression at a care facility in Iowa. For a control group, the researchers used randomly selected people of the same age and sex who also lived in Iowa. Follow-up studies began two years after the patients were released from the hospital and continued for fourteen years. Death rates among the depressed patients soared for the first two years following hospitalization and remained higher than average throughout the fourteen years of the study.[73]

In another important large-scale study, Dr. Richard Shekelle of the University of Chicago examined the health of about 2,000 men who were employed by Chicago's Western Electric Company. The men's personalities were first measured in 1958, then researchers tracked their health for the next two decades. During the next twenty years, those who had scored high on depression in 1958 were more likely than other men to die, including some of cancer. Others also found this cancer death link, sometimes from increased infections.[74] It's important to note that this increased risk remained even after the researchers took into account the men's age, occupation, cigarette smoking, and family history of cancer. Researchers found one interesting footnote to the study: The more time that elapsed since the measurement of depression, the weaker was its association with illness and death.[75] In other words, the link between depression and illness/death lessens over time.

Depression has also been linked to sudden death (usually from heart arrhythmias) in a number of studies. This is particularly true when they were also faced with situational stress. In one of the best-known studies, psychiatrist William Greene and colleagues at the University of Rochester studied twenty-six employees at Eastman Kodak Company who died suddenly and unexpectedly. Almost all of the employees who died had been depressed before their death—some for only a week, some for several months. Researchers found that the depressed employees suddenly underwent definite arousal; in other words, people who had been living in slow motion or depression became suddenly lurched into third gear. The "arousal" that occurred was in the form of an increased workload and the accompanying stress, a conflict in the workplace, or marital stress. The sudden shift from depression to arousal can produce incompatible reactions, leading to arrhythmia, myocardial infarction, or both.[76] The fact is, far and away the greatest cause of the increased deaths among depressed people is cardiovascular disease.[77]

## Depression and the Heart

Depression is now considered a major coronary risk factor, comparable in severity to smoking. In fact, much of cynical hostility, discussed for its heart toxicity in Chapter 4, is highly related to depression, and cynical hostility responds to many of the same treatments as depression. A number of impressive studies have proved that depression's biological abnormalities can lead to more cardiovascular disease.

Researchers in England examined 2,000 patients and an equal number of matched controls. They identified which ones were suffering from chronic mild depression. In prospectively following the study subjects, they found that new coronary artery disease was much more likely to later develop in those who suffered from depression than in those who did not.[78]

In fact, individual symptoms of depression can also predict future heart attacks. In a study of 1,300 graduates of Johns Hopkins Medical School, researchers isolated those for whom depression was a problem. Then they classified the depressed graduates according to their various symptoms of depression. They found that one particular symptom of depression, early-morning fatigue, was more often present among graduates who later suffered a myocardial infarction than among those who remained healthy.[79]

The effect of depression on the heart is so profound that researchers have been able to predict who would have a heart attack based solely on the presence of depression. In one such prediction, University of Oklahoma Medical School's Dr. Stewart Wolf examined sixty-five patients who had suffered documented myocardial infarctions, and sixty-five matched control subjects who were healthy and had not had any sign of heart disease.[80] To prove his theory, Wolf interviewed all 130 subjects once a month; he also gave each one a battery of psychological tests to determine how depressed each one was. After a series of interviews with each subject, Wolf made his predictions without knowing which ones had previously suffered a heart attack. He chose ten people who had failed to find meaningful satisfaction in their social and leisure activities, basically, the ten people who were the most depressed. He predicted (solely on the basis of depression) that they would be among the first to have a heart attack and die. All ten of the subjects Wolf pinpointed did, indeed, have a heart attack and die. In fact, those ten were among the first twenty-three who died during the four years following the predictions.[81]

In another prospective study, death due to heart disease was associated with depression. Robert Anda and his colleagues at the Centers for Disease Control and Prevention in Atlanta studied 2,832 adults ranging in age from forty-five to seventy-seven who entered the study healthy and free of heart disease. As they entered the study, volunteers were asked about their feelings of depression, discouragement, and hopelessness. Researchers then followed them for an average interval of twelve years. They found that those who felt depressed and hopeless suffered four times more deaths from heart disease.[82]

Other researchers studied heart disease in smokers. Findings showed that potentially fatal blood vessel disease progressed more rapidly among the smokers who were mildly to moderately depressed than among those who were not depressed.[83] One reason may be that depression appears to magnify risk factors associated with heart disease; in other words, depression makes risky behaviors even riskier. In a study reported at an American Heart Association meeting, researchers say that depression adds to the danger of all the standard risk factors for heart disease.

For example, diabetes increases coronary risk greatly, particularly if poorly controlled. Depression makes diabetic control much more erratic. This diabetes effect is in part because of the insulin resistance created by depression. This insulin resistance, creating "the Metabolic Syndrome" that puts people at very high cardiovascular risk, is worsened by depression in several studies.[84] The high cortisol and catecholamines seen with depression make people less responsive to insulin needed to get sugar into cells.[85] This insulin function is already poor in diabetics and gets twice as bad when they are depressed. In a ten-year study, depressed diabetics had over three times as many heart attacks as diabetics without depression.[86] Treating the depression corrects the insulin resistance created by the depression,[87] and can significantly lower the high blood sugars.[88]

The negative effects of smoking are 3.4 times greater for people who are depressed. Interestingly, in a study of 3,543 smokers, those who took antidepressant medication that improved serotonin function remarkably had 65 percent fewer heart attacks than the total group.[89] Similarly, an epidemiological study of 52,000 people showed that those taking serotonergic antidepressants had 20 percent fewer heart attacks than the overall community, despite the fact that they were being treated for depression that (when untreated) puts them at higher risk. All of this suggests that central nervous system serotonin abnormalities play a significant role in heart attacks. How that works is now beginning to be understood.

Three mechanisms are involved in creating myocardial infarction, or heart attack: plaque, arterial spasm, and finally a clot that finishes the job. All three are significantly accelerated in depression. Depression doubles the negative impact of low-density lipoproteins ("bad" cholesterol) on blood vessels. How could this be? Anxious depression causes an elevation of the stress chemical norepinephrine within peripheral blood vessels. Norepinephrine causes damage to the lining of blood vessels, in that it allows any cholesterol present in the blood vessel to create plaque (narrowing) at a much more rapid rate. This creates a synergy between chronic stress and cholesterol in causing more rapid onset of vascular damage.[90]

Depression creates an additional risk for cardiovascular events both by causing blood vessel (smooth muscle) spasm and by creating more blood clots. Depression's effect on serotonin in the brain is reflected in serotonin problems in the blood-clotting cells called platelets, making them adhere to each other more aggressively, setting off the clotting process that causes the final step in heart attacks and many strokes.[91] Most newer antidepressants act to improve serotonin levels in the brain and block this effect, producing an antiplatelet effect with less clotting[92] in a similar but different way than aspirin does, thus preventing heart attacks. Antidepressant medications that work by primarily improving norepinephrine levels do not have this platelet-protecting effect.[93] (Also see the discussion of these mechanisms in Chapter 5.)

Depression hits persons who already have coronary artery disease even harder than the general population. A striking example was provided by a study conducted by psychologist Robert M. Carney and his colleagues at the Washington University School of Medicine in St. Louis. The researchers followed fifty-two persons who had been diagnosed with coronary artery disease for one year.[94] Of the people in the study, 18 percent were seriously depressed before the diagnosis. The researchers used a strict definition for depression, too, taken from the *Diagnostic and Statistical Manual* (DSM IIIR). To qualify as "depressed," a person had to have suffered extreme sadness or hopelessness, loss of interest or pleasure in most activities, insomnia, loss of energy, or thoughts of suicide for at least two weeks.

Major depression was found to be the best single predictor of serious problems and complications among the heart patients, and it was an even stronger predictor than factors such as age, smoking, severity of artery damage, and levels of cholesterol in the bloodstream.[95] Researchers found that 78 percent of the depressed patients had some cardiac event during the twelve months after the diagnosis, and one died. Only a third of the nondepressed patients had problems.

Similarly, in a Canadian hospital study of more than 200 heart attack patients, patients were given diagnostic interviews a week after entering the hospital and again six months later. Forty percent of the patients had depression, starting before their heart attacks. All else being equal, say the researchers, depression raised the risk of death 3.4 times and the risk of recurrent coronary events 5.7 times.[96] Thus, the mechanisms described above do indeed create cardiovascular havoc.

According to researchers, the increased stress hormones and activity of the sympathetic nervous system present in depression create more arrythmias and thus sudden death. In a prospective study over one year, those depressed at the beginning had five times more ventricular tachycardia than the nondepressed.[97] (Ventricular tachycardia is a dangerous heart rhythm that often precedes sudden death, which is death that occurs unexpectedly in a person who previously seemed healthy and exhibited no symptoms of illness.)

A study in New York of 283 myocardial infarction patients found that 45 percent were depressed one week later; 18 percent had major depression, 27 percent had minor depression.[98] (Remember that to make a diagnosis of depression, the symptoms must be present for at least two weeks. That means that the above 45 percent were depressed *before* their myocardial infarction.) Depression was not associated with severity of heart disease, but those who were depressed did have a greater prevalence of other medical problems. Three to four months later, 33 percent were still depressed. After a heart attack, depression was even more predictive of cardiac disability than was the severity of heart damage. Among those who had been working before their heart attack, most who had major depression had not returned to work three months later; only 38 percent eventually returned, as compared with 63 percent of the heart attack victims who were not depressed. Minor depression was not as disabling.

Of interest in this study was the fact that medical problems masked the depression: Only 10 percent of those with major depression and 4 percent of all depressed patients had received treatment for depression. Another impressive finding is that, particularly in women, depression appears to predict death from heart disease more accurately than either hostility or Type A behavior; it may also be more important in accelerating atherosclerosis (see the related discussion in Chapter 4).[99] Some of the cardiotoxic Type A behaviors, such as cynical hostility (see Chapters 3–4), improve greatly with antidepressant medication. This response implies that some of the neurochemistry of depression (shown to increase heart attacks) probably also underlies the angry, cynical hostility that puts a person at higher risk for heart disease. People with that behavior pattern later develop more clinical depression. In fact, that cynical hostility may be more the way depression shows up in men.

With depression established as a major coronary risk factor, and based on preliminary results, longer term studies have now begun to determine the outcome of actively treating heart disease patients for depression, and the predicted better outcomes[100] with treatment are beginning to emerge in impressive ways. In two large studies published in recent years in the *Journal of the American Medical Association,* depressed heart attack patients who were treated with serotonergic antidepressants had 43 to 61 percent less cardiac death and fewer heart attacks than those who received a placebo.[101] Those treated with antidepressants that worked by nonserotonin mechanisms were not nearly as protected. These are striking numbers, as good as any cardiac medications used to prevent heart attacks. (The effects of nonpharmacological approaches to these problems will be discussed in Chapter 6.)

## Depression and the Immune System

Several years ago, the first phases of an unusually severe Asian influenza epidemic began to creep around the world. In a midwestern college community, people in an enterprising college health center wondered what effect preexisting mental distress would have on those exposed to the flu. Before the epidemic arrived, a large number of college students whose health care was provided by the clinic were screened with the Minnesota Multiphasic Personality Inventory (MMPI), a test that has become a standard for defining mental state. Then they waited for the flu to hit. Those who got influenza returned after three and six weeks to see who was still sick (most people recover well by three weeks). Those depressed before the epidemic were significantly more likely to still be sick at six weeks. The same results were found in a similar military study at Fort Dietrich, Maryland.[102]

Other physicians have noted that depressed (or sometimes chronically stressed) patients not infrequently complain of "getting everything that's going around," or of having trouble getting rid of their respiratory or intestinal infection. An interesting British study determined a "stress index" for a group of people, based on the presence or absence of depression symptoms or overwhelming stress. These people were then exposed to tiny amounts of cold viruses in nose drops to see who would actually get a viral infection. Sure enough, those with the high stress index got the colds at a much higher rate.[103] How could that be? What is it about depression and chronic stress that might affect the immunity that protects from such common infections? Are some of the same psychoneuroimmunology mechanisms discussed in Chapter 1 the culprit?

The increased infections noted above suggest that the immune changes seen in depression are clinically relevant. The immune system has two large components: cellular immunity (which primarily destroys challenging agents like viruses or bacteria) and humoral or antibody immunity (which attracts the cellular components and plays a role in allergies). Both are at times significantly impacted by depression. One of the most significant impacts of depression on immune function is on the activity of natural killer cells, the immune cells that assist the body in its surveillance against tumors and in its resistance to viral disease. A number of studies show that natural killer cell activity is reduced among people who are depressed. Researchers at Boston University School of Medicine, for example, reported lower natural killer cell activity in depressed persons.[104]

Dr. Michael Irwin and his colleagues at the University of California, San Diego, measured the natural killer cell activity of women whose husbands had recently died. The widows had significantly reduced levels of natural killer cell activity compared to women who were not bereaved. Among the bereaved women, the ones who were depressed had the greatest impairment in natural killer cell activity.[105]

It wasn't just the bereavement that curtailed immune function, then, because the more severely depressed the woman, the more reduced her natural killer cell activity. In reporting on his findings, Irwin commented, "Depression is qualitatively different from grief. People who are depressed feel down, blue, and gloomy persistently. Those who are grieving move in and out of those feelings." In summing up the study results, Irwin confirmed that it was "the severity of their depression," not merely their husbands' death, that seemed to be related to their weakened immune responses.[106]

Other components of the immune system are crippled by depression as well. Psychiatrists at the Mount Sinai School of Medicine in New York have been doing long-term studies in which they observe men whose wives have breast cancer. As early as two weeks after the wives die, the men show a "striking" drop in the white blood cell response when the immune system is challenged.[107]

Researchers working in the laboratory with animals have had similar results. Psychiatrist Martin Reite, University of Colorado, and his colleagues created depression in monkeys by separating them from their mothers at the age of six months. The baby monkeys, who were put into cages separate from their mothers, showed all the classic signs of depression. To test immune response, Reite took blood samples from the baby monkeys both before and after the separation; as part of the tests he ran, he checked the ability of white blood cells to proliferate. Following separation from their mothers, the baby monkeys showed a "significant reduction" in white blood cell activity.[108]

Researchers also suspect that depression interferes with the ratio of helper and suppressor cells. Helper and suppressor cells are two classes of lymphocytes; the helper cells turn on the immune response, and the suppressor cells turn off the immune response. If the immune system is to function normally, the two kinds of cells have to have a proper ratio. Neither too little immunity (getting infections) nor too much immunity (allergies and autoimmune diseases) is desirable. The higher the ratio of helpers to suppressors, the stronger the immune response; the lower the ratio, the weaker the cellular immunity response. When suppressors severely outnumber helpers, the immune system is considered to be suppressed (which is what happens in AIDS).

The results of a large number of studies show that depression definitely has an influence on the ratio, although the precise results vary. Test results differed somewhat for various reasons: Some of the studies involved patients who were hospitalized, though most did not; in some of the studies, patients were on antidepressant drugs; and so on. In some studies, depressed people had a normal number of suppressor cells but a small proportion of helper cells. In other studies, the people who were depressed had lower numbers of both kinds of cells.[109] When depression is treated, the abnormalities return toward normal.[110]

One study involving the helper-suppressor ratio was conducted by psychologist Margaret Kemeny and her colleagues at the University of California School of Medicine in San Francisco. To test the effect of depression on the immune system, they studied thirty-six subjects with genital herpes. Kemeny took regular blood samples over a six-month period and monitored outbreaks and recurrences. The people in the study who were depressed showed a drop in both helper and suppressor cells; they had significantly lower levels of suppressor cytotoxic T cells, which are thought to help keep outbreaks from occurring. The depressed people had more recurrences of symptoms and more outbreaks than did others in the study. Kemeny and her colleagues discovered that they could accurately predict which study subjects would have outbreaks based on how depressed they were.[111]

The hormones and chemicals produced in depression may also affect the immune system. One is cortisol. In depression, the adrenal gland often secretes far too much cortisol, which then acts to suppress the immune system.[112] When the adrenals manufacture and secrete these corticosteroids, having "no apparent biological brake,"[113] the immune system begins to slow down. University of Iowa psychiatrist Dr. Ziad Kronfol has done a series of studies in which he has subjected depressed people to standard immunity tests. One finding is consistent: The cellular immune systems of depressed people are less responsive than those of normal people—and even those of people with other mental illnesses.[114]

Now we come to an interesting paradox about the immune abnormality in depression. While decreased cellular immunity may lead to more infections, anxiously depressed patients often have excessive humoral immunity, that is, excessive antibodies, leading to more allergy problems and autoimmune diseases. Studies of people with multiple distressing allergies show that about two-thirds of these people are depressed.[115] And, interestingly, when the depression is treated, allergies begin to subside. In fact, in a large (12,058-person), prospective, thirty-one-year follow-up study in Finland, women who had the genetics for high allergy predicted later development of excessive allergy. If both the mother and the person were allergic, the risk for depression was four times normal.[116] And the severity of the allergies is worse if a person is depressed.[117]

For example, more hives occur when a person is anxiously depressed. Many people with hives experience worse symptoms when stressed. One study found that over one-third of those with hives were depressed.[118] When Japanese hive sufferers were studied not only for depression but for anxiety as well, the percent went up to 70 percent (compared to 26 percent of controls).[119]

Depression also is a significant factor in activating autoimmune disorders, such as lupus or rheumatoid arthritis.[120] Mental stress itself can activate rheumatoid arthritis[121] in about half the patients. In the other half, mental stress is not much of a factor. Depression is one form of chronic stress. Even animals under chronic stress will overrespond to materials (adjuvant) injected into joints to induce arthritis very much like rheumatoid arthritis. The onset of autoimmune diseases of the thyroid is often preceded by either major stressful events or clinical depression.[122]

Antidepressant medication and neural stabilizers like lithium can help to normalize the abnormal immunity of depression.[123] Both in animals and people, exercise also helps.[124] Those affecting other neurotransmitters in depression, such as dopamine, are not of much benefit for the immune abnormalities.[125] The brain, once again, seems to have great capacity to bring about that which is expected, all the way down to cellular levels (see the later discussions of the effect of optimism versus pessimism in Chapter 17, and of faith in Chapter 16). Immune responses and the well-proven placebo effect are involved in this phenomenon.

## Depression and Cancer

Until recently, scientists were convinced that depression could lead to cancer. While researchers argued about how great the effect was—and how strong the link—most agreed that there was a link between depression and cancer. Top medical researchers were convinced that depression either contributed to the development of cancer or caused it to be more severe once it did develop, and a variety of studies seemed to support that conviction.

Then researchers started to waffle. One report in *Science News* reported that the finding that depression "was associated more strongly with cancer mortality than with cancer incidence suggests that it may promote, rather than initiate, the disease process."[126]

Some research suggests the link between depression and cancer is much less likely. A study published by Zonderman in the *Journal of the American Medical Association*[127] says that many factors probably raise the risk of cancer, but depression isn't one of them.

Even with Zonderman's conclusive findings, some scientists think depression may at least contribute to some kinds of cancer (for example, cancers of the immune system, such as lymphoma, and cancers affected by hormones, such as breast cancer) that may be more susceptible to nervous system influence. This may in part be related to damage to DNA seen with depression.[128] University of Miami researcher Karl Goodkin says that depression might affect different types of cancer in different ways. Pointing out that Zonderman and his colleagues didn't specify which kinds of cancer cropped up among their study subjects, "We don't know whether their results are supportive of depression's effect on the incidence of viral tumors or not." Speaking of the danger of lumping together all types of cancer and drawing a single conclusion, he adds that "there may be two strong, opposite effects hidden by mixing all types of cancers."[129]

# Feeling Sad, Feeling Bad

The hopelessness, frustration, sadness, and dissatisfaction that constitute depression can quite literally make you feel bad physically. In many studies, the greater the depression, the higher the number of physical symptoms associated with any illness.[130] In fact, both the number of physical symptoms a patient has and the number of medical visits per year are directly proportional to the likelihood of being depressed.[131] The facts and figures from hosts of studies tell the story.[132] Physicians know that high utilizers of medical care (those in the top 10 percent of costs, number of visits, and hospitalizations) have an extremely high likelihood of being depressed (usually prior to all the medical need).

One-fourth to one-half of all patients who see primary care physicians are depressed. An estimated three-fourths of all depressed people see physicians because they are physically ill.

During depression, medical problems and discomfort become magnified. Depressed persons are apt to have multiple chronic medical illnesses. Depressed patients tend to do much more poorly on self-treatment and self-monitoring of chronic illnesses, such as making sure they inject insulin on schedule.

Depressed people tend to have more aches and pains, too, though researchers debate whether depression causes pain or pain causes depression. But the fact that the pain tends to greatly diminish, or even disappear, when the depression is treated suggests that the depression (and its associated endorphin and neurotransmitter deficiencies) underlies the pain. More accurately, both chronic pain and depression have the same underlying neurochemistry that magnifies both.

People who are depressed may not do as well in surgery, either. According to a study published in the *American Journal of Public Health,* depressed elderly women who had hip fractures did much more poorly following surgery than did the same type of patients who were not depressed.[133] Surgical complications, prolonged hospitalization, and costs were all significantly higher in those who were depressed.

The person experiencing depression is not the only one who may suffer physical illness as a result; studies show that family members may also have an increase of physical signs and symptoms. In one study, eighty-eight families that each had a depressed member were compared to eighty-eight families that did not; other than the factor of depression, there were no significant demographical differences between the families. The study clearly showed that depression in one member of the family is associated with physical illness in other family members. Before the family member became depressed, these people had no greater incidence of physical illness than those in comparison families, but their episodes of physical illness rose dramatically in the year following the occurrence of depression in the family.[134]

## What to Do About Depression?

At least part of feeling better appears to involve getting control over depression. That may not be as difficult as it seems. Experts estimate that 80 to 90 percent of persons who suffer from depression can be helped substantially. Because of the underlying neurochemical (and conditioned) vulnerability, however, depression tends to be a recurrent illness. Eight years after    ⨍ successful treatment of a first episode, three-fourths of the previously depressed patients will have had a recurrence. Treatment studies show that combined medication and counseling-behavioral treatment is best. If one must choose between one or the other, comparison studies confirm that longer term medication is superior to counseling in preventing recurrence.[135] Medication studies suggest that milder, anxious depression involves more serotonin abnormalities, but more severe, melancholic depression may involve more norepinephrine and dopamine abnormalities. Treatment is effective, and usually shows striking improvement in most of the medical problems associated with depression. Longer term outcome studies are needed to determine how much the treatment of depression substantially prevents many of these associated medical illnesses.

When depression is mild, counseling and learning relaxation coupled with stress resilience techniques can be very effective, even without medication. Giving up blame and thus taking back a personal sense of control of one's feelings and responses can improve central serotonin function. Loving relationships can improve dopamine function; and both exercise and meaningful work can improve norepinephrine function. Meditation and deep relaxation techniques can improve GABA function. So all these principles act chemically like antidepressant medications (perhaps not as profoundly). Adequate sleep (usually eight hours—see Chapter 7) is crucial, as is good nutrition (Chapter 22). If the depression primarily occurs in the winter, bright light exposure in the morning can be very useful. If all of these are inadequate, early medical treatment is far more effective than starting late (to avoid the kindling effect mentioned above). Keep in mind that even severe PMS can be a form of depression, and responds to the same methods of treatment. And common medical problems such as irritable bowel syndrome and migraine are rooted in the same neurochemical abnormalities, and usually respond to these same treatments. If all this is starting in childhood or teenage years, the chance of a bipolar depression is much higher, and usually needs neural stabilizer medications before any antidepressants are used.

Ongoing research is providing new clues about the malady we call depression, and scientists continue looking for even more effective treatments. One recent landmark study provides new evidence about how pervasive depression can be. The study, conducted by researchers at the University of Washington in Seattle, studied the infants of women who were classified as clinically depressed. According to research director Geraldine Dawson, the infants of mothers who are depressed showed changes in electrical brain activity that led to unusual responses.[136] Simply stated, the infants were prone to depression, too.

Dawson has called for further research to determine the exact reasons for the infants' depression. She theorizes that the infants may be reacting to nonresponsive mothers or that the depression may be genetic.[137] The mothers' stress hormones can also affect fetal brain development. Motherly neglect in childhood can also activate the genetic vulnerability, for example by turning on the gene for CRH, as noted above. What is clear, say researchers, is that depression may include a broad circle of influence. Such studies also raise the important question about how depression should be treated in pregnancy—is it *safer* for the child if a depressed, pregnant mother receives antidepressant medication if counseling is not enough? The evidence thus far suggests the answer may be yes.

While studies like these indicate that depression may be genetic, at least part of the cause of depression is cultural, says San Diego psychiatrist Dennis Gersten. As a response to years of practice, Gersten likens personalities to crystalline structures, like diamonds, quartz, ice, mica, and so on. "Each fractures under predictable lines when stressed," Gersten says. "When the stress is massive enough, each structure will collapse."[138]

It's important to remember that depression can be caused by physical factors—certain prescription drugs (e.g., heart medications, cortisone, glaucoma medication, and antihistamines), premenstrual syndrome, other female hormone disturbances (including oral contraceptives), diabetes, rapid-weight-loss diets, lack of exercise, sunlight deficiency, and inadequate nutrient intake (especially of iron, thiamine, and magnesium). Depression is also a common side effect of thyroid problems; researchers estimate that 10 to 15 percent of all depressed people have thyroid problems.[139] If these problems are present, correcting them is important.

The depression-prone personality, Gersten concludes, is one that can fracture under multiple stresses. Those stresses—genetic, psychological, chemical, allergic, and toxic—offer not only a clue to the causes of depression but also a valuable panorama of ways we may prevent it.

## ENDNOTES

1. Bernie S. Siegel, *Love, Medicine, and Miracles* (New York: Harper and Row, 1986).
2. Winifred Gallagher, "The Dark Affliction of Mind and Body," *Discover,* May 1986, 66–76.
3. Gallagher, "The Dark Affliction of Mind and Body," 66–76.

4. QuestionBuilder.com, "Patient Health Questionnaire," http://www.question builder.com/patient-health-questionnaire.html (accessed December 17, 2004).

5. R. Spitzer, J. Williams, and K. Kroenke, et al., "Discovering Depression in Medical Patients," *JAMA* (1999).

6. Depression Guideline Panel, *Depression in Primary Care: Volume 1, Detection and Diagnosis* (Rockville, Md.: U.S. Department of Health and Human Services, Agency for Healthcare Policy and Research, Publication no. 93–550, 1993), 23.

7. Joseph Alper, "Depression at an Early Age," *Science,* May 1986, 45–50.

8. W. Katon, M. Von Korff, E. Lin, T. Bush, and J. Ormel, "Adequacy and Duration of Antidepressant Treatment in Primary Care," *Medical Care* 30 (1992): 67–76.

9. J. E. Mezzich, K. J. Evanczuk, R. J. Mathias, and G. A. Coffman, "Admission Decisions and Multiaxial Diagnosis," *Archives of General Psychiatry* 41 (1989): 1001–4.

10. Depression Guideline Panel, *Depression,* 47–48.

11. Anna M. Bardone, Terrie E. Moffitt, Avshalom Caspi, Nigel Dickson, Warren R. Stanton, and Phil A. Silva, "Adult Physical Health Outcomes of Adolescent Girls with Conduct Disorder, Depression, and Anxiety," *Journal of the American Academy of Child and Adolescent Psychiatry* 37 no. 6: 594–601.

12. Martin E. P. Seligman, *Learned Optimism* (New York: Alfred A. Knopf, 1991), 75.

13. I. Grant, T. L. Patterson, and J. Yager, "Social Supports in Relation to Physical Health and Symptoms of Depression in the Elderly," *American Journal of Psychiatry* 145, no. 10: 1254–58.

14. Anne H. Rosenfeld, "Depression: Dispelling Despair," *Psychology Today,* June 1985, 28.

15. Rosenfeld, "Depression: Dispelling Despair," 28.

16. Alper, "Depression at an Early Age," 45–50.

17. G. J. Kennedy, H. R. Kelman, C. Thomas, W. Wisniewski, H. Metz, and P. E. Bijur, "Hierarchy of Characteristics Associated with Depressive Symptoms in an Urban Elderly Sample," *American Journal of Psychiatry* 146, no. 2: 220–25.

18. Kenneth B. Wells, Anita Stewart, Ron D. Hays, M. Audrey Burnam, William Rogers, Marcia Daniels, Sandra Berry, Sheldon Greenfield, and John Ware, "The Functioning and Well-Being of Depressed Patients," *Journal of the American Medical Association* 262, no. 7: 914–19.

19. Depression Guideline Panel, *Depression,* 24–25.

20. P. E. Greenberg, L. E. Stiglin, S. N. Finkelstein, and E. R. Berndt, "The Economic Burden of Depression in 1990," *Journal of Clinical Psychiatry* 54 (1993): 405–18.

21. P. E. Greenberg, R. C. Kessler, et al., "The Economic Burden of Depression in the United States: How Did It Change Between 1990 and 2000?" *J Clin Psychiatry* 64 (2003): 1465–75.

22. W. R. Coryell, R. Noyes, and J. Clancey, "Excess Mortality in Panic Disorder: A Comparison with Primary Unipolar Depression," *Archives of General Psychiatry* 39 (1982): 701–3.

23. Gallagher, "The Dark Affliction of Mind and Body," 66–76.

24. Ibid., 66–76.

25. M. Anguelova, C. Benkelfat, and G. Turecki, "A Systematic Review of Association Studies Investigating Genes Coding for Serotonin Receptors and the Serotonin Transporter: II. Suicidal Behavior," *Mol Psychiatry* 8, no. 7: 646–53.

26. D. A. Collier, G. Stober, T. Li, et al., "A Novel Functional Polymorphism Within the Promoter of the Serotonin Transporter Gene: Possible Role in Sus-

ceptibility to Affective Disorders," *Mol Psychiatry* 1, no. 6: 453–60; and V. E. Golimbet, M. V. Alfimova, T. V. Shchebatykh, L. I. Abramova, V. G. Kaleda, and E. I. Rogaev, "Serotonin Transporter Polymorphism and Depressive-Related Symptoms in Schizophrenia," *Am J Med Genet.* 126B, no. 1: 1–7.

27. Clive Wood, "Who Gets Depressed?" *Advances* 4, no. 2: 61–65.

28. G. W. Brown, A. Bifulco, and T. O. Harris, "Life Events, Vulnerability, and Onset of Depression: Some Refinements," *British Journal of Psychiatry* (1987).

29. C. Nemeroff, Amer. Psychosomatic Society Annual Meeting 2001.

30. R. M. Post, "Transduction of Psychosocial Stress into the Neurobiology of Recurrent Affective Disorder," *American Journal of Psychiatry* 149 (1992): 999–1010.

31. L. Capuron and R. Dantzer, "Cytokines and Depression: The Need for a New Paradigm," 2004.

32. P. Trzonkowski, J. Mysliwska, B. Godlewska, et al., "Immune Consequences of the Spontaneous Pro-Inflammatory Status in Depressed Elderly Patients," *Brain Behav Immun.* 18, no. 2: 135–48.

33. G. Fricchione, R. Daly, M. P. Rogers, and G. B. Stefano, "Neuroimmunologic Influences in Neuropsychiatric and Psychophysiologic Disorders," *Acta Pharmacol Sin.* 22, no. 7: 577–87.

34. Rosenfeld, "Depression: Dispelling Despair," 30.

35. A. Neumeister, "Tryptophan Depletion, Serotonin, and Depression: Where Do We Stand?" *Psychopharmacol Bull.* 37, no. 4: 99–115.

36. P. L. Delgado, *Biol Psychiatry* 1999; 46: 212–220.

37. D. L. Rosenhan and M. E. P. Seligman, *Abnormal Psychology* (New York: Norton, 1984), 307.

38. Kroenke et al., *Am J Med.* 1989;86:266–66.

39. Depression Guideline Panel, *Depression,* 18, 49, 50, 64, 80.

40. E. R. Braveman and C. C. Pfeiffer, "Suicide and Biochemistry," *Biological Psychiatry* 20 (1985): 123–24.

41. Christopher Vaughan, "The Depression-Stress Link," *Science News* 134 (1988): 155.

42. J. Bancroft, D. Rennie, and P. Warner, "Vulnerability to Perimenstrual Mood Change: The Relevance of a Past History of Depressive Disorder," *Psychosomatic Medicine* 56 (1994): 225–31.

43. T. Silverstone and C. Thompson, eds., *Seasonal Affective Disorder* (London: Clinical Neuroscience Publishers, 1989).

44. D. A. Oren and N. E. Rosenthal, "Seasonal Affective Disorders," in E. S. Paykel, ed., *Handbook of Affective Disorders,* 2nd ed. (London: Churchill Livingstone, 1992), 551–67; and M. Terman, "On the Question of Mechanism in Phototherapy for Seasonal Affective Disorder: Considerations of Clinical Efficacy and Epidemiology," *Journal of Biological Rhythms* 3 (1988): 155–72.

45. M. Terman et al., "Seasonal Symptom Patterns in New York: Patients and Population," in Silverstone and Thompson, eds., *Seasonal Affective Disorder* (London: Clinical Neuroscience Publishers, 1989), 77–95.

46. Michael Freeman, "Don't Be SAD," *Medical Self-Care,* January–February 1989.

47. S. Kasper, N. E. Rosenthal, S. Barberi, A. Williams, L. Tamarkin, S. L. B. Rogers, and S. R. Pillemer, "Immunological Correlates of Seasonal Fluctuations in Mood and Behavior and Their Relationship to Phototherapy," *Psychiatry Research* 36 (1991): 253–64.

48. Frederic Flach, *Resilience* (New York: Fawcett Columbine, 1988).

49. Vaughan, "The Depression-Stress Link," 155.

50. Nemeroff, American Psychosomatic Society.

51. Depression Guideline Panel, *Depression*.

52. Flach, *Resilience*.

53. Depression Guideline Panel, *Depression*, 23.

54. Blair Justice, *Who Gets Sick: Thinking and Health* (Houston, Tex.: Peak Press, 1987), 100, 102–3.

55. Depression Guideline Panel, *Depression*, 51–52.

56. I. J. Russell, *Fibrositis/Fibromyalgia Syndrome*, in B. M. Hyde, ed., *The Clinical and Scientific Basis of Myalgic Encephalitis/Chronic Fatigue Syndrome* (Ottawa: Nightingale Research Foundation, 1992); H. Vaeroy et al., "Elevated CSF Levels of Substance P and High Incidence of Raynaud Phenomenon in Patients with Fibromyalgia: New Features for Diagnosis," *Pain* 32 (1988): 21–26; and R. M. Murphy and F. P. Zemlan, "Differential Effects of Substance P on Serotonin-Modulated Spinal Nociceptive Reflexes," *Psychopharmacology* (Berlin) 93 (1987): 118.

57. J. I. Hudson, M. S. Hudson, L. F. Pliner, D. L. Goldenberg, and H. G. Pope, Jr., "Fibromyalgia and Major Affective Disorder: A Controlled Phenomenology and Family History Study," *American Journal of Psychiatry* 142 (1985): 441–46.

58. L. M. Arnold, P. E. Keck, Jr., and J. A. Welge, "Antidepressant Treatment of Fibromyalgia: A Meta-Analysis and Review, *Psychosomatics* 41, no. 2:104–13.

59. L. Crofford, American College of Rheumatology Annual Meeting 2003.

60. B. B. Singh, B. M. Berman, V. A. Hadhazy, and P. Creamer, "A Pilot Study of Cognitive Behavioral Therapy in Fibromyalgia," *Altern Ther Health Med* 4, no. 2: 67–70.

61. L. A. Rossy, S. P. Buckelew, N. Dorr, K. J. Hagglund, J. F. Thayer, M. J. McIntosh, J. E. Hewett, and J. C. Johnson, "A Meta-Analysis of Fibromyalgia Treatment Interventions," *Ann Behav Med* 21, no. 2: 180–91.

62. M. B. Scharf, M. Hauck, R. Stover, M. McDannold, and D. Berkowitz, "Effect of Gamma-Hydroxybutyrate on Pain, Fatigue, and the Alpha Sleep Anomaly in Patients with Fibromyalgia," *J Rheumatol* 25, no. 10: 1986–90.

63. I. Caruso, P. Sarzi Puttini, M. Cazzola, and V. Azzolini, "Double-Blind Study of 5-Hydroxytryptophan Versus Placebo in the Treatment of Primary Fibromyalgia Syndrome," *J Int Med Res* 18 no. 3: 201–9; and P. S. Puttini, and I. Caruso, "Primary Fibromyalgia Syndrome and 5-Hydroxy-L-Tryptophan: A 90-day Open Study, Rheumatology Unit, L Sacco Hospital, Milan, Italy," *J Int Med Res* 20, no. 2: 182–89.

64. Gregory Manov and William Guy, "Medical Disorders That May Present as Depression," *Physician and Patient*, January 1985, 46–51.

65. C. Blaum, 1999 Gerontological Society Annual Meeting, reported in *Medical Tribune*, December 1999, 26.

66. Ibid.

67. Linda C. Higgins, "Depression May Shorten Survival," *Medical World News*, July 10, 1989, 20.

68. G. I. Keitner, C. E. Ryan, L. W. Miller, R. Kohn, and N. B. Epstein, "12-Month Outcome of Patients with Major Depression and Comorbid Psychiatric or Mental Illness," *American Journal of Psychiatry* 148 (1991): 345–50; P. J. Lustman, L. S. Griffith, and R. E. Clouse, "Depression in Adults with Diabetes: Results of a Five-Year Follow-Up Study," *Diabetes Care* 11 (1988): 605–12; and R. M. Carney, M. W. Rich, K. E. Freedland, et al., 627–33.

69. Barry W. Rovner, Pearl S. German, Larry J. Brant, et al., "Depression and Mortality in Nursing Homes," *Journal of the American Medical Association*, 265 (1991): 993–96.

70. Higgins, "Depression May Shorten Survival," 21.
71. Ibid., 21.
72. A. Schins, A. Honig, H. Crijns, L. Baur, and K. Hamulyak, "Increased Coronary Events in Depressed Cardiovascular Patients: 5-HT2A Receptor as Missing Link?" *Psychosom Med.* 65, no. 5: 729–37.
73. D. W. Black, G. Winokur, and A. Nasrallah, "Mortality in Patients with Primary Unipolar Depression, Secondary Unipolar Depression, and Bipolar Affective Disorder: A Comparison with General Population Mortality," *International Journal of Psychiatric Medicine* 17 (1987): 351–60.
74. Janice K. Kiecolt-Glaser and Ronald Glaser, "Psychological Influences on Immunity," *Psychosomatics,* 624.
75. Howard S. Friedman, *The Self-Healing Personality* (New York: Henry Holt and Company, 1991), 61.
76. W. A. Greene, S. Goldstein, and A. J. Moss, "Psychosocial Aspects of Sudden Death," *Archives of Internal Medicine* 129 (1972): 725–31; R. M. Charney, K. E. Freedland, M. W. Rich, L. J. Smith, and A. S. Jaffe, "Ventricular Tachycardia and Psychiatric Depression in Patients with Coronary Artery Disease," *American Journal of Medicine* 95 (1993): 23–28; and E. M. Levy, D. J. Borelli, S. M. Mirin, P. Salt, P. H. Knapp, C. Peirce, B. H. Fox, and P. H. Black, "Biological Measures and Cellular Immunological Function in Depressed Psychiatric Inpatients," *Psychiatry Research* 36 (1991): 157–67.
77. L. R. Wulsin, *Psychosomatic Med* 2003.
78. Donald E. Girard, Ransom J. Arthur, and James B. Reuler, "Psychosocial Events and Subsequent Illness—A Review," *Western Journal of Medicine* 142, no. 3: 358–363.
79. Girard, Arthur, and Reuler, "Psychosocial Events and Subsequent Illness—A Review," 358–63.
80. James J. Lynch, *The Broken Heart: The Medical Consequences of Loneliness* (New York: Basic Books, 1977).
81. Lynch, *The Broken Heart.*
82. *Science News,* 144, no 5: 79.
83. *Science News,* 79.
84. F. Okamura, *Internal Med* 1999;38(3):257–60; also Stewart TD, *Conn Med* 2000 Jun; 64(6): 343–5; also Chiba M, *Metabolism* 2000 Sep; 49(9): 1145–9; also Bjorntorp P, Diabet Med. 1999 May; 16(5): 355–7; also Winokur A, *Am J Psychiatry* 1988 Mar; 145(3): 325–30.
85. G. P. Chrousos, *Int J Obes Relat Metab Disord* 2000 Jun; 24 Suppl 2: S50–5.
86. R. E. Clouse, *Psychosomatic Medicine* 2001; 63:103.
87. F. Okamura and S. M. Cheer, *Drugs* 61, no. 1: 81–110001.
88. P. J. Lustman, *Diabetes Care* 2000; 23(5): 618–23; also P. J. Goodnick *Ann Clin Psychiatry* 2001; 4101; 13:31–41.
89. Sauer, *Circulation* 2001;104:1894–1898.
90. S. B. Manuck, J. R. Kaplan, and K. A. Matthews, "Behavioral Antecedents of Coronary Artery Disease and Atherosclerosis," *Atherosclerosis* 6 (1986): 2–14.
91. J. I. Haft and Y. S. Arkel, "Effect of Emotional Stress on Platelet Aggregation in Humans," *Chest* 70 (1979):501–05; and S. Cohen, J. R. Kaplan, and S. B. Manuck, "Social Support and Coronary Heart Disease: Underlying Psychologic and Biologic Mechanisms," in S. A. Shumaker and S. M. Czajkowski, eds., *Social Support and Cardiovascular Disease* (New York: Plenum, 1992).
92. Serebruanny and Glassman, *Eur J Heart Function* 2003.
93. *Jl Clin Psychopharacology,* 2000; 20: 137–40.

94. R. M. Carney, M. W. Rich, K. E. Freedland, J. Saini, A. TeVelde, C. Simeone, and K. Clark, "Major Depressive Disorder Predicts Cardiac Events in Patients with Coronary Artery Disease," *Psychosomatic Medicine*, 50 (1988): 627–33.

95. Carney, et al., "Major Depressive Disorder," 627–32.

96. Nancy Frasure-Smith, Francois Lesperance, and Mario Talajic, "Depression Following Myocardial Infarction: Impact on Six-Month Survival," *Journal of the American Medical Association* 270 (1993): 1819–25. (See also the editorial by Williams and Chesney in the same issue.)

97. R. M. Carney, et al., "Ventricular Tachycardia and Psychiatric Depression in Patients with Coronary Artery Disease," *Am J Med* 95 (1993): 23–28.

98. Margaret A. Chesney, "Social Isolation, Depression, and Heart Disease: Research on Women Broadens the Agenda," *Psychosomatic Medicine* 55 (1993): 434–35.

99. Chesney, "Social Isolation."

100. R. B. Lydiard, "Effects of Sertraline on Quality of Life: A Double Blind Study," scientific exhibit at the American Academy of Family Physicians Annual Assembly, 1993; and Redford B. Williams and Margaret A. Chesney, "Psychosocial Factors and Prognosis in Established Coronary Artery Disease," *Journal of the American Medical Association* 270 (1993): 1860–61.

101. A. H. Glassman, et al., (The SADHART Trial), *JAMA* 288 (2002):701–09; and S. M. Czajkowski, (The ENRICHED Trial), *JAMA* 289 (2003): 3106–16.

102. J. B. Imboden, *Archives of Internal Medicine* 108 (1961): 393.

103. S. Cohen, D. A. Tyrell, and A. P. Smith, "Psychological Stress and Susceptibility to the Common Cold," *New England Journal of Medicine* 325 (1991): 606–12.

104. S. E. Locke, M. W. Hurst, J. S. Heisel, L. Kraus, and R. M. Williams, *Life Change Stress and Human Natural Killer Cell Activity*, research report (Boston: Department of Biological Sciences and Psychosomatic Medicine, Division of Psychiatry, Boston University School of Medicine, 1979).

105. "Bereavement: An Immune Reaction," *Mind/Body/Health Digest* 1, no. 2: 1987, 2.

106. "Bereavement: An Immune Reaction," 2.

107. From *Medical World News*, as summarized in Padus, 577.

108. Steven Locke and Douglas Colligan, *The Healer Within: The New Medicine of Mind and Body* (New York: E. P. Dutton, 1986), 68.

109. "Depression and Immunity," *Harvard Medical School Mental Health Letter*, 1986, 8.

110. A. V. Ravindran, J. Griffiths, Z. Merali, and H. Anisman, "Lymphocyte Subsets Associated with Major Depression and Dysthymia: Modification by Antidepressant Treatment," *Psychosomatic Medicine* 57, no. 6: 555–63.

111. Margaret Kemeny, "Clinical Psychoneuroimmunology in Genital Herpes Recurrence," paper presented at the Annual Meeting of the Society for Behavior Medicine, 1986; and Justice, *Who Gets Sick*, 157.

112. "Depression and Immunity," 8.

113. Locke and Colligan, *The Healer Within*, 66.

114. Ibid., 68.

115. A. I. Terr, "Environmental Illness: A Clinical Review of 50 Cases," *Arch Int Med* 146 (1986): 145–9.

116. M. Timonen, J. Jokelainen, A. Herva, P. Zitting, V. B. Meyer-Rochow, and P. Rasanen, "Presence of Atopy in first-degree Relatives as a Predictor of a Female Proband's Depression: Results from the Northern Finland 1966 Birth Cohort, *J Allergy Clin Immunol* 111, no. 6: 1249–54.

117. M. Kovacs, A. Stauder, and S. Szedmak, "Severity of Allergic Complaints: The Importance of Depressed Mood," *J Psychosom Res.* 54, no. 6: 549–57.

118. S. G. Consoli, "Psychological Factors in Chronic Urticaria," *Ann Dermatol Venereol* 130, spec. no. 1: 1S73–7.

119. M. Hashiro and M. Okumura, "Anxiety, Depression, Psychosomatic Symptoms and Autonomic Nervous Function in Patients with Chronic Urticaria," *J Dermatol Sci.* 8, no. 2: 129–35.

120. A. J. Zautra, D. C. Yocum, I. Villanueva, B. Smith, M. C. Davis, J. Attrep, and M. Irwin, "Immune Activation and Depression in Women with Rheumatoid Arthritis," *J Rheumatol.* 31, no. 3: 457–63.

121. A. J. Zautra, N. A. Hamilton, P. Potter, and B. Smith, "Field Research on the Relationship Between Stress and Disease Activity in Rheumatoid Arthritis," *Ann N Y Acad Sci.* 876:397–412.

122. V. J. Pop, L. H. Maartens, G. Leusink, M. J. van Son, A. A. Knottnerus, A. M. Ward, R. Metcalfe, and A. P. Weetman, "Are Autoimmune Thyroid Dysfunction and Depression Related?" *J Clin Endocrinol Metab.* 83, no. 9: 3194–7.

123. J. Lieb, "Lithium and Antidepressants: Inhibiting Eicosanoids, Stimulating Immunity, and Defeating Microorganisms," *Med Hypotheses* 59, no. 4: 429–32.

124. S. Kubesch, V. Bretschneider, et al., "Aerobic Endurance Exercise Improves Executive Functions in Depressed Patients," *J Clin Psychiatry* 64: 1005–12; and A. Moraska and M. Fleshner, "Voluntary Physical Activity Prevents Stress-Induced Behavioral Depression and Anti-KLH Antibody Suppression," *Am J Physiol Regul Integr Comp Physiol.* 281, no. 2: R484–89.

125. A. Mizruchin, I. Gold, I. Krasnov, G. Livshitz, R. Shahin, and A. I. Kook, "Comparison of the Effects of Dopaminergic and Serotonergic Activity in the CNS on the Activity of the Immune System," *Neuroimmunol.* 101, no. 2: 201–4.

126. B. Bower, "Science News of the Week/ Depression and Cancer: A Fatal Link," *Science News* 132 (1987): 244.

127. Alan B. Zonderman, Paul T. Costa, and Robert R. McCrae, "Depression as a Risk for Cancer Morbidity and Mortality in a Nationally Representative Sample," *Journal of the American Medical Association* 262, no. 9: 1191–200.

128. M. Irie, S. Asami, M. Ikeda, and H. Kasai, "Depressive State Relates to Female Oxidative DNA Damage via Neutrophil Activation," *Biochem Biophys Res Commun.* 311, no. 4: 1014–18.

129. Karl Goodkin, quoted in S. Hart, "Depression and Cancer: No Clear Connection," *Science News* 136 (1989): 150.

130. K. Bolla-Wilson and M. L. Bleecker, "Absence of Depression in Elderly Adults," *Journal of Gerontology* 44, no. 2: 53–55.

131. Smith, American Psychosomatic Society; and Shavers, *The Identification of Depression and Anxiety.*

132. Wayne Katon, "Depression: Somatization and Social Factors," *Journal of Family Practice* 27, no. 6: 579–80.

133. Jana M. Mossey, Elizabeth Mutran, Kathryn Knott, and Rebecca Craik, "Recovery After Hip Fractures: The Importance of Psychosocial Factors," *Advances* 6, no. 4: 23–25.

134. Magdalena Sobieraj, Jeanine Williams, John Marley, and Philip Ryan, "The Impact of Depression on the Physical Health of Family Members," *British Journal of General Practice* 48 (1998): 1653–55.

135. Frank et al., *Archives of General Psychiatry* 47 (1990): 1093ff.

136. "Infant Brains Reflect Moms' Depression," *Science News* 138 (1990): 28.

137. "Infant Brains."

138. Dennis Gersten, "Depression: Is It a Product of Our Culture?" *Brain/Mind Bulletin* 16, no. 6: 6–7.

139. "Ten Physical Reasons You May Be Depressed," *Prevention*, June 1992, 69–76.

# CHAPTER 7

# Insomnia and Sleep Deprivation: Health Effects and Treatment

*Not poppy, nor mandragora,*
*nor all the drowsy syrups of the world*
*shall ever medicine thee*
*to that sweet sleep which thou ow'dst yesterday.*

—William Shakespeare

## Learning Objectives

- Define insomnia and sleep deprivation.
- List the major types and causes of insomnia.
- Understand the factors in the development of chronic insomnia.
- List the behavioral, psychological, and physiological effects of insomnia.
- Understand the treatment of insomnia.
- List effective medications to treat insomnia.

A s often happens with new mothers, Maria found her sleep frequently interrupted after the birth of her baby; soon, she began to get irritable, and eventually she became depressed. Even after the baby finally began sleeping through the night, Maria continued to have trouble sleeping. To make matters worse, she also started having aching muscles and stomach problems. Thinking she could at least do something about her sleeping problems, she tried some over-the-counter sleeping aids (antihistamines), but was disappointed when they didn't seem to help much.

Months later, when seeking medical help for her muscle aches and stomach problems, she mentioned the insomnia to her physician. Maria was somewhat surprised when her physician focused on treating the insomnia, not the pain. He started with some short-term medication to help her sleep, but also taught her some long-term relaxation and stress resilience techniques. Maria was amazed: The techniques not only relieved her fatigue and irritability, but also resolved her physical problems as well.

Sleep needs vary greatly from person to person. Some people are "short sleepers," requiring less than six hours a night, though that is quite uncommon. Others are "long sleepers," requiring nine hours or more. Most people need seven to eight hours of sleep at night to feel good all the next day.

So, how do you determine how much sleep you need? You need enough sleep to provide full restoration and function for the next day. In other words, you need to feel fully rested and energized enough to meet the demands of the day. If you "hit the wall" in the afternoon, or need caffeine, you are clearly not getting enough sleep at night. And don't think you can simply make up for it with a couple of quick naps during the day: Napping during the day causes the quality of night sleep to deteriorate.

Tiredness is the number one reported symptom in general medical clinics. Tiredness can be either *fatigue*—an exhausted feeling not relieved well by rest—or *excess day sleepiness*—feeling drowsy when slowing down, which usually responds to adequate rest. It's important to make the distinction, because the two have different causes. Fatigue is usually caused by medical illness (about 10 percent), sleep deprivation (about 20 percent), or mental disorders like depression and anxiety disorders (about 70 percent). Excessive sleepiness is almost always caused by inadequate night sleep—either too few hours or poor quality sleep. Thus, much of the tiredness people experience today is due to *sleep deprivation*—simply, they don't spend enough time asleep in bed. About seventy years ago, Americans became hooked on the notion that a person's worth was based on their measurable productivity—the numbers they generate, hours worked, income, status, and so on—and thus the conundrum of "having too much to do." This notion has caused great distress. For example, old people are seen as of lesser value because they are "less productive" (compare some Asian cultures, where the measure of worth has more to do with wisdom, character, vision, and the insights necessary to nurture and empower the young in meaningful ways). It's possible we may be killing ourselves both mentally and spiritually, and even physically, with this excessive productivity notion. Too many tend to think that sleep is a waste of time, or that they have too many other "more important" things to do instead. That kind of thinking leads to sleep deprivation, and is likely to be very costly to both health and quality of life. The National Sleep Foundation surveys find that 50 percent of Americans are sleep deprived, with 30 percent averaging less than six ✓ hours sleep per night.

If you wonder if you are getting enough sleep, take the Epworth Sleepiness Scale in Table 7.1.

**Table 7.1**    Epworth Sleepiness Scale (ESS)

| Situation | Chance of dozing (0–3) | | | |
| --- | --- | --- | --- | --- |
| Sitting and reading | 0 | 1 | 2 | 3 |
| Watching television | 0 | 1 | 2 | 3 |
| Sitting inactive in a public place—for example, a theater or meeting | 0 | 1 | 2 | 3 |
| As a passenger in a car an hour without a break | 0 | 1 | 2 | 3 |
| Lying down to rest in the afternoon | 0 | 1 | 2 | 3 |
| Sitting and talking to someone | 0 | 1 | 2 | 3 |
| Sitting quietly after lunch (with no alcohol) | 0 | 1 | 2 | 3 |
| In a car, while stopped in traffic | 0 | 1 | 2 | 3 |
| Total score | | | | |

| | |
| --- | --- |
| 0=would never doze | 2=moderate chance of dozing |
| 1=slight chance of dozing | 3=high chance of dozing |

**ESS total score ≥10 indicates possible excessive sleepiness or sleep disorder.**

Source: M.W. Johns. *Sleep.* 1991; 14:540–545. Reprinted with permission from the American Academy of Sleep Medicine.

Getting enough sleep is far more important to physical health than many realize, yet far too many people *don't* get adequate sleep. More than one-third of all Americans complain of trouble sleeping, and half of those feel that their inability to get enough sleep interferes significantly with their health or their ability to function. The frequency of insomnia increases with age: After age fifty, more than half of all Americans are unable to get the sleep they need.[1] For one-fourth of the troubled sleepers—approximately 9 percent of the population—the insomnia is chronic and unrelenting. Twenty-four percent of young adults (age 18–29) doze off while driving. (Such dozing causes more accidents than alcohol.)

That's not all: The total annual cost of sleep problems to Americans is startling—one careful and conservative estimate places the total cost of insomnia in the United States between $92.5 and $107.5 billion per year.[2] To put that in perspective, that's more than the cost of heart disease (at $43 billion a year) and comparable to the cost of cancer (at $104 billion a year).[3]

As a society, Americans now sleep less than their counterparts of previous generations. A Stanford study spanning more than seventy years shows that since 1910, the average time of sleep among Americans has decreased nearly two hours per night.[4] (Presumably nighttime lighting, television, and the desire to be more productive have cut sleep hours from the natural amount needed to provide adequate rest.) That two hours may not seem like much, but other studies show that a sleep deficit of just two hours per night has significantly detrimental effects on health, as will be discussed later in this chapter.

When patients in two general internal medicine clinics were recently surveyed, physicians found that 43 percent have bothersome sleeping problems—and problems with sleep was the third most common medical symptom listed by the patients (fatigue was first). But while almost half of any patient population may have problems sleeping, few of those ever mention their sleep problems to their physician. Another survey found that 69 percent of people with chronic insomnia had never let a physician know about the problem. Only 5 percent of patients with insomnia came to the physician specifically to get help for their insomnia, and an additional 26 percent mentioned it only incidentally while being evaluated for other problems.[5] Obviously, a very common and significant problem often remains undetected!

Research shows that there is a significant gender difference when it comes to insomnia. Women are more prone to insomnia than men—and are more susceptible to the mood-altering effects of sleep loss. This gender difference is even truer at menopause, particularly among women who experience hot flashes.[6] Insomnia is the most common bothersome menopausal symptom, and experience shows that estrogen replacement therapy reduces the number of nighttime awakenings.

There are three general kinds of sleep disturbance:

1. Trouble falling asleep

2. Trouble staying asleep (either waking up too early or waking up multiple times during the night)

3. Perception of inadequate sleep (not feeling refreshed after sleep)

Each of these types of sleep disturbance has different causes, and each calls for different types of treatment.

## Types and Causes of Insomnia

Different patterns of insomnia tend to have varying causes:

- **Initiatory insomnia,** or trouble falling asleep, may be caused by anxiety disorders or poor "sleep hygiene." Poor "sleep hygiene" can occur when a person or an environment is not conducive to sleep—for example, the room may be noisy, too light, too warm, or too cold, or the person's core body temperature may be too high.

- **Early awakening**—waking up at 3 or 4 A.M. and not being able to go back to sleep—is most commonly caused by clinical depression. Aging can also contribute, particularly if there is a need to go to the bathroom during the night.

- **Multiple awakenings**—waking up numerous times during the night, often with difficulty going back to sleep—may be caused by a medical problem, such as heart failure, acid reflux, or obstructive sleep apnea (with loud snoring). Depression also commonly causes multiple awakenings.

- **Daytime sleepiness,** as opposed to simple fatigue, is often caused by inadequate time in bed, but can also be caused by poor sleep quality from primary sleep disorders, an underlying medical problem, or *sleep phase advance* (common in teenagers), which will be discussed later. These potential causes need to be ruled out before assuming that the sleepiness is simply caused by too little time in bed. (Primary medical sleep disorders are discussed briefly later in this chapter.)

Far more than half of the people who come to primary care medical clinics with sleep problems also have problems with anxiety or depression. It is important to remember that sleep deprivation itself can, in turn, precipitate or contribute to a major depression or anxiety episode in a person who is under stress or who is genetically predisposed to depression or anxiety problems.

## Factors in the Development of Chronic Insomnia

Three major types of factors play a role in the development of chronic insomnia:[7]

1. **Predisposing factors.** These include a genetic predisposition to depression, anxiety, or insomnia; psychological coping styles; learned habits; the inability to relax; and age.

2. **Precipitating factors.** Chronic insomnia may be caused by a series of stressful events, a psychiatric or medical illness, environmental disturbances, or certain kinds of drugs used to treat unrelated medical or psychiatric conditions (a number of drugs cause sleep disturbances as a side effect).

3. **Perpetuating factors.** Perpetuating factors include mentally conditioned anxiety or arousal upon going to bed, poor sleep hygiene, a chronically stressed lifestyle, drugs used to treat medical or psychiatric conditions, or certain psychiatric disorders.

Alcohol, sleeping pills, caffeine, and tobacco are also important perpetuating factors, especially in a person who is trying to self-medicate, or use these substances to promote sleep (or, in the case of caffeine, to overcome daytime drowsiness). These substances disturb sleep in various ways:

- Caffeine and other stimulants inhibit the neurochemistry of sleep, disturbing the natural chemical balances in the brain that promote sleep. If one is not sleeping well, these should not be taken after 2 P.M.

- Alcohol causes what's known as a "rebound"; initial drowsiness is followed by wakefulness, which persists until there is absolutely no alcohol left in the body.

- Nicotine has a two-phase effect on sleep; at low levels, it is relaxing, but at high levels, it inhibits sleep.

- Activating medications, such as some antidepressants or treatments for Parkinson's disease, can interfere with sleep if taken late in the day.

- Typical sleeping pills or herbs that have been on the market for several years and that are used over an extended period of time may create a rebound effect; instead of promoting sleep, they may actually cause arousal.

- Herbs used for energy often contain high doses of caffeine and other stimulants.

## Mental Conditioning and Perpetuating Factors

Regardless of which precipitating factor contributes to insomnia, other components quickly enter the equation to create a "learned" (conditioned) ✓ insomnia. In other words, cognitive and behavioral components soon pitch in to create chronic insomnia, independent of what originally caused the problem. If treatment is to be effective, it is critical to understand what goes into that "conditioning" or learned response, particularly if the insomnia is chronic.

Mental conditioning is an essential part of life and allows us all to be able to effectively function through the day. For example, automatic conditioned responses come into play every time you tie your shoes or drive a car; those responses are triggered by the situation. When you are exposed to a situation to which you have responded in a certain, repeated way—such as seeing your untied shoelaces—the expected automatic response is elicited once again, usually both behaviorally and physiologically.

That's what happens with "repetitively practiced" insomnia as well. An initial stressor, particularly in a predisposed individual, can cause a few days of sleeplessness. For example, you may be making an important presentation at the end of the week, and thoughts about what you need to do and how well you need to perform may be racing through your mind. The more frustrated you get—and the more you worry about your possible poor performance or lack of well-being the next day—the harder you "try to sleep."

(Remember: "Trying" to do anything is arousing—and anything that is arousing causes you to stay awake.) You may then decide to do something active in order to avoid wasting time—so you get up, go over your presentation a few times, then watch some television.

As this pattern repeats itself for a few nights, a mentally conditioned effect is created. Gradually, you create an expectation, or mental "picture," of what is going to happen when you go to bed—you will become anxious and be unable to sleep. Once this conditioning has been established, it automatically takes over. As soon as you see your bed at bedtime, your mind automatically elicits its established response: You are frustrated, anxious, and unable to sleep, even though you're no longer dealing with the upcoming presentation. That frustrated, anxious response is "just what happens" when you're exposed to the bed, even when you are extremely tired.

Approaches to treating chronic insomnia that neglect this conditioning effect, which has usually become the predominant perpetuating factor, will be less effective than those methods that include reconditioning—learning a different behavior in response to the bed and bedtime.

## Why Do We Sleep?

The National Sleep Foundation describes at least two reasons we sleep:

1. **Repair and restoration.** During deep stages of sleep is when most growth hormone is secreted. This is needed for repair of the microinjuries (for example, from muscle use) we all sustain daily. Growth hormone deficiency, which occurs with loss of deep stages of sleep, causes aches and symptoms similar to depression. Also during sleep is when restoration occurs for many of the neurotransmitters that keep the nervous system running well. For example, sleep deprivation causes falls in central nervous system serotonin, which then can also worsen pain, depression, and anxiety.

2. **Integration of experience.** Particularly during REM (rapid eye movement, or dream) sleep, we seem to organize new memory and to incorporate the day's experiences into our worldview. Deprivation of REM sleep can sometimes cause psychosis-like symptoms.

### Five Stages of Sleep

Stages one and two are light sleep—dozing. Brain waves here show moderate activity. Much of the night is spent in stage two.

Stages three and four are deep sleep, when much restoration occurs. Brain waves here consolidate into large "delta waves," indicating that many neurons are firing in rested synchrony with each other.

REM sleep is when we dream, and is almost the opposite of deep sleep. The brain waves look much like they do when we are awake, but we are paralyzed so as not to act out the dreams. "REM sleep disorders" are characterized by some loss of this paralysis: walking, talking, and even doing seemingly purposeful but often bizarre things while sleeping. Other significant sleep disorders will be discussed near the end of this chapter.

# Behavioral and Psychological Effects of Insomnia

Sleep deprivation leads to some significant reductions in functioning, particularly in concentration, memory, well-being, enjoyment, coping, and motivation. Persistent sleep loss also causes an increased number of mistakes and boosts the incidence of irritability and depression.[8]

## Accidents

When compared to people who do not have insomnia, chronic insomniacs have four times the incidence of automobile accidents—a rate comparable to that caused by alcohol.[9] Falling asleep at the wheel causes half of all accidents that result in fatal injuries, and insufficient sleep is the primary cause of falling asleep at the wheel.[10]

The problem isn't limited to the highways. A strikingly large percentage of catastrophes caused by human error—including the nuclear disasters at Chernobyl and Three Mile Island—and many accidents in the workplace occur when operators are sleep-deprived or working on night shifts. Night shifts aren't the only problem, either; more than half of sleepy day shift workers have accidents, too.[11]

People with sleep problems also have 2.4 times more alcoholism than average,[12] which in turn also increases the rate of both industrial and automobile accidents.

## Depression

There is a major link between depression and insomnia in both directions: 70 to 90 percent of all depressed patients have insomnia,[13] and people with insomnia have 35 times the rate of depression as people who sleep well.

Insomnia often precedes depression, rather than simply being a consequence of depression. A well-designed study of almost 8,000 adults found that those with successfully treated insomnia had only 1.6 times the risk of subsequently developing clinical depression when compared to people who had never suffered with insomnia. But those with unresolved, continuous insomnia had nearly *40 times* the likelihood of developing subsequent major depression.[14] Over time, about 40 percent of untreated, chronic insomniacs develop major depression or anxiety disorders.

It doesn't take months of full-blown insomnia to cause a problem. Symptoms of depression can be caused by depriving normal people of just two hours less sleep than they need to feel good for as few as five nights.[15] When the sleep problem is corrected, the depression is usually relieved. (Perhaps the current "epidemic" of clinical depression may be compounded by the fact that the average American now gets one and one half to two hours less sleep than Americans did in 1910, as was mentioned earlier.)

Part of the reason for depression among those with sleep problems is that changes in day-night sleep cycles affect the brain chemicals that regulate mood. Research shows that people who have lived for months without clocks or external cues to light and dark cycles become depressed.[16] These mechanisms may account in part for the symptoms of depression that occur with jet lag and that often happen with changes in work schedules. Findings of some compelling research suggest that those who tend to get depressed should avoid jobs that require changes in work shifts. Shift work can indeed become hazardous to health, because it increases not only accident risk but also cardiovascular disease and mood disorders.

## Quality of Life and Function Issues

Lack of sleep has a significant impact on function, especially in the workplace.[17] People who suffer from insomnia are often simply too tired to perform their assigned tasks effectively. When workers are tired, mistakes occur and the rate of industrial accidents soars.

People who chronically don't get the sleep they need may also simply not show up at work—and if they do, they are generally far less productive than their colleagues. Insomnia is the second most powerful predictor of job absenteeism and lost productivity, and is an even more powerful predictor of absenteeism than job dissatisfaction.

The effects of insomnia spill over into most aspects of life, affecting both the quality of life and the stability of relationships. A study of 691 untreated insomniacs revealed that:[18]

- 83 percent were "easily upset, irritated, or annoyed."
- 78 percent were "too tired to do things."
- 59 percent had "trouble remembering things."
- 43 percent were "confused in their thinking."

Other proven complications of insomnia include reduced life satisfaction, unsatisfying relationships, reduced ability to cope, and reduced enjoyment of life.[19] Quality of sleep is also a powerful predictor of academic performance.[20]

Economists have known for decades about the "point of diminishing returns," which comes from studies of productivity in workers relative to the time and effort spent on the job. With more effort, productivity goes steadily up—to a certain point. And then, with more time and effort, productivity goes back down. When that happens—because of fatigue, burnout, and mental clumsiness—the point of diminishing returns has been reached. One then becomes *more* productive by reducing the time spent working back to where adequate rest allows for renewed energy, sharpness, and creativity. All these enhance the joy of life. And perhaps much of the purpose of life has to do with discovering what brings joy. One occasionally needs to ask, "Is all this I'm doing enhancing the joy, or getting in the way of it?"

# Physiological Effects of Insomnia[21]

Studies involving animals have shown that sleep deprivation causes malnutrition and weight loss.[22] Malnutrition may also occur in humans, along with increased pain and changes in other body systems. Compared to good sleepers, people with insomnia are hospitalized twice as often, are admitted to nursing homes twice as often, and have more than twice as many medical office visits.[23]

## Pain

Pain increases significantly as sleep decreases. In one study that has since been repeated twice with the same result, normal volunteers who were deprived of deep-stage sleep for a period of only several days developed muscle aches and pains similar to those of fibromyalgia,[24] a common muscular pain disorder caused by hypersensitivity of the pain system. Those aches and pains were relieved when the volunteers' sleep was allowed to return to normal.

The study was prompted by the fact that most people with fibromyalgia have sleep disturbance characterized by loss of deep-stage sleep, which also occurs in people with depression and those with chronic fatigue syndrome.[25] Researchers and physicians have noted that when sleep problems are corrected, patients with fibromyalgia usually experience improvement of muscle pain.[26] Exercise also reduced the increased pain caused by sleep loss, as did some medications that improve deep sleep.

Loss of deep-stage sleep also often accompanies other chronic pain problems. Insomniacs have two to three times the incidence of headaches, gastrointestinal pain, muscle pain, and back and neck pain as noninsomniacs.[27]

There is also a strong link between pain and depression in both directions: When depressed people are persistently deprived of deep sleep, they experience greater aches and pain, and two-thirds of chronic pain patients have major depression.

Some people become obsessed with cause and effect: Which comes first, the pain or the insomnia? Does the pain cause the insomnia, or does the insomnia cause the pain? Focusing on the result may be more appropriate: Clinical experience shows that treating the insomnia (or the underlying anxiety/depression, if present) *significantly* relieves pain and reduces other medical problems. Clinical experience also shows that attempts at treating chronic pain without restoring deep-stage sleep are likely to fail.

## Immune System Function

When people in experiments are deprived of sleep, the immune system stops functioning as it should.[28] When that happens, the body is not able to defend itself against invasion by bacteria, viruses, and other microorganisms—and illness, disease, and infection can result.[29] This may account in part for the fact that the body wants more sleep when infected—and why colds and other infections are more readily picked up when people have not had enough sleep.

Studies also show that sleep deprivation reduces the protective response provided by immunization.

## Hormonal Changes

Research also demonstrates that when people are chronically deprived of the sleep they need, hormonal changes occur in the body.[30] Especially impacted are thyroid and growth hormones, which are necessary for the repair of body tissues. Insulin resistance occurs, causing less blood sugar control (see Chapter 22).

## Nervous System Changes

The nervous system changes that occur with inadequate sleep are usually mild, but they can include tremors and increased gag and deep tendon reflexes. There is also an increased potential for seizures, and a worrisome loss of respiratory response to low oxygen levels.[31] As noted above, sleep deprivation also creates neurochemical changes in the brain (such as a fall in norepinephrine and serotonin) that can lead to depression and anxiety disorders, which in turn can cause a multitude of medical problems. (See Chapters 5 and 6.)

## Mortality

Mortality is 30 percent higher among people who sleep less than six hours a night (compared to those who sleep seven to eight hours a night). Inadequate sleep (less than six hours of sleep a night) also diminishes the protective effects of other good health practices, such as not smoking and getting regular exercise. A study of health-oriented churchgoers in California showed that the protective effects of avoiding smoking, alcohol, and unhealthy foods were lost when people did not get enough sleep.[32]

# Treatment of Insomnia

Appropriate treatment depends on the pattern of insomnia and how long the insomnia has been a problem.

**Transient insomnia** is insomnia that has lasted for only a few nights. It can usually be successfully treated by improving sleep hygiene (as detailed below) and using a short-term sleep medication. For example, a short-acting sedative used by night shift workers creates both better function and improved daytime sleep.[33]

**Short-term insomnia** is insomnia that has lasted for as long as three weeks. It should be treated the same as transient insomnia—by improving sleep hygiene and using short-term sleep medication—as well as by identifying and dealing with the precipitating stressor. Active treatment in the early stages of short-term insomnia can successfully prevent the conditioning that leads to chronic insomnia, which is much more difficult to treat.

**Chronic insomnia** is defined as sleep problems that have consistently occurred for more than three weeks. The treatment of chronic insomnia, which is much more difficult than the treatment of shorter-term sleep problems, involves treating the underlying psychological or medical condition, improving sleep hygiene, and undergoing behavioral reconditioning. A sleep medication may be used for as little as a few days to as long as three weeks to facilitate the mental reconditioning process. The downside of using medication, however, is that it can be tempting to continue the medication without doing the work of the behavioral reconditioning.

The integrated approach to chronic insomnia involves combining both medication and behavioral reconditioning. Older sleep medications generally work well during the first three weeks, then tend to lose effectiveness. Behavioral methods work more slowly at first, as they are being learned, but then increase substantially in effectiveness after the first two weeks— just as the effectiveness of the medication is declining. Some newer sleep medications are less likely to lose effect or show habituation (to create a habit, as in a dependency).[34]

In a study of older patients, researchers compared three groups of people with insomnia: those who were treated with medication alone, those who were treated with behavioral reconditioning alone, and those who were treated with a combination of medication and behavioral reconditioning.[35] After eight weeks, patients who underwent only the behavioral reconditioning were doing better than those who received only the medication. But the patients who had the most significant improvement were those who had a combined treatment of both behavioral reconditioning and medication.

One plausible explanation for these results makes a lot of sense: Behavioral therapies recondition what happens when the person goes to bed, promoting relaxation and sleep. Medication facilitates the reconditioning by causing sleepiness; after a few days of taking the medication, the person *expects* to be sleepy and get deeply relaxed when going to bed. The new behavioral reconditioning (particularly regularly practiced deep relaxation techniques) then maintains the improved sleeping pattern.

Successful treatment of chronic insomnia generally requires several types of behavioral reconditioning. Some behavioral therapies, such as stimulus control, are more effective for helping people get to sleep. Other types of behavioral therapies, such as progressive muscle relaxation, work better to deepen the quality of sleep.[36] Both types are explained in greater detail below.

When stress is a significant component of the sleep trouble, **cognitive behavioral therapy** can be highly effective, even more so than the progressive muscle relaxation described below. This therapeutic approach uses some of the behavioral techniques described below, but focuses on coming to think in more rational, productive ways about the situational stressors.

## Specific Behavioral Strategies for Treating Insomnia[37]

Some of the more effective behavioral strategies for treating insomnia include sleep hygiene, stimulus control, relaxation methods, thought stopping, exercise, and paradoxical intention.

### Sleep Hygiene

All people with insomnia can benefit from improving their sleep hygiene, which includes some of the following techniques:

- Do something enjoyable and relaxing before you go to bed in a routine, ritualistic way.

- Set your troubles and concerns aside. For example, if you're facing a hectic day, plan out on paper how you'll tackle all your demands well before going to bed, then forget about it. If you're afraid you might forget an important detail, call your own voice mail and leave yourself a reminder.

- Wake up at the same time seven days a week, and go to bed on time so that you get enough hours of sleep. Use an alarm to get up on time, no matter how much sleep you get that night.

- Avoid taking naps; naps almost always disturb the pattern of night sleeping.

- Expose yourself to plenty of bright light early in the day, particularly as soon as you wake up.

- Avoid caffeine after noon.

- Warm your body by taking a bath or exercising four to six hours before you go to bed.

- Avoid going to bed either hungry or full. A *small* snack can help promote sleep. Starches and foods containing tryptophan (such as walnuts and milk) increase the amount of the brain chemical serotonin, which promotes sleep. Avoid fluids after supper.

## Stimulus Control

Reinforce your bed as a sleep stimulus by limiting any nonsleep behaviors in or around bed. For example:

- Use the bed *only* for sleep and sex. Don't read, eat, watch television, study, or catch up on work from the office in bed (or in the bedroom).

- Go to bed only when you are feeling drowsy.

- If you haven't fallen asleep within ten to fifteen minutes after you get into bed, get out of bed, leave the bedroom, and read something dull somewhere else in the house until drowsy.

- Make sure the conditions in your bedroom are optimal for sleep. Your room should be dark and quiet, your room should be the right temperature (a room that is either too warm or too cool can interfere with sleep), your nightclothes should not be binding, and your bed should be comfortable and supportive (a mattress that is either too firm or too soft can also interfere with sleep).

## Relaxation Methods

Any kind of stress arouses both the mind and the body. Relaxation methods train you to mentally quiet the arousal of stress, inducing the relaxation response. With practice, you can produce deep relaxation rather quickly; this ability not only helps you fall asleep quickly, but also helps to quiet stress responses that occur during the day.

Some relaxation methods can be learned within a few days; others may take as long as three or more weeks to learn. Different people respond differently to each method, and each person will likely have a preference for a particular method that is based on the way he or she mentally processes information. For example, some people process information best if they have visual cues; others do best if they hear or feel the information. If you have difficulty learning a particular method after three weeks, your practitioner should have you learn a different method.

The relaxation methods most commonly used in the treatment of insomnia include the following:

- **Progressive muscle relaxation.** This helps people stay asleep and feel more refreshed. Specific muscle groups are tightened and then relaxed, with the tightening and relaxing of muscle groups progressing over the entire body. For example, using the in-breath to tense and the out-breath to relax, start at one foot, then one leg, then the other side, and slowly progress up each part of the body to the face and head. By focusing attention on the difference between how tension and relaxation feel, you can learn how to create relaxation from tension. This then can become a metaphor for life's stresses.

- **Imagery.** A beautiful, relaxing setting is experienced mentally in great detail; ideally, all the senses are involved in creating this mental image. When all the senses (sounds, smells, temperature, texture, and sights) are involved in creating and maintaining the mental image, the entire mind and body relax.

- **Self-hypnosis.** Progressively deepening relaxation is used to help the body "let go" of the tension it uses for protection. Some common methods of self-hypnosis include using a mental escalator, slowly counting, or imagining a heavy and warm feeling in the arms and legs.

- **Mindfulness.** Total attention is focused on one specific thing. For example, complete attention may be focused on a pattern of breathing, a harmonious sound (even music), slow and progressive counting, or the details of an image.[38]

- **Meditation.** Similar to mindfulness, meditation involves focusing on a word, a phrase, or a thought that has symbolic meaning.[39]

## Thought Stopping[40]

Thought stopping is a technique that helps people whose minds are crowded with "racing" or worrisome thoughts. Its foundation lies in the understanding that mental distress is caused not so much by events themselves as by the *thoughts* about those events. With simple training, you can learn to control those kinds of thoughts.

A technique called cognitive psychotherapy can help you change thoughts about underlying anxieties, and requires professional work over a period of time. A simpler technique that can help improve your sleep involves what is called "rapid thought stopping":

- As soon as your thoughts start to race or you have an unwanted thought, mentally say with definitive emphasis, "Stop!" Redirect your attention instead to a relaxing thought that you've planned for ahead of time. You might use meditation, mindfulness, or imagery to redirect your thoughts.

- If the unwanted thoughts reappear, repeat the process as needed, saying, "Stop!" more softly each time.

- Keep in mind that racing thoughts could be a symptom of a mood disorder (such as bipolar) that might need medical attention.

## Exercise

Exercise has a double benefit: It improves your ability to handle stress, which can interfere with sleep, and it changes your core body temperature in a way that promotes sleep.[41] When compared to people who are not fit and do not exercise, those who are physically fit get to sleep more quickly, wake up less often during the night, have more slow-wave sleep, and feel more rested when they wake up in the morning.[42]

Here's what happens: Normally, core body temperature falls at bedtime, and this drop in core body temperature causes a feeling of sleepiness. Exercise (or a hot bath) raises the core body temperature at first, but then induces a rebound drop in temperature approximately four to six hours later. This means that if you want to improve your sleep, you should exercise (or take a hot bath) about four to six hours before you want to go to bed and fall asleep (about 3 to 6 P.M. for most people). Be careful: If you exercise in the morning, you will get drowsy in the afternoon.

Rhythmic aerobic exercise is best for inducing sleep. Avoid any rigorous or hostile competition, which may undermine the stress-reduction effect of the exercise. As far as exercise is concerned, there's an important caveat to remember: Exercise increases deep sleep, but only if you are careful to replace body fluids after you exercise.[43]

## Paradoxical Intention

Oddly enough, *trying to stay awake* can make you sleepy. Why? The act of trying to stay awake apparently reduces the anxiety that is associated with trying to fall asleep.

## Sleep Restriction

This is surprisingly effective at times. First, the number of hours actually slept on an average night are calculated, then on following nights, a person is allowed to stay in bed only that number of hours. As drowsiness increases, each night the amount of sleep is slowly increased, until a full night's sleep is achieved.

## Sleep Hygiene Techniques

How does one choose which of these behavioral techniques to use? All sleep problems can benefit from good sleep hygiene. If the problem is trouble falling asleep:

- If you feel awake as soon as you go to bed: Use stimulus control and perhaps sleep restriction.
- If you are physically tense and anxious: Use cognitive behavioral therapy and progressive muscle relaxation.
- For mind racing: Use thought stopping and mindfulness practice.

If the problem is staying asleep:

- Use stimulus control and sleep restriction.

# Using Medication to Treat Insomnia

The studies that compared the effectiveness of behavioral and drug treatment (described earlier) suggest that medication is best used for periods of less than three to four weeks. For one thing, sleep medications tend to lose effectiveness after about three weeks. Additionally, using some of the older sleep medications for a long period can perpetuate the insomnia because of habituation, rebound anxiety, or insomnia when the medication is stopped. Some of the newer sleep medications, however, cause no drowsiness or impairment the next day and pose little risk of withdrawal or rebound insomnia. Nevertheless, if really necessary, such medications are best used in the short term to prevent or help solve the conditioning problems of insomnia.

Several kinds of medications are used to treat sleep problems, with varying success.

**Over-the-counter sleep aids** that contain antihistamines are generally not a good idea because of side effects, which can include:

- daytime drowsiness
- drying and slowing of the bowels
- dizziness
- reduced coordination

- weight gain
- paradoxical agitation or delirium (particularly in the young)

**Herbal sleeping medications** act like tranquilizing drugs, and need to be treated as such.

**Antidepressants** can be very useful if sleep problems are accompanied by anxiety or depression. In addition, antidepressants are not habit forming. They work better for awakening-type insomnia.

**Melatonin** is a natural, sedating neurotransmitter that the body secretes in response to darkness as part of normal sleep cycling and body rhythms. Studies have found that people with insomnia, especially the elderly, often have low blood levels of melatonin—often half that of people without insomnia.[44]

When melatonin supplements are used therapeutically, the melatonin can reset the timing of sleep rhythms when needed. While there are few well-controlled studies on the long-term use of melatonin for treatment of routine insomnia, studies *have* shown that short-term use of melatonin can be very useful for people with phase-shifting problems such as jet lag, changes in shift work, or delayed sleep phase. The usual dose used in these studies is 2 to 3 mg at bedtime, but that is 7 to 10 times the normal amount that is secreted by the brain. Taking such a dosage is probably not wise over a prolonged period of time, because it may disrupt necessary normal body cycles. Long-term side effects of even low doses are not known. Higher doses of melatonin can cause depression, and studies show that it contributes to the winter depression known as seasonal affective disorder (SAD).[45]

**Herbal sedatives and tranquilizers** need to be used with the same caution as any other drug. Unfortunately, the side effects of these preparations are often not known, and in some cases information about quality controls in manufacturing is not available.

**Amino acids** such as tryptophan (or SHTP), together with vitamin $B_6$ to help convert it to serotonin, can occasionally be helpful.

# Primary Medical Sleep Disorders

It's important to differentiate between the kind of insomnia that has been discussed in this chapter and *primary sleep disorders*, which are characterized by excessive daytime sleepiness.

Two of the characteristic hallmarks of primary medical sleep disorders are:

- Loud snoring accompanied by pauses in breathing while asleep (known as **sleep apnea**). **Obstructive sleep apnea** (OSA) can cause a multitude of serious health problems, including hypertension, cardiovascular disease, and swelling of the legs. When a person with OSA becomes deeply relaxed, the airways also relax and close off, obstructing air flow into the lungs. The resulting low oxygen causes recurrent arousals in the nervous system all night, blocking deep sleep and resulting in a system that starts to overrespond to stimuli, including pain. Anyone who snores and feels sleepy in the day should consider testing for this very common condition of sleep apnea.

- A crawling, creeping sensation in the legs that causes the legs to be constantly moving (called **restless legs syndrome**). Restless legs syndrome can also interfere with deep sleep, and is readily treatable medically. It seems to be caused by low central dopamine function.

People with primary medical sleep disorders need to be evaluated in a sleep lab, usually in a hospital setting, and require different kinds of treatment than those described above as effective for insomnia.

### Circadian Rhythm Disorders

In addition to shift work problems, these include sleep phase delay (often seen in teenagers) and sleep phase advance (often seen in the elderly).

Sleep phase delay is important to distinguish from insomnia, because its treatment is quite different and usually fairly simple. This disorder consists of the whole sleep cycle being shifted back a few hours—for example, feeling naturally inclined to fall asleep about 2 or 3 A.M. and to wake up around 10 or 11 A.M. if allowed to stay in bed (and usually sleeping well in between). This is treated for one to two weeks with melatonin, usually 1 mg at supper and 3 mg at the new, desired bedtime, followed by using bright light (sunlight or a light box) for sixty minutes at the desired wake-up time. The sleep phase will usually shift to a more socially acceptable time frame following this treatment.

Sleep phase advance (e.g., falling asleep at 7–8 P.M. and awakening at 4 A.M.) is treated in the opposite way: bright light in the evening and melatonin on awakening in the early morning. Light stimulates the tiny suprachiasmatic nucleus (about 20,000 neurons in the hypothalamus of the brain) to shut off melatonin secretion by the pineal gland. When melatonin falls, people wake up.

Such simple corrections of sleep cycles pay big dividends in quality of life.

## Conclusions

Insomnia and sleep deprivation are significant medical problems that need to be taken seriously. If you start having sleep problems that can't be resolved by fairly simple measures, tell your physician right away—the longer you struggle with sleep problems, the more likely you are to develop long-term or chronic insomnia as the brain becomes "conditioned" to expect them. Make sure you share any depression or anxiety problems with your physician as well; these problems exist in about half of all cases of chronic insomnia, can cause significant health problems if untreated, and are usually very treatable.

The most effective treatment for insomnia is usually an integrated approach that uses both short-term medication and behavioral reconditioning. Both medication and behavioral treatment are effective regardless of the duration of the insomnia, but behavioral reconditioning is especially important in the treatment of chronic insomnia.

In nature, insomnia is often a protective mechanism. Dolphins, for example, are able to let only half of their brain sleep at any given time; the "awake" half of the brain watches for sharks while the other half sleeps. We can learn a tremendous lesson from nature: As humans, we often create our own "sharks" out of the stresses we are faced with on a daily basis. The lesson? A deep sense of inner peace may be one of the most effective ways to promote restful sleep.

## ENDNOTES

1. G. D. Mellinger, M. D. Balter, and E. H. Uhlenhuth, "Insomnia and Its Treatment: Prevalence and Correlates," *Arch Gen Psychiatry* 42 (1985): 225–32.
2. M. K. Stoller, "Economic Effects of Insomnia," *Clinical Therapeutics* 16 (1994): 263–87.
3. P. E. Greenberg, L. E. Stiglin, S. N. Finkelstein, and E. R. Berndt, "The Economic Burden of Depression in 1990," *J Clin Psychiatry* 54 (1993): 405–18 (also 419–24).
4. Reported in the National Commission on Sleep Research, *Wake Up America: A National Sleep Alert,* vol. 1 of *Executive Summary and Executive Report* (Washington, DC: National Commission on Sleep Research, 1993), 17–37; and see also H. S. Friedman, J. S. Tucker, J. E. Schwartz, et al., "Psychosocial Predictors of Longevity: The Aging and Death of the Termites," *Am Psychol* 50 (1995): 69–78.
5. Gallup Organization, *Sleep in America: A National Survey of U.S. Adults* (Washington, D.C.: National Sleep Foundation, 1991).
6. J. Shaver, E. Giblin, M. Lentz, and K. Lee, "Sleep Patterns and Stability in Perimenopausal Women," *Sleep* 11 (1988): 560–61.
7. A. J. Spielman, L. S. Caruso, and P. V. Glovinsky, "A Behavioral Perspective on Insomnia Treatment," *Psych Clin No Amer* 10 (1987): 541–53; and see also H. M. Bearpark, "Insomnia: Causes, Effects and Treatment," in *Sleep,* edited by R. Cooper, 588–613 (London: Chapman and Hall Medical, 1994).
8. M. Kuppermann, D. P. Lubeck, P. D. Mazonson, et al., "Sleep Problems and Their Correlates in a Working Population," *J Gen Int Med* 10 (1995): 25–32.
9. A. I. Pack. "The Prevalence of Work-Related Sleep Problems," *J1 Gen Int Med* 10 (1995): 57; also see Gallup Organization, *Sleep in America,* M. B. Balter and E. H. Uhlenhuth, "New Epidemiological Findings About Insomnia and Its Treatment," *J Clin Psychiatry* 53, suppl. (1992): 34–39; P. K. Schweitzer, C. L. Engelhardt,

N. A. Hilliker, et al., "Consequences of Reported Poor Sleep," *Sleep Res.* 21 (1992): 2, abstract; and M. S. Aldrich, "Automobile Accidents in Patients with Sleep Disorders," *Sleep* 12 (1989): 487–94.

10. D. Leger, "The Cost of Sleep-Related Accidents: A Report for the National Commission on Sleep Disorders Research," *Sleep* 17 (1994): 84–93; and A. I. Pack, "The Prevalence of Work-Related Sleep Problems."

11. P. Lavie, "Sleep Habits and Sleep Disturbances in Industrial Workers in Israel: Main Findings and Some Characteristics of Workers Complaining of Excessive Daytime Sleepiness," *Sleep* 4 (1981): 147–58.

12. D. E. Ford and D. B. Kamerow, "Epidemiologic Study of Sleep Disturbances and Psychiatric Disorder: An Opportunity for Prevention?" *JAMA* 263 (1989): 1479–84.

13. F. Hohagen, K. Rink, C. Kappler, et al., "Prevalence and Treatment of Insomnia in General Practice: A Longitudinal Study," *Eur Arch Psych Clin Neurosci* 242 (1993): 329–36.

14. Hohagen et al., "Prevalence and Treatment."

15. T. Wehr, "Manipulations of Sleep and Phototherapy: Nonpharmacological Alternatives in the Treatment of Depression," *Clin. Neuropharmacol.* 13, suppl. 1(1990): S54–65.

16. S. H. Onen, F. Onen, D. Bailley, P. Parquet, "Prevention and Treatment of Sleep Disorders Through Regulation of Sleeping Habits," *Presse Med* 23 (1994): 485–89.

17. P. V. Leigh, "Employee and Job Attributes as Predictors of Absenteeism in a National Sample of Workers: The Importance of Health and Dangerous Working Conditions," *Soc Sci Med* 33 (1991): 127–37.

18. M. B. Balter, E. H. Uhlenhuth, "The Beneficial and Adverse Effects of Hypnotics," *J Clin Psychiatry* 52, suppl. (1991): 16–23.

19. Stoller, "Economic Effects of Insomnia."

20. M. W. Johns, H. A. F. Dudley, and J. P. Masterson, "The Sleep Habits, Personality and Academic Performance of Medical Students," *Med Educ* 10 (1976): 158–62; and D. Blum, A. Kahn, M. J. Morin, et al., "Relation Between Chronic Insomnia and School Failure in Preadolescents," *Sleep Res* 19 (1990): 1, abstract.

21. D. E. Ford and D. B. Kamerow, "Epidemiologic Study of Sleep Disturbances and Psychiatric Disorder," and M. H. Bonnet, "Sleep Deprivation ," in *Principles and Practice of Sleep Medicine,* edited by M. H. Kryger, T. Roth, and W. C. Dement, 55–68 (Philadelphia: W. B. Saunders, 1994).

22. C. A. Everson and T. A. Wehr, "Nutritional and Metabolic Adaptations in Prolonged Sleep Deprivation in the Rat," *Am J Physiol* 264, 2 pt. 2 (1993): R376–87.

23. Stoller, "Economic Effects of Insomnia", S. Weyerer and H. Dilling, "Prevalence and Treatment of Insomnia in the Community: Results Form the Upper Bavarian Field Study," *Sleep* 14 (1991): 392–98; J. D. Kales, A. Kales, E. O. Bixler, et al., "Biopsychobehavioral Correlates of Insomnia. V. Clinical Characteristics and Behavioral Correlates," *Am J Psychiatry* 141 (1984): 1371–76; and similar results were found in L. C. Johnson and C. L. Spinweber, "Quality of Sleep and Performance in the Navy: A Longitudinal Study of Poor Sleepers," in *Sleep/Wake Disorders: Natural History, Epidemiology and Long Term Evolution,* edited by C. Guilleminault and E. Lugaresi, 13–28 (New York: Raven Press, 1983).

24. H. Moldofsky, P. Scarsbrick, et al., "Induction of Neurasthenic Musculoskele-

tal Pain Syndrome by Selective Deep Sleep Stage Deprivation," *Psychosom Med* 38 (1976): 35–44.

25. C. L. Whelton, I. Salit, and H. Moldofsky, "Sleep, Epstein-Barr Virus Infection, Musculoskeletal Pain and Depressive Symptoms in Chronic Fatigue Syndrome," *J Rheumatol* 19 (1992): 939–43.

26. H. Moldofsky, "Sleep and Fibrositis Syndrome," *Rheum Dis Clin No Amer* 15 (1989): 91–103; also see H. Moldofsky, "Fibromyalgia, Sleep Disorder and Chronic Fatigue Syndrome," *Ciba Found Symp* 173 (1993): 262–79; and H. Moldofsky, P. Scarsbrick, R. England, and H. Smythe, "Musculoskeletal Symptoms and Non-REM Sleep Disturbance in Patients with 'Fibrositis Syndrome' and Healthy Subjects," *Psychosom Med* 37(1975): 341–51.

27. Kupperman, "Sleep Problems and Their Correlates in a Working Population."

28. Bonnet, "Sleep Deprivation," 57.

29. C. A. Everson, "Sustained Sleep Deprivation Impairs Host Defense," *Am J Physiol* 265, 5pt.2 (1993): R1148–54.

30. A. Baumgartner, K. J. Graf, I. Kurten, et al., "Neuroendocrinological Evaluations During Sleep Deprivation in Depression. I. Early Morning Levels of Thyrotropin, TH, Cortisol, Prolactin, LH, FSH, Estradiol, and Testosterone," *Biol Psychiatry* 28 (1990): 556–68; A. Baumgartner, D. Riemann, and M. Berger, "Neuroendocrinological Evaluations During Sleep Deprivation in Depression. II. Longitudinal Measurement of Thyrotropin, TH, Cortisol, Prolactin, GH and LH During Sleep and Sleep Deprivation," *Biol Psychiatry* 28 (1990): 569–87; and Bonnet, "Sleep Deprivation," 56–57.

31. Bonnet, "Sleep Deprivation," 56–68.

32. J. E. Enstrom, "Health Practices and Cancer Mortality Among Active California Mormons," *J National Cancer Institute* 81 (1989): 1807–14.

33. M. H. Kryger, *Principles and Practice of Sleep Medicine* (Philadelphia: Saunders, 1994).

34. H. Y. McClusky, J. B. Milby, P. K. Switzer, et al., "Efficacy of Behavioral Versus Triazolam Treatment in Persistent Sleep Onset Insomnia," *Am J Psychiatry* 148 (1991): 121–26.

35. C. Morin, J. Stone, C. Maghakian, et al., "Cognitive-Behavioral Therapy and Pharmacotherapy for Late-Life Insomnia: A Placebo-Controlled Trial," *Sleep Research* 22 (1993): abstract 21.

36. C. A. Espie, W. R. Lindsay, D. N. Brooks, E. M. Hood, and T. Turvey, "A Controlled Comparative Investigation of Psychological Treatments for Chronic Sleep-Onset Insomnia," *Behav Res Ther* 27 (1989): 79–88.

37. D. J. Buysse and C. F. Reynolds, "Insomnia," in *Handbook of Sleep Disorders,* edited by M. J. Thorpe, 375–433 (New York: Marcel Dekker, 1990); and A. J. Spielman, et al., "A Behavioral Perspective on Insomnia Treatment."

38. J. Kabat-Zinn, L. Lipworth, and R. Burney, "The Clinical Use of Mindfulness Meditation for the Self-Regulation of Chronic Pain," *J Behav Med* 8 (1985): 163–90; and J. Kabat-Zinn, *Full Catastrophe Living* (New York: Delacorte Press, 1990): 362–67.

39. J. Kabat-Zinn, L. Lipworth, R. Burney, and W. Sellers, "Four Year Follow-Up of a Meditation-Based Program for the Self-Regulation of Chronic Pain: Treatment Outcomes and Compliance," *Clin J Pain* 2 (1986): 159–73.

40. M. Davis, E. R. Eshelman, and M. McKay, "Thought Stopping," in *The Relaxation and Stress Reduction Workbook* (Oakland, CA: New Harbinger Public, 1988): 91–97.

41. P. Hauri and S. Linde, *No More Sleepless Nights* (New York: John Wiley,

1991): 130–31.

42. J. D. Edinger, M. C. Morey, R. J. Sullivan, et al., "Aerobic Fitness, Acute Exercise and Sleep in Older Men," *Sleep* 16 (1993): 351–59.

43. A. Montmayeur, A. Buguet, H. Sollin, and J. R. Lacour, "Exercise and Sleep in Four African Sportsmen Living in the Sahel: A Pilot Study," *Int J Sports Med* 15 (1994): 42–45.

44. I. Haimov, M. Laudon, N. Zisapel, et al., "Sleep Disorders and Melatonin Rhythms in Elderly People," *British Med J.* 309 (1994): 167.

45. J. S. Carman, R. M. Post, R. Buswell, and F. K. Goodwin, "Negative Effects of Melatonin on Depression," *Am J Psychiatry* 133 (1976): 1181–86; and A. J. Lewis, N. A. Kerenyi, and G. Feuer, "Neuropharmacology of Pineal Secretions," *Drug Metabol Drug Interact* 8 (1990): 247–312.

# CHAPTER 8

# The Disease-Resistant Personality

*The mind is its own place, and in itself can make
a heaven of hell, a hell of heaven.*

—John Milton

## Learning Objectives

- Understand the role of stress in health.
- Define the basic mechanisms of stress and how they impact health.
- Identify major stress buffers.
- Define the personality traits that help people resist disease.
- Identify healthful choices that will promote disease resistance.

Too often we ask ourselves why someone became ill instead of how someone has managed to stay well. As Pennsylvania State University's Evan G. Pattishall reflected, if we study twenty-five people who are exposed to the influenza virus and five of them get sick, "we tend to study the five who developed influenza, when we should be exerting even more effort studying the twenty who didn't become ill."[1]

Howard S. Friedman echoed that sentiment when he wrote, "Each week the prestigious *New England Journal of Medicine* publishes a 'Case Record of the Massachusetts General Hospital,' detailing the pathology of an unusual or informative patient's case. There is no corresponding 'Case History of a Person Who Remained Well Throughout a Long Life.'"[2]

Researchers have long known that certain groups of people enjoy "remarkable good health and longevity." Among them are "Mormons, nuns, symphony conductors, and women who are listed in *Who's Who*. This suggests that something in the way these people live, possibly even such abstractions as faith, pride of accomplishment, or productivity, plays a role in diminishing the ill effects of stress."[3]

**251**

The way we behave influences health. Whether we smoke cigarettes, sip wine before dinner, start the day with a brisk walk, and eat fatty foods all affect our health. But could something other than behavior play a role in our ability to withstand stress and stay healthy? Researchers believe so. And the key may lie in personality, because apparently personality is a major determinant in how well we are able to resist stress.

## The Role of Stress in Health

Medically speaking, stress is a fairly new concept. Only in the last fifty years or so have researchers been able to pinpoint some of the effects of stress on the human body. And much of what we know about stress today originated with pioneer researcher Hans Selye. Early in this century, physicians believed that each disease was caused by a distinct and separate agent. But Selye, then a medical student in Prague, was puzzled by something he observed in the hospital: Patients with a wide variety of illnesses shared a number of symptoms (especially fatigue, joint pains, and weight loss). If distinct organisms caused each disease, Selye wondered, how could patients with so many different diseases all have the same symptoms?[4]

Unable to solve the mystery, Selye moved on, largely forgetting the puzzling patients in the hospital. Ten years later, a totally unrelated experiment with rats focused Selye's mind sharply back on those hospital patients.

Selye set out to test a chemical extract that he believed contained a new ovarian hormone. The experiment required that the laboratory rats be injected at frequent intervals with the extract; a control group of rats was injected at the same frequency, but with ordinary saline. After days of being jabbed with the needle, the rats who were receiving the chemical extract started developing an unexpected set of symptoms: enlarged and overactive adrenal glands, withered thymuses (a sign of a deteriorating immune system), and gastric ulcers. The rats who were injected with the saline solution developed the same set of symptoms.

Selye thought back to the hospital where he had worked ten years earlier. What occurred to him then became the cornerstone of stress research: He realized that both the patients and the rats were reacting to stress. And he believed that no matter what causes distress (whether it's a terminal illness, an overdrawn checking account, or a fight with a spouse), the body's reaction is the same. Selye called that reaction "the stress response," and it has become well documented during the ensuing decades of medical research.

The decades of research that have focused on the human stress response and its associated ills have also posed a fascinating question: Why do some people who undergo chronic stress fall ill while others sail through unscathed? One of the researchers most intrigued by that question was

Suzanne Ouellette Kobasa, who teaches psychology in the City University of New York's graduate school. She was familiar with all the state-of-the-art research that drew definite connections between stress and illness—but she believed there had to be a middle ground. It is impossible to avoid stress altogether; some stressful events (such as the death of a loved one) are completely beyond control. And, she concluded, even if it were possible to completely avoid stress, that would be "a prescription for staying away from opportunities as well as trouble. Since any change can be stressful, a person who wanted to be completely free of stress would never marry, have a child, take a new job, or move."[5]

Kobasa had other concerns, too. The popular notion regarding stress and illness, she believed, ignored "a lot of what we know about people. It assumes we're all vulnerable and passive in the face of adversity. But what about human resilience, initiative, and creativity? Many come through periods of stress with more physical and mental vigor than they had before."[6]

The more she pondered the stress-illness connection, the more engrossed Kobasa became with the people who didn't get sick under stress—and the more intent she became on discovering why. In 1975, she mobilized a group of her colleagues and went to work on a study of what she calls "the walking wounded of the stress war"—a group of high-powered business executives faced with personal and career upheaval.

## The Mechanisms of Stress

The American Academy of Family Physicians has estimated that 60 percent of all problems brought to physicians in this country are stress-related, and the problems that aren't directly caused by stress are made worse—or last longer—because of it.[7] Every week, some 95 million Americans suffer a stress-related problem and take medication for their aches and pains. And there's a greater toll than just the personal one; American businesses lose an estimated $150 billion each year to its employees' stress-related problems.[8]

Hosts of experiments have shown that people are susceptible to the ravages of stress. In one particularly interesting study, pediatricians wanted to determine why some children get sick when they are exposed to a certain bacteria while others stay healthy. Pediatricians Roger Meyer and Robert Haggerty chose the streptococcus bacteria, a variety that was usually harmless, not the virulent form that causes strep throat, ear infections, and scarlet fever, noting that "peaceful coexistence between this organism and its human host is the rule, while disease is the exception."[9] Many children harbor the bacteria—but only a few get sick as a result. The researchers wanted to figure out why.

To get some answers, they watched sixteen families, each with two or more children, for a year. They noted every possible factor: the child's age, sex, family health history, antibody response, size of family, housing conditions (such as type of heating system and number of rooms), type of medical treatment received, whether the child had had a tonsillectomy, weather conditions throughout the study, and special stresses at home. Every three weeks, the two doctors checked on the family's health and took throat cultures from everyone.

After monitoring the rates of infection for a year, the doctors started to look for patterns. One was age: School-aged children got sick the most often, probably because they are continually exposed to a wider range of bacteria. Also, children who shared rooms with infected people had a higher rate of infection. And time of year seemed to have a role: Most outbreaks were in the early spring (March or April).

Throughout the study, family members were asked to keep diaries in which they noted particular stresses. Crises were noted, ranging from a grandmother dying in one family to the house burning in another. As researchers noted increases in stress in the diaries, they saw a corresponding increase in strep illness among affected family members.

The results were specific and astonishing. In one family, a visiting uncle with tonsillitis exposed the entire family to infection at the beginning of a month. Of the family of six (four children and the parents), only one was ill by the end of the month—the oldest daughter, who was under tremendous pressure at the time of her uncle's visit to learn her catechism in time for her confirmation.

The researchers concluded that stress was four times as likely to precede an infection as to follow it. Throughout the year of the study, only about one-fifth of the low-stress families had any infection, whereas half of the high-stress families did. Does stress cause infection? Researchers don't think so. They are convinced, however, that stress compromises the immune system enough for infection to take hold.[10]

If stress research has shown one thing, it is that stress alone won't cause illness. How a person reacts to stress does. Your personality, your unique way of viewing things, will determine what impact stress has on you.

Watching general population groups during stress demonstrates this principle well. The Irish are one example. When the Irish were transplanted by the thousands to the eastern seaboards of America during the last century, their standard of living improved dramatically. Conditions were much cleaner, and they had plenty of food to eat (while they faced starvation in Ireland). But the death rate from tuberculosis soared. While the transplanted Dubliners were better housed and better fed, the tuberculosis death rate was 100 percent higher than it was during the same period in Dublin, where the conditions were much worse. Why did the Irish die of tuberculosis despite such dramatically improved conditions? Many did not want to migrate to America—and they were unprepared for the discrimination they faced.[11]

For example, when the American Indians were forced off the Plains and onto reservations (often within only a few miles of where they had lived), they had much better sanitation and a higher standard of living. Considering physical conditions alone, they should have enjoyed much better health. But that was not the case. Again, deaths from tuberculosis increased.[12] They were being uprooted from the land of their forefathers. Their traditions were in danger. They felt powerless—and they gave in.

A third example is the Bantu natives in South Africa. They were moved in droves from their native villages into Johannesburg, where sanitation was dramatically better and where food and housing were vastly improved. Thousands became ill with tuberculosis. When hundreds of the dying were permitted to return to their native villages to die, the tuberculosis bacillus was then spread throughout the villages. But the people who had remained in the villages didn't get sick.[13]

Was it the move alone that made these populations sick? Chinese and Hungarian refugees overcame great odds and dangerous political upheaval to immigrate to the United States. Although their new home represented a place vastly different than the one they left, they thrived. They viewed their new lives as an opportunity and a challenge, not as a negative.[14]

The effect is even more pronounced in populations in which one segment has a different outlook than another. Take, for example, a group of Portuguese who immigrated to Canada for employment reasons. The men who immigrated saw the move as a chance for a better job and a new future—and their health actually improved after their move to Canada. Their wives saw the move as a disruption of their valued family ties in Portugal—and they were more likely to get sick.[15]

## Stress Buffers

Some things have been identified as "stress buffers," or elements that alleviate the deleterious effects of stress. Controversy surrounds some of these findings, but researchers have generally shown that social support, a sense of control, physical fitness, a sense of humor, self-esteem, optimism, coping styles, and Kobasa's "hardiness" personality all help to buffer stress.[16] Most important may be what's within a person—how a person reacts to and views the situation that has created stress. Dr. N. Lee Smith defines the components of stress resilience as caring love (committed to the fulfillment of the other), responsible free will (able to create your own life experience and influence events), integrity (being true to core values), challenge (enjoying growth), and hope (feeling positive expectation).

In her revolutionary studies on stress and illness, Kobasa and her colleague Salvatore Maddi commented, "We could not believe that the same human imagination responsible for urbanization and industrialization was somehow incapable of coping with the . . . ensuing pressures and disruptions. It seemed obvious that the individual differences in response to stress were important."[17]

With that attitude, Kobasa and her colleagues decided to expand their stress and illness studies beyond the original group of Illinois telephone company executives. Would the same principles hold true in other populations?

Others have done similar studies, and their findings have been remarkably consistent with Kobasa's. Lawrence Hinkle and his associates in the departments of medicine and psychiatry at New York Hospital's Cornell Medical Center conducted a series of studies over a twenty-year period. They found that personality traits had a definite bearing on health. They concluded that those with "a good attitude and an ability to get along with other people" enjoyed the lowest frequency of illness.[18]

In another study, two psychiatrists, an endocrinologist, and a cancer specialist in New York teamed up to determine the stress reactions and hormonal changes that occurred when people were faced with a truly life-threatening situation. To test their theories, they picked a group who did face a life-threatening situation: Thirty women who were undergoing biopsies for breast tumors at Montefiore Hospital and Medical Center.

To determine the amount of "distress" each woman was suffering, researchers did tests to measure how much hydrocortisone each woman secreted per day. (Hydrocortisone is a hormone secreted by the adrenal gland in response to stress. The researchers measured it each day for the three days preceding each woman's biopsy.) At the end of the study, the researchers concluded that the crisis of possibly having cancer wasn't what determined how much or how little distress each woman experienced. The determining factor was each woman's "psychological defenses" or coping style—especially her outlooks and beliefs. The lowest amount of adrenal hormone was secreted by a forty-five-year-old woman who consistently used faith and prayer to deal with life's stressful events. The woman who fared the next best was a fifty-four-year-old who had a healthy philosophical acceptance of adversity.

## Gender Differences

Interestingly, there appear to be differences in the way men and women handle stresses—and the differences appear to be tied much more to emotion, personality, and sociology than to biology, especially to gender role socialization among men.[19]

According to researchers, emotions are largely learned behaviors, and—as discussed elsewhere in this book—the efficient handling of emotions is a key to good health. It is generally accepted among those who study disease resistance and proneness that men are not as efficient as women in dealing with emotions, and that ineffective emotion management is implicated in each of the four causes of death for which men's death rates are twice as high as women's: accidents, suicide, cirrhosis of the liver, and homicide.[20] Those same researchers suggest that significant reductions in death rates among men could be achieved if men learned healthier ways of handling their feelings.[21]

There are particular areas of emotion that men are socialized toward that can harm health—and areas in which changes could promote disease resistance.

## Anger and Hostility

Studies show that men are more likely than women to have cynical hostility and poorly controlled anger.[22] Unfortunately, boys tend to learn harmful lessons about anger and aggression in childhood. First, parents tend to be more accepting of expressed anger in their sons than in their daughters.[23] That's not all: The gender role socialization for boys actually encourages them to be aggressive when they get angry.[24] Boys are often given "messages" from the media—as well as their peers and often their parents—that it is appropriate to settle arguments by wrestling, hitting, kicking, pushing, or shoving. In many cases, physical aggression is required for boys to earn respect from peers both at school and in the neighborhood.[25] During a time that girls are learning that it's good to express emotions (other than anger), boys are learning that anger shows masculinity and toughness—but that other emotions demonstrate weakness and cowardice. As shown in Chapter 4, the health effects of anger and hostility are devastating, and men who are not able to overcome early socialization are at risk as a result.

## Depression and Grief

Most of the major studies on depression have focused on women—possibly because only an estimated 13 percent of men struggle with major depression at some time during their lives.[26] Many now believe, however, that depression among men is undiagnosed and underreported, probably because men are socialized not to complain about (or admit to) sadness or guilt.[27] Instead, men are prone to see their physicians about the less stigmatized symptoms of depression, such as fatigue or irritability. One large study found that physicians failed to properly diagnose depression in almost two-thirds of men who actually were depressed.[28]

The cause of depression in men is much the same as that in women: the unfinished mourning of a loss, including death, divorce, the end of a significant relationship, the loss of a job, or retirement (which often represents the loss of status or financial security). Unfortunately, though, men are taught as boys to "keep a stiff upper lip" and to avoid crying—at least in public. They are much less likely to reach out and discuss their feelings with their male friends;[29] in fact, one prominent scholar contends that *alexithymia* (having no words for emotions) is so common among men that it is considered normal.[30] If it is a factor, alexithymia obviously prevents men from successfully completing grief work after a major loss.

## Substance Abuse and Misuse

Studies consistently show that men have much higher rates of substance abuse and misuse than do women.[31] Studies also show that men turn to substance abuse/misuse to assuage difficult or painful feelings, and the type of substance they use depends on the feelings or type of pain they are trying to deal with.[32]

There are other factors as well. For example, drinking alcohol is considered an integral part of becoming a man in the United States; in most areas, there is a firm association between alcohol use and manliness. Because there is such widespread acceptance of alcohol use among men, they rely on alcohol more often than women to cope with stressors. As a result, in the United States men are twice as likely to engage in heavy drinking episodes (more than five drinks in one sitting),[33] and heavy episodic drinking is the leading cause of death among America's college undergraduate students.[34]

# Personality Traits That Keep Us Well

The cumulative results of studies conducted over the past three or four decades—Kobasa's as well as others—show beyond a doubt that certain personality traits keep us well, boost our immunity, and improve our immune systems. Perhaps most convincing was a study of 650 children in Hawaii.

In their book *Vulnerable but Invincible,* researchers Emmy Werner and Ruth Smith report their study of the 650 children, born and reared on the island of Kauai in Hawaii. The children in the study were followed from a few months before their birth until they were in their early twenties. They were assessed at regular intervals with a battery of interviews, questionnaires, and examinations; researchers monitored their health records closely.[35]

By all standards, these children were at high risk. All were born into poor families and lived in chronic poverty. Many were born to single mothers, some of whom were depressed or schizophrenic. The fathers of those who did have fathers in the home were semiskilled or unskilled laborers. The children were born prematurely at higher than average rates; many were victims of severe perinatal stress. The mothers had little formal education (none had graduated from high school). The families themselves were plagued by a multitude of problems.

The stresses didn't end there. As psychologist Robert Ornstein and physician David Sobel put it:

*They came of age in the years 1955 to 1979—a time of unprecedented social change. They had to deal with the influx of many newcomers from the U.S. mainland during the long war in Southeast Asia and later with the burgeoning of tourism. They witnessed the assassination of one president and the resignation of another. They were the first generation to deal with the invasion of the home by television. They faced unprecedented choices since they had access to contraceptive pills and mind-altering drugs.[36]*

The combination of these biological and social stresses took their toll on some of the children. By the age of ten (the first major interval the researchers used), at least half of the children were in serious trouble. They were in physical ill health, had serious behavioral problems, and had learning disabilities that impacted their ability to progress through the school system.

By the age of eighteen, the next major follow-up period, an additional 25 percent—or three-fourths of all the children in the study—had very serious problems. Those who didn't have profound psychological problems did have learning disabilities, behavioral problems, and poor health.

That didn't surprise anyone. After all, these kids had started out under the most dreadful conditions and had grown up in an environment charged with unrelenting stress. What did surprise researchers was the group of kids—approximately one-fourth of the group studied—who, despite all the stress, rallied. They prevailed with strong psychological adjustment, good health, and enviable school records. Ornstein and Sobel describe three of them:

*Life did not start out well for Michael. His mother was sixteen years old, unwed, and lived with her mother and grandmother. She managed to hide her pregnancy from her own mother until the third trimester when she married a nineteen-year-old boy. The child's biological father was very much against the marriage. The mother did not receive any medical care until the seventh month of pregnancy, and Michael was born prematurely and weighed only four pounds ten ounces. Michael spent the first three weeks of his life in an army hospital. At two, Michael's adoptive father was sent with the army to Korea, where he remained for two years. At age eight, Michael's parents divorced and his mother left, leaving him with his father and three younger siblings.*

*Early life was also not easy for Kay. She was born to seventeen-year-old unmarried parents. They had both been asked to leave school because of the pregnancy, and the father was without a job. Family Court sent Kay's mother to a Salvation Army Home to have her baby; placing her for adoption was considered but rejected, and the parents were eventually married when Kay was six months old despite objections from their parents. Kay's parents later separated.*

*Mary got off to a rough start as well. Her mother's pregnancy occurred after many unsuccessful attempts to conceive and a previous miscarriage. Her mother was very much overweight and had various minor medical problems during pregnancy. She was hospitalized three times for severe false labor and eventually was in labor for more than twenty hours. During Mary's childhood her parents experienced financial difficulties, and her mother found it necessary to work outside the home for short periods. Between Mary's fifth and tenth birthdays, her mother had several major illnesses, surgeries, and two hospitalizations for "unbearable tension," nervousness, annoyance with her children, and fears that she might harm them.[37]*

How did things turn out for the three? Despite everything, they grew up to be healthy, well-adjusted, successful adults. Michael ranked at the top of his class and was awarded a college scholarship. Well-liked by his peers, he was described as confident, persistent, self-assured, dependable, and realistic. Kay did well throughout life. She was an alert, healthy, affectionate, and robust baby; as a child, she had above-normal grades in school and was described as agreeable, relaxed, and mentally normal. As an adult, she was described as poised, sociable, self-assured, respectful and accepting of others, and a person who made good use of the abilities she had. She planned to go into the entertainment field and to marry. Mary was described as having high self-esteem, persistence, concern for others, and an outgoing personality; she was willing to open herself up to new possibilities after only initial hesitancy. She planned to enroll in college, and was keeping her future career goals open. At eighteen, Mary described herself this way:

*If I say how I am it sounds like bragging—I have a good personality and people like me. . . . I don't like it when people think they can run my own life—I like to be my own judge. I know right from wrong, but I feel I have a lot more to learn and go through. Generally, I hope I can make it—I hope.[38]*

Hope seemed to be a key attitude with the children who prevailed over their difficult circumstances. So did perseverance. They were what Indiana psychiatric social worker Katherine Northcraft calls transcenders—people who, "in the worst of times, envision themselves as elsewhere, imagining that they can do great things despite their surroundings."[39] Despite difficult family situations, these resilient children developed strong bonds with a parent, grandparent, sibling, or other caretaker, usually early in life (almost always during the first year). When they felt confused or troubled, they sought help—but they were also children who eagerly accepted challenge. These children had personalities that kept them healthy, and enabled them to overcome adversity. They were, in Kobasa's terms, "hardy."

Where do resilient traits come from? No one knows for sure. Some of them may be inborn. Werner found that most of the resilient children in her study had been alert, sociable, even-tempered, responsive infants. "There seems to be a group of children who temperamentally and probably constitutionally have a better chance of making lemonade out of lemons," she believes. Does that doom the rest—those who are introverted, shy, or difficult? Not necessarily, she says—it's just that "it's easier for those who are more outgoing to find support."[40]

According to psychologist Ann Masten, associate director of the University of Minnesota's Institute of Child Development, the fact that Werner's resilient children had a strong adult figure is important. "When resilient adults talk about how they made it, virtually everyone mentions a key adult," she explains. But that adult doesn't have to be a parent. In fact, in her study of more than 200 resilient children, many found inner strength through bonds they developed with a neighbor, family friend, teacher, minister, or other respected adult.[41]

A similar study—started by one researcher in the early 1920s and continued by others over a period spanning seven decades—provides what scientists call "the first evidence of its kind" and may give further information about the concept of disease resistance. In the early 1920s, Stanford researcher Lewis Terman recruited 1,178 eleven-year-old gifted children who had been recommended for the study by their teachers.

At the outset, Terman had parents and teachers rate the children on more than two dozen psychological and intellectual traits. Terman himself then used a set of scales—called "remarkably modern" by University of California, Riverside, researcher Howard Friedman—to rate the children. Terman's scales included sociability, energy level, self-esteem/motivation, conscientiousness/dependability, moodiness, and cheerfulness. Terman began the study, and his successors continued to track the volunteers over the next seventy years.

According to the researchers, two clear patterns emerged. First, conscientious, dependable people who showed permanence and stability of mood lived significantly longer than the others. Second, in a surprise to researchers, cheery optimists lived substantially shorter than normal.

Why? One reason might be the tendency of an optimist to underestimate the gravity of certain risks—and the tendency of the conscientious to stay organized, plan ahead, and be prepared for the unexpected.[42]

### Hardiness

Hardiness is "a set of beliefs about oneself, the world, and how they interact. It takes shape as a sense of personal commitment to what you are doing, a sense of control over your life, and a feeling of challenge."[43]

Kobasa defines the personality traits of hardiness as "the three Cs": commitment, control, and challenge. Commitment is an attitude of curiosity and involvement in what is happening around you, control is the belief that you can influence events instead of becoming a victim, and challenge is the belief that change brings a chance for growth instead of the fear that change is threatening.[44]

## Commitment

Commitment—an attitude of curiosity and involvement in what is happening around you—means a commitment to yourself, your work, your family, and the other important values in your life. This is not a fleeting involvement, but a deep and abiding interest. People who are committed in this way have a deep involvement with their work and their families, a deep sense of meaning, and a pervasive sense of direction in their lives. In one study involving students at Harvard Medical School, students best able to withstand stress were personally committed to a goal of some kind.[45]

A sense of challenge often drives us to a hectic pace filled with plenty of pressures—but it is healthy, because there is a drive to live life to its fullest. The important element, say some researchers, is commitment to an ideal greater than oneself.[46] For some people, that commitment comes in the form of commitment to a religion; for others, it's a commitment to political reform or to a certain philosophy. And some healthy people have a deep sense of commitment to something as simple as a hobby.

A perfect example is Mohandas K. Gandhi, a man who by all standards was a driven workaholic. He went on countless fasts, depriving himself of nourishment, and spent months in prison—one of the most stressful scenarios possible. Yet he was strong and healthy until his assassination at the age of seventy-seven. Many believe it was because of his unwavering commitment to become one of the world's great leaders and to win political freedom for his homeland.

## Control

As defined by psychologist S. C. Thompson in 1981, control is "a belief that one has at one's disposal a response that can influence the aversiveness of an event. . . ." It's the belief that you can cushion the hurtful impact of a situation by the way you look at it and react to it. The kind of control that keeps you healthy is the opposite of helplessness. It is the firm belief that you can influence how you'll react, and the willingness to act on that basis. It's the refusal to be victimized. It is not the erroneous belief that you can control your environment, your circumstances, or other people; that kind of an attitude leads to illness, not health. The control that keeps you healthy is a belief that you can control yourself and your own reactions to what life hands you.

The healthiest Harvard Medical School students were the ones who approached problem solving with a sense of control; the least healthy were those who were passive.[47] The healthiest and hardiest people are those who focus on what they can control, ignoring the rest. Through skill, planning, and diligent attention to detail, they believe that every problem has a solution.

We all want to be able to predict what will happen to us. We all crave a sense of mastery. No one wants to feel responsible without being in control.[48] A sense of control—a belief that you can control your own behavior, not necessarily control the people and events around you—promotes health. It endows you with the belief that even if everything around you gets bad, you will still be fine.

### Challenge

Challenge means the ability to see change as an opportunity for growth and excitement. Excitement is critical, because boredom puts people at a high risk for disease.[49] People who are constructively challenged are more healthy—and a German philosopher mused that one of the two biggest foes of human happiness is boredom.

A person who is not healthy and hardy views change with helplessness and alienation. A healthy, hardy person can face change with confidence, self-determination, eagerness, and excitement. Change becomes an eagerly sought-after challenge, not a threat. Joan C. Post-Gorden, psychologist at the University of Southern Colorado, says that healthy people don't even see the negatives, because they thoroughly expect a positive outcome.[50]

That healthy view of challenge is exemplified by Mary Decker Slaney, the world-class runner who has broken four world records.[51] The stress of competition is crushing—yet she has stayed healthy, and keeps competing. When asked why, she responded, "I love it. Running is something I do for myself more than anything else." Those positive emotions and personal triumph demonstrate a great sense of healthy challenge. And since every life is filled with obstacles, it stands to reason that the way we view those obstacles—whether as crushing problems or as challenges to be eagerly met—determines in part how healthy we are.

Research showed that among more than sixty HIV-positive gay men, those who treated their HIV-positive status as a challenge—and then developed strategies to fight it—had improved natural killer cell activity. University of Miami psychiatrist Karl Goodkin, who spearheaded the study, said that an active coping style, along with fewer life burdens and good social support, led to improvement of natural killer cell activity and immunity.[52]

### Coherence

Adding to Kobasa's "three C's" is coherence—a "pervasive, enduring though dynamic feeling that one's internal and external environments are predictable and that there is a high probability that all things will work out as well as can be reasonably expected."[53] Other research verifies that stress-resistant personality traits include involvement in work or other tasks that have great meaning, the ability to relate well to others, and the ability to interact in a strong social network. The most vulnerable people are those who are socially isolated. The healthiest Harvard Medical School graduates sought out other people, were actively and empathically engaged with other people, and had strong social networks.[54]

## Healthful Choices

People with a disease-resistant personality tend to exercise regularly; 80 percent of the healthiest Harvard Medical School students engaged in regular aerobic exercise, while only 20 percent of the ill students did.[55] They relax for at least fifteen minutes a day.[56] They limit refined sugars in their diet, and limit stimulants (such as nicotine and caffeine).[57] In the Harvard study, healthy students used a minimum of "substances"—things they considered to be drugs or drug-like, including nicotine and caffeine.[58] "Hardy" people also tend to engage in more consistent health behaviors—"and, therefore, when under stress are physically more resistant to disease and illness."[59]

Hardiness or stress-resistant personality traits may combine with healthy behaviors to result in enhanced resistance to disease. "When individuals have high health concern they are more likely to engage in appropriate health behavior if they are at the same time high in hardiness," one researcher concluded. "When hardy people become concerned about their health, they are more likely than nonhardy people to engage in appropriate health-protective behaviors."[60]

The hardy (or disease-resistant) personality is summed up in a profile provided by Ornstein and Sobel:

> A small, neat man in his mid-50s, Chuck L. introduced himself as someone who enjoys solving problems. In the company, his specialty is customer relations, even though he was trained as an engineer. His eyes light up as he describes the intricacies of investigating customer needs and complaints, determining the company's service capabilities and obligations, formulating possible solutions that appear fair to all parties, and persuading these parties to agree. He thinks customer relations work is more demanding as the company streamlines and approaches reorganization. Asked in a sympathetic manner whether this is making his job unmanageable, he notes an increase in stress but adds that the work is becoming all the more interesting and challenging as well. He assumes that the role he plays will become even more central as the company's

*reorganization accelerates. He looks forward to this and has already formu-
lated plans for a more comprehensive approach to customer relations.*

*Chuck doesn't seem to neglect family life for all his imaginative and ener-
getic involvement at work. He married in college, and the couple has two
grown children. His wife has returned to school to finish a college degree long
ago interrupted. Although her absence from the home causes Chuck some
inconvenience, it is clear that he encouraged her. He is full of plans about how
he can preserve a close home life. Should he find too much time to himself, he
imagines he will get involved in useful community activities.*

*In the past, Chuck's family life has hardly been uneventful. His daughter's
two-year-old son died; then her husband divorced her, and she returned home
for a year. This was a difficult time not only for her but for Chuck and his wife,
who felt their daughter's pain and sense of failure in a very personal way.
Chuck describes the long talks they had. Although he mentions their crying
together, it is also clear that he was always searching for a way, a formula, to
relieve mutual pain. He encouraged his daughter to pick up the pieces of her
life, learn from what had happened, and begin again. He tried to help his wife
see that she had little responsibility in what had happened and that it was not
the end of the world. He told himself the same thing. This difficult time, in his
view, drew the three of them closer together.[61]*

In a comprehensive year-long study of college students, researchers at
Boston University School of Medicine concluded that there's a definite
series of events that precedes illness. Here's what they believe happens:[62]
A person perceives a distressing life situation. For whatever reason, he or
she is not able to resolve the distressing situation effectively. As a result, the
person feels helpless and anxious; those feelings of helplessness weaken the
immune system and the resistance to disease, and the person becomes more
vulnerable to disease-causing agents that are always in the environment.

The traits of a disease-resistant personality interrupt this cycle, and
therefore help prevent illness. A study of women with breast cancer shows
that personality and behavior can help protect against cancer and can help
improve survival.[63] There's a real difference between the way healthy people and ill people look at things.[64] Healthy people, for example, tend to
maintain reasonable personal control in their lives. If a problem crops up,
they look for resources and try out solutions. If one doesn't work, they try
another one. People who are frequently ill, on the other hand, leave decisions up to others and try to get other people to solve their problems. Their
approach tends to be passive.

Furthermore, those researchers say healthy people are generally committed to a goal of some kind—and they typically spend at least a few hours
every week doing something that provides a sense of challenge or enhances
their sense of meaningful participation in life. What they do holds personal
significance for them. People who are ill, on the other hand, often report

being bored; they are not able to find things that interest them. Healthy people generally seek out other people and are actively involved with them. Ill people, on the other hand, tend to be more socially isolated.

In discussing people who were able to overcome disease and heal themselves, *Psychology Today* editor Marc Barasch said that if "there is a thread that stands out, it is that each person, some readily, some reluctantly, wound up doing the opposite of what sick people are supposed to: Rather than only trying to 'get back to normal,' they embarked on a voyage of self-discovery. Like early circumnavigators, they seemed to cling to an instinctive faith that the only way home was forward, into the round but unknown world of the self."[65]

"One reason people can undergo tremendous stress and not get sick," says Yale surgeon Bernie Siegel, ". . . has a lot to do with meeting your own needs, expressing your own feelings, learning to say 'no' without guilt. Now, I'm not suggesting that people blame themselves for an illness. Rather, they should see the illness as a message to redirect their life accordingly—to resolve conflicts with other people, express anger and resentment and other negative emotions they've been bottling up inside, to begin looking out for their own needs. And, in so doing, the immune system becomes stimulated and healing takes place."[66]

In part, Siegel is describing the hardy personality. And hardiness promotes health. Following the initial phase of their landmark study at Illinois Bell, Kobasa and Maddi began training the telephone executives in hardiness—began helping them develop disease-resistant personalities. Specific health benefits came to the people who received the training. They not only enjoyed more job satisfaction, but also had reduced anxiety, less depression, fewer physical ills (such as headaches), lower blood pressure, and better sleep.[67]

An entire spectrum of studies verifies the findings: People with the traits of a "disease-resistant" personality do, indeed, enjoy better health. They have fewer episodes of illness, even when people around them have contagious diseases. The results of preliminary studies show that a resilient personality may even help boost recovery from illness. In fact, scientists have identified what they call a "self-healing personality"—and they say it's characterized by enthusiasm, alertness, responsiveness, energy, curiosity, security, and contentment. Scientists say "self-healing" people have a continual sense of growth and resilience; achieve balance in meeting their biological needs, gaining affection, and having self-respect; are good problem solvers; have a playful sense of humor; and have good relationships with others.[68]

With all the research and the scientific backup, disease resistance emerges as an extremely individual thing. What works for one person might not necessarily work for another, so we must exercise great caution and resist the tendency to create fool-proof universal "formulas." In expressing that thought, Friedman wrote, "Self-healing personalities have an inherent resilience, but they are not identical. They share an emotional equilibrium that comes from doing the right combinations of activities appropriate for the individual."[69]

Siegel sums up the entire personality/wellness picture by advising people to take control over their own lives and to have hope:

> *If there's one thing I learned from my years of working with cancer patients, it's that there is no such thing as false hope . . . hope is real and physiological. It's something I feel perfectly comfortable giving people—no matter what their situation. I know people are alive today because I said to them, "You don't have to die."*
>
> *If statistics say that nine out of ten people die from this disease, many physicians will tell their patients, "The odds are against you. Prepare to die." I tell my patients, "You can be the one who gets well. Let's teach you how."*[70]

Is it possible to develop hardiness? Researchers believe so. Kobasa herself has two exercises she recommends to people who are trying to develop a more disease-resistant personality.

The first is called compensating through self-improvement. What it entails, she says, is an important strategy that helps you overcome stressful situations that you can't control by experiencing personal growth in an area you can control. Here's how it works: Say the company you work for is purchased by a larger corporation, and your division is abolished as part of the merger. Or say a favorite brother-in-law is killed in a traffic accident. You can't control either of those things—so, says Kobasa, you compensate. How? You might learn to pilot a small-engine plane, write the family history you've been researching for a decade, or learn a difficult foreign language that has always interested you. Simply stated, you focus your energies on a new challenge instead of on the stress you can't control. This strategy, she says, helps you feel confident and in control.

Kobasa's second strategy is what she calls reconstructing stressful situations. In essence, it's a clever way of "rewriting" your own history—only this time, you come out the winner. Here's how: Start by mentally recalling a stressful event that happened to you—the more stressful the better, the more recent the better. Rehearse the whole thing in your mind, and concentrate on remembering as many details as you can. Now, write down three ways the event could have been worse. Finally, write down three ways it could have been better—in other words, what could you have done to improve the situation?

This kind of an exercise does three things for you, says Kobasa. First, it helps you realize that things weren't as bad as they could have been (a realization that, in itself, can help change your perspective on stress). Second, it gives you ideas about what to do better next time (ideas that can help relieve stress about the future). Third, and most important, it gives you a sense of control by teaching you that you can influence the way things turn out.

Following are some additional suggestions on what you can do to increase your resilience:

- Do whatever you can to develop creativity, to find new ways of looking at things, or to transform confusion into order. The creative expressions you make through writing, playing a musical instrument, dancing, or painting can also help you work through inner strife.

- When confronted with a challenge, rely on keen insight. Ask tough questions; be a careful observer; use brainstorming techniques to come up with as many ways as possible to look at the situation. Learn to trust your own interpretation of things instead of relying on what other people tell you.

- If you start to feel stressed, break your problems down into smaller "chunks" that you can face more easily. Take on the easiest challenges first; those help you gain confidence and make the next problem easier to solve.

- Try to change your perspective on problems: Instead of seeing them as negatives, try finding the positives—the exciting challenges that can result. An upcoming professional examination is an undisputed stress; however, look at studying for it as a chance to hone your skills, increase your knowledge, and give yourself an edge over competitors in the job market.

- Do whatever you can to build your network of social support. If a friend has failed you, that's okay—start now to cultivate a circle of even better friends. Develop a sense of humor, a sense of compassion, and empathy. Whatever happens, stay involved with the people around you—start a study group, join a church committee, get involved in a political campaign, or volunteer at your child's school.

Developing resilience means developing a sense of control—of recognizing that you are ultimately the one in charge of what happens to you. One of the best tips comes from psychiatrist Steven Wolin and developmental psychologist Sybil Wolin: "Get revenge by living well instead of squandering your energy by blaming and faultfinding."[71]

## ENDNOTES

1. Evan G. Pattishall, "The Development of Behavioral Medicine: Historical Models," *Annals of Behavioral Medicine* (November 1989): 43–48.
2. Howard S. Friedman, *The Self-Healing Personality* (New York: Henry Holt and Company, 1991), 99.

3.  Claudia Wallis, "Stress: Can We Cope?" *Time,* June 6, 1983, 48–54.
4.  Robert M. Sapolsky, "Lessons of the Serengeti," n.s., n.d.
5.  Suzanne Ouellette Kobasa, "How Much Stress Can You Survive?" *American Health* (September: 1984): 67.
6.  Kobasa, 67.
7.  Ronald G. Nathan, Thomas E. Staats, and Paul J. Rosch, *The Doctors' Guide to Instant Stress Relief* (New York: G. P. Putnam's Sons, 1987), 39.
8.  Nathan et al., *The Doctor's Guide.*
9.  Steven Locke and Douglas Colligan, *The Healer Within: The New Medicine of Mind and Body* (New York: E. P. Dutton, 1986), 127.
10.  Locke and Colligan, *The Healer Within,* 127–28.
11.  W. F. Adams, *Ireland and Irish Emigration to the New World* (New Haven, Conn.: Yale University Press, 1932); and G. J. Drolet, "Epidemiology of Tuberculosis," in B. Goldberg, ed., *Clinical Tuberculosis* (Philadelphia: F. A. Davis, 1946).
12.  L. J. Moorman, "Tuberculosis on the Navajo Reservation," *American Review of Tuberculosis* 61 (1950): 586.
13.  J. B. McDougal, *Tuberculosis—A Global Study in Social Pathology* (Baltimore: Williams & Wilkins, 1949).
14.  L. E. Hinkle, "The Effect of Exposure to Culture Change, Social Change, and Changes in Interpersonal Relationships on Health," in B. S. Dohrenwend and B. P. Dohrenwend, eds., *Stressful Life Events: Their Nature and Effects* (New York: Wiley, 1974), 9–44.
15.  E. Roskies, M. Iida-Miranda, and M. G. Strobel, "Life Changes as Predictors of Illness in Immigrants," in C. D. Spielberger and I. G. Sarason, eds., *Stress and Anxiety* (Washington, D.C.: Hemisphere, 1977), 3–21.
16.  Robert J. Wheeler and Monica A. Frank, "Identification of Stress Buffers," *Behavioral Medicine* (Summer 1988): 78–79.
17.  Joshua Fischman, "Getting Tough," *Psychology Today* (December 1987): 26–28.
18.  Blair Justice, *Who Gets Sick: Thinking and Health* (Houston, Texas: Peak Press, 1987).
19.  W. H. Courtenay, "Counseling Men in Medical Settings in the Six-Point HEALTH Plan," in G. R. Brooks and G. E. Good, eds., *The New Handbook of Psychotherapy and Counseling with Men* (San Francisco: Jossey-Bass, 2001), 59–91.
20.  D. R. Williams, "The Health of Men: Structured Inequalities and Opportunities," *American Journal of Public Health* 93, no. 5: 724–31.
21.  Sandra P. Thomas, "Men's Health and Psychosocial Issues Affecting Men," *Nurs Clin N Am,* 39 (2004): 259–70.
22.  J. C. Barefoot, B. L. Peterson, W. G. Dahlstrom, I. C. Siegler, N. B. Anderson, and R. B. Williams, "Hostility Patterns and Health Implications: Correlates of Cook-Medley Hostility Scale Scores in a National Survey," *Health Psychology* 10 (1991): 18–24.
23.  D. W. Birnbaum and W. L. Croll, "The Etiology of Children's Stereotypes About Sex Differences in Emotionality," *Sex Roles* 10 (1984): 677–91.
24.  H. Lytton and D. M. Romney, "Parents' Differential Socialization of Boys and Girls: A Meta-Analysis," *Psychology Bulletin* 109 (1991): 267–96.
25.  B. Murray, "Boys to Men: Emotional Miseducation," *Am Psych Assoc Monitor* 30, no. 7: 38–39.
26.  G. E. Good and N. B. Sherrod, "Men's Problems and Effective Treatments: Theory and Empirical Support," in G. R. Brooks and G. E. Good, eds., *The New Handbook of Psychotherapy and Counseling with Men* (San Francisco: Jossey-Bass, 2001), 22–40.

27. M. C. Miller, "Stop Pretending Nothing's Wrong," *Newsweek* 24, no. 141: 71–72.

28. M. K. Potts, M. A. Burnam, and K. B. Wells, "Gender Differences in Depression Detection: A Comparison of Clinician Diagnosis and Standardized Assessments," *Psychol Assessment* 3, no. 4: 609–15.

29. C. C. Cooper, "Men and Divorce," in G. R. Brooks and G. E. Good, eds. *The New Handbook of Psychotherapy and Counseling with Men* (San Francisco: Jossey-Bass, 2001), 335–52.

30. R. F. Levant, "Toward the Reconstruction of Masculinity," in R. F. Levant and W. S. Pollack, eds. *A New Psychology of Men* (New York: Basic Books, 1995), 229–51.

31. R. C. Kesler, K. A. McGonagle, S. Zhao, C. B. Nelson, M. Hughes, S. Eshelman, et al., "Lifetime and 12-Month Prevalence of DSM-III-R Psychiatric Disorders in the United States: Results from the National Comorbidity Survey," *Arch Gen Psych* 51 (1994): 8–19.

32. B. Schaub and R. Schaub, *Healing Addictions: The Vulnerability Model of Recovery* (Albany, N. Y.: Delmar, 1997).

33. Williams, "The Health of Men."

34. Wechsler, G. W. Dowdall, A. Davenport, and S. Castillo, "Correlates of College Student Binge Drinking," *American Journal of Public Health* 85 (1995): 921–26.

35. Robert Ornstein and David Sobel, *The Healing Brain* (New York: Simon & Schuster, 1987), 230.

36. Ornstein and Sobel, *The Healing Brain*.

37. Ibid., 228–29.

38. Ibid., 229.

39. Kenneth Pelletier, *Sound Mind, Sound Body: A New Model for Lifelong Health* (New York: Simon & Schuster, 1994), 57.

40. Susan Chollar, "The Miracle of Resilience," *American Health,* April 1994, 74.

41. Chollar, "The Miracle of Resilience," 74.

42. *Journal of Personality and Social Psychology,* as reported in *The Meninger Letter,* March 1994, 6.

43. Fischman, "Getting Tough."

44. Joan Borysenko, *Minding the Body, Mending the Mind* (Reading, Massachusetts: Addison-Wesley, 1987), 24.

45. Raymond B. Flannery, "The Stress-Resistant Person," *Harvard Medical School Health Letter,* February 1989, 1–3.

46. Friedman, *The Self-Healing Personality,* 110.

47. Flannery, "The Stress-Resistant Person."

48. Friedman, *The Self-Healing Personality,* 106.

49. Friedman, *The Self-Healing Personality,* 111.

50. Darius Razavi, Christine Farvaques, Nicole Delvaux, Tania Beffort, Marianne Paesmans, Guy Leclercq, Paul Van Houtte, and Robert Paridaens, "Psychosocial Correlates of Estrogen and Progesterone Receptors in Breast Cancer," *The Lancet,* 335: 1990, 931–33.

51. Friedman, *The Self-Healing Personality,* 114.

52. *Journal of Psychosomatic Research,* 635–50.

53. Paula Tedesco-Carreras, "Maintaining Mental Wellness," *NSNA/ Imprint,* February/March 1988, 38.

54. Flannery, "The Stress-Resistant Person."

55. Flannery, "The Stress-Resistant Person."

56. Flannery, "The Stress-Resistant Person."

57. Raymond E. Flannery, Jr., "Towards Stress-Resistant Persons: A Stress Management Approach to the Treatment of Anxiety," *American Journal of Preventive Medicine* 3(1): 1987, 26.

58. Flannery, "The Stress-Resistant Person."

59. T. Edward Hannah, "Hardiness and Health Behavior: The Role of Health Concern as a Moderator Variable," *Behavioral Medicine,* Summer 1988, 59–62.

60. Hannah, "Hardiness and Health Behavior."

61. Robert Ornstein and David Sobel, *Healthy Pleasures* (Reading, Massachusetts: Addison-Wesley, 1989), 280–81.

62. M. A. Jacobs, A. Spilken, and M. Norman, "Relationship of Life Change, Maladaptive Aggression, and Upper Respiratory Infection in Male College Students," *Psychosomatic Medicine* 31(1) 1969: 31–44.

63. Darius Razavi, Christine Farvaques, Nicole Delvaux, Tania Beffort, Marianne Paesmans, Guy Leclercq, Paul Van Houtte, and Robert Paridaens, "Psychosocial Correlates of Estrogen and Progesterone Receptors in Breast Cancer," *The Lancet,* 335: 1990, 931–33.

64. Flannery, "The Stress-Resistant Person," 5–6.

65. Marc Ian Barasch, "The Healing Path: A Soul Approach to Illness," in *Proceedings of the Sixth International Conference of the National Institute for the Clinical Application of Behavioral Medicine, The Psychology of Health, Immunity, and Disease,* vol. B, 9.

66. Bernie Siegel, "Mind Over Cancer," *Prevention* (March 1988): 61–62.

67. Fischman, "Getting Tough."

68. Howard S. Friedman and Gary R. VandenBos, "Disease-Prone and Self-Healing Personalities," *Hospital and Community Psychiatry* 23(12): 1992, 1178.

69. Friedman, "Disease-Prone and Self-Healing Personalities."

70. Siegel, "Mind Over Cancer," 64.

71. Chollar, "The Miracle of Resilience," 75.

# Part III

# Social Support and Health

The chapters that comprise this section of the book examine the impact of social connections, or the lack thereof, on health. They explore the positive health effects of marriage and families and the detrimental health effects of loneliness. The importance of social support versus loneliness in grieving gives credence to the power of social support on health. The chapters and topics presented in this section are:

**Chapter  9**   *Social Support, Relationships, and Health*

**Chapter 10**   *Loneliness and Health*

**Chapter 11**   *Marriage and Health*

**Chapter 12**   *Families and Health*

**Chapter 13**   *Grief, Bereavement, and Health*

# Social Support, Relationships, and Health

*Help thy brother's boat across, and lo!*
*thine own has reached the shore.*

—Hindu Proverb

## Learning Objectives

- Define social support.
- Identify the sources of social support.
- Understand how social support protects health and how isolation has the potential to harm health.
- Discuss the implications of social support on the health of the cardiovascular system.
- Understand the importance of touch to health.

A group of researchers went to Alameda County, California, and gathered data on more than 7,000 people over a nine-year period. At the end of the study, they found the common denominator that most often led to good health and long life: the amount of social support a person enjoys.

Researchers who conducted the study concluded that people with social ties—regardless of their source—lived longer than people who were isolated. And people who have a close network of ties with other people seem to maintain better health, resist disease, and deal more successfully with problems they encounter. The strength of social relationships, in fact, has been called "a major source of happiness, relief from distress, and health," and the importance of social relations to human happiness has been declared a "deep truth."[1]

The people with many social contacts—a spouse, a close-knit family, a network of friends, church, or other group affiliations—lived longer and had better health. People who were socially isolated had poorer health and died earlier. In fact, those who had few ties with other people died at rates two to five times higher than those with good social ties.[2] The link between social ties and death rate held up regardless of gender, race, ethnic background, or socioeconomic status.[3] "Some well-loved people fall ill and die prematurely," researchers concluded; "Some isolates live long and healthy lives. But these occurrences are infrequent. For the most part, people tied closely to others are better able to stay well."[4]

The importance of social relationships actually begins at birth, as infants are cared for and develop attachment to their parents and other consistent caregivers. An important determinant of both physical and mental health is demonstrated in the bond between an infant and a caregiver: The healthiest infants have a secure bond with at least one caregiver, express distress when separated from the caregiver, and receive appropriate attention from the caregiver in response to that distress—and those are the infants who are most likely to survive to adulthood. The security of that relationship enables a child to develop a sense of self-worth, to see others as supportive, and to accept others as a source of affection and comfort. On the other hand, when a caregiver's response is chronically inadequate or is poorly matched to the infant's needs, the attachment disorder that develops impacts the child's emotional and physical health and can lead to premature death.[5]

Writing in *The Sciences*, the journal of the New York Academy of Sciences, California physician and epidemiologist Leonard Sagan made a sobering observation of the state of social connectedness in our nation. The United States, he wrote, spends far more per capita on health care—but has far lower life expectancies than Greece, Spain, and Italy. The difference, he believes, "exists because of the decreasing level of natural family support in America. Many of us badly need an activity that boosts our sense of social support and our connections with other people."[6]

Nobel Prize–winning author Saul Bellow agrees. In commenting on life in the United States today, he says that "something is wrong, something is missing. There is ice in the heart—the ice of self-interest—which has to be thawed out by anyone who really wants anything human from himself or from others."[7]

In talking about the impact of social ties on health, one doctor commented that all diseases seem related to breakdowns in the body that are in turn related to a breakdown in social support.

Dr. Kenneth Pelletier of the Stanford Center for Research in Disease Prevention says that "a sense of belonging and connection to other people appears to be a basic human need—as basic as food and shelter. In fact, social support may be one of the critical elements distinguishing those who remain healthy from those who become ill."[8]

Studies involving large samples demonstrate that the protection of social support comes in many different forms and through a number of different channels: marriage and family, ties to friends and neighbors, civic engagement (both individually and collectively), relationships with coworkers, and trust all seem to be independently and robustly related to happiness, health, and life satisfaction.[9] Although researchers aren't sure why, it has become apparent that social support affects physical health—both in terms of mortality and in the onset and progression of disease.[10] As a positive influence, social support and personality are considered the two best predictors of recovery from illness or other assault to the body's ability to defend itself.[11] According to the research, social support influences behaviors that impact health—such as diet, the amount of exercise you get, whether you smoke cigarettes, and whether you drink alcohol (as well as how much you drink). The amount of social support you enjoy also appears to have an impact on biological processes, such as neuroendocrine responses, immune responses, and changes in blood flow. In their negative influence, these behavioral and biological influences together may directly or indirectly lead to stroke, coronary heart disease, coronary artery disease, cancer, infectious diseases, allergies, autoimmune diseases, and liver disease.

Sidney Cobb, president of the Society of Psychosomatic Medicine, claims that the notion of social support as an element of health is not new. What is new, he says, is the collection of hard evidence that proves the case—proof positive that social support can indeed protect people in crisis from what he calls a "wide variety" of diseases. Adequate social support, Cobb says, has been proven to protect against conditions "from low birth weight to death, from arthritis through tuberculosis to depression, alcoholism, and other psychiatric illness. Furthermore, social support can reduce the amount of medication required, accelerate recovery, and facilitate compliance with prescribed medical regimens."[12]

## Social Support Defined

As defined by most researchers, social support is the degree to which a person's basic social needs are met through interaction with other people. It's the resources—both tangible and intangible—that other people provide. It's a person's perception that he or she can count on other people for help with a problem or for help in a time of crisis.

Leading researchers who have studied the effect of social support on heart disease say it involves five components.[13]

- Being cared for and loved, with the opportunity for shared intimacy
- Being esteemed and valued; having a sense of personal worth
- Sharing companionship, communication, and mutual obligations with others; having a sense of belonging
- Having "informational" support—access to information, appraisal, advice, and guidance from others
- Having access to physical or material assistance

The resources that your social network provides may come in the form of tangible, instrumental aid—lending you money, driving you to your doctor's appointment, doing your grocery shopping, or helping assume responsibility for your children while you are sick. But another kind of resource is equally important: It's the emotional, "intangible" kind of help such as affection, understanding, acceptance, and esteem.[14]

According to research, you don't necessarily derive health benefits from a single, isolated, personal encounter or relationship. More likely, the health benefits of social support are cumulative, resulting from recurring patterns of love, affection, nurturance, and the other positive effects and emotions that stem from social ties.[15] And the greater the number of positive social relationships you have over a prolonged period of time, the greater the benefit to your health and longevity. In a similar way, it is a *recurrent* pattern of stress, isolation, and negative interaction that is most likely to impact health in a negative way, not a single episode or relationship.[16]

According to University of Michigan researchers James S. House and Robert L. Kahn, three factors comprise social resources:[17]

1. *Social network*—the size, density, durability, intensity, and frequency of your social contacts
2. *Social relationships*—the existence of relationships, number of relationships, and type of relationships
3. *Social support*—the type, source, number, and quality of your resources

## Sources of Social Support

Social support can come from family members, friends, professional associates, members of the church congregation, neighbors, people who belong to the same bowling league or bridge club, and so on. The people who make up one's social support network are the people with whom one associates and to whom one could turn in time of need.

Sources of social support vary, depending on gender, age, and other factors. In one study, 900 people selected at random from six states were interviewed. All were aged sixty-five and older; none was living in an institution. Almost half were married, and more than half—64 percent—were retired.[18]

The main source of social support for married men was their wives—but the same didn't hold true for women. The married women in the study relied more heavily on other family members and friends than they did on their husbands. According to the results of the study and the findings of other researchers, women seem to get their greatest health benefits from contact with other women. Those with the best health had close female friends or relatives. There may be a number of reasons why, and one of them, according to sociologists at the University of Texas at Austin, may be evidence showing that "women are just more effective at providing support" than are men.[19] When it came to "instrumental" support—the rendering of physical help and the sharing of responsibilities—women used family helpers, agency personnel, and paid helpers more than men did.[20]

Research has also exploded some long-held myths about elderly people and social support. For years, the elderly were often regarded as being "takers"—being the ones who gained from a network of social support. Recent research, however, dispels that myth. A national survey involving more than 700 elderly adults demonstrated that their health and vitality have more to do with what they contribute to their social support network than what they receive from it.[21]

It's also important to consider both gender *and* age in considering the importance of specific kinds of social support. An Australian study looked at more than 11,000 men and women between the ages of eighteen and ninety-five, all of whom were twins. The study found that seven kinds of social support were consistently important: support from spouse, twin, children, parents, other relatives, friends, and helpers. The importance of support from a twin remained constant across ages and for both men and women. As they grew older, the women found support from spouse, parents, and friends slightly less important than did the men; the men found support from relatives and helpers to be more important as they got older. Both men and women relied substantially on support from children as they grew older. Interestingly, women were more likely to have an important confidant when young, but the importance of that relationship grew less significant as they got older. Not so for the men in the study: The importance of having a confidant grew *more* important for the men.[22]

An important source of social support for both men and women of all ages is the sense of belonging to a neighborhood. "Belonging" to a neighborhood can encompass factors like interaction with other people in the neighborhood and/or community, the nature and quality of social contacts in the neighborhood, emotional attachment to neighbors and/or the community, the belief that people in the neighborhood can be effective in making positive changes, participation in community organizations, feelings of safety and security, and a positive environment (such as a neighborhood or community with low crime rates). A sense of belonging to a neighborhood generally increases the longer a person lives in one place and is more likely in rural or remote areas and suburbs—and least likely in urban areas. Research shows that a strong sense of belonging to a neighborhood reduces stress, improves mental and physical health, and increases the likelihood that people are physically active.[23] Neighborhood quality is especially important in promoting the well-being, both physical and mental, of children.[24]

## How Does Social Support Protect Health?

No one knows for certain how social support works to protect health, but some theories by prominent researchers who have done the most specialized work in the field of social support seem to be standing up to close scrutiny:[25]

1. Social support enhances health and well-being no matter how much stress a person is under; the enhancement may result from an overall positive feeling and a sense of self-esteem, stability, and control over one's environment.

2. Social support acts as a buffer against stress by protecting a person from the diseases that stress often causes.

Still other researchers believe that a strong social network and healthy social ties gradually lead to a greater, more generalized sense of control. An impressive array of studies has shown that a sense of control improves and protects health, whereas a feeling of little control can have serious health consequences.

Regardless of how social support protects health, we know that it does. Psychologist Joan Borysenko writes, "The consequences of emotional abandonment are no less serious than those of physical abandonment. Babies in foundling homes that are fed and changed on schedule but starved emotionally often develop a syndrome called hospitalism or failure to thrive. No one is present to coo when the baby coos, to smile when the baby smiles, to mirror back its existence to the child. As a result of this loneliness, the babies' pituitary glands fail to produce sufficient growth hormone and the children wither away despite adequate nutrition. Many of these children die before reaching toddlerhood, and those who do survive are often severely damaged psychologically."[26]

Early researchers who struggled to determine what sort of patient has disease found striking similarities in the circumstances of people with conditions as diverse as depression, tuberculosis, high blood pressure, multiple accidents, and even complications in pregnancy. The people who were ill usually lacked a strong supportive network or had experienced a recent disruption in their traditional sources of social support.[27]

Unfortunately, the number of people in that category seem to be increasing. In comparing people in the United States today with those of earlier generations, a disturbing trend is evident. People today are more likely to live alone, less likely to be married, and less likely to belong to a social organization.[28] The result is a generation of people with weaker social ties—and poorer health.

Besides buffering the effects of stress and protecting health, strong social ties might give people still another edge in good health. The range of problems people bring to friends and neighbors is much broader than those brought to doctors, says Dr. Eva Salber, professor emeritus of Duke University's School of Medicine. Fewer than 5 percent of all physician visits are for psychological problems, she says, "because we learn that if we want a doctor's attention, we must focus on a physical symptom. A woman might tell her doctor she has a bladder infection," but she'll tell a friend "that she's lost her job, had a fight with her husband, and has a bladder infection." What it boils down to, says Dr. Salber, is that "the great majority of human ills are never seen by a doctor. The real primary care is provided by one's family, close friends, and neighbors."[29] These natural helpers—friends, family, and neighbors—may "very well prove to be our most important untapped resource," she adds.

The act of confiding may be one of the most important health boosts of all. Research into the importance of various kinds of social support to health found that interactions with confidants mattered the most—in other words, had the greatest impact on health.[30] Southern Methodist University psychologist James W. Pennebaker has done some of the most impressive research in the area of confiding. Apparently all kinds of health benefits are associated with confiding. In his pioneering book, *Opening Up: The Healing Power of Confiding in Others,*[31] Pennebaker sums it up simply by saying, "Not disclosing our thoughts and feelings can be unhealthy. Divulging them can be healthy."

As mentioned earlier, there is a difference between the genders when it comes to the importance of confidants. Both men and women report feeling less lonely when their interactions with confidants are more intimate and satisfying. Interestingly, women report confiding in both men and women—but men overwhelmingly report intimate and satisfying confidant relationships with women and significantly less intimate relationships with other men.[32]

In recounting more than two decades of specialized research into the health benefits of confiding, Pennebaker says his initial interest was piqued by a polygrapher in San Francisco.[33] The polygrapher, who was examining a forty-five-year-old bank vice president for embezzlement, explained to Pennebaker that the banker's physiological signs—such as heart rate and blood pressure—were very high at first, which is normal for both guilty and innocent people confronted by the threatening dilemma of taking a polygraph test. When quizzed about the details of the embezzlement, however, his vital signs skyrocketed so dramatically that he broke down and confessed to embezzling $74,000 over six months.

That in itself was not dramatic, says Pennebaker. The surprise came later, when the bank official was retested—standard procedure to test the possible deception of a confession. This time the man was completely relaxed. His breathing was slow and relaxed; his heart rate and blood pressure were not only normal, but extraordinarily low; and his palms were dry.

"You can appreciate the irony of this situation," Pennebaker writes. "This man had come into the polygrapher's office a free man, safe in the knowledge that polygraph evidence was not allowed in court. Nevertheless, he confessed. Now, his professional, financial, and personal lives were on the brink of ruin. He was virtually assured of a prison term. Despite these realities, he was relaxed and at ease with himself. Indeed, when a policeman came to handcuff and escort him to jail, he warmly shook the polygrapher's hand and thanked him for all he had done. This last December, the polygrapher received a chatty Christmas card written by the former bank vice president with a federal penitentiary as the return address." "Even when the costs are high," Pennebaker concludes, "the confession of actions that violate our personal values can reduce anxiety and physiological stress. . . . Revealing pent-up thoughts and feelings can be liberating, even if they send you to prison."[34]

The healthful aspects of confiding can also occur when the confession is written, says Pennebaker. In an experiment that demonstrated the power of written confession, Pennebaker and his colleagues at Southern Methodist University asked a group of student volunteers to write about their experiences for fifteen minutes a day over a total of four days.

The students could choose to write either about superficial topics or about a traumatic experience. The students who chose to write about a traumatic experience were instructed to describe their emotions about the event, describe the facts surrounding the event, or write about both the facts and their emotions. Researchers then attempted to determine how often the students got sick by noting how often they visited the student health center. Researchers compared the number of visits in the two and a half months before the students wrote with the number of visits in the five and a half months after they wrote.

All of the students who participated in the experiment visited the health center at the same rate before writing. After writing, those who wrote both the facts and their feelings about a traumatic experience visited the health center 50 percent less often than those who simply wrote about a superficial topic—or those who wrote either the facts or their feelings.

Interestingly, says Pennebaker, writing about a traumatic experience didn't make the students feel better right away. In fact, just the opposite was true—at first, they were depressed."[35]

In a subsequent study, Pennebaker and Martha E. Francis recruited forty-one university employees to write for twenty minutes once a week for four consecutive weeks.[36] The employees wrote about personal experiences, either traumatic or nontraumatic.

During the month that the employees were writing, those who wrote about traumatic experiences had a 28.6 percent decrease in absentee rates; those who wrote about nontraumatic experiences had a 48.5 percent increase in absentee rates. Pennebaker and Francis followed up with blood tests that showed significant health benefits from writing about traumatic experiences.

Although heart rate and blood pressure almost always increase significantly during the act of confiding, they decrease significantly afterward. It's a long-lasting effect, too: People who confide continue to show smaller increases in blood pressure when under stress or when confronted with a challenging task—a benefit that can make big differences in overall health.

There are other health benefits associated with confiding, says Pennebaker, but perhaps the one most associated with good health is immunity.[37] People who confide enjoy better functioning of the immune system. Those who don't face a myriad of immune system disorders; their white blood cell counts are "seriously disturbed." Natural killer cells are weakened and decrease in number; T lymphocytes can't do their job. Almost without exception, Pennebaker says, the people in his studies who began confiding enjoyed enhanced immune function. They showed improvement in physical symptoms; they visited the doctor less often.

Best of all, Pennebaker says, immune system enhancement related to confiding lingers. In one test, students who wrote about troubling experiences they had never before confided experienced significant improvement in immune function as a result—and the improvement from that one session tended to persist for six weeks following the confiding experience.[38]

Part of the benefit from writing about feelings is that it doesn't require feedback—in other words, we're not restricted by how others react. "One reason why writing is so potent is that usually when we start to tell somebody about some personal thing," Pennebaker explains, "we're watching their face very closely to see how they react. If we see any sign that the other person is shocked or disapproving, we immediately start to change the story."[39]

Want to try it yourself? To get started, follow Pennebaker's guidelines for effective written confession:

- To get started, write continuously about the most upsetting or traumatic experience of your entire life. Keep writing until you can't think of anything else to say.

- Don't worry about spelling, grammar, or sentence structure; work on a free flow of your feelings and the facts as you remember them.

- Go beyond the surface—discuss your deepest thoughts and feelings about the experience.

"You can write about anything you want," says Pennebaker. "But ideally, it should be about something you have not talked about with others in detail. It is critical, however, that you let yourself go and touch those deepest emotions and thoughts that you have. In other words, write about what happened and how you felt about it, and how you feel about it now."[40]

## The Ties That Bind

According to one researcher:

> Despite the potential for stress in close personal relationships, it's becoming increasingly clear that healthy, long lives depend on strengthening our bonds with others. A full and rewarding social life can nourish the mind, the emotions, and the spirit, and good physical health depends as much on these aspects of ourselves as it does on a strong and well-functioning body.[41]

Social ties—good friendships, good relationships with family members, the presence of people we know we can lean on—play an important part in our good health. A scientific panel convened by the U.S. government found that social support not only reduced mortality, but was key in protecting health as well. According to the panel, there is a close relationship between the number and strength of an individual's social relationships and an individual's health and longevity. Panel experts say that strong social support can be shown to reduce complications in pregnancy, aid in recovery from surgery, reduce the need for medications in some chronic illnesses, combat the symptoms of stress, protect against a variety of emotional and psychological problems, and help to keep patients in needed medical treatment and promote adherence to needed medical treatment regimens.[42] Social support has also been shown in several studies to promote positive health practices.[43]

Dr. James Lynch, a specialist in psychosomatic medicine at the University of Maryland's School of Medicine and a well-known researcher in the field of social support, concludes that "those individuals who lack the comfort of another human being may very well lack one of nature's most powerful antidotes to stress."[44] One of the reasons may be the impact of social support on cortisol, one of the hormones the body secretes in response to stress: Strong social support results in less cortisol production, which would help protect the body from some of the harmful effects of stress.[45] In summing up the results of his research, Lynch remarked, "The mandate to 'Love your neighbor as you love yourself' is not just a moral mandate. It's a physiological mandate. Caring is biological. One thing you get from caring for others is you're not lonely; and the more connected you are to life, the healthier you are."[46]

Leonard Syme, a professor of epidemiology at the University of California, Berkeley, echoed scientific frustration with the subject as well as realization of its impact on health when he said, "Statistically, this is one of the strongest areas under study. What isn't clear is how it works. How does a relationship get into the body and influence biological processes? All we know at this point is, something very important is happening."[47]

Information continues to pour in as studies are completed that prove that, indeed, something very important is happening. "The ties that bind," as we so often call them, are also apparently the ties that can keep us healthy and help us live a long, happy life.

In a long-term study, almost 3,000 adults in Tecumseh, Michigan, were studied for ten years. At the beginning of the study, each adult was given a thorough physical examination to rule out any existing illness that would force a person to become isolated. Researchers then watched these people closely for the next ten years, making special note of their social relationships and group activities. Those who were socially involved were found to have the best health. When social ties were interrupted or broken, the incidence of disease increased significantly. Researchers particularly noticed that certain conditions seemed related to marginal social ties. Among them were coronary heart disease, cancer, arthritis, strokes, upper respiratory infections, and mental illness. In fact, researchers concluded, interrupted social ties actually seemed to suppress the body's immune system.[48]

Those who conducted the study called close personal relationships a "safety net." They stated that people without such a safety net fall vulnerable to a wide variety of diseases far more frequently than people who are surrounded by the comfort of good social relationships.

Apparently, the impact of social relationships on immunity may be affected by how early in life the social support occurs and how long-lasting social relationships are. A brief disruption in social support (such as a brief separation) may have impact on immunity, but it is likely to be a short-term effect. Disruption in social support that occurs early in life (stress on the fetus during pregnancy or separation from the mother at birth, for example) or that is more long-lasting causes more long-term impact on immunity—sometimes lasting longer than two years. Studies show that it is often difficult to restore normal immunity after that kind of serious impact.[49]

We seem to derive an odd sort of comfort from other people—a comfort that can literally influence us biologically. One researcher observed that the menstrual cycles of close friends and roommates in a college dormitory appeared to be related—but randomly selected girls on the same campus showed no similarities in cycles.[50]

In another experiment, researchers from Walter Reed Army Institute studied a group of three crewmen who worked closely together on a lengthy B-52 flight. The crew members were studied for both physical and emotional symptoms and disorders, and blood tests were taken as part of the study. Researchers found that the levels of seventeen stress-related hormones peaked in all three crewmen at the same time each day.[51]

Dr. Stanley Schachter and his colleagues at Columbia University tested the importance of social relationships with a group of volunteers.[52] Each had agreed to be part of a study in which they would receive a series of electric shocks. Some of the subjects were told that they would receive mild electric shocks, while the others were threatened with receiving painful electric shocks. Dr. Schachter and his colleagues then gave the volunteers the choice of waiting alone or in the presence of other volunteers.

The volunteers who were threatened with only a mild shock chose most often to be alone. Those who were threatened with a painful electric shock most often asked to wait with others—probably, say researchers, because being with other people helped reduce the stress of waiting for an electric shock. "People do serve a direct anxiety-reducing function for one another," Dr. Schachter concluded. "They comfort and support, they reassure one another and attempt to bolster courage. There can be little doubt that the state of anxiety leads," he said, "to the volunteers' desire to be with other people."[53]

## Battle Stress

That support factor was demonstrated even more clearly in a comprehensive study conducted by the U.S. Office of the Surgeon General. In 1973, twenty-eight years after the end of World War II, the office finally completed its thorough analysis of American war casualties.[54] As part of the study, researchers looked at the way troops reacted to the intense stress of battle. Researchers decided that the sustaining influence of other people, the strength imparted by social ties, was what kept troops from crumbling under the stress of battle. Soldiers who benefited from "group identification," "group cohesiveness," or "the buddy system"—those who had strong social support—were able to withstand even intense battle stress. Those in the small combat groups who were sustained by other members suffered the lowest casualties.

Those who did not feel the cohesiveness of a small group, who were not encouraged to come together in "the buddy system," or whose small group was disrupted during combat were the ones who mainly suffered psychiatric breakdown in battle. These soldiers—the lonely, isolated ones—were the ones who suffered the greatest casualties.[55]

Epidemiologist Leonard Syme, who was one of the researchers instrumental in the study of the 7,000 Alameda County, California, residents, confirmed the importance of social support in helping people deal with "battle stress"—not the kind encountered in combat, but the kind real people contend with every day. He remarked that "people who have a close-knit network of intimate personal ties with other people seem to be able to avoid disease, maintain higher levels of health, and in general, to deal more successfully with life's difficulties."[56]

## Unemployment

Can social support help ease the problems associated with unemployment? Apparently it can. In one study, researchers looked at 110 men who were forcibly unemployed when a plant closed.[57] The men were given thorough examinations at various times before and after the plant closing. Examiners measured levels of serum cholesterol, symptoms of illness, symptoms of depression, and the degree of social support each man had from his family and his friends.

The result was a firm testimony of social support. The men who had little social support during the study were significantly more likely to get sick, become depressed, and suffer from elevated levels of serum cholesterol. The men who had good social support from their friends and family members and who had plenty of opportunity for social interaction were significantly more healthy, despite the stress of losing their jobs.

## Pregnant Women Under Stress

Another study looked at pregnant women who were undergoing stressful life events. Researchers studied the 170 women, assessed how stressful the life events were both before and during pregnancy, and also determined how much social support each woman had. (A number of other "psychosocial assets" were also measured.) Researchers then recorded the outcome of each of the pregnancies.

Again, social support seemed to be the key: Only 33 percent of the women under stress had complications during pregnancy if they felt they had strong social support. Among the stressed women who perceived that their social support was weak, 91 percent had complications during pregnancy.[58]

## Relocation and Disruption

Part of the stress from relocation is connected to unfamiliar geographic territory, but another (and perhaps even more significant) part is related to the loss of familiar friends. It is, in a real sense, a loss of social support.

Experiments in the animal world have demonstrated how important it is to be surrounded by friends. In one experiment, chickens were injected with neoplasms (which would have been expected to cause cancer). The chickens that remained in their familiar pecking order stayed healthy; the chickens that were housed with unfamiliar chickens developed cancer.[59]

In another study, mice were put in a situation where there was intense competition for food. The mice that were kept with their familiar litter mates handled the stress of competing for food well—without getting sick over it. The mice that were placed with unfamiliar mice, however, developed high blood pressure.

In yet another experiment, young goats were repeatedly subjected to harmful stimuli in a laboratory. Those that received the stimuli while they were isolated became neurotic; those that were allowed to remain with their mothers while they were stimulated showed no symptoms.

The same thing holds true for people. When people are uprooted and forced to move away from familiar people or places, they often get sick. People who have moved or who have otherwise experienced great disruption in their situations are sicker more often and absent from work at a higher rate than their coworkers.

Researchers were able to observe the effect of disruption by watching the coal miners and their families who moved from small valleys in Appalachia to the company towns created when coal mines were reopened. By looking at the family names of the workers, it was possible to determine how many had relatives living in the towns to which they had come.

Researchers found that those who moved to towns where they did not have family members had a significantly higher rate of absenteeism due to sickness. The coal miners who moved to towns where they had kinfolk were able to stay significantly healthier. The only real factor that distinguished the two groups was the amount of social support they had.[60]

These findings have particular significance for the elderly, whose disrupted social ties are a common part of daily life associated with bereavement, retirement, or a change in residence. Researchers have noted that these changes tend to cause severe depression among the elderly—but that people are able to maintain good health and avoid depression if they have even one close supportive confidante.[61]

A fascinating study conducted on the Sinai peninsula in Israel sheds light on social support in general, but gives particular insight into the phenomenon of relocation, disrupted ties, friendships, and the presence of kinfolk.[62] In 1972, a civilian community named Ophira (Sharm-el-Sheik in Arabic) was established at the southernmost tip of the Sinai peninsula, primarily by families with a pioneering spirit who had wanted to build a town in the desert. Geographically, Ophira was quite isolated. The closest Israeli town of any size, Eilat, was more than 200 miles away.

Because of its distance from Eilat, the town of Ophira quickly became self-contained and self-sufficient, both physically and psychologically. Not only were residents of the town self-sufficient, but they were also unusually similar to each other, partly because the living conditions in the community were so uniform. All the people in town lived in a single housing complex. There was only one shopping center, one school, and one medical center with one doctor and one nurse, so everyone in town also shared the same support services.

Ten years after it was established, Ophira was disbanded as part of the Camp David accords with Egypt that ordered evacuation of the Sinai peninsula. The residents of Ophira, who had lived as such a tightly knit group for ten years, were forced to evacuate—and were relocated over a widely scattered area throughout Israel. Some of the Ophira residents were relocated to rural areas, and others moved to urban areas.

Researchers interested in the effect of the relocation assessed the residents six weeks before the final evacuation and again two years later. A questionnaire and a variety of tests were given to the residents who participated in the study; researchers focused on eighteen husband/wife pairs (a total of thirty-six people) similar in age, ethnic background, educational level, and occupational status.

Several interesting findings emerged:

1. The demoralization and distress that stem from stressful life events (such as relocation) are long-lasting, not temporary. Sophisticated psychological tests given to Ophira residents showed that the stress associated with the relocation was basically as severe after two years as it was six weeks before the actual evacuation. Researchers concluded from their findings that an individual's adjustment to stress at the time it occurs is a good predictor of how adjusted he or she will be two years later.

2. Each individual in the study was asked to list his or her friends, both six weeks before evacuation and two years later. As could be predicted, the

first list of friends—the one made six weeks before the relocation—consisted almost entirely of other Ophira residents. The list made two years later, predictably, contained an entirely new group of friends, with only one or two Ophira residents still included.

In almost all cases, the lists were almost exactly the same size at two years as they had been at six weeks! Even though the friends themselves changed, the size of the network remained about the same, which led researchers to conclude that people actively work to shape their own friendship networks. (Previous theories had suggested that the size of one's friendship network is largely dependent on environment and circumstances, not the result of any effort.)

3. A strong social relationship with kinfolk (or family members) seemed to be a better predictor of health and adjustment than a strong relationship with friends. Few of the couples in the study had kinfolk in Ophira. Likewise, few of the couples moved to areas where their kinfolk were. But those who had strong ties with their kinfolk tended to maintain them and gain strength from them regardless of where they lived. Unlike friends, family members seem to be a source of strength even at distances.

Although the example of Ophira provided researchers with a case in which entire family units were relocated, scientists have also been interested in what has happened when children are separated from their parents in a forced evacuation. To determine how such relocation would affect the children, researchers studied children in England during World War II who were separated from their parents and relocated to safer areas.[63]

As expected, children in both situations were under a tremendous amount of stress: The children who remained with their parents lived with the constant stress of physical danger from the war; the children who had been moved to safer areas to escape the danger of physical injury suffered the stress of being separated from their parents.

Which group fared the best? The children who stayed with their parents exhibited the fewest signs of stress—even though they lived with the daily threat of injury from the enemy blitz. The children who exhibited the greatest signs of stress were those who were separated from their parents—those who lost their most meaningful source of social support—even though they were physically safer.

In summing up the general protective nature of social ties, California psychiatrist Robert Taylor said, "When people have close relationships, they feel less threatened, less alone, more confident, and more in control. Knowing you have people you can turn to in times of need can provide some very important feelings of security, optimism, and hope—all of which can be great antidotes to stress."[64]

# Love Stronger, Live Longer

Larry Dossey, M.D., co-chair of the newly established Panel on Mind/Body Interventions at the National Institutes of Health, says about one of the most celebrated emotions, "The power of love to change bodies is legendary, built into folklore, common sense, and everyday experience. Love moves the flesh, it pushes matter around—as the blushing and palpitations experienced by lovers attest. Throughout history, 'tender, loving care' has uniformly been recognized as a valuable element in healing."[65]

The results of a variety of studies prove that if we want to live longer, we surround ourselves with at least a few good people who can act as friends and confidants. That finding has consistently held true across the board, regardless of how studies have been set up or what population was studied. Healthy people with good social support are at consistently lower risk for mortality than are their isolated counterparts.[66] Again, that finding holds true across the board. Some studies show results for both men and women. Others have studied only women and show that women with good social support have much less disease than those who are more isolated.

Social support is such a powerful factor in mortality that it even lowers mortality among those who are unhealthy (such as survivors of heart attacks). In one study of more than 2,500 elderly men and women, researchers asked each how many sources of social support they had. The researchers then observed those who were eventually hospitalized for heart attack.

The differences were stark. Only 12 percent of those with two or more sources of social support died in the hospital, but 23 percent of those with only one source of social support died while still in the hospital. And 38 percent of those who said they had no source of social support died in the hospital. The results applied to both men and women even after taking into account differences in the severity of the heart attack, illness due to other diseases, the presence of traditional risk factors (such as cigarette smoking and high blood pressure), and symptoms of depression.

"It appears that being married or unmarried, living with someone or living alone, are not as critical to surviving a heart attack as just having someone to turn to for emotional support," the researchers concluded. "And this support seems to work like a drug—the higher the dose, the greater the protective effect."[67]

In a paper presented by residents from Portland's Kaiser Permanente Center for Health Research at the Society of Behavioral Health Meetings, the strength of social networks was shown to predict mortality at two-, five-, ten-, and fifteen-year follow-up visits.

## The Alameda County Study

During the 1980s and 1990s, a number of studies involving large populations showed a distinct relationship between longevity and strong social support.

In the Alameda County, California, study discussed at the beginning of this chapter, the residents were initially studied for nine years.[68] First, researchers separated people into two groups: those who lived lonely lives (without many friends or relatives) and those who had rich resources of family and friends. To determine which category a person fit into, researchers looked at marital status, a person's contact with friends and relatives, church membership, organizational affiliations, political activities, and group activities (such as membership in a garden club or bridge club or participation on a bowling league).

Then researchers wanted to make sure they were comparing the right set of statistics, so they accounted for things that might artificially shorten life. They made allowances for factors such as obesity, cigarette smoking, alcohol consumption, lack of exercise, harmful health practices, and poor health at the beginning of the study.

Researchers then painstakingly sifted through all the data, examining the records of the state health department and cross-checking death certificates. As a final check, the researchers checked each name to determine which category the individual had initially been classified in—lonely or friendly.

The results were convincing: The people who had been classified as lonely and isolated were dying at three times the rate of those who had stronger social ties.[69] To put it simply, people with many social contacts had the lowest mortality rates; those with the fewest contacts had the highest rates.

The results of that study, as well as many others, show that people with social ties—no matter what the source—live longer than isolated people. This holds true regardless of cigarette smoking, alcohol consumption, obesity, sleeping and eating habits, and medical care.[70]

As part of the follow-up to the initial Alameda County study, researchers continued to monitor health and death records for the next eight years; as a result, they had access to complete records for a seventeen-year period. When later analyses of the data were made, the same results held true: People with the strongest social ties had the lowest mortality rates. Those rates were lowest for the people with the best social contacts even after allowances were made for age, sex, race, health status at the beginning of the study, depression, health practices, and the way people viewed their own health.[71]

According to the researchers who analyzed the data from the study, the types of social ties seemed to vary in importance to health depending on the person's age. At the beginning of the study, the participants ranged in age from thirty-eight to ninety-four years. For those under sixty, marital status seemed the best way to predict health and mortality. For those over sixty, ties with close friends or relatives, or both, seemed to be more important to health and long life than did marital status.[72]

## The Michigan Study

In a study constructed similarly to the Alameda County study, psychologists and other researchers studied 2,754 adults in the small community of Tecumseh, Michigan. Each person in the study underwent a thorough medical examination to rule out any existing illness that might force a person to become isolated, such as any communicable disease or any chronic disease that limits or prevents mobility. They then participated in elaborate psychological tests and were rated according to their personal relationships. Researchers took special note of each person's number of friends, degree of closeness to relatives, participation in group activities, and choice of activity.[73]

Researchers then carefully watched the adults in the study for ten years (from the early 1970s to the early 1980s). Those who had the strongest social ties and who were the most socially involved had the best health. Those who were the most socially isolated had four times the mortality rate of those who were more socially involved.

## The North Carolina Study

In another study involving more than 100 communities in North Carolina, researchers looked at black men of all ages. The highest death rates—regardless of the men's age—occurred among those who were "socially disorganized." Social disorganization in the study was characterized by family instability, separation, divorce, single-parent families, and many illegitimate children.[74]

## The Swedish Study

A study of Swedish men who were all fifty years old at the beginning of the study showed that good social support and strong social networks decreased mortality from all causes.[75] In the study, the men who did the worst were those who felt a lack of social and emotional support, those who were dissatisfied with their social activities, and those who lived alone.

## The Japanese Studies

Some of the most fascinating evidence regarding social ties and mortality involved a group of studies of Japanese people. A number of studies showed that people in Japan—even though they smoke cigarettes, have high blood pressure, endure crushing stress, and live in polluted and crowded cities— live longer than we do. In fact, despite those normally unhealthy factors, they enjoy the longest life expectancy in the world. And, even though those factors—cigarette smoking, high blood pressure, stress, and crowding—are characteristically considered to be factors leading to heart disease, the Japanese enjoy relative immunity from heart disease. Researchers who strived to figure out why finally decided that the Japanese are protected from ill health and death by their unusually close ties to friends, family members, and community. University of California, San Francisco, School of Medicine researcher Ken Pelletier believes that the longevity of the Japanese is due to the emphasis they place on the community. The social aspect of human companionship, Pelletier believes, is one of the most important factors in health.[76]

Dr. S. Leonard Syme of the Department of Epidemiology and Public Health at Yale University teamed up with researchers from the University of California, Berkeley, to study the situation in greater depth. Syme and his colleagues studied 12,000 Japanese men in three different groups: (1) men who still lived in southwestern Japan, (2) men who had immigrated from Japan to Hawaii and who had resisted a Westernized lifestyle, and (3) men who had immigrated from Japan to the San Francisco Bay area.[77]

To their surprise, researchers found the highest life expectancy and the lowest rate of heart disease among the group in which they least expected it: the men who had immigrated to San Francisco. The men who had immigrated to San Francisco had formed the closest social ties, the closest family ties, and the strongest social networks. Researchers found that the Japanese men in the San Francisco area stayed heavily involved with Japanese people, moved into Japanese neighborhoods, formed close friendships with other Japanese people, attended Japanese-language schools in addition to English-language schools, and returned to Japan for further schooling.

Research from a variety of studies shows, in essence, that people who are socially isolated—the unmarried, divorced, and widowed; people with few friends; and people who have few church or social contacts—are three times as likely to die of a wide variety of diseases than those who have happy, fulfilling social lives.[78]

A number of studies shows that social support may even increase the longevity of people with AIDS. Long-term survivors of AIDS have been studied to determine what nutritional, medicinal, and other factors may contribute to the ability of the immune system to resist the onslaught of the disease for a prolonged period of time. Research has found that those with low social support are much more prone to depression, other mental health problems, and poorer physical health, while those who maintain strong social support have much better physical health. Some of the ways AIDS patients are able to maintain strong social support include positive ways of dealing with family, renegotiating the friendship group, helping others with HIV infection, and developing a relationship with a higher power.[79]

# Social Connections and the Heart

Researchers who studied the Japanese men found that those who had immigrated to the San Francisco Bay area were the ones with the lowest incidence of heart disease. The unique and intense social ties they formed in San Francisco seemed to offer protection against heart disease. The Japanese men had significantly lower heart disease, even though they had the same high serum cholesterol level as their Western counterparts, often ate Western foods, smoked cigarettes, and had high blood pressure.[80]

Social support—even the most simple social support—appears to affect the heart. In one ambitious study—the Enhancing Recovery in Coronary Heart Disease Patients, reported in the *Journal of the American Medical Association*—it was determined that social isolation is a "special hazard" for people with heart disease, according to Harvard University's Lisa Berkman, one of the study's lead investigators.[81] One particular study shows how simple that support can be. Researchers at the University of Pennsylvania gave a series of college women stressful tasks to do. As the students struggled to complete the stressful tasks, researchers measured their blood pressure and heart rates. The women who brought a friend along had significantly lower blood pressure and heart rates while under stress than the women who faced doing the stressful task by themselves.[82]

## The Roseto Study

A landmark study in Roseto, Pennsylvania, confirms other research and theories that social support and social ties protect the heart. Roseto is a close-knit Italian-American community nestled among other traditional eastern communities. Researchers interested in the lifestyle of the community residents followed their health status and rates of death for years. They found that the residents of Roseto had average incidences of exercise, cigarette smoking, obesity, high blood pressure, and stress. In addition, their diets were higher in fat, cholesterol, and red meat than the average American diet. But the men in Roseto had only about one-sixth the incidence of heart disease and deaths from heart disease as random population groups in the United States. The rates for Roseto's women were even better.

Researchers concluded that the protective factor was the people's strong sense of community and their strong social ties. Stewart Wolf, a professor of medicine at Temple University School of Medicine in Philadelphia and one of the study's researchers, said:

> More than any other town we studied, Roseto's social structure reflected old-world values and traditions. There was a remarkable cohesiveness and sense of unconditional support within the community. Family ties were very strong. And what impressed us most was the attitude toward the elderly. In Roseto, the older residents weren't put on a shelf; they were promoted to "supreme court." No one was ever abandoned.[83]

Researchers continued to watch the residents of Roseto, and they found that when the younger generations began changing—moving away, marrying "outsiders," severing the close emotional ties to the "old neighborhood"— the physical health of the Rosetans began to deteriorate. By the mid-1970s, the mortality and heart disease rates of the Rosetans were comparable to that in surrounding Pennsylvania communities.

Community members had tremendously strong social ties, and their hearts were protected. When the social ties started to vanish, so did the protection. "The experience clearly demonstrates that the most important factors in health are the intangibles—things like trust, honesty, loyalty, team spirit," Wolf concluded. "In terms of preventing heart disease, it's just possible that morale is more important than jogging or not eating butter."[84]

Indeed, studies have shown that human interaction itself has a biological value: Human interaction causes changes in blood pressure, heart rate, and blood chemistry. Those changes promote good health for the heart.

Dr. James Lynch, who has become renowned for his research involving social support, says that "nowhere is the power of human contact more readily apparent than in the period of emotional crisis that follows the sudden occurrence of a heart attack. Warm, interpersonal support is a critical element in the recovery process of such a patient."[85] Lynch explains that the therapeutic power of human contact begins immediately after a heart attack with the physician and nurse; strong contact throughout the recovery process can, he says, lead to a fuller and more complete recovery.

## Swedish Studies

Supporting research was conducted by Dr. Gunnar Biorck, who studied more than 200 cardiac patients in the town of Malmo, Sweden. Biorck found that the patients gained physical and psychological strength in the hospital where teams of nurses and physicians were at close hand and where there was plenty of human contact. The most serious medical problems among Biorck's study patients occurred after the patients left the hospital—a time when "many patients feel deserted and very lonely." When the social support drops off, the protection is often lost.[86]

In another Swedish study, 150 middle-aged Swedish men were studied for ten years to determine the effects of various factors on ischemic heart disease.[87] The men were divided into three groups: (1) men with clinically manifest ischemic heart disease (men who were already sick), (2) men with risk factors for ischemic heart disease, and (3) healthy men. Each man was given standardized interviews and answered questionnaires; researchers recorded factors such as socioeconomic factors, marital status, educational level, occupational status, social class, cigarette smoking, alcohol consumption, Type A behavior, social activities, and social integration. Each was then given a complete physical examination, which included an electrocardiogram and fasting serum lipids.

During the ten-year follow-up, thirty-seven of the men died—twenty of them from ischemic heart disease. The greatest factor in who lived and who died was not necessarily the presence of disease or the presence of risk factors, but social isolation. The men who had the greatest social isolation also had the poorest survival rates.[88]

## Type A Studies

The Swedish study, a Finnish study,[89] and others show that social support may actually help reduce or modify risk factors. One well-known risk factor for heart disease is the Type A personality—a person who is time-oriented, hard-driving, stressed, and competitive. In an attempt to find out what factors might help modify the risk to people with Type A personality, researchers at Duke Medical Center interviewed 113 patients (most of them men) who had come to the hospital for coronary angiography (X-rays of the heart that reveal how much blockage exists in coronary arteries).[90]

All the men in the study were given psychological tests to determine if they were Type A personality or Type B personality (a much more easy-going, relaxed type of personality, much less prone to coronary heart disease). The patients were also given a questionnaire to help determine whether they had strong or weak social support. Finally, patients had a coronary angiography.

When researchers analyzed data from all of the tests and questionnaires, they found that the Type A personalities who had strong social support were on a par with the Type B personalities. The Type A personalities who were isolated or who had weak social support had the most severe coronary artery disease. The study indicates "that social support moderates the long-term health consequences of the Type A behavior pattern."[91]

## Other Studies

Even with established heart disease, social support can be a healing and protective factor. The National Heart and Lung Institute did a five-year study of angina pectoris among men at the Sackler School of Medicine at Tel Aviv University. Even when coronary risk factors were present, the men who had loving wives and strong social relationships did significantly better than those who did not have good social relationships.[92]

In another study, researchers at Yale studied men with coronary heart disease; they looked at how much social support the men in the study enjoyed and focused their interest on men who had survived myocardial infarction. Their findings add dramatically to the evidence that strong social support can help prevent heart disease. They found that good social support actually reversed the effects of stress and distress on cardiac symptoms. Social support acted not only as a powerful preventive, but, also as a healer. The effects of social support were greatest in the first six months following myocardial infarction.[93]

A series of studies that spanned more than a decade demonstrates that social support is an important factor to recovery following heart attack. The first study showed that socially isolated men had a greater risk of death during the recovery period following myocardial infarction. The second study showed that those who were unmarried and did not have a confidant had substantially worse survival rates in the five years following a heart attack. And the last study showed that people who lived alone were significantly more likely to have follow-up coronary events—both fatal and nonfatal— during the four years after the initial heart attack.[94]

Two new studies[95] show the benefits of social support for people with coronary disease. In the first, 1,234 people who survived for the first few days after a heart attack were observed by researchers. Only 5.7 percent of those who lived with other people died during the first year after the heart attack—but more than twice as many (12.4 percent) of those who lived alone died during that first year.

According to researchers, the risk was highest during the first six months. People living alone had a 16 percent probability of dying during that period compared with a 9 percent probability for those who lived with others.

In the second study, researchers at Duke University interviewed 1,368 patients who underwent cardiac catheterization, were found to have coronary disease, and were treated with medication. They tracked the patients for nine years. Those who were married fared better than those who were unmarried. But those who fared the worst were unmarried people who also had no confidant—their five-year survival rate was only 50 percent compared with 82 percent for those with either a spouse or a confidant. When researchers accounted for other factors that affect mortality, the unmarried people who had no confidant had more than a threefold increase in the risk of death within five years.

## The Best Health Bet—Good Social Ties

Perhaps one reason that social support is so conducive to good health is that it appears to improve immune function. A review of a number of studies shows that interpersonal relationships reverse the adverse effects of both short- and long-term stress. Well-documented studies show that stress generally decreases the number and function of natural killer cells and lowers the percentage of T lymphocytes. Strong interpersonal relationships, however, protect the functioning of the immune system—even in the face of stress.[96]

In several studies of college students, researchers measured the rate of immunoglobulin A (s-IgA) secreted in the students' saliva; s-IgA is an important immune defense against upper respiratory infections caused by both viruses and bacteria. In one part of the study, researchers found that students under stress secreted significantly less s-IgA than students not under stress. Students under stress were not as able to resist or fight infection. But researchers also found that students who had good social ties and valued warm personal relationships secreted more s-IgA at all points than did the other students in the study. The students who were socially connected were always in a better position to fight infection, regardless of whether they were under stress.[97]

Ohio State University psychologist Janice Kiecolt-Glaser tested groups of people with psychological profiles designed to determine how lonely they were. Those who were lonelier—those with the lowest levels of social support—also suffered in other ways: Their immune systems did not function as well as their counterparts who had good social support. The lonelier people in the studies had significantly lower levels of natural killer cells, an important part of the immune system that helps control viruses and cancerous tumor formation. Kiecolt-Glaser reported that the lonelier people in her study were less capable of fighting cancer because of immune system weakness.[98]

Increasing social support and reducing loneliness seem to help strengthen the immune system significantly. In a study of thirty elderly patients in retirement homes, researchers took blood tests at the beginning of the study and continued to measure immune system components throughout the test. Volunteers visited the patients in the retirement home three times a week for one month. There was a significant increase in both antibodies and natural killer cell activity, proving that there had been a real boost in the immune system.[99]

Possibly because of the immune system boost, social support seems to have significant impact on a number of disease conditions. Take cancer, for example. Some studies show no correlation between isolation and cancer, but others show a link between social isolation or disruption and cancer.

Lawrence LeShan studied the personalities and emotional life histories of more than 300 cancer patients. When he compared the life histories and emotional circumstances of cancer patients with those of healthy patients, he noticed a pattern in more than 60 percent of the cancer victims—but in only 10 percent of the healthy people: Early in life, these patients learned to perceive relationships as dangerous, to be invested in only at the risk of much pain and rejection. To protect themselves, they kept relationships with others on a superficial basis. They held back emotionally and felt isolated and different from others, though they appeared to be functioning well.[100]

Usually in adolescence or early adulthood, "A relationship came along that seemed relatively safe. Slowly this new relationship became the central focus of life. Then, for one reason or another, the loved one was lost. A spouse died, children grew up and moved away, or a divorce occurred. Cancer developed following the loss."[101]

Social support may even help determine the outcome of cancer. One study that supports that theory was conducted at the Stanford University Medical School and was reported to professionals gathered for annual meetings of the American Psychiatric Association; similar studies in Michigan, Georgia, Sweden, and Finland have produced comparable results.

For the Stanford study, professor of psychiatry David Spiegel followed eighty-six breast cancer patients for ten years.[102] During the first year, the women were randomly divided into two groups. The first group of thirty-six received traditional medical treatment. The second group of fifty received weekly ninety-minute group therapy sessions in addition to traditional medical treatment. At the end of ten years, those who had received therapy lived for approximately thirty-seven months following diagnosis, whereas those who did not receive therapy lived an average of only nineteen months.

Spiegel originally designed the research to refute the notion that the mind plays a role in the course of disease. What he did find was the powerful effect of social support. Taking care to describe his findings, Spiegel commented that "we did not find that any psychological variables—like mood—were associated with survival time. It was only participation in the groups that seemed to make a difference."[103]

Describing himself as "stunned" at the study results, Spiegel said the magnitude of the effects on the body was "much greater than anything I expected."[104] William Breitbart, assistant professor of psychiatry at Memorial Sloan-Kettering Cancer Center, says the important factor is "an intervention addressing two factors: social support and feelings of hopelessness and isolation."[105]

Spiegel says that social support may influence health because of the "grandmother effect": People who feel that others care about them are more likely to eat well, sleep well, exercise, and avoid harmful habits, thus maximizing the body's ability to cope with illness. It's also possible, he says, that people who interact well with family and friends also have better relationships with their healthcare providers.[106]

In commenting on the study, Spiegel expressed concern that some cancer patients might be made to feel "responsible" for their illnesses or be labeled a "failure" because they did not defeat the disease. The effect of the social support, he maintains, "comes not by denying the illness or wishing it away, but by more successfully managing one's life in terms of family relationships, relationships with physicians, and one's own feelings about having a terminal illness, and dealing with these factors as directly as possible."[107]

In fact, Spiegel says, it's important to face the issues head-on. "It doesn't demoralize patients to talk about these things," he says. "The less hidden the problem, the better. Isolation is a symbol of death. The more isolated patients feel, the more helpless and already dead they feel. This is a time to strengthen social networks, not let them wither."[108]

In a similar study headed by UCLA psychiatrist Fawzy I. Fawzy, researchers provided a ninety-minute weekly group therapy session for one group of malignant melanoma patients; the other group received no therapy.[109] The therapy sessions, which continued for six weeks, focused on education about melanoma, stress management, coping and problem-solving skills, and psychological support.

Six years after their initial diagnosis and treatment, the people in the support group had a 60 percent reduction in death rate as compared with the other patients—and approximately half as many recurrences of the melanoma.[110]

Similar findings emerged from separate studies involving people with breast, lung, and colorectal cancer. Researchers in each of the studies found that social support and a sense of control were important to coping with serious illness.[111]

And an interesting new study shows that social support may impact patients differently depending on the cancer site and the extent of the disease. In the seventeen-year study, socially isolated women were shown to have a significantly higher risk of dying of cancer of all sites and of smoking-related cancers. Cancer incidence was not associated with social connections among men, but men with few social connections had significantly poorer survival rates from cancer.[112]

Social support has been found to impact recovery from stroke. In a longitudinal study conducted in New Haven, Connecticut, those who were isolated or who did not have good social support *before* experiencing the stroke had significantly poorer function six months after having the stroke. They also suffered greater impairments in daily living activities and were more likely to be placed in a nursing home. Other studies have found that good social support *following* a stroke makes a substantial difference in recovery from the stroke.[113]

Social support can even affect the unborn. To test what kind of impact social support had on newborns, researchers studied single adolescent Navajo mothers at the University of Arizona. Questionnaires and detailed interviews enabled researchers to categorize the mothers-to-be into three different groups—those who had low social support, medium social support, and high social support. Researchers then followed the women through their pregnancies and deliveries.[114]

The teenagers who had only medium or low social support delivered babies who were significantly more prone to complications. The mothers with medium or low social support also had four times the rate of neonatal complications when compared with the mothers with high levels of social support![115]

Controlled tests by researchers at Baylor College of Medicine showed that the presence of a female companion who provided continuous emotional support throughout labor and delivery was a significant benefit. When such a woman was present, Caesarean section rates dropped from 18 percent to 8 percent. The need for epidural anesthesia dropped from 55 percent to 8 percent, and the average labor was shortened by about two hours. Finally, the need for prolonged hospitalization of the babies after birth was significantly decreased.[116]

In another study, researchers measured the perceived availability of emotional and tangible support among expectant mothers—how much support they believed they had, and whether that support actually did or did not exist. Researchers found that the mothers who perceived that they had good support had fewer premature births and fewer infant complications than those who believed their support to be scant.[117]

The amount of social support given to a mother can even influence the way she bonds to her infant. In one study, researchers evaluated how much social support mothers had from family members and friends; they then rated how well the mothers and infants had become attached to each other. Among the women with good social support, only 10 percent had problems bonding with their infants. But among the women with poor social support, more than half—55 percent—had inadequate or insecure bonding with their infants.[118]

Convinced of the need for good social support? If you need to strengthen your own social connectedness, try the following suggestions:

- Start by making your needs known; let others know that you're interested in strengthening your friendships and your circle of support.

- Look for groups to join. Many corporations offer groups for people who share the same interests (such as stress management); also, you can often find groups through your community or church. Find a group that you feel comfortable in and that deals with a subject you're interested in learning more about.

- Consider enrolling in special classes (such as how to create furniture from willows), special courses (such as how to administer cardiopulmonary resuscitation), or adult education classes offered through your local school district. These classes are usually widely varied in subject— almost everyone can find something of real interest.

- Find a cause you're committed to, and volunteer. You'll find more information about all aspects of volunteer work in Chapter 19.

- Plan now for what you'll be doing a year from now, ten years from now, and during your retirement years. Too often, people restrict their social connections to the workplace; once they retire, they become isolated and lonely. Make active decisions now to help you stay involved.

## Touch: A Crucial Aspect of Social Support

As important as social support is to health, perhaps one of its most powerful components is also one of its simplest: People who touch others and are touched themselves seem to enjoy the best health!

Observations made by researchers nearly four decades ago as they watched groups of monkeys provided us with some of the best information we have on the power of touch. University of Wisconsin researchers Harry and Margaret Harlow compared monkeys who were raised together in cages with monkeys whose only social contact came through seeing, hearing, and smelling other monkeys.[119]

The Harlows found that the monkeys who did not have touch, or actual body contact with other monkeys, grew up with a variety of emotional abnormalities. While young, the monkeys seemed especially prone to self-mutilation; as they grew older, their self-aggression turned into aggression against other monkeys. Perhaps most striking was the example of how mothers behaved toward their young: The mothers who grew up without touch showed less warmth and affection toward their offspring. Some even killed their own babies.

The same thing happens with humans. Countless studies have borne out the deleterious effects on people who are deprived of touch. One landmark study of victims of child abuse spanned three generations of families in which child abuse had occurred. The most powerful predictor of child abuse was not necessarily whether the abuser had himself been abused—but, instead, whether the abuser had been deprived of touch and its associated pleasure.[120]

The skin is the earliest sensory organ to develop. Many researchers argue that it is also the most important.[121] According to one health journal,[122] a piece of skin the size of a quarter contains more than 3 million cells, 12 feet of nerves, 100 sweat glands, 50 nerve endings, and 3 feet of blood vessels. Overall, the skin has about 50 receptors per 100 $cm^2$, or a total of 900,000 sensory receptors. "Viewed from this perspective," reports the journal, "the skin is a giant communication system that, through the sense of touch, brings messages from the external environment to the attention of [the body and the mind]."[123]

Some researchers have shown that touch is stronger than either verbal or emotional contact—and that touch affects nearly everything we do.[124] Cornell University researcher Diane Ackerman points out that "massage therapy"—the act of reaching through the holes in isolettes to stroke and massage premature babies—literally saves their lives. Ackerman cites a previously published article in *Science News* confirming that preemies who are touched are "better able to calm and console themselves." Eight months after being released from the hospital, the preemies who benefited from massage therapy, says Ackerman, are healthier, have better weight gain, and have fewer physical problems than the infants who were not touched regularly.[125]

Although the research linking touch to emotional behavior occurred nearly four decades ago, the first research linking touch to physical health happened—by accident—nearly seventy years ago. Anatomist Frederick Hammett did an experiment in which he removed rats' thyroid and parathyroid glands—and he was astonished when some of the rats survived. Careful research led him to the discovery that the rats who survived the surgery came from colonies where they had been regularly "petted and gentled" by their keepers. They were six times as likely to survive the operation than were rats who had not been touched regularly—and were also much less timid, apprehensive, and high-strung.[126]

According to researchers, touch has both physical and emotional benefits. For example, studies show that touch subdues heart irregularities; people who have a certain type of irregular heartbeat have a more normal heartbeat in the minute after they are touched as their pulse is being taken. And touch can relieve depression; in one study, daily massage improved depression and anxiety scores in children and adolescents who were hospitalized for depression.[127]

What does all of this mean? People who enjoy regular, satisfying touch—a pat on the back, a hug—enjoy health benefits as a result. Their hearts are stronger, their blood pressure is lower, their stress levels are decreased, and their overall tension is reduced. So try these simple ways to add more touch to your life: Acknowledge your children with a hug, kiss, or gentle squeeze of the arm; shake hands when greeting someone; hold a friend's hand while you talk; have a massage; get a manicure; have someone else wash your hair; or volunteer to rock babies at a local hospital.[128] Having good relationships with other people seems to help us resist infection. It seems to protect us against disease. It helps protect us against stress, and it makes us healthier physically and mentally. It can even help us live longer.

Truly, no man is an island. Only by surrounding ourselves and becoming involved with others can we live the longest, healthiest, happiest life possible.

## ENDNOTES

1. Harry T. Rcis, "Relationship Experiences and Emotional Well-Being," in Carol D. Ryff and Burton H. Singer, eds., *Emotion, Social Relationships, and Health* (New York: Oxford University Press, 2001).
2. Sheldon Cohen, "Social Relationships and Susceptibility to the Common Cold," in Ryff and Singer, *Emotion, Social Relationships, and Health.*
3. Cohen, "Social Relationships."
4. Marc Pilisuk and Susan Hillier Parks, *The Healing Web* (Hanover, N. H.: University Press of New England, 1986).
5. Reis, "Relationship Experiences."
6. Allan Luks and Peggy Payne, *The Healing Power of Doing Good* (New York: Fawcett Columbine, 1992).
7. Susan Bell, "Thawing the Ice in the Heart: An Interview with Saul Bellow," *The Writer,* May 1988, 15.
8. Kenneth Pelletier, *Sound Mind, Sound Body: A New Model for Lifelong Health* (New York: Simon & Schuster, 1994), 137–38.
9. J. F. Helliwell and R. D. Putnam, "The Social Context of Well-Being," *Philos Trans R Soc Lond B Biol Sci.* 359, no. 1149 (September 2004): 1435–36.
10. Sheldon Cohen, "Social Support and Physical Illness," *Advances* 7, no. 1: 35–48; original source, *Health Psychology* 7 no. 3: 269–97.
11. "Up Close and Personal," *British Medical Journal* 321, no. 7253 (July 8, 2000): 92.
12. Pilisuk and Parks, *The Healing Web.*
13. Terrence L. Amick and Judith K. Ockene, "The Role of Social Support in the Modification of Risk Factors for Cardiovascular Disease," in Sally A. Shumaker and Susan M. Czajkowski, eds., *Social Support and Cardiovascular Disease* (New York: Plenum Press, 1994), 260–61.
14. Deborah Preston and Jorge Grimes, "A Study of Differences in Social Support," *Journal of Gerontological Nursing* 13, no. 2: 36–40.

15. Carol D. Ryff and Burton H. Singer, "Introduction: Integrating Emotion into the Study of Social Relationships and Health," in Ryff and Singer, *Emotion, Social Relationships, and Health*.
16. Reis, "Relationship Experiences."
17. Cohen, "Social Support."
18. Preston and Grimes, "A Study of Differences."
19. Editors of *Prevention* magazine and the Center for Positive Living, *Positive Living and Health: The Complete Guide to Brain/Body Healing and Mental Empowerment* (Emmaus, Pa.: Rodale Press, 1990), 165.
20. Preston and Grimes, "A Study of Differences."
21. C. E. Depner and B. Ingersoll-Dayton, "Supportive Relationships in Later Life," *Psychology and Aging* 3, no. 4: 348–57.
22. W. L. Coventry, N. A. Gillespie, A. C. Heath, and N. G. Martin, "Perceived Social Support in a Large Community Sample," *Psychiatry Psychiatr Epidemiol* 39 (2004): 625–26.
23. Anne F. Young, Anne Russell, and Jennifer R. Powers, "The Sense of Belonging to a Neighbourhood: Can It Be Measured and Is It Related to Health and Well Being in Older Women?" *Social Sciences and Medicine* 59, no. 12 (December 2004): 2627–37.
24. Lori J. Curtis, Martin D. Dooley, and Shelley A. Phipps, "Child Well-Being and Neighbourhood Quality: Evidence from the Canadian National Longitudinal Survey of Children and Youth," *Social Sciences and Medicine* 58, no. 10 (May 2004): 1917–27.
25. Sheldon Cohen and S. Leonard Syme, eds., *Social Support and Health* (London: Academic Press, 1985).
26. Joan Borysenko, *Fire in the Soul* (New York: Warner Books, 1993), 83.
27. Meredith Minkler, "The Social Component of Health," *American Journal of Health Promotion*, Fall 1986, 33–38.
28. "Social Isolation Pessimism: Link to Poor Health," *Medical Abstracts Newsletter*, October 1988, 5.
29. Tom Ferguson, "The Invisible Health Care System," n.s., January–February 1988.
30. Reis, "Relationship Experiences."
31. James W. Pennebaker, *Opening Up: The Healing Power of Confiding in Others* (New York: William Morrow and Company, 1990).
32. Ryff and Singer, "Introduction."
33. Pennebaker, *Opening Up*.
34. Ibid.
35. Martha E. Francis and James W. Pennebaker, "Putting Stress into Words: The Impact of Writing on Physiological, Absentee, and Self-Reported Emotional Well-Being Measures," *American Journal of Health Promotion* 6, no. 4: 280–87.
36. Francis and Pennebaker, "Putting Stress into Words."
37. Pennebaker, *Opening Up*.
38. Ibid.
39. "Writing as a Means of Healing," *HealthFacts* 16, no. 145: 1.
40. Henry Dreher, "The Healing Power of Confession," *Natural Health*, July–August 1992, 80.
41. Barbara Powell, *Good Relationships Are Good Medicine* (Emmaus, Pa.: Rodale Press, 1987).
42. Leonard A. Sagan, *The Health of Nations* (New York: Basic Books, 1987).
43. N. E. Mahon, A. Yarcheski, and T. J. Yarcheski, "Social Support and Positive Health Practices in Early Adolescents: A Test of Mediating Variables," *Clinical Nursing Research* 13, no. 3 (August 2004): 216–36.

44. James J. Lynch, *The Broken Heart: The Medical Consequences of Loneliness* (New York: Basic Books, 1977).
45. M. C. Rosal, J. King, Y. Ma, and G. W. Reed, "Stress, Social Support, and Cortisol: Inverse Associations?" *Behavioral Medicine* 30, no. 1 (Spring 2004): 11–21.
46. Brent Q. Hafen and Kathryn J. Frandsen, *People Who Need People Are the Healthiest People: The Importance of Relationships* (Provo, Utah: Behavioral Health Associates, n.d.).
47. Jeff Meade, "How to Enrich Your Relationships," *Prevention,* March 1988, 86–89.
48. Hafen and Frandsen, *People Who Need People.*
49. Ryff and Singer, "Introduction."
50. Lynch, *The Broken Heart.*
51. Ibid.
52. Ibid.
53. Ibid.
54. Ibid.
55. Ibid.
56. Padus.
57. Minkler, "The Social Component of Health."
58. Ibid.
59. Animal studies from Pilisuk and Parks.
60. Pilisuk and Parks, *The Healing Web.*
61. Pilisuk and Parks, *The Healing Web.*
62. From Peter Steinglass, Eli Weisstub, and Atara Kaplan De-Nour, "Perceived Personal Networks as Mediators of Stress Reactions," *American Journal of Psychiatry* 145, no. 10: 1259–63.
63. Blair Justice, *Who Gets Sick: Thinking and Health* (Houston, Texas: Peak Press, 1987), 128.
64. Hafen and Frandsen, *People Who Need People.*
65. Larry Dossey, *Healing Words* (San Francisco: Harper San Francisco, 1993), 109.
66. Cohen, "Social Support."
67. "Surviving a Heart Attack: Emotional Support Is Key," *Mental Medicine Update,* spring 1993, 2.
68. S. Leonard Syme, "Coronary Artery Disease: A Sociocultural Perspective," *Circulation* 76, suppl. I, I–112; and Steven Locke and Douglas Colligan, *The Healer Within* (New York: E. P. Dutton, 1986), 89.
69. Ibid.
70. Cohen, "Social Support."
71. Seeman, Kaplan, Knudsen, Cohen, and Guralnik, "Social Network Ties and Mortality Among the Elderly in the Alameda County Study," *American Journal of Epidemiology* 126, no. 4: 714–23.
72. Seeman et al., "Social Network Ties."
73. Locke and Colligan, *The Healer Within,* 89.
74. Robert Ornstein and David Sobel, *The Healing Brain* (New York: Simon & Schuster, 1987), 121.
75. Teresa Seeman, "How Do Others Get Under Our Skin? Social Relationships and Health," in Ryff and Singer, *Emotion, Social Relationships, and Health.*
76. Editors of *Prevention* magazine and the Center for Positive Living, *Positive Living and Health,* 163.
77. Hafen and Frandsen, *People Who Need People.*
78. Meade, "How to Enrich Your Relationships," 86–89.
79. Julie Barroso, "Social Support and Long-Term Survivors of AIDS," *Western Journal of Nursing Research* 19 no. 5: 554–82.

80. Hafen and Frandsen, *People Who Need People.*
81. "Enriching Mental Health Good for the Heart," *Harvard Health Letter* 14, no. 1, (September 1, 2003).
82. Thomas W. Kamarck, Stephen B. Manuck, and J. Richard Jennings, "Social Support Reduces Cardiovascular Reactivity to Psychological Challenge: A Laboratory Model," *Psychosomatic Medicine* 52 (1990), 42–58.
83. Hafen and Frandsen, *People Who Need People.*
84. Ibid.
85. Lynch, *The Broken Heart.*
86. Ibid.
87. Kristina Orth-Gomer and Anna Lena Unden, "Type A Behavior, Social Support, and Coronary Risk: Interaction and Significance for Mortality in Cardiac Patients," *Psychosomatic Medicine* 52: (1990): 59–72.
88. Orth-Gomer and Unden, "Type A Behavior."
89. G. A. Kaplan, J. T. Salonen, R. D. Cohen, R. J. Brand, S. L. Syme, and P. Puska, "Social Connections and Mortality from All Causes and from Cardiovascular Disease: Prospective Evidence from Eastern Finland," *American Journal of Epidemiology* 128, no. 2: 370–80.
90. "Friendship: Heart Saver for Type A's," *Men's Health,* November 1987, 4.
91. "Friendship."
92. Hafen and Frandsen, *People Who Need People.*
93. Alan F. Fontana, Robert D. Kerns, Roberta L. Rosenberg, and Kathleen L. Colonese, "Support, Stress, and Recovery from CHD: A Longitudinal Causal Model," *Health Psychology* 8, no. 2: 175–93.
94. Seeman, "How Do Others."
95. "The Lonely Heart," *Harvard Heart Letter* 3, no. 4: reporting on studies in the *Journal of the American Medical Association,* January 1992.
96. S. Kennedy, J. Kiecolt-Glaser, and R. Glaser, "Immunological Consequences of Acute and Chronic Stressors: Mediating Role of Interpersonal Relationships," *British Journal of Medical Psychology* 61 (1988): 77–85.
97. Cohen, "Social Relationships."
98. Editors of *Prevention* magazine and the Center for Positive Living, *Positive Living and Health.*
99. Justice, *Who Gets Sick,* 134.
100. Powell, *Good Relationships.*
101. Ibid.
102. David Spiegel and Rachel Kimerling, "Group Psychotherapy for Women with Breast Cancer: Relationships Among Social Support, Emotional Expression, and Survival," in Ryff and Singer, *Emotion, Social Relationships, and Health.*
103. Spiegel and Kimerling, "Group Psychotherapy."
104. Ibid.
105. "Can the Right Attitude Cure Cancer?" *Patient Care,* June 15, 1991, 208–9.
106. "A Strong Circle of Friends," *Consumer Reports,* February 1993.
107. Spiegel, "A Psychosocial Inervention."
108. "Can the Right Attitude Cure Cancer?"
109. Fawzy I. Fawzy, "Malignant Melanoma: Effects of an Early Structured Psychiatric Intervention, Coping, and Affective State of Recurrence and Survival Six Years Later," *Archives of General Psychiatry* 50 (1993): 681–89.
110. Fawzy, "Malignant Melanoma."
111. K. O. Ell, J. E. Mantell, M. B. Hamovitch, and R. H. Nishimoto, "Social Support, Sense of Control, and Coping Among Patients with Breast, Lung, or Colorectal Cancer," n.s., 7, no. 3: 63–89.

112. Kathleen Ell, Robert Nishimoto, Linda Mediansky, Joanne Mantell, and Maurice Hamovitch, "Social Relations, Social Support and Survival Among Patients with Cancer," *Journal of Psychosomatic Research* 36, no. 6: 531–41.

113. Seeman, "How Do Others."

114. W. Thomas Boyce, "Stress and Child Health: An Overview," *Pediatric Annals* 14, no. 8: 539–42.

115. Boyce, "Stress and Child Health."

116. J. Kennell et al., "Continuous Emotional Support During Labor in a U.S. Hospital: A Randomized Controlled Trial," *Journal of the American Medical Association* 265 (1991): 2197–201.

117. Cohen, "Social Support."

118. Boyce, "Stress and Child Health."

119. Albert L. Huebner, "The Pleasure Principle," *East/West*, May 1989, 14–19.

120. Huebner, "The Pleasure Principle."

121. Ibid.

122. Barbara Montgomery Dossey, Lynn Keegan, Leslie Gooding Kolkmeier, and Cathie E. Guzzetta, *Holistic Health Promotion: A Guide for Practice* (Rockville, Md.: Aspen, 1989), 255.

123. Diane Ackerman, "The Power of Touch," *Parade Magazine*, March 25, 1990, 4–6.

124. Ackerman, "The Power of Touch."

125. Ibid.

126. Robert Ornstein and David Sobel, *Healthy Pleasures* (Reading, Mass.: Addison-Wesley, 1989).

127. *Mayo Clinic Health Letter*, June 1994, 7.

128. *Mayo Clinic Health Letter*.

# CHAPTER 10

# Loneliness and Health

*We are, most of us, very lonely in this world; you who have*
*any who love you, cling to them and thank God.*

—Author Unknown

## Learning Objectives

- Define loneliness and distinguish how it is different from being alone.
- Identify national trends in being alone.
- Understand the factors that contribute to loneliness.
- Identify the health consequences of loneliness.
- Understand the importance of good friends.
- Discuss the health benefits of pet ownership in alleviating loneliness.

The dayroom on the fourth floor of the nursing home was sparkling clean. The television was on. The sun streamed in. There were only two patients in the room, each in a wheelchair. The woman slumped in her chair. Her hair was dull; I could hardly see her face. She rolled her chair toward where I sat on a couch talking with the psychiatrist, stopped, looked us over, turned, and wheeled away.

The man, who, I was told, was over a hundred years old, was dressed in a blue polka-dot shirt and gray pants. Nurses came in to check on him from time to time, touching his shoulder, adjusting his wheelchair. He didn't come near us. From afar, he tapped out a rhythm with his hand on the arm of the chair. Every once in a while, he let out a sound. At first, I thought he was whining.

Did he feel fatherless?

Was his freedom unbearably curtailed?

Not this man. He had been kissed and stroked and fussed over.

"Loneliness," Dr. Cath had said, "has to do with an individual's failure to create an inner, soothing presence." This man, for whatever reasons, had not failed. He was not whining. As I came closer, I heard, distinctly, the rhythm and the pitch.

He was singing.[1]

## What Is Loneliness?

Loneliness—a condition that has been shown to affect both health and long life—can be present when we're surrounded by people. As the popular saying goes, a person can be "lonely in a crowd." Loneliness is generally defined as the failure to attain satisfying levels of social involvement—and, as such, it is one of the most common types of distress people feel.[2] According to psychologist and cell biologist Joan Borysenko, "To be isolated is the greatest tragedy for a human being and the most generic form of stress."[3] According to research at Kent State University, loneliness is connected less with the number of people in our lives than to satisfaction with those relationships. Loneliness occurs when we believe that current relationships fall short of our ideal.[4]

Feelings of loneliness are worse when the lonely person is surrounded by people who don't seem to be lonely—people who seem to have secure interpersonal attachments—or when the lonely person suffers from a sense of low self-esteem.[5] And, although loneliness can stem from lack of attachment to someone else, loneliness can be just as intense if there is a sense of not belonging within an accepting community.[6] Loneliness is not the same as being alone—you can feel lonely when surrounded by people if those people don't meet your expectations.

Loneliness has been characterized as an "unpleasant experience that occurs when a person's network of social relationships is significantly deficient in either quality or quantity."[7] And loneliness can be more than just unpleasant; it can be profound. One prisoner during the Korean War endured extreme physical torture and starvation with surprising stamina. His worst point came, however, when he was placed in solitary confinement and separated from the friends he had made during his confinement in the prison camp. "I was captured and tortured," he remembers, "and after a while I could stand it. But I couldn't stand even a few days of this," he said, referring to his loneliness.[8]

A questionnaire about loneliness that appeared in five U.S. newspapers was answered by more than 22,000 people over the age of eighteen. The survey confirmed that feeling lonely is associated with greater health risks. What was a little surprising was that loneliness is not necessarily a consequence of living alone. In fact, almost one-fourth of the survey respondents who lived alone fell into the "least lonely" category. (Survey results, however, showed that they had more friends on average than people who lived with other people.) The loneliest respondents were people who lived with their parents, possibly because of psychological conflict or social stigma that leads to feelings of rejection.

## Loneliness Versus Aloneness

Loneliness is quite different from merely being alone. The number of persons with whom we surround ourselves is not what counts—what counts is the satisfaction we get from our relationships and whether we perceive that we are isolated.[9] Many feel lonely within a marriage or when surrounded by a group of people if they are unsatisfied with the sense of connection they get from others. On the other hand, people who are alone much of the time may not necessarily feel "lonely" because of the fulfillment they get from the relationships they do have in their lives.

These are some of the factors that help determine whether someone who is "alone" is also "lonely":

- **General attitude.**  People either react to being alone by being sad and passive or by developing "creative solitude": spending time reading, listening to music, working on a hobby, studying, writing, playing a musical instrument, or some other creative endeavor.
- **Boredom.**  Researchers concluded from the survey that some loneliness stems from simple boredom.
- **Attitude toward self.**  Researchers concluded that a person must feel secure with the self in order to be content when alone.

Associate Professor of Psychology David A. Chiriboga has this advice: "When you find yourself alone, see it as an opportunity to discover yourself. Take it as a challenge. Find out what you want to be, where you want to go, and what gives you pleasure. Anyone can be an interesting person. All you have to do is look inside yourself." And, he concludes, people who are loving—who completely accept themselves and others—can be happy and content whether they are in a crowd of people or quietly at home by themselves. In a study of more than 9,000 people reported in the *Journal of Community and Applied Social Psychology*, researchers found that living alone can be healthy if those who live alone seek outside contacts (such as friends and extended family members) and limit their alcohol intake.

Anne Morrow Lindbergh wrote in *Gift from the Sea:*

*I find there is a quality to being alone that is incredibly precious. Life rushes back into the void, richer, more vivid, fuller than before. It is as if in parting one did actually lose an arm. And then, like starfish, one grows it anew; one is whole again, complete and round—more whole, even, than before, when the other people had pieces of one.*

## Trends in Being Alone

Although being alone doesn't necessarily mean people are lonely, many people who are alone are lonely. And there are more people than ever living alone—in 1999, more than 25 million in the United States alone, with a third of all noninstitutionalized adults over the age of sixty-five living alone.[10] Between 1950 and 1980, the figure rose by 385 percent. And the most radical change has been in the number of men living alone: twice as many now as ten years ago.[11]

In 1985 there were more than 35 million households in the United States headed by singles. Estimates at the time suggested that by the first few years of the 1990s there will be almost as many American households headed by divorced, separated, and widowed people as by married ones.[12] That prediction is now a reality.

A number of trends and factors help explain why so many Americans in such increasing numbers are living alone.

1. The divorce rate is rising.

2. In the United States, there has been a trend away from marriage. People are waiting longer to get married, and many are not marrying at all. Today, almost one-fifth of all women in their early thirties have never married, one-fourth of the women in their later twenties have never married, and more than one-half of those in their early twenties are unmarried. Not too long ago, most women were married by the time they were twenty-two.

   The older women get, the less their chance of getting married, says a study conducted by researchers at Yale and Harvard. For women in their late twenties and thirties, the prospects can be dim. Never-married, college-educated Caucasian women have a 50 percent chance of eventually marrying if they are twenty-five. The chance dips to 20 percent by age thirty, 5 percent by age thirty-five, and only 1 percent by age forty. The study is based on averages; obviously, women in these age groups are still getting married, although their chances decrease with each passing year.[13]

3. Household size is getting smaller. The average household size in the United States was 4.1 members in 1930; that figure dropped to 2.8 in 1980.[14] Today, 42 percent of all households are composed of only one person.

4. Mobility is increasing. In the United States, one in five persons changes residence every year; almost half the U.S. population relocates within any five-year period. Young, educated people move—often long distances—in search of employment and more favorable environments. Poor people move—usually short distances—as the economic and ethnic characteristics of their neighborhoods force them out. We are free—free to relocate to another area, free to quit our job, free to quit our family, free to move on. The changing face of America reflects this "freedom"; the individual is in many ways replacing the family as the basic unit of society.[15]

Other trends have led to the alone and lonely trend in the United States. Fewer face-to-face business transactions are completed; computers write letters, make telephone calls, and handle all financial transactions. People sit alone in front of the television set and video machine instead of going out into the community to watch movies, go to the theatre, attend plays, or patronize the arts. Our larger cities, especially, have become impersonal—and the high crime rate in many cities discourages people from leaving home for purely social reasons.[16]

## Reasons for Loneliness

There are very personal reasons for being lonely. Researchers have divided these into five separate categories:

1. Being alone (coming home to an empty house)

2. Needing friends (feeling different, being misunderstood)

3. Forced isolation (being housebound, being hospitalized, having no transportation)

4. Being unattached (having no spouse, having no sexual partner)

5. Dislocation (being far from home, being in a new job or school, moving too often, traveling often)[17]

Whatever the reason, many Americans feel lonely. Estimates reveal that more than 35 million are lonely each month. According to a national survey completed by the U.S. Department of Health and Human Services, more than one-fourth of all Americans—an estimated 50 million—have been lonely recently.[18] Nearly one-fifth of the U.S. adult population feels lonely at least once a month, and one in ten feels overwhelming loneliness at least once a week.

Recent research also shows that education may play a role in loneliness. In a study involving the effects of loneliness on heart attack, Dr. William Ruberman and his colleagues found that the best-educated people had the least amount of social isolation. On the other hand, poorly educated people had the most job stress and the most social isolation—and the highest risk of dying.

Although Ruberman and his associates considered social isolation to be the most potent factor in the increased death rate among their study subjects, they believe that poor education may also result in less access to good health care and the tendency to neglect self-care practices.[19]

# Causes of Loneliness

According to researchers with the Department of Health and Human Services, loneliness has two basic causes: (1) predisposing (general cultural values, the characteristics of the situation, or the characteristics of the individual), and (2) precipitating (what happens following a specific event, such as a move to a new community or the breakup of a love relationship). The following causes are the most common.[20]

## Personal Characteristics

Many lonely people have distinctive social characteristics that make it difficult for them to form and maintain relationships. They may be extremely shy, for example, and may find it very difficult to introduce themselves, participate in groups, enjoy parties, make phone calls to initiate social activities, and so on. They may lack self-esteem or may be excruciatingly self-conscious. Researchers have found a strong relationship between loneliness and self-concept, as well as the individual's concept about his or her relationships with both same-gender and opposite-gender peers: the lower that belief in self and the ability to relate to others, the greater the loneliness.[21] Many lonely people are unable to be assertive, and some feel they are controlled by others.

Lonely people also tend to have distinct patterns of interaction. When they are conversing with someone else, they respond slowly to the other person's statements, change the subject often, talk more about themselves, and ask few questions of the other person. A researcher who studied these patterns says that lonely people are "self-focused and nonresponsive." Lonely people tend to spend less time with confidants, and often have trouble developing the kind of intimacy that helps them build those deeply connected types of relationships.

Lonely people often had problems relating to their parents, too. Many lonely people say their parents did not give emotional nurturance, failed to give guidance or support, and did not encourage their children to strive for relationships or popularity. Many lonely people remember their parents as remote, untrustworthy, and disagreeable.

## Characteristics of the Situation

Certain situations have everything working against them as far as fostering relationships and becoming involved in meaningful social networks. Some constraints are very basic—time, distance, and money. The student who carries a full course load and a heavy work schedule may have little time for sleep, let alone for making friends. The fire spotter who lives in a remote part of the forest has few opportunities to socialize. The single parent on a tight budget may not be able to afford the babysitter who would allow time for social activities.

Constraints can also limit the number of "eligible" people. For example, a person may not be surrounded by people considered appropriate as friends. An elderly person may live in an apartment building full of young married couples, or a Hispanic family may be the only one of that ethnic group on the block. This kind of "situational" isolation sometimes makes it difficult to initiate relationships.

## Cultural Values

American culture encourages us to be independent, individualistic, and eager to travel our own paths. In addition, as mentioned, we have become a highly mobile, urban society; many people who live in condominiums or townhouses in crowded urban areas could not tell you the name of their next-door neighbors.

## The Nature of Social Relationships

Lonely people tend to have fewer social contacts and relationships than people who are not lonely. They spend less time with other people, and are likely to spend their time with people they are not close to rather than with good friends. Children who are lonely often have poor relationships with their mothers; adults who are lonely are apt to lack meaningful relationships with other adults.

The quality of relationships is important as well. People who have shallow, withdrawn relationships are much more likely to feel lonely (even when surrounded by throngs of people) than those who have deep, intense, and close friendships with others.

## Relationships That Don't Meet Needs

A person might have ten close relationships with others and still be lonely. For most people, relationships have to provide a feeling of personal attachment and social integration; they have to provide nurturance, reassurance of one's worth, a sense of reliable alliance, and guidance. Relationships that meet those needs are more likely to keep a person from feeling lonely.

## Precipitating Events

Countless events in life (many of which are beyond our control) can make us feel lonely, rejected, alone, and inadequate. The most frequent precipitators of loneliness are the death of a spouse, divorce, geographical moves, leaving family and friends to begin college or start a new job, the breakup of a romantic relationship, and a fight with a good friend or family member.

# Risk Factors for Loneliness

No one is immune from loneliness. Depending on one's needs, relationships, and life circumstances at any given time, anyone may fall prey to loneliness. However, two groups are at higher risk for loneliness overall: teenagers and people over age eighty.

It shouldn't surprise many that people over eighty are at risk. As people mature, they tend to become more satisfied with their relationships, and loneliness is not as common—until people experience the death of friends, loved ones, and spouses. As people age, they typically suffer more losses; besides the death of friends and family members, they suffer losses such as the stress of relocating after spending years in a community, the loneliness that results when children leave home, and the isolation that can result when friends become seriously ill.[22]

Some think that teenagers are the most socially active. It's true that they usually have more opportunity for social interaction, but many teenagers also have unrealistic expectations about what friendships should involve. Therefore, their needs aren't met, and they feel lonely. Teenagers who get pregnant may have an especially difficult time with loneliness. A twelve-year longitudinal study looked at the social relationships and psychological status of young adult women who had been pregnant as teenagers as compared to similar young adults who did not have their first child until in their twenties. Those who had their first child as a teenager struggled with greater loneliness, depression, and lack of self-esteem.[23] Another study had similar findings: adolescent mothers recruited from primary health care practices in various Midwestern cities found a strong correlation between early pregnancy, loneliness, and depression.[24]

Also, people who are happily married are less lonely than people who are single. Among single people, those who have never been married are less lonely than those who have been divorced or widowed.

Loneliness tends to be less of a problem for women—although women are more willing to admit they are lonely. Women fare slightly better because they tend to form deep and intimate relationships; they generally remain friends with people, even though time and distance separate them. Their conversations are more personal and intimate; women tend to discuss feelings, whereas men tend to discuss things (such as the structure at the office or the results of last night's football game).

As one researcher put it, "In public, the loneliness of men is more visible than the loneliness of women. Men make friends less easily as they grow older; women seem to continue to replace the friends they have lost. Most older men lack what social scientists call the social skills for making friends with other men and have had little experience in making friends with women."[25]

People with certain kinds of family structure are also more prone to loneliness than others. In doing research on loneliness, psychologists commented on many people who described a family life in which:

> The parents clung tightly to one another and shut out both the world and the child. The parents had no friends; there were no models in the home of what it meant to have friends. There was a sense of being stranded, both shut out from the clinging marriage and alone in the rest of the world. Nobody ever came to dinner. Nobody ever called or went to the movies. Nobody confided in anyone. The family seems, to people who talk this way, the most antisocial unit imaginable, less a haven than a dungeon. Some children growing up in families like these become compensatory—filling their lives with other people, looking for other families to "adopt" themselves into, marrying young. Others repeat the patterns they learned at home, isolating themselves, walling themselves off from intimate connections, ignoring the thirst.[26]

People with lower incomes are more likely to be lonely than those at middle- or high-income levels, probably because there are fewer opportunities for socializing due to economic restrictions.

Other groups at higher risk for loneliness are recent widows, couples who are separating or getting a divorce, students changing schools, people starting new jobs, people who are moving, unemployed people, people who live alone, prison inmates, patients with chronic or terminal illness, children of divorced parents, and women whose children have left home (commonly called the "empty nest syndrome").[27] Research shows that childlessness itself is not as great a factor as marital status, however: Those in middle and old age who are married demonstrate far less loneliness, regardless of whether they have children.[28] Other studies also show that those middle-aged people who are single or divorced not only have a higher risk of loneliness than those who are married, but also suffer greater social isolation, more frequent depression, more pronounced hopelessness, and lower emotional support than those who are married.[29]

## The Health Consequences of Loneliness

Loneliness carries with it a big risk for health problems. Both short-term and chronic loneliness are major risk factors for illness and premature death from a number of causes; they have been shown in studies to be linked to unhealthy behaviors, major depression, and diminished immune function.[30] Psychologist James J. Lynch, scientific director of the Psychophysiological Clinic at the University of Maryland Medical School, says loneliness is "the greatest unrecognized contributor to premature death in the United States."[31] Widespread evidence indicates that those who are lonely are less healthy and die earlier than those with strong social involvement;[32] those who are socially isolated are twice as likely to die during any given period than those who enjoy good social relationships.[33] In a 1992 study by researchers at Duke University Medical Center, scientists studied patients with coronary artery disease. Those who were isolated—unmarried, and without a close friend or confidant— had a 50 percent death rate within five years, as compared to only a 17 percent death rate among the heart disease patients who had a spouse, a close friend, or both.[34]

Loneliness—and the stress that accompanies it—has been connected to not only premature death,[35] but a host of physical and mental disorders as well. Loneliness has been shown to be important in three factors that can cause disease: unhealthy behaviors, excessive reaction to stress, and inadequate or inefficient ability of the body to repair and maintain its normal physiological processes.[36] Good social support has been linked to a lower risk of depression, heart disease, and alcoholism.[37] Loneliness, on the other hand, has been definitely linked to disease; people who are not lonely have a better chance of staying healthy or recovering from disease than people who are lonely. Studies have shown that those who are lonely are more likely to get sick in the first place when exposed to pathogens, like bacteria and viruses, presumably because of the impact of loneliness on the immune system. Those who have only one to three satisfying relationships run more than four times the risk of getting ill when exposed to pathogens than those with less loneliness and more social relationships.[38]

Researcher Louise Bernikow reports:

*Loneliness can, indeed, make you sick. Heart disease and hypertension are now generally thought of as loneliness diseases, exacerbated by a person's sense of abandonment by the world, separation from the rest of humanity. Most addictions are also considered loneliness diseases, which the medical profession is beginning to recognize but which recovering alcoholics, drug addicts, even smokers have been long aware of. Most addicts admit that their best friends have been booze, drugs, or tobacco.*[39]

Apparently one of the crucial factors in determining whether loneliness will make you sick is what it means to you to be lonely; one study of immigrants to Israel from the former Soviet Union showed that those who suffered distressing effects of loneliness were the ones who saw their loneliness as negative.[40] Research shows that the effects of loneliness on the immune system, which can lead to the development of cancer, not only depend on how an individual perceives the loneliness but also appear to unfold over a relatively long period of time.[41] In one study, California Department of Health Services epidemiologists Peggy Reynolds and George A. Kaplan used data from the Alameda County study, which involved 7,000 healthy adults. What they found was that socially isolated women had a significantly greater chance of developing cancer and dying from it.[42]

But what interested the researchers most was the fact that the determining factor seemed to be the women's perception of loneliness—what being lonely meant. Some of the women had many social contacts, but still felt isolated; Reynolds and Kaplan found those women had 2.4 times the normal risk of dying from cancers of the ovary, uterus, and breast. Then there were the women who had few social contacts and felt isolated: They were five times as likely to die from the same cancers.[43]

In a comprehensive study that shed light on the health impact of loneliness, Dr. Caroline Thomas and Dr. Karen Duszynski of the Johns Hopkins School of Medicine examined 1,185 Johns Hopkins medical students who had attended medical school between the years 1948 and 1964.[44] While they were still in medical school, all the students were given a questionnaire that probed into their attitudes and behaviors. All of the students were healthy at the time they completed the questionnaires.

The researchers then followed the progress of the medical students who had completed questionnaires. In 1974, they began reporting on the relationship between a variety of attitudes and behaviors and the health problems that students subsequently developed.

Thomas and Duszynski found that the physicians who eventually committed suicide, were hospitalized for mental illness, or developed malignant tumors had initially reported similar feelings: They had significantly greater problems in interpersonal relationships and had suffered significantly more from loneliness.[45]

Interestingly, those who later developed cancer not only reported a lack of closeness to parents in childhood, but also were found—based on the

Rorschach test—to have the poorest "relationship potential." When researchers recently reviewed personality test findings for 972 of the physicians in the study, they found that those who were "loners" and who suppressed their emotions were sixteen times more likely to develop cancer.[46]

Lynch, who has done intensive research into the Johns Hopkins study, says that much of the loneliness reported by the students stemmed from an absence of "closeness" to parents early in life. In commenting on the parent-child relationship, Thomas and Duszynski remarked:

> *Early in life damage is done to the child's developing ability to relate to others, resulting in marked feelings of isolation, a sense that intense and meaningful relationships bring pain and rejection, and a sense of deep hopelessness and despair. Later, a meaningful relationship is formed in which the individual invests a great deal of energy. For a time, he enjoys a sense of acceptance by others and a meaningful life, although the feeling of loneliness never is completely dispelled. Finally, with the loss of a central relationship, whether the death of a spouse, forced job retirement, or children leaving home, comes a sense of utter despair and a conviction that life holds nothing more for him.*[47]

That early attachment is critical to the health and well-being of infants and children. Infants who fail to develop attachments sometimes do not survive. Those who do survive are believed to be more likely to develop psychopathic personalities (personalities that render them unable to care and be responsible for others).[48] The resulting loneliness leads to a variety of physical and mental health problems, and sometimes premature death. People with strong attachments, on the other hand, suffer far less loneliness—and are less vulnerable, less helpless, more likely to have the confidence to take risks, more likely to have the confidence to move in new directions, and more creative.[49]

Attachment—the social ties it brings, and the loneliness in its absence—appears to be an extremely important health factor. Dr. James House, a sociologist at the Institute of Gerontology at the University of Michigan, has done an in-depth review of a series of studies conducted in the United States, Sweden, and Finland. The studies examined various health issues in relationship to how lonely people were—with loneliness calculated in terms of whether a person was or was not married, had contacts with extended family, had a strong network of friends, was active in a church, or had any other social affiliations. In cooperation with a team of two other researchers who also examined the studies, House concluded that loneliness constitutes a "major risk factor" for health—rivaling the effects of "well-established health risk factors such as cigarette smoking, blood pressure, blood lipids (fats), obesity, and physical activity."[50]

Even research in the laboratory with animals shows the health risks of loneliness and the health benefits of companionship. House and his colleagues point out that "the mere presence of a familiar member of the same species can lessen physiological impact of stress in producing ulcers, hypertension, and neurosis."[51] House says that affectionate petting by humans—or even their mere presence—can reduce stress (as measured by heartbeat and other cardiovascular symptoms) in dogs, cats, horses, and rabbits. Research shows that the opposite may be true, too: Humans may benefit from the companionship of pets (discussed in greater detail later in this chapter).[52]

The effects of loneliness may be even greater than originally thought, as researchers look into a variety of situations. In one fascinating study, researchers decided to find out whether companionship that alleviated loneliness could make a difference in the outcome of labor and delivery. To test their notion, researchers randomly divided first-time mothers into two groups. In the first group, each mother went through labor alone, except for occasional checks by the hospital staff; in the second group, each had the companionship of an untrained woman throughout labor. The mothers in the second group had never met their companions; the support provided during labor varied from mere companionship to holding hands, talking, or rubbing the mother's back during labor.[53]

The results were striking. Among the mothers who underwent labor alone, 75 percent developed complications during labor or birth, including induced labor, fetal distress, stillbirths, or Caesarean section deliveries. Only 12 percent of the mothers with companions developed complications. When researchers looked at just the uncomplicated labors, there was still a marked difference. The unsupported mothers had an average length of labor of 19.3 hours; the mothers who enjoyed support averaged 8.7 hours—less than half as long.[54] The differences continued even after birth. When physicians and researchers observed the mothers for the first hour after the babies were born, the supported mothers were more awake and alert, talked to their babies more, stroked their babies more, and smiled more at their babies.[55]

In a new study that involved 616 women, research director John Kennell of Case Western Reserve University estimated that emotional support during labor could save the health industry $2 billion a year. In his study, Kennell compared women who went through labor and delivery alone to those who were given emotional support and companionship by another woman. Those who were less lonely during labor and delivery required fewer Caesarean sections, less anesthesia, and fewer induced deliveries. Those with companionship delivered their babies faster, and the babies required shorter hospital stays than those born to women who went through the experience alone.[56]

## Loneliness and Longevity

University of Maryland psychologist James J. Lynch says that all the available data from hundreds of in-depth studies point to several factors, including lack of human companionship, chronic loneliness, and social isolation, as "among the leading causes of premature death."[57] And, says Lynch, although the effects of human loneliness are related to "virtually every disease," they are particularly strong in heart disease, the leading cause of death in the United States.

Samuel Silverman, associate clinical professor of psychiatry at Harvard University, claims a person can add up to fifteen years to life simply by reducing two "emotional aging factors," one of which is loneliness.[58]

A study by University of Michigan researchers followed 2,754 men and women to determine which behavioral factors influenced health and longevity. Loneliness turned out to be a substantial health risk—and an apparent cause of premature death. According to researchers, women who were lonely and isolated were one-and-a-half times more likely to die prematurely than women with close social ties. For men, the risk was double.[59]

In the study conducted on residents of Alameda County, California (detailed in Chapter 9), researchers followed 7,000 men and women for nine years, looking for clues on what leads to health and long life. Again, loneliness was strongly implicated as being detrimental. In that study the genders seemed to "switch risk": Lonely women had a nearly three times greater risk and lonely men had a doubled risk of illness and premature death than men and women who had close ties with family and friends.

## Loneliness and Immune Function

A host of studies has shown that loneliness has a considerable effect on immune system function. In one study, University of Denver psychologist Mark Laudenslager and his colleagues separated two baby macaque monkeys from their peers and two others from their mothers. At the time of separation, the baby monkeys were about six months old—comparable to two or three years old in a human child. And, even though the separations were brief, the stress they caused was high; the monkeys didn't know that they'd soon be reunited with their loved ones. Later, when the monkeys were three or four—comparable to adolescence in humans—researchers compared their immune systems with those of five monkeys who had never been isolated during childhood. All the lonely monkeys, those who had been separated, showed lower levels of both B-cell and T-cell activity. The monkeys were at a higher risk for disease.[60]

In another measure of loneliness, researchers at Harvard Medical School studied 111 students—78 men and 33 women. All students in the study were physically healthy, and none was taking drugs that would have suppressed the immune system. Students were given the Minnesota Multiphasic Personality Inventory, a questionnaire-form test that rates, among other things, depression, loneliness, social isolation, and maladjustment. They were also given blood tests that measured the activity of natural killer cells, white blood cells that attack tumors and viruses even without being previously exposed to them. There was a definite correlation in the study: Students who showed high levels of loneliness also had significantly low functioning of the immune system. Researchers found that their natural killer cells were not as active and that they were less able to fight off the Epstein-Barr virus.[61]

A closely related study yielded the same results. Researchers administered a blood test and the UCLA Loneliness Scale—a psychological test measuring loneliness—to a group of first-year medical students and a group of psychiatric inpatients. When researchers measured immune system function, they found that the lonelier medical students and the lonelier psychiatric patients both had significantly lower levels of natural killer cell activity than those who were not lonely.[62]

Apparently there's a medical reason for the reduction in immune system functioning: Lonely people secrete an excessive amount of the hormone cortisol, which suppresses the immune system. And when loneliness is coupled with stress—another condition that stimulates cortisol production—the results can be particularly crippling.

A study that measured the effects of loneliness coupled with stress was carried out at Harvard Medical School; researchers measured the levels and activity of natural killer cells in students both before and after they took exams. As expected, the activity of natural killer cells declined under the stress of taking an exam. But the students who were also lonely had the lowest natural killer cell activity.[63]

Researchers at Ohio State University carried the tests a step further by involving a specific disease: herpes.[64] Researchers looked at herpes simplex Type I, which causes common cold sores, and herpes Type II (genital, or venereal, herpes). Those who were lonely were not able to fight against herpes viruses of either type. Their immune systems were compromised.

In a similar study, psychologist Margaret Kemeny and her colleagues at the University of California School of Medicine in San Francisco studied thirty-six people with Type II (genital) herpes. Those who were lonely—whose immune systems were not functioning well—had significantly more recurrences of the disease than those who were not lonely. The critical element in averting loneliness seemed to be at least one frank and confiding relationship—having at least one person with whom to share open and honest thoughts and feelings. At least one person in whom to confide, researchers summed, is better than an entire network of more superficial relationships.[65]

## Loneliness and Heart Function

Researchers looked for ways in which the mind had an influence over the heart. One of the brain's perceptions—that a person is lonely—apparently has a significant effect on that individual's heart. In the largest study yet attempted of the impact of loneliness on cardiac health, Dr. Kristina Orth-Gomer of the Karolinska Institute in Sweden and Dr. Jeffrey Johnson of the Johns Hopkins School of Public Health studied 17,433 Swedes. Orth-Gomer and Johnson looked at how lonely the Swedes were—as measured by how much they interacted with family, friends, neighbors, and coworkers—and compared the loneliest with those who were not lonely for a period of six years. Then the researchers made allowances for typical heart disease risks, such as age, smoking, physical inactivity, and a family history of heart disease. After making these allowances, they reasoned, they should be able to determine what actual impact loneliness had. They found that those who were lonely had a 40 percent greater risk of dying from cardiovascular disease than the rest of the people in the study.[66]

Orth-Gomer and her colleagues followed up with a second study that zeroed in even more carefully on loneliness and its impact on heart disease. She and her colleagues studied 150 middle-aged men between the ages of forty and sixty-five, observing them for ten years beginning in 1976. One-third of the men were healthy, one-third had heart disease, and the last third were at high risk for developing heart disease. The researchers tested the men's physical health in a variety of ways and examined a range of psychosocial factors to determine which factors were most strongly associated with those who eventually died of heart disease. After ten years, thirty-seven men had died from heart disease. Of those who died, almost all had been initially categorized as socially isolated and lonely. In fact, loneliness was as strong a factor as the strongest physical factor—having an irregular heartbeat—in determining who would eventually die from heart disease.[67]

Another interesting finding stemmed from the study at Karolinska Institute: Researchers found that there is apparently an actual physiological link between loneliness and heart disease. According to the researchers, loneliness creates neuroendocrine changes that lead to atherosclerosis.[68] Some studies indicate that there may be differences between the genders when it comes to the effect of loneliness on the cardiovascular system. In one study of middle-aged working men and women, loneliness was shown to compound the effect of stress on high blood pressure—but only among the women. The authors of the study concluded that loneliness has potentially adverse effects on how well people adjust to and cope with stress.[69]

In still another study of more than 1,700 elderly men and women in Odense, Denmark, a feeling of loneliness was found to be associated with death from cardiovascular disease. That association was especially true for the men.[70]

One of the most comprehensive retrospective studies of early predictors of disease and premature death involved 50,000 former students from the University of Pennsylvania and Harvard University who attended college between the years of 1921 and 1950. Dr. Ralph Paffenbarger and his colleagues carefully studied the records of the first 590 men who had died of coronary heart disease and compared them with 1,180 randomly selected classmates of equivalent age who were still alive.[71]

Nine factors distinguished the men who died of heart disease: heavy cigarette smoking, high blood pressure, increased body weight, shortness of body height, early parental death, absence of siblings, nonparticipation in sports, a higher emotional index, and scarlet fever in childhood. Researchers said several of those factors, including early parental death, absence of siblings, and nonparticipation in sports, were clear and accurate indicators of which were the loneliest. And, researchers say, those who were loneliest and most socially isolated were the ones most at risk to die of heart disease.[72]

Paffenbarger and his colleagues then did a second study involving 40,000 students. In the years following graduation, 225 of them had committed suicide. When researchers compared the suicides with a large number of randomly selected students, they found that the students who committed suicide were lonely, socially isolated, and came from homes in which the parents had separated early or in which the father had died early. The students who committed suicide tended to have fathers who had a professional status and parents who were college-trained.[73]

All of these factors worked together to bring about loneliness, researchers say. As Paffenbarger commented, "Lack of participation in extra-curricular activities seems to acquire meaning in loneliness, fear, hostility, or frustration. Wealth or success of the father may have an adverse influence on the son through paternal absence, deprivation of companionship and counsel, overbearing demand for emulation, possible lack of interest or lack of need for individual success or effort in the son."[74]

An opposite scenario is the case study provided by the city of Seattle, Washington, where an unusually high percentage of its population—almost 40 percent—is trained in cardiopulmonary resuscitation (CPR). In Seattle, say observers, it's considered a "civic virtue" to know what to do for possible cardiac arrest; it's considered important to care, to be prepared to save someone else. Seattle has the highest rate in the country for recovery from cardiac arrest, in part because it addresses the question of loneliness.[75]

## Loneliness and Cancer

A number of studies have correlated loneliness with unusually high incidences of cancer, and researchers now believe that a great deal of the increased cancer rate among the lonely may have to do with the fact that loneliness cripples the immune system. As years of research have shown, a compromised immune system is not as adept at fighting off cancers.

A significant study that showed the link between loneliness and cancer was conducted by the Johns Hopkins University School of Medicine. Researchers collected psychological data between 1948 and 1964 on nearly 1,000 male medical students who attended Johns Hopkins. The men were divided into five groups based on their personality traits. They then collected medical records each year through 1987 and examined the records carefully. Only 1 percent of the "acting out/emotional" cluster—the group who were anxious, easily upset, and prone to depression—developed cancer during the years of the medical follow-up. Nearly one in five of the "loner" cluster—a group who felt lonely and faced the world with bland, unemotional exteriors—developed cancer.[76]

# The Importance of Good Friends

One of the greatest benefits provided by friends is that they avert the distress of loneliness. As Robert Louis Stevenson said, "A friend is a present you give yourself." People without friends are lonelier. Studies involving neurotic people have noted that they have far fewer friends (usually no more than one).[77]

And, even though friends are clearly less important in terms of social support than are spouses, it's also clear that close friendships help buffer stress and help overcome the health effects of loneliness. In the study of 7,000 residents of Alameda County, California, it was concluded that a "larger network size and greater frequency of contact was related to decreased mortality for both men and women at all ages, even when other factors, such as socioeconomic status, initial health status, and health practices," were taken into account.[78]

Researchers stress that although having a few close friends is critical to health, it's also wise to have a large social support network. A larger network gives a greater likelihood of finding someone who can provide the kind of support needed when things get tough.

In some cases, the support of close friends may be even more important than the support of family. One study looked at persons aged fifty-five and older in three North Carolina communities. The researchers first determined who had the greatest satisfaction with life—who were the happiest, healthiest, and generally most satisfied. Then they searched to determine what kinds of social support seemed to contribute most to that satisfaction. For this elderly population, at least, the frequency of contacts with family and the satisfaction with contacts from family weren't what made people happiest in life. It was contact with close friends that made the biggest difference.[79]

In a study conducted at Ohio State University, researchers reviewed how many visitors the patients had and how strong their immune systems were. Researchers measured the immune systems by taking blood samples and measuring both antibodies and natural killer cell activity. The elderly residents who had visitors three times a week or more had significantly stronger immune systems than did the elderly residents who had fewer visitors.

Friends contribute to health by providing all the functions of the family. In some cases, friends may be closer confidants than family members are. And people who are able to build close relationships with friends have greater health protection against stress.[80]

A study of working-class women in London demonstrates the point. Women who were under severe stress were much more likely to be depressed. The women who had close friendships still suffered stress, but the effects of the stress were four times less severe. In summing up the results of the study, researchers said that the difference was due to the "protective effect of confidants," and that those with fewer close friends were more vulnerable to both psychiatric and physical illness.

In one of the Johns Hopkins studies, researchers developed an inkblot test and a method for scoring it. They then showed more than 1,000 graduates the test and evaluated them psychologically based on test results. In the ensuing years, the graduates who developed cancer were the ones who were withdrawn. The ones who remained cancer-free were judged to be congenial, more easily able to interact with others and make friends, and better able to express affection to their friends.[81]

## Types of Friends

Judith Viorst has categorized friends by the five different functions they fulfill in our lives:[82]

1. **Convenience friends.** These are the neighbors or the office mates with whom we exchange pleasantries. We engage in "pleasant chitchat," but don't really share our intimate feelings with them. They are important enough to us that we want to keep up a pleasant face

with them. We might occasionally ask them for help—such as with a carpool—but don't lean on them for intense support in times of need.

2. **Special-interest friends.** With these friends we share some interest or activity: members of the bowling team, someone we meet on Saturdays for a game of tennis, the people in a ceramics class. We do things with these people, but we don't share our feelings with them.

3. **Historical friends.** These are people with whom we have been close at one time or another, but because of any of a number of reasons, we've drifted apart. We enjoy an occasional telephone call with these friends, perhaps exchange Christmas cards or other infrequent correspondence, and maybe even meet for occasional nostalgic reunions. These friends are important—not because they offer ongoing support, but because they help us maintain a link with the past.

4. **Cross-generational friends.** This type of friendship is between members of different generations. It could be an eighteen-year-old neighbor who used to babysit your children or an elderly man on the corner who brings you bags of tomatoes and onions from his garden. These friendships can be close, and even intimate, but they don't usually provide intensive support. There's almost always an inequality involved: The older partner usually gives advice, and the younger one is expected to take it.

5. **Close friends.** These are the gems—the friends we see the most often, the people who are most important to us. They are the ones in whom we confide our deepest feelings, the ones we see and talk with most often, and the ones whose advice and confidence are most important to us. They are the ones who provide the greatest protection from illness and premature death.

Close friendships seem more common among women than among men. Friendship patterns tend to vary a little, too: Women have closer friendships with other women and fewer friendships with men, whereas men tend to have closer friendships with women. There could be a variety of reasons, but researchers think it might have to do with the confiding nature of women. A variety of studies has shown that conversations with women tend to do more to relieve loneliness for members of both sexes. Women's conversations are generally more pleasant, are more intimate, tend to involve more self-disclosure, and are likely to be more meaningful than the conversations of men.[83]

## Specific Health Benefits of Friends

One loneliness study found that female students visited their physicians less often if they had close contacts with good friends. If the women had friends who were pleasant, intimate, and encouraged them to confide, they had a considerably lower rate of illness than women students with fewer close friends.[84]

Friends can also help buffer the effects of stress—and it's well established that stress can make people sick. Friends help one to weather stress. From the results of two separate studies, researchers believe the harmful consequences of stress can be significantly reduced through an active network of friends and family members. Based on studies, psychologists and other researchers say that people with a number of close friends and confidants, people with a "high capacity for intimacy," and people who can openly discuss their deepest feelings are better able to cope with stress in general. Whereas stress overwhelms and exhausts some, people with friends tend to be challenged and stimulated instead.

Good friends can even help alleviate the stress of something as serious as layoffs and unemployment. When a manufacturing plant shut down, researchers looked at the health effects on 100 married men who no longer had jobs. Those who had few friends and felt that they had little support from their wives became ill. Those who felt support from their wives and relatives and who had a strong network of close friends fared much better: They suffered less depression, had less illness, and had lower levels of cholesterol than their former coworkers.[85]

Lillian B. Rubin, a psychologist who has studied the health benefits of friends, says that "people who have others with whom they can communicate about the tensions in their lives often find relief for those tensions."[86] Other psychologists agree—and some go so far as to say that a good friend who is willing to listen in confidence is as good as professional counseling when facing a problem.[87]

Friendship protects health because it provides a natural outlet for confiding feelings to others. Researchers have found that openly discussing a traumatic event with someone else—such as a friend—can actually improve physical health even when the traumatic event occurred many years previous.[88] In his research, Southern Methodist University psychologist James Pennebaker found that immune system function is boosted by confiding upsetting events. And the health benefits of confiding in a friend are longlasting: Pennebaker's research shows that immune function improvement lasts as long as six weeks afterward![89]

According to a study conducted by the California Department of Mental Health, close, confiding personal relationships—good friends—have been found to buffer the stress not only from life's major changes (such as death of a loved one), but from life's daily hassles as well. People in crisis—whether from a major life change or from an accumulation of daily hassles—have higher morale, fewer physical symptoms, and less illness if they have support from and contact with close friends.[90]

In addition to the factor of social support, friends may help protect health because they are familiar. They are comforting because we are used to them. What is familiar is often less threatening because it seems more predictable and manageable.

Experiments with animals have proven the point. Those who have the benefit of the familiar are able to withstand the effects of stress; those who don't are crippled by it. In one of a series of animal experiments, researchers induced coronary occlussions—blockages of the heart arteries—in a group of pigs. Researchers then randomly split the group of pigs in half. One group of pigs was housed in a laboratory and tended by staff members with whom the pigs were familiar. These staff members were in essence friends. None of the pigs in the group suffered lethal, irregular contractions of heart muscles—contractions that would have been expected following the inducement of coronary occlusions. The pigs in the other group were housed in a new, unfamiliar laboratory and were tended by strangers—laboratory crew members they had never seen before. Many of those pigs suffered fatal arrhythmias of the heart.[91]

Other experiments proved the same thing. At the UCLA School of Medicine, researchers tried to create high blood pressure in mice by severely overcrowding them in their cages. Only the mice that were surrounded by stranger mice—mice with whom they were unfamiliar—developed the high blood pressure the researchers expected. The mice surrounded by litter mice and other familiar mice had little trouble adjusting to the crowded conditions and did not develop high blood pressure.[92]

## The Importance of Pets

Research into the health benefits of pet ownership has shown beyond a doubt that comfort does not always have to come only from people.[93] There are an estimated 100 million pets in the United States—pets who are sheltered, groomed, petted, talked to, babied, and showered with toys. More than half of all American homes have one or more pets. Those pets may return a health benefit to the owners who care for them.

According to research,[94] pets fulfill a variety of needs for their human owners. They provide a chance for interaction with another living thing and fulfill the natural craving for companionship and emotional relationships. They provide for our need to care and our desire to be loved. They act as a stimulus for exercise. As anyone who owns a pet knows, they also give love in return.

The discovery that pets benefit health came quite by accident at first and was due to three landmark events. The first occurred in 1959, when New York child psychiatrist Boris Levinson happened to have his dog Jingles with him when a patient paid an unexpected visit. The young patient had been withdrawn and isolated, and had failed to respond to the repeated attempts to help. Jingles suddenly ran up to the boy and licked his face. The child broke out of his usual withdrawal and started to play with the dog. Levinson began using pets as a way to break the ice with his young patients.[95]

The second landmark event also occurred quite by accident. In the mid-1970s, Ohio State University psychologist Samuel A. Corson kept a kennel of dogs on the grounds for use in his research. When mental patients in an adjoining hospital heard the dogs barking, they insisted on seeing the dogs. They began to visit, they developed relationships filled with trust and affection, and as a result they were able to trust their physicians and make great progress in their treatment.[96]

The final landmark event in pet studies occurred in 1980 when University of Pennsylvania researchers Aaron Katcher and Erika Friedmann found that people with pets lived longer after experiencing heart attacks than those without pets,[97] and that pet ownership may facilitate both physical and mental fitness. Subsequent research has shown that among people who have heart attacks, pet owners have one-fifth the death rate of those who do not have pets.[98]

The benefits of pet ownership even extend to a population that is traditionally the most prone to health problems: the elderly. A study by Judith M. Siegel and her colleagues at UCLA followed 1,000 Medicare enrollees for one year. The elderly were interviewed at the beginning of the study and then every two months throughout the year of the study. In addition, they were assessed for psychological distress at six months and twelve months. Siegel found that more than one-third of the people involved in the study owned pets—cats, dogs, birds, and fish.[99]

She found that pet owners enjoyed better health and had fewer visits to the doctor than did those without pets. Even among those under the most stress during the year of the study, the pet owners had 16 percent fewer physician visits.

Of interest was the finding that the greatest benefit seemed to come from dog ownership—perhaps because those who owned dogs "spent more time outdoors with them, spent more time talking to them, felt more attached to them, and, during the course of the study, had fewer physician contacts than other pet owners."[100] Researchers found that even the most highly stressed dog owners in the study had 21 percent fewer physician contacts than people without pets.[101]

People who own pets have better health, recover more quickly from all kinds of illness and surgery, and live longer lives than those who don't have pets.

As the title of Shelley Levitt's article says, "Pet Two Poodles and Call Me in the Morning."[102]

## Why Pets Benefit Health

Pets, among other things, alleviate loneliness. They provide companionship. They make us feel safe. They help us feel calm. No matter what else may happen around us, they are a constant amid the change. And they can exert an overall good influence. University of California, Davis, researchers found that elderly people with pets not only enjoyed an improvement in their well-being, but worked actively to improve their overall living conditions, too.[103]

As mentioned, the first notice of the health benefits of pets on a scientific level was quite by accident. A team of medical researchers from the University of Maryland and the University of Pennsylvania designed and carried out a study between 1977 and 1979 to determine how social conditions affect heart disease.[104] They delved into the backgrounds and living conditions of people who had been hospitalized with heart disease. They checked out income, marital status, lifestyle, and a number of other "social" factors. A year after the patients were released from the hospital, researchers followed up to see which ones were still alive. They also did detailed computer analyses to figure out which factors had helped keep those patients alive.

People who owned pets had fared much better than people who didn't. In fact, three times as many of the nonowners had died in the year since they had been released from the hospital![105] One of the reasons may be, simply, that pets enhance social interactions between *people,* and pet owners are more likely to have strong social interactions—which have been shown in numerous studies to benefit both health and longevity.[106]

## The Cardiovascular System

One of the studies almost exactly duplicated the initial, accidental study. At the University of Pennsylvania's Center for Interaction of Animals and Society, researchers studied ninety-two patients who had been hospitalized for coronary disease. Those with pets had one-third the death rate of the people who did not have pets. In that study, researchers discovered one possible reason for the coronary survivals: Patients actually had lower heart rates when they were with their pets. Friedmann maintains that's an important result because "even small reductions in the heart rate repeated thousands of times per week could provide direct health benefits by decreasing the frequency of arterial damage, and thus slowing the arteriosclerotic process. The results of this research may have important implications for middle-aged and elderly individuals with a variety of stress-related chronic diseases."[107] Subsequent research at Brooklyn College showed that pets do, indeed, slow the heart rate—even among high-stressed, high-intensity, Type A personalities.

Studies show that pet owners tend to have lower blood pressure, lower levels of triglycerides in the blood, and lower cholesterol—findings that are especially pronounced in men over the age of forty. Other studies have shown that pet owners have better survival rates after heart attack, and that simply getting a pet is associated with an elevated sense of psychological well-being.[108]

Pets have another important effect on the cardiovascular system: They help reduce blood pressure. In a number of studies, pets of all kinds have been shown to lower blood pressure. Petting a dog decreased blood pressure among healthy college students, hospitalized elderly, and adults with hypertension. The blood pressure of bird owners dropped an average of ten points when they were talking to their birds. Watching fish in an aquarium brought blood pressure to below resting levels.[109]

One of the least sterile and most clinical studies was carried out by researcher James Lynch in the recreation room of his home—and with the help of his three children. For the study, Lynch and his kids invited neighborhood children to come over and read in the recreation room. Each child's blood pressure was measured both while sitting quietly and while reading aloud—and both while alone and while a dog was in the room. The kids had lower blood pressure while the dog was in the room, whether they were sitting quietly or reading aloud. The dog seemed to be what made the difference.[110] Some researchers think pets help lower blood pressure because of their calming influence and because most people slow down and become more calm and gentle when talking to their pets.

People in hospitals, including mental hospitals, recover more completely and more quickly and are discharged sooner if they have pets waiting for them at home. The patients might feel a responsibility for the pet and want to get home to resume caring for the pet. Some hospitals have started allowing pets to visit patients, a practice that has been found to speed recovery. Swedish-American Hospital in Rockford, Illinois, initiated use of a "pet visiting room," where pets can be brought to visit their hospitalized owners. Researchers in charge of the project have found that visits from pets calm the patient, boost patient morale, and improve and speed postsurgical recovery.[111] Many believe that for the patients, the pet represents an important source of companionship and love and an alleviation of loneliness. And study results still point to the effect of reducing blood pressure.

Effects of reducing blood pressure have been most profound among elderly people and children, even though it seems to work regardless of age. In one experiment, children at the University of Pennsylvania School of Veterinary Medicine were brought into a room and interviewed by a stranger. The reaction of the children was predictable: They experienced stress, and their blood pressure increased. When a friendly dog was brought into the room, the children relaxed and their blood pressure dropped.[112]

## Stress

Pets also help alleviate the effects of stress. To test that notion, researchers at the University of Oklahoma decided to try it against one of life's most stressful situations: the death of a spouse.[113] Researchers compared two groups of recent widows; one group had pets and the other did not. The two groups were studied to see how they responded in terms of physical complaints, lifestyles, interactions with others, and feelings toward self. The widows with pets did "significantly" better than the widows who did not have pets. Those with pets were healthier, had fewer illnesses and physical complaints, and were able to interact with others better. The widows without pets had more persistent fears, headaches, and feelings of panic—and they tended to take more medications than did the pet owners.

In another study, psychologists Karen M. Allen and James J. Blascovich of the State University of New York at Buffalo gave forty-five women a challenge that's often used in the laboratory to create stress—performing mental arithmetic.[114] The women had to rapidly count backwards by threes from a four-digit number. During the test, the researchers measured the women's pulse rate, blood pressure, and electrical skin conductance—all measures that can indicate how stressed someone is feeling.

What happened? The women who had a human friend at their side during the test had poor performance and a lot of stress. But the women who had their pet dogs at their side during the test did much better on the arithmetic—and they did it with lower blood pressure and fewer other physical responses to stress.[115]

## Pet-Facilitated Therapy

Pets have been shown to have such a benefit on both physical and mental health that they are now being used in a whole new field of therapy called pet-facilitated therapy. They are being used with hospitalized patients, with mental patients, with the elderly in convalescent centers, and even in prisons.

In one of the most successful programs of its kind, social worker David Lee of Lima State Hospital for the Criminally Insane in Ohio introduced small animals—fish, parakeets, and so on—to the prisoners as "mascots." Among the prisoners were murderers, rapists, and others who had committed violent crimes. Allowing the criminals to care for the animals almost completely stopped fighting among prisoners and suicide attempts.[116]

## ENDNOTES

1. Louise Bernikow, *Alone in America* (New York: Harper & Row, 1986).
2. Harry T. Reis, "Relationship Experiences and Emotional Well-Being," in Carol D. Ryff and Burton H. Singer, eds., *Emotion, Social Relationships, and Health* (New York: Oxford University Press, 2001).

3. Joan Borysenko, *Fire in the Soul* (New York: Warner Books, 1993), 83.
4. "Loneliness: A Healthy Approach," *Longevity,* April 1990, 22.
5. Boris Blai, "Health Consequences of Loneliness: A Review of the Literature," *JACH* 37 (1989): 162.
6. Blai, "Health Consequences."
7. Ibid., 163.
8. Robert Ornstein and David Sobel, *Healthy Pleasures* (Reading, Mass.: Addison-Wesley, 1989), 222–23.
9. "You're Not Alone When It Comes to Loneliness," *Harvard Health Letter* 24, no. 7: 4.
10. "You're Not Alone," 4.
11. Bernikow, *Alone in America.*
12. Barbara Powell, *Alone, Alive and Well* (Emmaus, Pa.: Rodale Press, 1985).
13. Brent Q. Hafen and Kathryn J. Frandsen, *People Need People: The Importance of Relationships to Health and Wellness* (Evergreen, Colo.: Cordillera Press, 1987).
14. Marc Pilisuk and Susan Hillier Parks, *The Healing Web* (Hanover, N. H.: University Press of New England, 1986).
15. Pilisuk and Parks, *The Healing Web.*
16. Carin Rubenstein and Phillip Shaver, "Are You Lonely? How to Find Intimacy, Love, and Happiness," *Shape,* August 1987, 72.
17. Rubenstein and Shaver, "Are You Lonely?" 75.
18. Hafen and Frandsen, *People Need People,* 29–31.
19. Dossey, 70.
20. Hafen and Frandsen, *People Need People.*
21. S. Lau and C. K. Kong, "The Acceptance of Lonely Others: Effects of Loneliness and Gender of the Target Person and Loneliness of the Perceiver," *Journal of Social Psychology* 139, no. 2 (April 1999): 229–41.
22. "You're Not Alone."
23. J. R. Vicary and D. A. Corneal, "A Comparison of Young Women's Psychosocial Status Based on Age of Their First Childbirth," *Family Community Health* 24, no. 2 (July 2001): 73–84.
24. D. B. Hudson, S. M. Elek, and C. Campbell-Gorssman, "Depression, Self-Esteem, Loneliness, and Social Support Among Adolescent Mothers Participating in the New Parents Project," *Adolescence* 35, no. 139 (Autumn 2000): 445–53.
25. Bernikow, *Alone in America.*
26. Ibid.
27. Hafen and Frandsen, *People Need People,* 32.
28. T. Koropeckyj-Cox, "Loneliness and Depression in Middle and Old Age: Are the Childless More Vulnerable?" *J Gerontol B Psychol Sci Soc Sci* 53, no. 6 (November 1998): S303–12.
29. A. Steptoe, N. Owen, S. R. Kunz-Ebrecht, and L. Brydon, "Loneliness and Neuroendocrine, Cardiovascular, and Inflammatory Stress Responses in Middle-Aged Men and Women," *Psychoneuroendocrinology* 29, no. 5 (June 2004): 593–611.
30. Reis, "Relationship Experiences."
31. Ibid., 33.
32. Ibid.
33. Sheldon Cohen, "Social Relationships and Susceptibility to the Common Cold," in Ryff and Singer, *Emotion, Social Relationships, and Health.*
34. "You're Not Alone."
35. Ibid.

36. L. C. Hawkley and J. T. Cacioppo, "Loneliness and Pathways to Disease," *Brain, Behavior, and Immunity* 17, suppl. 1 (February 2003): S98–105.

37. Ibid.

38. Cohen, ."Social Relationships."

39. Bernikow, *Alone in America.*

40. A. M. Ponizovsky and M. S. Ritsner, "Patterns of Loneliness in an Immigrant Population," *Compr Psychiatry* 45, no. 5 (September–October 2004): 408–14.

41. Hawkley and Cacioppo, "Loneliness."

42. Dossey, 94.

43. Ibid.

44. James J. Lynch, *The Broken Heart: Medical Consequences of Loneliness* (New York: Basic Books, 1977).

45. Lynch, *The Broken Heart.*

46. Henry Dreher, "The Type C Connection: A Powerful New Tool in the Fight Against Cancer," presented to the National Institute for the Clinical Application of Behavioral Medicine, December 1992.

47. Lynch, *The Broken Heart.*

48. Pilisuk and Parks, *The Healing Web.*

49. Ibid.

50. "Lack of Social Relationships Increases Risk of Illness and Death," *Wellness Newsletter,* November–December 1988, 4.

51. "Lack of Social Relationships," 5.

52. Ibid., 5.

53. Robert Ornstein and David Sobel, *The Healing Brain* (New York: Simon & Schuster, 1987), 195–96.

54. Ornstein and Sobel, *The Healing Brain.*

55. Ibid.

56. Bruce Bower, "Emotional Aid Delivers Labor-Saving Results," *Science News* 139 (1991): 277.

57. Sharon Faelten, David Diamond, and the editors of *Prevention* magazine, *Take Control of Your Life: A Complete Guide to Stress Relief* (Emmaus, Pa.: Rodale Press, 1988), 58.

58. Frances Sheridan Goulart, "How to Live a Longer, Healthier Life," n.p., n.d.

59. "Lack of Social Relationships," 4.

60. Nan Silver, "Lonely Child, Sick Adult?" *American Health*, April 1986, 20.

61. Barbara R. Sarason, Irwin G. Sarason, and Gregory R. Pierce, *Social Support: An Interactional View* (New York: John Wiley & Sons, 1990), 256; and J. Stephen Heisel, Steven E. Locke, Linda J. Kraus, and R. Michael Williams, "Natural Killer Cell Activity and MMPI Scores of a Cohort of College Students," *American Journal of Psychiatry* 143 (1986): 1382–86.

62. Janice Kiecolt-Glaser and Ronald Glaser, "Q & A," *Medical Aspects of Human Sexuality* 19, no. 12: 56–57.

63. "Depression and Immunity," *Harvard Medical School Mental Health Letter,* n.d., 8.

64. "Depression and Immunity."

65. Blair Justice, "Think Yourself Healthy," *Prevention,* May 1988, 27–32, 102, 107.

66. Alix Kerr, "Heart Need Friends," *Physician's Weekly,* n.d.

67. "Social Isolation Tied to Heart Attack Deaths," *Deseret News,* May 1, 1988, A10.

68. The editors of *Prevention* magazine, *Positive Living and Health: The Complete Guide to Brain/Body Healing and Mental Empowerment* (Emmaus, Pa.: Rodale Press, 1990), 154.

69. Ibid.

70. Rolf Bang Olsen, Jorn Olsen, Finn Gunner-Svennsson, and Bodil Waldstrom,

"Social Networks and Longevity: A 14-Year Follow-up Study Among Elderly in Denmark," *Social Science Medicine* 33, no. 10: 1189–95.

71. Lynch, *The Broken Heart.*
72. Ibid.
73. Ibid.
74. Ibid.
75. Bernikow, *Alone in America.*
76. Eleanor Smith, "Fighting Cancerous Feelings," *Psychology Today,* May 1988, 22–23.
77. Michael Argyle, *The Psychology of Happiness* (New York: Methuen and Company, 1987).
78. Sheldon Cohen and S. Leonard Syme, *Social Support and Health* (Orlando, Fl.: Academic Press, 1985).
79. Cohen and Syme, *Social Support.*
80. Leonard A. Sagan, *The Health of Nations* (New York: Basic Books, 1987).
81. Dan Zevin, "Blotting Out Cancer with a Smile," *Health,* May 1987, 14.
82. Sagan, *The Health of Nations.*
83. Argyle, *The Psychology of Happiness.*
84. Ibid., 182–83.
85. Blair Justice, *Who Gets Sick: Thinking and Health* (Houston, Texas: Peak Press, 1987), 133.
86. Faelten, Diamond, and the editors of *Prevention* magazine, *Take Control of Your Life,* 272.
87. Ibid.
88. J. W. Pennebaker et al., *Psychosomatic Medicine* 51 (1989): 577.
89. Sarah Hoying, "Confess for Your Health?" *Self,* September 1990, 96.
90. Faelten, Diamond, and the editors of *Prevention* magazine, *Take Control of Your Life,* 273.
91. Justice, *Who Gets Sick,* 139–40.
92. Ibid., 140.
93. Robert Ornstein and Charles Swencionis, *The Healing Brain: A Scientific Reader* (New York: Guilford Press, 1990), 93.
94. Lea B. Jennings, "Potential Benefits of Pet Ownership in Health Promotion,"*Journal of Holistic Nursing* 15, 0 no. 4: 358–72.
95. Editors of *Prevention* magazine, *Positive Living and Health,* 298.
96. Ornstein and Sobel, *The Healing Brain,* 229.
97. Jennings, "Potential Benefits."
98. Ibid.
99. *Journal of Personality and Social Psychology,* June 1990.
100. "Pet Ownership Reduces Stress and Physician Visits Among Elderly," *Healthline,* October 1990, 8, originally cited by the American Psychological Association.
101. *Journal of Personality and Social Psychology.*
102. Title of an article by Shelley Levitt in *50 Plus,* July 1988, 56–61.
103. Editors of *Prevention* magazine, *Positive Living and Health,* 157.
104. To come.
105. Lynne Lohmeier, "The Healing Power of Pets," *East/West,* June 1988, 52.
106. June McNicholas and Glyn M. Collis, "Dogs as Catalysts for Social Interactions: Robustness of the Effect," *British Journal of Psychology* 19, no. 1 (February 2000): 61.
107. Leavitt, 57.
108. McNicholas and Collis, "Dogs as Catalysts."

109.  Lohmeier, "The Healing Power of Pets," 58.
110.  Ornstein and Sobel, *The Healing Brain,* 166.
111.  Editors of *Prevention* magazine, 235.
112.  Hafen and Frandsen, *People Need People,* 78.
113.  Bruce Bower, "Stress Goes to the Dogs," *Science News* 140 (1992): 285.
114.  Bower, "Stress."
115.  Ibid.
116.  Karen M. Allen, "The Human-Animal Bond," *Insights,* n.d., 5.

# CHAPTER 11

# Marriage and Health

*To be happy at home is the ultimate result of all ambition.*

—Samuel Johnson

## Learning Objectives

- Understand the health hazards related to divorce for both adults and children.
- Identify how divorce differs from an unhappy marriage in impacting health.
- Understand the health benefits of a happy marriage.

Marriage—a good one, that is—can help protect people from illness and disease, help them bounce back more quickly if they do get sick, and even help people live longer! If current research is accurate, divorced people and those who are unhappily married don't fare nearly as well in terms of health and long life. And the impact seems to vary depending on age and gender (the health impact of dissolving a marriage seems to be greatest on men).[1]

According to the latest census figures, marriage demographics have changed dramatically over the last decade. Today, 25 million American adults live alone, and married couples make up the smallest percentage of the nation's households in two centuries—only 55 percent of the nation's households include married couples. Households designated by the census as "nonfamily" make up 30 percent of the nation's households; 85 percent of them are single, and the rest are roommates and nontraditional families, such as unmarried heterosexual couples and gay couples.[2]

## The Health Hazards of Divorce

Divorce rates have been on a roller coaster in this country since the end of World War I, when family life was pretty stable and the divorce rate was relatively low. Following World War II, when soldiers started coming back from the war, the divorce rate soared—temporarily. For a period of time after World War II, the divorce rates fell back to their prewar level. Since the postwar period, divorce rates have steadily increased—from about 10 percent in the early 1950s to a rate that approaches 50 percent today. In one disturbing trend, increasing numbers of couples are ending longtime marriages. The percentage of divorces among people over the age of sixty-five more than doubled in the past two decades. Research Associate Professor Marjorie A. Pett of the University of Utah pinpointed five basic reasons for divorce among older couples: They had grown apart and no longer shared dreams, they had personal differences, there was an extramarital relationship, the couples had poor communication, and the marriage was plagued by financial difficulty.

Overall, as a country, the United States has the highest divorce rate in the world.[3] According to statistics, the parents of more than 1 million children divorce in the United States every year.[4] Those same statistics tell us that 30 percent of America's white children and 40 percent of black children spend at least part of their formative years in postdivorce, single-parent families. More than 90 percent of all postdivorce children live with their mother—and only one in three children see their noncustodial parent as often as once a month.

Increasingly, children are being subjected to a second divorce during their childhood. In fact, statistics from the 1980 census indicate that a child born in 1983 will have a 40 percent chance of experiencing a parent's second divorce by the time he or she is eighteen years old. The custodial parent of more than 70 percent of all white children involved in divorce remarries within five years—and more than half of those divorce a second time.[5] According to researchers, the children of these "twice-divorced parents are often seriously disturbed."[6]

## Effects on Children

The effect of divorce on children is perhaps a good starting point in the discussion of how divorce impacts health because it is often the children who suffer the most profoundly. And the suffering is long-lasting as well as deep, according to a study that followed more than 100 children for fifteen years following their parents' divorce.[7]

Researcher Ann S. Masten points out:

*A stressful event rarely occurs in isolation. Divorce is not a single event, but a series of related events embedded in the ongoing lives of people. It often occurs in the context of extreme family conflict and emotional crisis. It can precipitate recurrent financial problems and separations, custodial conflicts, changes of school, home, and daily routine. Above all, divorce can be so devastating to the parents that the children temporarily lose the most important protective factor in their lives, a healthy, well-functioning caregiver.[8]*

The numbers of children affected by divorce and the profile of those caregivers have changed steadily over the past few decades. The number of one-parent families has more than doubled since 1978, and the percentage of children living in one-parent families rose from 12.9 to 25.7 percent in just fifteen years. Although the largest category of single-parent families is that headed by a divorced mother, the number of children living with the father alone has more than doubled since 1970.[9] Even children living in two-parent families are not immune from the stresses involved in divorce. Many are living with one parent who is not their natural parent. The often hostile relationships that exist between stepparents and stepchildren are well known.

And parents of conventional two-parent families can't be too smug about their children being protected from the damaging consequences of divorce. With the increasing frequency and visibility of divorce, even children in stable families are anxious about the possibility of it affecting them.

A ten-year-old in New York saw the movie *Kramer vs. Kramer,* an emotional portrayal of a couple going through a divorce. A few days later her parents had a fight. "My mother walked out of the house," she remembers. "I thought to myself, 'This is it!' and cried and cried. But she had just gone next door to the neighbor's."[10] In the same study, a fifth grader proudly told researchers that "we're one of those families that aren't divorced." After a pause, he added, ". . . at least, not yet."[11]

For children, divorce is one of the most disruptive life events possible—and it leads to changes in biological health. Children almost universally experience divorce as a profound personal, familial, and social loss.[12] In addition to health problems, most children involved in divorce suffer emotional and behavioral changes that can also impact health. Adding insult to injury, most divorced families end up with less affluence—forcing children along with the rest of the family to adjust to a whole new spectrum of reduced economic advantages.

In terms of financial loss, women suffer the most profoundly following a divorce. Studies show that a woman's standard of living declines an average of 73 percent in the first year after divorce. Income levels after divorce depend on how long a couple was married, too. Among those married less than ten years, women have only 51 percent of their former income, whereas men have 195 percent. Among those married ten to seventeen years, women have only 64 percent of their predivorce income, whereas men have 222 percent.[13]

There is a wide range of social, academic, and health problems associated with the children of divorce. They visit health clinics and physicians more often; some childhood cancer and other alterations in physical health as a result of injury have been strongly associated with divorce.[14] On the emotional side, children are prone to become depressed and aggressive and to suffer regression in development; some develop psychosomatic disorders. Many adopt delinquent behavior. Boys especially seem to bear the brunt of divorce. Studies have shown that following a divorce, boys, more than girls, suffer from poor self-image, loss of self-concept, bedwetting, a sense of sorrow, below-average academic performance, anger, withdrawal, delinquent-like behavior, aggression, and frequent fighting.[15]

The propensity for school problems following divorce is well established. Children of divorce are more likely to be lower achievers in school. Among two-parent children, 30 percent were ranked as high achievers and only 2 percent were ranked as low achievers. The figures do a complete turnaround when divorce enters the picture: Among one-parent children, only 1 percent are ranked as high achievers, and a dismal 40 percent are ranked as low achievers.[16]

There are other school problems, too. Children of divorce are more likely to be truant, late, and subject to disciplinary action at school. Absence rates are much higher. Most children involved in divorce attain less education than children of two-parent families, and studies show they are more than twice as likely to give up on school altogether.

Divorce is particularly damaging to a child's emotional and physical health if it involves a move. Moves have been implicated in "a variety of childhood disorders," and, coupled with the stress of a divorce, can be very damaging to a child. "For children especially," researchers say, "stable identification with a place and home seems to represent an important predictor of health."[17]

## Effect on Adults

Children aren't the only ones who face health risks following divorce. Every major study agrees that divorced people—and others who are separated from their spouses—experience more physical and mental illness than those who are married. Divorced people visit physicians significantly more often than do married or single people.[18] Through in-depth studies, divorce has been significantly related to depression,[19] alcoholism, increased traffic accidents, admission to psychiatric facilities, homicides, and death from disease in general.[20] According to research, divorce has the same impact on health as smoking a pack of cigarettes a day.[21] And most therapists agree that divorced people have higher rates of cancer, heart disease, pneumonia, high blood pressure, and accidental death than do married, single, or widowed persons.[22]

Many theories have been extended to explain why. Perhaps it is because a person who has just been through a divorce all too often loses a major source of protecting social support: the family. The family of origin may not approve of the divorce, or may be going through its own crises at the time, unable to spare the considerable emotional strength to be of real support. Access to needed resources may also play a role: Women have low relative income compared to men, and divorce has been solidly shown to increase female poverty.[23] The difficulty of coping with divorce is considerable. According to one prominent researcher, new evidence suggests that divorce may be even more devastating to many people than losing a spouse to death, "since it's harder to accept that the relationship is really over."[24]

Various studies give insight into the specific health hazards of divorce. In one study, divorced Caucasian men under age seventy who live alone have twice the death rate from heart disease, stomach cancer, and cirrhosis of the liver, and three times the incidence of high blood pressure. James Lynch, who has done extensive research into the phenomenon of divorce and loneliness, says those facts are true for both men and women of all ages.[25]

In another study,[26] British researchers looked at two groups of people in their forties from the MRC National Survey of Health and Development. The people in one group were married and had never been divorced or separated. The people in the second group had been divorced or separated at least once. A total of 2,085 people participated in the study. After all other traditional risk factors were considered, researchers found that divorce and separation were strongly associated with depression and anxiety and increased the risk of alcohol abuse. These risks were true even for those who were remarried or who had reunited with their spouses at the time of the study.

Statistics from a variety of nations reveal a significantly higher death rate among divorced men and women than among the married. The divorced die much more frequently from suicide, homicide, and accidental death. The death rate among the divorced is also significantly higher for alcoholism, diabetes, tuberculosis, and lung cancer.[27]

Research has shown that divorce can actually compromise the immune system, which helps explain why there is an increase in illness and death among the divorced. Immune system compromise is especially apparent the first year following divorce. A study of divorced or separated women during the first year following divorce or separation showed that they had poor cellular immune function, a lower number of natural killer cells, and a deficit in their ability to fight disease with responsive lymphocytes.[28]

Research shows that age at the time of divorce may significantly influence how the divorce impacts health. In one study,[29] researchers from the University of Pennsylvania did two successive five-year studies on a large national sample of women (originally derived from the National Longitudinal

Surveys of Young Women). When the study started, all women were between the ages of twenty-four and thirty-four; researchers compared those who had never been married with those who had been divorced or separated. At the conclusion of the first study, the women who had never married had worse health trends and worse overall health than those who had been divorced or separated. But at the conclusion of the second study, when the women were older, it was the divorced and separated women who had experienced the more harmful health effects—findings that were exactly reversed when compared to the first study.

For some reason, divorce also seems to have its most deleterious effects on men. Divorced men suffer significantly more disease and die in far greater numbers before the age of sixty-four than do their married counterparts. The statistics are sobering. Ten times as many die of tuberculosis; seven times as many die of pneumonia and are killed in homicides. More than twice as many die of heart disease, and almost three times as many die of lung cancer. More than twice as many die of complications of strokes, of cancer of the digestive system, and of high blood pressure. More than three times as many commit suicide, and almost eight times as many die of cirrhosis of the liver. Almost four times as many are killed in motor vehicle accidents.[30]

Dr. Robert Seagraves of the University of Chicago Medical School points out:

> *It is difficult for happily married individuals to appreciate the extent of disruption caused by divorce. The individual has lost a social network as well as a spouse. Typically, close friends of married couples are themselves married, and many of these friendships are lost following divorce. The divorced individual reenters the world of dating, feeling rusty in middle age, and facing the same insecurities experienced as a teenager.*[31]

While it has been shown in numerous studies that those who are separated and divorced have greater risk of mental health problems, few studies have determined the causal effect. In other words, did mental health issues possibly *cause* the separation and divorce? It's clear that separation and divorce *do* increase mental health problems, but one study compared the mental health issues of separated and divorced people with those who were widowed. All had problems with mental health after the marriage ended, regardless of whether by separation, divorce, or death—but the study showed that those who were separated or divorced also had mental health problems (though less pronounced) *prior* to the end of the marriage, suggesting that mental health issues could have contributed to the separation or divorce.[32]

Studies show that in all psychiatric hospitals, divorced people are overrepresented—and married people are underrepresented. Risks of disease in almost every category soar with divorce. And, apparently, divorce even affects longevity—clearly evidenced by the fact that the state of Nevada had the second highest death rate from all causes in the United States during the years when it was the divorce center of the country.[33]

Divorce has also been shown to have a particular result on the aging: Those older people who divorce are often forced to live with adult children, get financial assistance from adult children, rely on adult children for informal care, or pay for help from nonrelated caregivers. The effects are most pronounced for elderly men, and remarriage can often cause even more deleterious effects, especially for stepchildren.[34]

## The Divorced Versus the Unhappily Married

New evidence shows that unhappily married people may be the worst off in terms of good health and long life! United Press International recently reported on a collection of studies indicating that among those married in the mid-1970s who are still married, only about one-third are still happy with their spouses. Those studies indicate that women are more unhappy than men, and blacks are less happy than whites. "The outlook for the institution of marriage is bleak," reports the University of Texas sociologist who compiled the study results. And, he says, the study results say "something very negative about marriage"—or at least about the state of the nation's marriages.[35]

All social relationships involve some level of stress—and involve *both* wanted and unwanted demands, gratification, conflict, irritation, and pleasure.[36] The stress this creates is even more intense in an intimate relationship as important as marriage. While the health benefits of a good marriage are well recognized and documented, negative impact on health can occur when the marriage involves things like frequent conflict, anger, jealousy, criticism, moodiness, extreme financial problems, abuse, emotional or physical violence, or sexual assault.[37] According to research, the bad effects of a *negative* marriage are significantly stronger than the good effects from a *positive* marriage.[38]

Research results from a number of cross-sectional studies are all showing that unhappily married people have poorer health than their single counterparts—even the ones who are divorced. Apparently, a major variable in marriage and health is happiness: It isn't just being married that gives you a better chance of being psychologically well-adjusted and physically healthier, but being happily married.[39] According to research, unhappily married people are, healthwise, worse off than anyone else.[40]

Studies now offer preliminary evidence that actual physical changes occur during marital conflict. According to researchers at Stanford University, blood pressure is strongly correlated to positive and negative interactions: During positive interactions, blood pressure is lower, but during negative interactions—fights—it can skyrocket.[41] Similar research at the University of Washington and the University of California, Berkeley, shows that marital conflict affects the heart rate, pulse, and skin resistance.[42]

New studies show that marital fights actually weaken the immune system (especially in women), raise blood pressure, and speed up heart rate. A host of studies shows that marital stress plays a significant role in overall health, increasing the risk for everything from chronic pain to heart attack. Research, in fact, has shown that the risk of a bad marriage is as strong as other medical risks.[43] For women, simply discussing their angry feelings leads to these stressed-out body reactions. For men, the stress seems to accompany the act of talking louder and faster.

In one study, researchers brought ninety newlywed couples into the laboratory—those you would normally expect to have the least amount of conflict. The researchers gave each couple a role-play and asked them to resolve the disagreement involved. Interestingly, researchers noted a number of hostile behaviors—including criticizing, denying responsibility, interrupting, disagreeing, making excuses, and trying to coerce each other into accepting their point of view—even among what researchers considered to be mild disputes.[44]

Scientists monitored the couples' blood continuously for the next twenty-four hours to determine immune response, including measures of natural killer cells, which fight off infection.

"There was a far stronger effect on the immune system than we ever anticipated," said psychologist Janice Kiecolt-Glaser and immunologist Ronald Glaser, both of Ohio State University. "Those couples who expressed the most hostility during the discussions showed a drop of eight measures [of immunity] for the next twenty-four hours."[45]

In reporting on a large study conducted by the Human Population Laboratory of the California Department of Public Health, researchers believe that in terms of health and longevity, it's better to be single than unhappily married. Unhappy marriage has been implicated in a number of specific health problems by teams of researchers who have studied large groups of people. Coronary disease is among the most prevalent among the unhappily married. In one revealing study, researchers screened 10,000 Israeli men before any symptoms of coronary heart disease had appeared. They then observed this population for five years. The men who later had a myocardial infarction reported far more dissatisfaction with their marital life than those men who remained healthy.[46]

Separate studies seem to confirm these findings. Patients with coronary heart disease reported far more frequent dissatisfaction in their marriages than did those without heart disease—and they reported far more marital problems. A series of recent reports has revealed a trend: The occurrence of marital dissatisfaction and a sense of personal rejection stemming from unhappy marriage is the apparent trigger for a surprising number of acute myocardial infarctions.

Psychologist Vicki Helgeson of Carnegie-Mellon University found in a recent study that male cardiac patients were far less prone to follow-up heart attacks if they were able to discuss matters easily with their wives. Married men in the study who reported poor communication with their wives fared even worse than those who were not married. According to Helgeson, "The strong influence of good marriages has caused a general misappraisal of marriage's role in preserving health. A poor marriage may be worse than none at all."[47]

Marital problems apparently can also drive up blood pressure. Researchers at the Department of Psychology at the University of Michigan and at the university's School of Public Health studied almost 700 men and women for twelve years.[48] They found that people with unhappy marriages—especially those who can't easily express their anger—are at twice the risk of death. One key appears to be the way they deal with anger and conflict. Those who suppress anger suffer the greatest consequence of all among the unhappily married. The risks of high blood pressure are greatest for women between the ages of forty-five and sixty-nine, who are the most likely to suppress their anger, and for unhappily married women between the ages of thirty and forty-four, who are apt to feel guilty about expressing anger toward their husbands.

Those who are unhappily married are at a much higher risk for all kinds of illness. A reason could be reduced functioning in the immune system.[49]

Interestingly, preliminary data from new research show that women may bear the greatest health brunt of unhappy marriages. Psychologist Robert W. Levenson of the University of California, Berkeley, studied married couples to determine the health effects of unhappiness in marriage.[50] In Levenson's study, there was no correlation between unhappiness in marriage and the well-being of the husbands. On the other hand, the wives in those unhappy marriages suffered from anxiety, depression, and other stress-related illnesses.

In commenting on the study, psychologist Lynn Fainsilber Katz said that our culture makes emotional work "more of a woman's job. Women take on more of the responsibility for regulating the marriage, and in a distressed marriage, this takes a toll."[51]

Finally, marital satisfaction has a real bearing on not just physical, but also mental, health. Researchers have found a definite relationship between depression and dissatisfaction with one's marriage; the marriage relationship has such an impact on mental health because it is such an important and valued social tie.[52] In a study on depression conducted by the National Institute of Mental Health, 15,000 adults were given personality surveys and other tests that helped determine their level of depression. Only 2.4 percent of single men and 3.9 percent of single women reported major episodes of depression. But the figures changed drastically when researchers looked at those who were unhappily married: Almost one-fifth of all unhappily married men and nearly half of all unhappily married women had major episodes of depression.[53]

In a survey conducted several years ago by researchers at Vanderbilt University, sociologists quizzed 1,100 people nationwide about their feelings and followed up by giving these people personality tests. Those who said they were "not too happy" or "not at all happy" with their marriages were in poorer mental health than were people who were single, divorced, or widowed.[54]

Results of a separate study were the same: In the more than 5,000 people who were extensively studied, people who were unhappy or dissatisfied with their marriages were in poorer mental health than any of the people who were single—whether they had never married, had divorced, or had been widowed. Results of a recent study on marital stress indicate that unhappy marriages have an even greater impact on mental health than on physical well-being, and the researchers from Rutgers University who authored the study call for further studies examining how marriage affects mental health.[55]

## The Health Benefits of a Happy Marriage

The greatest benefits regarding health and long life come to those who are happily married. Those who are happily married seem healthier overall than any other group, according to government researchers with the National Center for Health Statistics. The center, which recently completed a survey of 122,859 people in 47,240 families nationwide, found that married people have fewer health problems than unmarried people.[56] Charlotte Schoenborn, who was instrumental in conducting the study for the government, said that the results "demonstrate that in spite of the recent changes in American marital patterns, there is still a clear association between being well and being married."[57]

Indeed, statistics dating back to the nineteenth century show that married couples have lower death rates from a whole range of diseases. Researchers with the Framingham Heart Study, which tracked the health of more than 5,000 people for more than three decades, reported that getting—and staying—married was a predictor for a long, healthy life.[58]

According to one researcher, "Studies consistently find that the married are in better mental and physical health than the unmarried. On the whole, married people live longer than the unmarried, and they make fewer demands on health care services."[59]

Why would being married help people be healthier and live longer? There are probably a number of factors at work—social, emotional, and economic, to name a few. One study sponsored by the Department of Health and Human Services showed that part of the reason why women, in particular, have better health when married is due to economic reasons. When married, women generally have access to income in excess of personal income, home ownership, and private health insurance.[60] And as research data come in, people who are studying the health effects of marriage believe it can probably be traced at least in part to the strong social support most people receive in marriage.[61] (That would help explain why unhappy marriages, in which social support would probably be absent, are not good protectors of health.)

That theory was borne from a study that followed up on more than 1,000 fifty-five-year-olds in Scotland and explored which factors caused the married to live longer and have better health. The researchers considered four possible factors: the tendency of the married to have less stress, to have better material resources, to indulge in fewer risky behaviors, and to have better social support.

The factors that seemed to make the difference were better material resources and better social support. According to the researchers who conducted the study, "Married people benefit compared with nonmarried people in the availability, amount, and quality of the social support available to them."[62]

## Social Support

Married couples are usually better integrated into the community than are single people. Although single people, especially in large cities, struggle to make friends and meet new people, married couples generally have a much easier time developing a strong social network. It may not be only the marriage, then, but also the entire spectrum of social networking that is enhanced or made easier by marriage.

One researcher believes that the health benefits of married life might be because married people seem to follow through better—maybe because each partner has someone to remind him or her. Married couples, she says, have a tendency "to eat more balanced, regular meals or to be more willing to see a doctor when they suspect something's wrong. Maybe it's having someone around to nag them, but married couples also seem to follow through more completely on taking medicines than do singles."[63]

The health benefits of marriage also might be due to economic factors, as previously mentioned. Many married couples have the benefit of double incomes, and married couples are less likely than singles or single-parent families to be living at or below poverty levels. And statistics have established that the more money you make and the more educated you are, the more healthy you will generally be.[64]

The health benefits of marriage seem to be even greater for men than for women, as previously discussed. (Some studies, in fact, indicate that single women who have never married may fare almost as well as married women in terms of health and longevity.) One reason may be the nature of the friendships outside the marriage. A man's friendships are traditionally "situational"—men have friends at work, friends they fish with, sports buddies, and so on. Women's friendships, on the other hand, are traditionally much longer and more permanent, serving as a source of great emotional strength. Women, unlike men, tend to maintain close confidants with whom they stay in regular contact after marriage. Friendships are important, even in marriage. Research shows that single people with strong networks of friends run fewer risks healthwise than do married people who are relatively isolated.

Social support and the socialization aspects of marriage may indeed play a strong role in health—and some researchers are trying to duplicate it or create a stronger social network for high-risk people, those who have separated or divorced. Results are lending credence to the belief that the social support of marriage is at least partially what helps keep marrieds healthy.

## Injuries and Medical Insurance

According to the earlier-cited National Health Interview Survey, married people report fewer injuries per year than single and divorced people (but, interestingly, more than widowed people). The survey, which studied 122,859 Americans, showed that divorced people had "by far" the highest rate of injuries, with divorced women having more than twice as many as married women.[65]

The same survey showed an interesting trend about insurance: Married people are more likely to be insured than single people, probably—according to a National Center for Health Statistics researcher—because spouses "share each other's employment benefits."[66] According to the center, about 84.5 percent of married women had private health insurance, compared with 66.9 percent of divorced women, 66.5 percent of widows, and 46.5 percent of those who were separated. According to government statisticians, women who are separated are the most likely to be uninsured; even though about 23 percent have public coverage, almost one-third are completely uninsured.

Marital status of parents also affects the health coverage of children. Approximately 80 percent of children who live with both parents are covered by private health insurance. Contrast that with children in single-parent families: Close to two-thirds of children living with their father only are covered by private health insurance, and fewer than one-half of children living with their mother only are covered. Even with public coverage taken into consideration, approximately 29 percent of the children living with fathers and 19.5 percent of the children living with mothers are completely uninsured.

## Coronary Heart Disease/High Blood Pressure

Detailed studies conducted by several researchers have carefully compared deaths from coronary heart disease between people who are married and those who are single, widowed, and divorced. Marriage seems to be a definite protecting factor. Coronary heart disease deaths in the United States per 100,000 population are 176 among the married and 362 among the divorced. Death rates for single, divorced, and widowed individuals are significantly higher than the rates for married individuals; this holds true for coronary heart disease deaths among both men and women and for both whites and nonwhites. Marriage seems to provide an even greater protection for some groups: Divorced white men between the ages of twenty-five and thirty-four have 2.83 times higher death rate from coronary heart disease than do married men of the same age.[67]

One researcher who has specialized in the study of heart disease says that "the magnitudes of some of the increases in death rates in the nonmarried groups are most impressive, sometimes exceeding the married death rates by as much as five times. The differences are greatest at younger ages and tend to diminish somewhat with age. But never do the death rates of the unmarried groups ever fall below those for married individuals."[68]

And, the researcher adds, differences are sometimes even more pronounced. "The excess risk in the widowed under age thirty-five, compared to the married, was greater than tenfold for at least one of the specific age-sex groups, involving several leading causes of death, including arteriosclerotic heart diseases," a degenerative disease that can begin in childhood and that generally progresses very slowly throughout life.[69] Bereavement and other emotions connected with the breakup of a marriage, the researcher says, can hasten the progress of arteriosclerotic heart disease—a disease that generally develops at an "imperceptibly slow pace" over the course of decades.[70]

Data from the Israel Ischemic Heart Disease Project[71] indicate another benefit of marriage in relationship to heart disease. Among men with angina, a wife's love and support appear to protect against the disease, particularly in men who also suffer from high levels of anxiety. University of Rochester School of Medicine researcher Thomas Campbell, in fact, believes that angina is an "illness behavior" rather than a sign of underlying coronary heart disease—and he says that statistics show it is much more common in unhappy marriages.[72]

As far as high blood pressure goes, married men and women are 20 percent less likely to have high blood pressure than people who are single, separated, divorced, or widowed.[73] Married men and women are also more likely to be aware of high blood pressure and to get help when they do develop it, according to researchers who studied a group of more than 4,000 people. In summing up the study, a University of Texas epidemiologist said, "Married people with high blood pressure were 59 percent more likely to be receiving treatment for it, and 78 percent more likely to have it under control."[74]

## Cancer

Earlier research has shown that married people statistically have a lower incidence of cancer at many sites. Only recently, however, has careful study shown that marriage itself actually has an influence on survival rates from cancer.

In one energetic study, researchers collected data on 27,779 cases of cancer on file at the New Mexico Tumor Registry, part of the National Cancer Institute's surveillance program. All the cancer victims in the study were older than twenty years. Researchers did not consider cancers that were diagnosed only from a death certificate or autopsy, cancers on which there was incomplete information, or cancer patients with unknown marital status. Researchers wanted to find out how marital status affected the diagnosis, treatment, and survival of people who had been diagnosed with cancer.[75]

Marital status at the time of diagnosis was used in the study. Patients were coded as single (never married), currently married, divorced, separated, or widowed. Follow-up information and updated files were obtained from the patients' private physicians. At the time of the study, more than one-half of the patients had died; almost two-thirds of the patients who were still alive had been diagnosed more than five years earlier.

In analyzing the results, being unmarried was associated with decreased survival for patients diagnosed with cancer. And the percentage of persons surviving at least five years was greater for married persons than for unmarried persons in almost every category of age, gender, and stage of cancer. Being unmarried was associated with poorer survival at all stages of cancer. All three categories of unmarried people—single (never married), divorced/separated, and widowed—were more likely to develop cancers that had spread beyond a local site, were less likely to receive definitive treatment, and had poorer survival after the diagnosis of cancer.

Researchers point out that the improved survival rate of married persons might be because married people have better health habits—and they are prone to seek medical help at an earlier stage. As stated earlier, marriage also provides important social support, which is widely accepted as buffering the effects of many diseases. And, finally, researchers note that survival from cancer increases as socioeconomic status increases—probably because cancer victims with more money can seek earlier and better medical care and are not apt to delay treatment. As discussed earlier, married people tend to be in higher socioeconomic classes and are more likely to have health insurance coverage, which would lead to earlier medical care.

The most controversial finding of the study was this: Even when the disease was diagnosed at a more advanced stage, the best odds for survival seemed to lie with those who were married. James Goodwin, director of the study, summed it up by saying that "the protective impact of being married affected every stage of cancer care."[76]

"Treatment for cancer often involves frequent trips to the hospital for chemotherapy or radiation. If you're married, you're twice as likely to have help getting there, and to have support when your motivation is waning," said Dr. Goodwin. "Sometimes health care is complex, and if there's no one there to say, 'Hey, wait a minute—that doesn't make sense,' you may ignore information you don't quite understand."[77]

A separate study that had similar results involved researchers who combed through information at the M.D. Anderson Hospital and Tumor Institute in Houston, Texas. Researchers studied 910 married white women with breast cancer and 351 widowed white women with breast cancer. They considered a number of factors, such as how old the women were, what their socioeconomic status was, what stage the disease was in at the time of diagnosis, and whether the women delayed in seeking medical treatment. Again, marriage came out a winner: Widowed patients were less likely to survive than married patients with similar histories. According to the researchers, marital status was "the strongest predictor" of survival among the breast cancer patients.[78]

In still another study, Medical College of Wisconsin researcher James Goodwin showed that the married have much better cancer survival rates. The difference, he says, is probably due to social support and/or better financial conditions among the married, both of which can enable a married person to seek a higher quality of medical care.[79]

## Immune System Function

A number of tests and several careful studies have shown that marriage helps keep the immune system strong—one possible reason why married people enjoy better health than their single, divorced, or widowed counterparts. According to measures of the immune system function—determined by blood tests that measure the level of immune cells in the bloodstream—married people fare the best. Next are singles—those who have never been married. Singles are followed by those who have been widowed. The group of people with the lowest immune system function are those who are divorced or separated.

Researchers at Ohio State University compared the immune function of thirty-eight separated or divorced women with that of thirty-eight married women.[80] Their findings confirm the belief that a happy, stable marriage provides health benefits. Researchers found the following:

- Women within the first year of separation had significantly poorer immune function than very well-matched counterparts in the community who were married.

- Among the married women, those who described their marriage as better had better immune function.

- The longer separated or divorced women had been separated or divorced (the less they were still attached to their ex-husbands), the better their immune systems were working.

A separate group of researchers at Ohio State University's College of Medicine decided to take a look at men with herpes, an infection that tends to directly mirror the strength of the immune system.[81] (When the immune system is compromised, the herpes infection flares up; when the immune system is strong, the infection is kept in check.) All the men in the study had active herpes infection. All were given psychological and immunological tests, and researchers compared the married men with the ones who were separated or divorced.

Again, strong marriages were demonstrated to be the best protection as far as a boost in immune function. The researchers found that:

- The separated or divorced men were more anxious, depressed, and lonely than were their married counterparts—and, not surprisingly, their immune systems were significantly weaker.

- Among the married men, the ones who were happy with their marriages had the strongest immune functioning. Those who had unhappy or unsatisfying relationships with their wives had higher levels of active herpes antibodies as well as lower ratios of T helper cells to suppressor cells.

In another study, researchers studied women, comparing married women to divorced women. In tests measuring the strength of the immune system, the married women came out on top. Those who had been separated or divorced for less than a year—and were still attached to their ex-husbands—fared the worst.[82]

## Mental Health

A growing body of evidence seems to indicate that the married are in better mental health than the unmarried—and that the married are happier, less likely to commit suicide, and less likely to be institutionalized for psychiatric illness.[83] Hosts of studies show that married people are less likely to have all kinds of mental disorders than the never married, separated, divorced, and widowed. Research shows that being married or having a marriage-like relationship even acts as a protective factor in reducing the impact of inherited liability to symptoms of depression.[84] Research shows that a man who has never married is 3.13 times more likely to have a mental disorder than is his married counterpart. Those who are widowed are more than twice as likely to have a mental disorder. But the most devastating risk is for a divorced man: He is more than five times as likely to have a mental disorder than is a married man of similar age and circumstance.[85] In this study, as in others, marriage seems to provide even greater protection to men than women: Single and widowed women are only about one and a half times as likely to have mental disorders as married women, and divorced women are nearly three times as likely to have mental disorders.[86]

Interestingly, recent studies show that the protective factor of marriage does not apply equally across ethnic lines. A study conducted by researchers in Hawaii compared four ethnic groups—white Americans, Japanese Americans, Filipino Americans, and native Hawaiians—to determine whether single people suffered more psychiatric symptoms than married people.[87]

The researchers concluded that marriage definitely seemed to provide protection from psychiatric symptoms among white Americans and native Hawaiians, but not among Japanese and Filipino Americans. Marriage simply did not seem to be as important to mental health among these two groups. There could be many reasons why, said the researchers, but a main, likely reason is that people in those cultures derive a great deal of good social support from sources outside of marriage.

People who are not married are also more likely to have alcoholism, sometimes considered a manifestation of mental illness. In a Swedish study of middle-aged men, researchers compared alcoholism rates between the married men in the study and the divorced men in the study. More than one-fourth of all the divorced men in the study were registered with the

Social Services as having alcohol problems; only 5 percent of the married men were so registered.[88]

A great deal of marriage's protection probably has to do with the fact that it provides "instant" social support: People with a supportive spouse are much less likely to become depressed following stressful incidents in their lives. Among women with stress, almost half who get little or no support from their husbands become deeply depressed. When married women have a high level of support from their husbands, only about 10 percent become depressed.[89]

## Marriage and Life Expectancy

As study results poured in, researchers reached the same conclusion: Happy marriage dramatically increases life expectancy. In fact, a man who marries can expect to automatically add about nine years and seven months to his life.[90] In one large-scale study of Swedish men, married men had a mortality rate of only 9 percent during the three years of the study; their divorced counterparts had a rate of 20 percent.[91]

One recent study of unmarried middle-aged men and women showed that they faced twice the risk of dying within ten years as did those still living with their spouses.[92] The study—which involved more than 7,600 people nationwide—was conducted by researchers at the University of California, San Francisco. They found a significant gap between the married and the unmarried—and divorce is a key factor in putting people at risk.

Marriage itself, they concluded, seems to be the key factor. "Of particular interest is that both men who live alone and those who live with someone other than a spouse are equally disadvantaged for survival," said epidemiologist Maradee Davis, who led the study. "The critical factor seems to be the presence of a spouse."[93]

Researchers agree: The unmarried have higher death rates from all causes of death. The differences are greatest at younger ages, and the differences are the most apparent among men. U.S. mortality rates for all causes of death are consistently higher for divorced, single, and widowed individuals of both sexes and all races.[94] In fact, according to one researcher who has specialized in the study of heart disease and other causes of death, some of the increased death rates in unmarried individuals are "astounding," rising as high as ten times the rates for married individuals of comparable ages.[95] The researcher sums up:

> *The overall death rate for divorced individuals in the United States is almost double that of married individuals. For every major cause of death, rates for divorced males range anywhere from two to six times higher than those of their married counterparts. Single and widowed males show similarly high death rates when compared to those who were married.*[96]

# ENDNOTES

1. K. Williams and D. Umberson, "Marital Status, Marital Transitions, and Health: A Gendered Life Course Perspective," *J Health Soc Behav* 45, no. 1 (March 2004): 81–98.

2. Mimi Hall, "Percentage of Marrieds Is Smallest in 200 Years," *USA Today,* June 11, 1991.

3. Leonard A. Sagan, *The Health of Nations* (New York: Basic Books, 1987).

4. Neil Kalter, "Effects of Divorce on Boys Versus Girls," *Medical Aspects of Human Sexuality,* November 1989, 26–34.

5. Kalter, "Effects of Divorce."

6. Sagan, *The Health of Nations.*

7. Judith Wallerstein and Sandra Blakeslee, "A Family Divided: Time Bombs of Divorce," *American Health,* June 1989, 49–59.

8. Ann S. Masten, "Stress, Coping, and Children's Health," *Pediatric Annals* 14, no. 8: 544–47.

9. Sagan, *The Health of Nations.*

10. Ibid.

11. Ibid.

12. Sheldon Cohen and S. Leonard Syme, eds., *Social Support and Health* (London: Academic Press, 1985).

13. Kalter, "Effects of Divorce."

14. Cohen and Syme, *Social Support.*

15. Kalter, "Effects of Divorce."

16. Sagan, *The Health of Nations.*

17. Cohen and Syme, *Social Support.*

18. Barbara R. Sarason, Irwin G. Sarason, and Gregory R. Pierce, *Social Support: An Interactional View* (New York: John Wiley and Sons, 1990), 257.

19. Sarason et al., *Social Support.*

20. Marc Pilisuk and Susan Hillier Parks, *The Healing Web* (Hanover, N. H.: University Press of New England, 1986).

21. H. Morowitz, "Hiding in the Hammond Report," *Hospital Practice,* August 1975, 35–39.

22. Bernie S. Siegel, *Love, Medicine, and Miracles* (New York: Harper & Row, 1986).

23. C. A. Heath and D. H. Ciscel, "Patriarchy, Family Structure and the Exploitation of Women's Labor," *Journal of Economic Issues* 22, no. 3 (September 1988): 781–94.

24. Siegel, *Love, Medicine, and Miracles.*

25. Brent Q. Hafen and Kathryn J. Frandsen, *People Need People: The Importance of Relationships to Health and Wellness* (Evergreen, Colo.: Cordillera Press, 1987), 33–34.

26. M. Richards, R. Hardy, and M. Wadsworth, "The Effects of Divorce and Separation on Mental Health in a National UK Birth Cohort," *Psychological Medicine* 72 (1997): 1121–28.

27. R. Taylor Segraves, "Divorce and Health Problems," *Medical Aspects of Human Sexuality,* June 1989, 106.

28. Sarason et al., *Social Support.*

29. Ingrid Waldron, Christopher C. Weiss, and Mary Elizabeth Hughes, "Marital Status Effects on Health: Are There Differences Between Never Married Women and Divorced and Separated Women?" *Social Sciences and Medicine* 45, no. 9: 1387–97.

30. Hafen and Frandsen, *People Need People,* 35.

31. Ibid.

32. T. J. Wade and D. J. Pevalin, "Marital Transitions and Mental Health," *J Health Soc Behav* 45, no. 2 (June 2004): 155–70.

33. Barbara Powell, *Alone, Alive, and Well* (Emmaus, Pa.: Rodale Press, 1985).

34. L. E. Pezzin and B. S. Schone, "Parental Marital Disruption and Intergenerational Transfers: An Analysis of Lone Elderly Parents and Their Children," *Demography* 36, no. 3(August 1999): 287–97.

35. "Just 1 in 3 Married in '70s Is Still Contented," *Deseret News,* January 27, 1989.

36. Allan V. Horwitz, Julie McLaughlin, and Helen Raskin White, "How the Negative and Positive Aspects of Partner Relationships Affect the Mental Health of Young Married People," *Journal of Health and Social Behavior* 39, no. 2: 124–36; and George Homans, *Social Behavior,* 2nd ed. (New York: Harcourt Brace Jovanovich, 1974).

37. Horwitz et al., "How the Negative"; and Paul R. Amato and Stacey J. Rogers, "A Longitudinal Study of Marital Problems and Subsequent Divorce," *Journal of Marriage and the Family* 59 (1997): 612–24.

38. Tracy A. Revenson, Kathleen M. Schiaffino, S. Deborah Majerovitz, and Allan Giborsky, "Social Support As a Double-Edged Sword: The Relation of Positive and Problematic Support to Depression Among Rheumatoid Arthritis Patients," *Social Science and Medicine* 33 (1991): 807–13; Heather A. Turner, "Gender and Social Support: Taking the Bad with the Good?" *Sex Roles* 30 (1994): 521–41; and Debra Umberson, Meichu D. Chen, James S. House, Kristine Hopkins, and Ellen Slaten, "The Effect of Social Relationships on Psychological Well-Being: Are Men and Women Really So Different?" *American Sociological Review* 61 (1996): 837–57.

39. Sarason et al., *Social Support,* 258.

40. Powell, *Alone, Alive, and Well.*

41. Bonnie Burman and Gayla Margolin, "Marriage and Health," *Advances* 6, no. 4: 51–58.

42. Burman and Margolin, *Marriage and Health.*

43. Tara Parker-Pope, "When Your Spouse Makes You Sick: Research Probes Toll of Marital Stress," *Wall Street Journal,* May 4, 2004, D1.

44. *Psychosomatic Medicine,* 55 (1993): 395–409.

45. Linda Murray, "Mad Marriages: Arguing Your Way to Better Health," *Longevity,* October 1993, 30.

46. James J. Lynch, *The Broken Heart: The Medical Consequences of Loneliness* (New York: Basic Books, 1977).

47. "Communication with Spouse Reduces Cardiac Risk," *Brain/Mind and Common Sense* 17, no. 12: 1.

48. Sharon Faelten, David Diamond, and the editors of *Prevention* Magazine, *Take Control of Your Life: A Complete Guide to Stress Relief* (Emmaus, Pa.: Rodale Press, 1988), 143–44.

49. Sarason et al., *Social Support.*

50. Linda Murray, "Love and Longevity," *Longevity,* January 1993, 56.

51. Murray, "Love and Longevity."

52. Horwitz et al., "How the Negative."

53. Catherine Houck, "Uncovering the Secrets of Happiness," *Cosmopolitan,* n.d., 236–40.

54. Powell, *Alone, Alive, and Well.*

55. Horwitz et al., "How the Negative."

56. "Marriage and Wellness Linked," *Deseret News,* November 15, 1988, 4A.
57. "Marriage and Wellness Linked."
58. Carol Turkington, "Have You Hugged Your Immune System Today?" *Self,* October 1988, 184.
59. Powell, *Alone, Alive, and Well.*
60. Beth A. Hahn, "Marital Status and Women's Health: The Effect of Economic Marital Acquisitions," *Journal of Marriage and the Family* 55(1993): 495–504.
61. Burman and Margolin, *Marriage and Health.*
62. Sally Wyke and Graeme Rod, "Competing Explanations for Associations Between Marital Status and Health," *Social Science and Medicine* 34, no. 5: 523–32.
63. Turkington, "Have You Hugged," 184.
64. Ibid.
65. Emily Friedman, "Marriage May Promote Health," *Medical World News,* December 26, 1988, 34.
66. Friedman, "Marriage May Promote Health."
67. Lynch, *The Broken Heart.*
68. Ibid.
69. Ibid.
70. Ibid.
71. J. H. Medalie and U. Goldbourt, "Angina Pectoris Among 10,000: II. Psychosocial and Other Risk Factors as Evidenced by a Multivariate Analysis of a Five-Year Incidence Study," *American Journal of Medicine* 60 (1976): 10–21.
72. Burman and Margolin, *Marriage and Health.*
73. Sally Squires, "Marriage—Good for the Heart," *American Health,* July 1987, 111.
74. Squires, "Marriage."
75. James S. Goodwin, William C. Hunt, Charles R. Key, and Jonathan M. Samet, "The Effect of Marital Status on Stage, Treatment, and Survival of Cancer Patients," *Journal of the American Medical Association* 258, no. 21: 3125–30.
76. Turkington, "Have You Hugged," 184.
77. Ibid.
78. Neale, Tilley, and Vernon, "Marital Status, Delay in Seeking Treatment, and Survival from Breast Cancer," *Social Science and Medicine* 23, no. 3: 305–12.
79. The editors of *Prevention* magazine and the Center for Positive Living, *Positive Living and Health: The Complete Guide to Brain/Body Healing and Mental Empowerment* (Emmaus, Pa.: Rodale Press, 1990), 337.
80. "Is Marriage Good for Your Health? An Interview with Janice Kiecolt-Glaser," *Mind/Body/Health Digest* 1, no. 2: 1.
81. Rick Weiss, "Worried Sick: Hassles and Herpes," *Science News* 132 (1987): 360.
82. J. K. Kiecolt-Glaser, L. A. Fisher, P. Olgrocki, J. C. Stout, C. E. Speicher, and R. Glaser, "Marital Quality, Marital Disruption, and Immune Function," *Psychosomatic Medicine* 49 (1987): 13–34.
83. Powell, *Alone, Alive, and Well.*
84. A. C. Heath, L. J. Eaves, and N. G. Martin, "Interaction of Marital Status and Genetic Risk for Symptoms of Depression," *Twin Research* 1, no. 3 (September 1998): 119–22.
85. Michael Argyle, *The Psychology of Happiness* (New York: Methuen and Company, 1987).
86. Argyle, *The Psychology of Happiness.*
87. From D. T. Takeuchi and K. N. Speechley, "Ethnic Differences in the Marital

Status and Psychosocial Relationship," *Social Psychiatry and Psychiatric Epidemiology* 24 (1989): 288–94.

88. A. Rosengren, H. Wedel, and L. Wilhelmsen, "Marital Status and Mortality in Middle-Aged Swedish Men," *American Journal of Epidemiology* 129, no. 1: 54–64.

89. Argyle, *The Psychology of Happiness,* 27.

90. Jo Ann Tooley and Lynn Y. Anderson, "Living Is Risky," *U.S. News and World Report,* January 25, 1988, 77.

91. Rosengren et al., "Marital Status."

92. Morton Hunt, "Long-Life Insurance: For Men, It's Marriage," *Longevity,* February 1991, 10.

93. Hunt, "Long-Life Insurance."

94. Lynch, *The Broken Heart.*

95. Ibid.

96. Ibid.

# CHAPTER 12

# Families and Health

*The happiest moments of my life have been the few which I
have passed at home in the bosom of my family.*

—Thomas Jefferson

## Learning Objectives

- Define the concept of *family.*
- Explain how the early influence of parents impacts the health and longevity of their children.
- Discuss the traits of weak or stressed families and their negative impact on health.
- Understand the traits of strong families and know how those families contribute to the health and longevity of their members.
- Explain the importance of family reunions and other traditions that keep families close.

In an October 1965 speech delivered at New York's Abbott House, the Reverend Martin Luther King, Jr., summarized the role of the family this way:

> *Family life not only educates in general, but its quality ultimately determines the individual's capacity to love. The institution of the family is decisive in determining not only if a person has the capacity to love another individual, but, in the larger sense, whether he is capable of loving his fellow men collectively. The whole of society rests on this foundation for stability, understanding, and social peace.*[1]

## What Is a Family?

The term *family* describes a "unique cluster of people who enjoy a special relationship by reason of love, marriage, procreation, and mutual dependence."[2] During the past three decades, Americans have virtually remade society—and, along with it, the family. The statistics tell at least part of the story: According to a special issue of *Newsweek,* today's American family is likely to be very different from Ozzie and Harriet or the Cleavers.

The divorce rate has doubled since 1965 . . . and demographers project that half of all first marriages made today will end in divorce. Six out of ten second marriages will probably collapse. One-third of all children born in the past decade will probably live in a stepfamily before they are eighteen. One out of every four children today is being raised by a single parent. About 22 percent of children today were born out of wedlock; of those, about a third were born to a teenage mother. One out of every five children lives in poverty; the rate is twice as high among blacks and Hispanics.[3]

But the image of Ozzie and Harriet is still with us, say researchers who are studying the family, and it still has a great deal of impact on today's family unit, regardless of how many changes take place. According to Yale historian John Demos, "In a time when parents seem to feel a great deal of change in family experience, that image is comfortingly solid and secure, a counterpoint to what we think is threatening for the future."[4]

Whatever the family unit, a family is a group that shares common goals and values, and they work together to achieve those goals. What goes on in a family—the network of relationships between its members—can have a profound influence on the health and longevity of its members. In fact, the health of each member of the family can be influenced by many factors: how big the family is, how many fights the family engages in, whether one or both parents work, whether family members can effectively communicate with each other, and more. A family member's health can even be affected by whether the family holds regular family reunions!

## The Early Influence of Parents

Parents have an incredible impact on the health and development of children. The way parents treat their children determines in large part the way the children will feel about themselves—while they are children and when they become adults. Parents can endow them with a healthy self-image or engender feelings of low self-esteem. Children react to parents' emotions, moods, and behavior. If the parents are stressed, they can rear children who are stressed—and, therefore, children who are prone to disease.

Relationships in early childhood seem to play a huge role in the development and health of family members, and the impact of the mother appears to be especially important. For example, monkeys who are raised by their peers instead of by their mothers have reduced function of serotonin in the central nervous system—a condition that has been linked in humans to violence, alienation, social isolation, and suicide.[5] There seems to be other impact on the brain as well: Adult rats that were handled and nurtured as infants experience slower aging of the hippocampus, the center in the brain that shows the earlier degeneration in Alzheimer's disease.[6] And those rats that were raised in a toy-filled "complex" with other rats had 30 percent more nerve cell connections in their brains, which are associated with better performance on difficult learning and problem-solving tasks.[7]

The impact of early relationships also seems to have an effect on how well we respond to stress. In one study, researchers subjected adult rats from nine litters to twenty minutes of restraint; the rats that were licked and groomed more as pups showed much lower response to the stress of being restrained.[8] And infants who lived for at least eight months amid the emotional and physical deprivation of Romanian orphanages were still producing much higher levels of stress hormones six years later when compared to children who had not lived in the orphanages.[9]

## Experiments with Monkeys

Other experiments have shown the importance of a parent's presence and touch. Dr. Harry F. Harlow at the University of Wisconsin noticed that baby monkeys that had cloth pads on the floor of their wire cages were stronger and huskier than the baby monkeys with no cloth pad. The babies treated the cloth pad much as a child treats a teddy bear; they cuddled it, caressed it, and played with it. That observation prompted Harlow to construct a kind of surrogate "mother" for the monkeys—a wire monkey covered with terry cloth that had a light bulb inside (to radiate heat) and a rubber nipple (to dispense milk). The baby monkeys were enthusiastic in their acceptance.

His success with the surrogate "mother" prompted him to examine whether the babies really needed a mother that was so touchable. He constructed a second "mother," this time of wire alone. There was no terry cloth and no light bulb to provide warmth. There was a rubber nipple and a supply of milk, but that was all. Of the eight baby monkeys, four were allowed to nurse from the terry cloth mother while the other four were allowed to nurse only from the wire mother. All eight of the monkeys spent most of their time cuddling the terry cloth mother. At feeding time, the four would go to the wire mother for their milk, but they would instantly return to the terrycloth mother as soon as they were finished eating. Whenever they were frightened, all eight would climb onto the terrycloth mother for solace.

In still other experiments, monkeys were placed in cages with nothing but a wire mother. Although they took their nourishment from her, many of them did not survive. Those who did had poor coping mechanisms. When placed under stress, they cowered in a corner, hid their faces under their arms, or screamed. Their deprived development occurred even though they could see, hear, and smell other baby monkeys.

Results of the study and its implications about early attachment between mothers and infants "reflects [*sic*] millions of years of evolutionary history," says Dr. Stephen Suomi, chief of the Laboratory of Comparative Ethology at the National Institute of Child Health and Human Development in Bethesda, Maryland, who worked with Harlow on the monkey experiments. "The mother buffers the child from the big, scary world. How she does that can have profound impact on her youngster's ability to function socially, as well as on their basic biology."[10]

## Studies with Babies

The same thing seems to apply to human beings. Twenty-five years ago Dr. Rene Spitz, now at the University of Colorado Medical Center, first described "marasmus"—the physical wasting away of infants who suddenly lost their mothers. Some infants who suddenly lost their mothers refused to eat and, even when force-fed, would eventually die.[11]

In studies conducted by Dr. Spitz and Katherine Wolf, ninety-one infants in foundling homes throughout the United States and Canada were carefully observed. Even though all of the babies were well cared for physically, they didn't grow as rapidly as normal babies; none gained the weight they should have, and some even lost weight. There were effects other than the physical ones, too; the babies seemed depressed and anxious. A little more than one-third of the babies in the foundling hospitals—thirty-four of the babies—died despite what researchers said was "good food and meticulous medical care."[12]

In one study of orphaned infants, half of the orphans were placed in foster homes and half were placed in institutions. After one year, researchers studied both sets of babies. The children who had been placed in foster homes did better in every way, both mentally and physically. At that point, when all the children were one year old, those who had been originally placed in institutions were placed in foster homes. Researchers then took another look when the children were five. Although the institutionalized children had improved in both behavior and performance, they were, five years later, still behind in development when compared with the children who had been placed in foster homes at birth. The researchers concluded that the psychic trauma "of the first year of neglect was never overcome."[13]

## The Effects of Neglect

Other experiments had similar results. Researchers studied a group of one-year-old children who had been born to mothers with an average IQ of 70 and who were unable to care for their children. Half of the children were routinely placed in institutions. The other half, who had been randomly selected from the group, were placed in a hospital ward of mentally retarded adults where each was assigned a one-to-one relationship with an individual woman who assumed a motherly role. Three years later researchers took a look at the children. Those in the routine institutional care hadn't fared very well: They had deteriorated and were significantly retarded. As a group, they had lost an average of 26 IQ points each. The group of children who had been cared for by the retarded women had gained an average of 29 IQ points each.[14]

Researchers didn't stop there. Thirty years later, they followed up on each child who had been part of the study. Again, the institutionalized children presented a bleak picture. All were still institutionalized; a number were dead. The most advanced among them had completed the third grade. In sharp contrast, the children who had been cared for by a "mother" in the hospital had made impressive gains. Most had completed high school. A few had even completed a year of college. All were self-supporting. The children in the study clearly illustrated "the debilitating effect of neglect during childhood, and of the benefit to intellectual development of affectionate care even by retarded mothers."[15]

Apparently the importance of a parent's influence is present at the moment of birth. The animal world presents many examples. Researchers at Cornell Animal Behavior Farm noted that when mother sheep were prevented from licking their newborn after birth, the lambs were unable to stand on their legs—and subsequently died. Almost the opposite occurs when mother animals are allowed "gentling" of their young—the baby animals show an increased immune response when they are experimentally exposed to vaccinations later in life. In one experiment, in fact, the enhanced immune response proved true in every animal tested![16]

Again, similar results have been obtained with human babies. In one study, mothers who had extra contact with a child during the first hours after birth demonstrated significantly more fondling, soothing, and eye contact with the child one month later. Two years later, these same mothers spoke to their children with more questions, fewer commands, and more words per proposition.[17]

In a separate study, 301 new mothers were randomly assigned to different postpartum nursing schedules: 134 of the infants were roomed with their mothers; the other 143 were roomed in the nursery and given routine visits to their mothers. Researchers kept track of the infants' progress during the next twenty-one months. Of the 143 babies roomed in the nursery, away from their mothers, 9 were hospitalized because of "parenting disturbances"—for abuse, neglect, abandonment, or failure to thrive. Of the 134 babies who had been roomed with their mothers, only 1 required hospitalization during the subsequent twenty-one months. The study should not only have an impact in setting hospital policy, but should also "demonstrate the extreme sensitivity of the infant to the care given in the first hours of life."[18]

Dr. Mary D. Salter Ainsworth, recognized as one of the top researchers in infant-mother attachment, believes that a parent's influence is significant from the moment of birth—and she's conducted studies to prove her point. In one study, she examined groups of babies who had been treated differently during their first year of life. Some had been virtually ignored, having little physical contact with their mothers; these mothers typically felt that by not "coddling" their babies, they were allowing their babies to develop a sense of independence and were avoiding what they felt to be an unhealthy "attachment." The second group of babies had been occasionally cuddled and held by their mothers—but, for the most part, they had been encouraged to be independent. The third group had mothers who consistently responded to their signals—especially their crying—by picking them up and comforting them.

At one year of age, the most secure, well-adjusted babies were the ones in the third group—the ones whose mothers had comforted them consistently. The babies in the second group—the ones whose mothers had occasionally responded to them—had a form of "anxious attachment." They seemed anxious and worried when separated from their mothers, and yet were not able to relate normally to their mothers, either. The worst of the babies were those in the first group—the ones whose mothers gave them little physical contact during the first year and who did not respond to their signals, such as crying. These babies were anxious and resistant. When researchers first separated them from their mothers by placing them in a strange room and then returning them to their mothers, the babies avoided contact with their mothers and resisted being held.

Ainsworth's conclusion speaks strongly about the influence of parents in a child's early life: "Babies under a year need a certain kind of tender, responsive holding when they're upset. If they don't get it, they learn to count on not having their needs met"—a situation that makes them hostile, angry, and rejecting. The influence of parents and the quality of relationship that a child has with the parents apparently continues to be a strong factor in both physical and mental health—even beyond the first few critical years.

## Parental Styles

The influence is great, too, for parental style when it comes to disciplining children. University of California psychologist Diana Baumrind reported findings to the American Psychological Association that were surprising even to her after she studied teenagers, their parents, and their health. Baumrind and her colleagues were looking for evidence that would validate one parenting style over another in terms of producing children who were healthy both physically and emotionally. "We expected that at puberty, some imbalance in favor of freedom over control would have become desirable, but that did not happen," she reports.[19] In fact, the healthiest children came from families in which the parents were authoritative, placing restrictions and demands on children but providing good support as well. These children did better academically, used fewer drugs and less alcohol, and showed the most social competence, maturity, and optimism.

In discussing the study results, Baumrind stressed the importance of support. Authoritative parents, she explains, "are not bossy. They make it their business to know their children, how they're doing in school, and who their friends are. Their control reflects a high level of commitment to the child, and they are not afraid to confront the child."[20]

Another long-range study of medical school graduates followed more than 900 of them from 1948 through 1964. At various intervals these graduates were given personality tests—tests that measured, among other things, how close they felt to their parents. By the middle of 1973, twenty-six of the graduates had developed malignant tumors. Researchers were curious about what those graduates might have had in common, so they poured over the personality tests the graduates had taken when they were healthy. Twenty of the cancer victims had scored extremely low on questions determining closeness to their parents.

Dr. Sidney Cobb, former president of the American Psychosomatic Society and professor emeritus of community health and psychiatry at Brown University, stated that there is "a great need for a family environment that allows us to be ourselves and to express ourselves openly."[21] Researcher Leonard Sagan adds, "Children raised in an affectionate environment grow more rapidly and reach greater size as adults. On the other hand, there is ample evidence that emotional deprivation can have a deleterious effect on growth.[22]

The affection style of parents also seems to have an impact on the health and development of the children in the family, especially on their emotional development. Those from families in which both parents were affectionate show less neuroticism as well as significantly less anxiety and depression. Here again, the mother may have the greatest influence: Those who had affectionate fathers but not affectionate mothers suffered greater emotional problems—and those families were marked by greater conflict, separation/divorce of the parents, emotional problems in the parents, and mistreatment by the parents.[23]

## Parental Loss

Even more devastating is the loss of a parent, especially during childhood. Early parental loss is directly related to a wide variety of physical, emotional, and intellectual problems in the child—and children deprived of one parent during childhood have a greatly increased risk of many individual diseases, as well as suicide and alcoholism.

A research group at Rochester Medical School decided to look into the backgrounds of the patients at the hospital. They found that a significant number of the adult patients hospitalized with physical disease had lost one or both parents when they were children. And data from two prominent heart studies showed that a significant number of coronary patients had lost their father to death, usually between ages five and seventeen.

# Traits of Weak or Stressed Families

Health problems can be traced to weak or stressed families—and many of those families share certain characteristics that help us identify them. Many of those families are also a product of the times. America is no longer a nation of extended families. Fifty years ago almost three-fourths of all households in the United States included at least one grandparent as an active, full-time member of the household. Today, fewer than 2 percent have a grandparent as a resource. Families have lost that important outlet, a person to lean on in times of stress.

In 1930 children spent an estimated four hours a day in close personal contact with members of the extended family: parents, grandparents, aunts, uncles, and cousins who lived nearby. Today, in a mobile society, chances are great that a child's grandparents, aunts, uncles, and cousins are spread across the state, if not across the nation. Few live in the same neighborhood. Extended families are not living under the same roof anymore. Americans have been reduced to what is called the "nuclear" family, consisting of parents and children.

Interaction within the nuclear family does not approach the three or four hours of intensive daily interaction in families earlier in the last century. Experts estimate that interaction in most nuclear families is limited to a few minutes a day—and those aren't necessarily positive. "Of those few minutes, more than half are used in one-way, negatively toned communications of parents issuing warnings or reproaching children for things done wrong."[24]

Then there's the trend toward two-career families. In 1940, more than 90 percent of all households in the United States had a full-time homemaker who spent approximately thirty-nine hours a week doing domestic chores. Even with time-saving appliances and methods, it still takes about thirty-seven hours a week to successfully run a household. Today, nearly 88 percent of all children who return home from school in the United States enter a household where every living member has been gone the best ten hours of the day. The scenario is vastly different: Everyone comes home at the end of an exhausting day, still faced with the routine business of the household. Little wonder that no one has lots of spare time for meaningful family interaction![25]

And team up those trends with the ten top stresses for today's families:

1. Economics, finances, and budgeting
2. Children's behavior, discipline, and sibling fighting
3. Insufficient couple time
4. Lack of shared responsibility in the family
5. Communicating with children
6. Insufficient "me" time
7. Guilt for not accomplishing more
8. Poor spousal relationships
9. Insufficient family play time
10. An overscheduled family calendar[26]

No wonder families experience breakdown!

A number of traits signify tension and distress in a family:

1. **Physical symptoms.** Children may bite their nails, stutter, or have other nervous habits usually associated with tension. Those over age six may still wet the bed. When children are placed under stress, they may react by throwing violent tantrums. Parents and children alike may have frequent and unexplainable illnesses, often hallmarked by a collection of vague symptoms that persist for months (such as chronic headache, indigestion, or fatigue).

2. **Signs of stress.** In problem families, molehills often do become mountains. Small disagreements or conflicts often escalate into major battlefields. There are far too many quarrels and misunderstandings, not to mention conflicts between husband and wife. Nobody seems able to relax. There never seems to be enough time to accomplish even basic goals. As a consequence, family members try to escape from each other— at the office, in a room with a locked door, anywhere they don't have to deal with the pressures of the family.

3. **Burnout.** Instead of being a joy, family life becomes a burden. Parents get to the point at which they no longer enjoy their children; they feel as though they are standing by helplessly while the children dominate

the family. This is the same kind of burnout that renders executives and medical personnel helpless.

4. **Lack of communication.** Children in troubled families don't feel free to approach their parents about difficult subjects, such as drug or alcohol use or premarital sex. Instead of depending on their parents for help, they try to cope with things on their own. These problem families have trouble talking about simple things as well. Too much of the time, confusion reigns—and, in the meantime, nobody explores ideas, talks about feelings, or reaches solutions. Nobody really listens to anybody else.

5. **"Controlled" arguments.** A few good shouting matches between family members are okay. In fact, this is desirable—if family members use good communication skills to patch things up afterward. That's what happens in healthy families. In troubled families, arguments are quite different. Troubled families often have an unwritten or unspoken rule that all anger must be controlled. Disagreements are buried in silence. Instead of getting things out in the open, these families let disagreements smoulder beneath the surface for weeks. When somebody finally gets around to talking about what's happened, no one seems to care (or hear) what is being said. Instead of negotiating and compromising, family members become absorbed with who is in control and who is right.

6. **Interaction with others.** In healthy families, members have a deep sense of loyalty and concern for members of the family, but they also have rich and rewarding relationships outside the family. No one in the family is threatened by these. Troubled families seem to be at one of two extremes. At one end of the spectrum, family members belong to a tight-knit group; parents insist that children have no outside friends, interests, or activities. All family members are forced into doing things only with other members of the family. At the other end of the spectrum are the families that are extremely loosely constructed; each family member has his or her own interests and activities, and very little interaction occurs between family members.

7. **Lack of affection.** Even if family members were able to share affection when children were young, they stop at some point, and in most troubled families, parents stay a "safe" distance from their children. Little, if any, hugging and kissing go on—which the children come to interpret as a lack of concern.

8. **Infidelity.** Many troubled families are characterized by sexual infidelity—but there is other infidelity, too. Some spouses become "unfaithful" by having an "affair" with their work, a hobby, an outside interest, or another relationship so that no time or effort is invested in the marriage.

Clinical psychologist Harriet B. Braiker defines the seven deadly sins of toxic relationships as anxiety, helplessness, hostility, frustration, depression, cynicism, and low self-worth.[27]

# Health Problems in Weak or Stressed Families

Results of studies gathered over many years demonstrate soundly that a healthy family and supportive family members have a great deal to do with the health of individuals in the family unit. On the other side of the coin, marital stress and tension, troubled family life, and other problems in the family unit can contribute to illness and stress in individual family members. Research has even shown that problems in the family unit can lead to greater chronic anger among family members.[28]

Criticism from family members can be especially detrimental on both physical and mental health. While a great deal of research has focused on the mental and emotional impact of criticism in the family, several recent studies have shown the impact of criticism on the physical health of family members as well. In one study, conducted at a primary medical care facility in upstate New York, almost 900 patients answered questionnaires about the amount of criticism in their families. Two scientifically accepted measurement tools were then used to assess the results. Researchers found that those who had the highest amount of criticism from family members also had the most harmful health behaviors, including smoking, lack of exercise, and high-fat diets. Those who were criticized the most not only had the most negative outlook, but also had the poorest physical health.[29]

## Learned Pain

Something as basic as pain, for example, may be learned from the family you grow up in. Psychologist Patrick Edwards of North Dakota State University believes that pain can be something children learn, something parents help them "rehearse." In a survey of 288 college students, he asked them to catalog the length, intensity, and frequency of their own pain experiences—pain from things like backache, toothache, headache, muscle ache, abdominal pain, and neck soreness. Then he asked the college students to recall how much and what types of pain their families suffered. He found that children who grew up in pain-plagued households were more likely to experience pain themselves. Girls seemed to be more influenced by the way other family members felt than were boys. Some of the college students who grew up in families with lots of physical pain developed an attitude of helplessness; they believed that pain was beyond their control and would happen no matter what.[30]

Edwards followed up with another study, which again showed the profound influence of families on pain. He asked 224 college students to describe their own pains and the pains of their families—and to describe how much time their parents took off from work because of pain. The findings showed that the students who felt the most pain—and whose parents apparently were in the most pain—were also the ones whose parents missed quite a bit of work. Children interpreted pain as a way to gain—and the "gains of pain" became special attention, sympathy, or a way out of difficult tasks. These children had learned to use pain as a way to miss school, a way to get out of doing chores, or a way to escape other things they wanted to get out of. An additional result was that these children tended to focus on pain more than was necessary. In some cases, they were conditioned to look for pain when it scarcely existed.[31]

Other researchers agree with Edwards that families can encourage or discourage physical distress and suffering. Some believe a family's response to a family member's complaints will influence how sick he or she feels, the way he or she feels about the symptoms, and, in the end, even how disabled he or she becomes.

A few researchers think family reaction can cause a sick person to "use" an illness to gain power and position in the family. At first glance, a sick person may seem to be "the weakest and most defenseless member of the family," one researcher says. But, in reality, "He is often the most powerful member, because his illness entitles him to special consideration, and his needs now have top priority: A sick family member can cause routine family life to grind to a halt and center on him."[32] Because illness confers this kind of power, it sometimes becomes a solution to family problems. In families that are rigid, enmeshed, and unable to openly acknowledge their difficulties, a family member's suffering may temporarily stabilize the family.

## Strep Infections

Aside from the issue of learned pain or illness used to gain power or attention, stress or weakness in the family unit can actually lead to illness. Two Harvard Medical School researchers decided to test that theory by doing extensive examinations of sixteen families—consisting of 100 people—for a year. Every three weeks, these two pediatricians performed throat cultures on each family member in addition to other clinical tests to determine whether the family members had any signs of streptococcal illness. Because of their situations, each of the families had about the same chance as the others to pick up a streptococcal infection: They all had a similar number of school-aged children, lived in similar degrees of neighborhood crowding, and had fathers with similar occupations.[33]

A number of the family members did acquire strep infections during the study period—but most of the time the acquisition of strep bacteria did not result in illness. Families that had high levels of chronic stress not only got infected more often but their infections developed into illness four times more frequently than in families without chronic stress.[34]

## Cancer

At Jefferson Medical College in Philadelphia, many cancer patients described their parents as "aloof, cold people." Their own emotional rigidity, which may lead to cancer, seemed a product of their strict upbringing.[35] When cancer patients were asked about childhood traumas, they tended to gloss over the death of a parent or sibling; some had to be prodded to even remember that a parent had died when they were very young. Perhaps they repressed the death, or perhaps they were not really emotionally attached to the person who died—but the researchers agreed that cancer patients tended to "bottle up" their emotions.

In a number of studies, cancer patients described themselves as "emotionally detached" from their parents—and they described their parents as having been disagreeable to each other. In the study involving Johns Hopkins graduates, more negative attitudes about the family prevailed among the cancer patients than among any other group in the study.[36]

## Asthma

Problems in the family may contribute to asthma. Studies of people with asthma reveal that many consider their parents to be rejecting or overbearing. In one study, researchers sent the parents of asthmatic children on paid vacations and left trained observers to care for the children. Without any other treatment, about half of the children improved.[37]

A similar experiment also pointed a finger at the family. In research done nearly thirty years ago, a physician studied a group of children who were genuinely allergic to house dust; inhaling the dust in their homes brought on violent asthma attacks. Then the doctor hospitalized each of the children. Next, he secretly took dust from each child's home and sprayed it into each child's hospital room. Only one of the twenty children had an asthma attack. Away from home and family, the remainder of the children were healthy.[38]

## Diabetes

Almost twenty years ago, a psychiatrist from Albert Einstein College of Medicine in New York wondered why diabetes strikes certain people at certain times in their lives. He decided to do some investigating at a local clinic where he had been counseling adolescents with diabetes. The clinic had kept detailed records of the age at which each adolescent became ill, as well as personal information about the family: deaths, divorces, family disturbances, and the like.[39]

In carefully studying these records, the doctor found that well over two-thirds of the diabetes patients had experienced the loss of a parent or a disturbed family life (characterized by serious illness of a parent, parental fighting, chaotic atmosphere, and so on). Only about one-fifth of a diabetes-free control group had experienced similar family problems. In about half of the diabetic teens, the parental loss had occurred before the onset of diabetes, suggesting a possible connection between the two.[40]

A separate study involved three girls who were members of apparently stable, pleasant, and cooperative families—but each girl frequently lost control of her treatment and ended up in the hospital. Doctors associated with the cases decided to take a closer look at the families. In each case, the girl had become enmeshed in family conflict. In each case, a parent had insisted that the girl ally herself with one of them, mediate, or in some other way become a party to the family feud.[41]

Apparently the health of the family has a great deal to do with the way children adapt to and cope with the stress of their own chronic illness. Researchers at Case Western Reserve University School of Medicine compiled the results of fifty-seven studies of children with chronic illness.[42] Those studies clearly show that children who come from weak, stressed families characterized by conflict and psychological distress in the mother were *consistently* less capable of adjusting to and coping with their illness. Those children who came from strong, healthy families were significantly better able to adjust to and cope with chronic illness, such as asthma and diabetes.

## Anorexia Nervosa

The same pattern seems to hold true for victims of anorexia nervosa. Some professionals think the development of anorexia nervosa is closely related to abnormal patterns of interaction between the patient and her family (anorexia nervosa usually occurs in girls), mostly involving overly restrictive or suffocating relationships. A leading family therapist who has worked extensively with anorectic victims claims that "the boundaries that keep family members over-involved with each other and separated from the world are well defined and strong. The boundaries within the family, however, are diffuse and weak."[43]

A study conducted at Duke University Medical Center indicated that people from weak families also tended to have weak health. The study showed that families weak in structure and support produced people with more symptoms, impaired physical health, and weakened emotional health.[44]

# Traits of Strong Families

Just as weak or stressed families can contribute to illness, strong families can contribute to good health and long lives. Children reared in a healthy, happy family have a better than average chance of enjoying a healthy, long life.

What are the hallmarks of a healthy family? Different researchers have different answers, and they have different ways of arriving at an opinion. One, for example, sent out questionnaires to more than 500 family professionals: teachers, pastors, pediatricians, social workers, counselors, and leaders of volunteer organizations. In the end the lists look much the same. Number one, according to all the experts, is the family's ability to communicate. The lists have the following traits in common.[45]

## Communication and Listening

Strong families gather around the table at mealtime and talk about what happened during the day and also about feelings. A lot of listening goes on, too. Parents listen in a way that encourages more communication. Instead of jumping to conclusions and reacting based on scanty information, they listen attentively and draw out more information. They know each family member well enough that they can read nonverbal messages. They know when a child feels inadequate, ugly, clumsy, stupid, unloved, or just plain worthless. Family members use positive words and phrases, and they stay away from sensitive subjects (like a brother's carrot-red hair or a sister's orthodontic braces).

There's a proper perspective on television watching. Family members enjoy it, but it doesn't take the place of fun family activities. Parents use what is on television to stimulate family discussions on subjects such as ethics, politics, sportsmanship, fidelity, or sexuality.

When parents communicate, there is clearly an equality. No one communicates in a way that indicates power or submission. Healthy families resist the urge to use silence as a "weapon" or punishment. When arguments take place, as they inevitably do, there's a reconciliation soon afterward. Things are talked out, and feelings are explored.

## Affirmation and Support

Everyone hungers after love and support—and members of healthy families give it freely to other family members. In a healthy family, members develop good self-esteem; they feel good about themselves, and they genuinely like the other members of the family. The parents are positive, confident, and secure; they have the esteem and courage to face the world, knowing that a defeat may be disappointing but not devastating. The family's basic outlook is positive, too: Family members help each other, support each other, and forget their own interests temporarily if someone in the family needs a hand. Each family member takes an active interest in every other family member.

## Respect

Children in healthy families are taught self-respect—both verbally and by example. Children are taught to respect each other—and, since individuality is valued, the family teaches respect for individual differences (the two children who love to get up early on Saturday morning, for example, have learned to be relatively quiet so they don't disturb the child who likes to sleep in). Respect isn't a "special-occasion-only" quality, either; it's a universal value meant for all people of all persuasions. Children are encouraged to associate with a broad spectrum of people—people of all religions, races, and philosophies. Because a child has learned self-respect, his or her parents need not fear losing their own sense of values.

Parents in healthy families respect a child's individual decisions (a father who always hoped his daughter would attend college gave her his full support when she enrolled instead in a nursing program at a local technical college). Children in healthy families, too, are taught to respect others and the property of others (a seven-year-old who shoplifts a candy bar is accompanied back to the store by his mother, who stands by him while he returns the candy bar and apologizes to the store manager).

## Trust

Members of healthy families trust each other because they have earned that trust. Children are gradually given opportunities to earn trust—and if a trust is broken, family members realize that it can be mended. Having trust is so important that members of healthy families constantly work to help all family members develop it. Family confidences are kept confidential. Nobody breaks a trust by betraying another family member. Trust isn't just for the children. In healthy families, the parents demonstrate that they can be trusted, too. They follow through on commitments, and keep promises.

## Enjoyment

Healthy families enjoy each other—and they work together to get enjoyment out of life. They get away from the problems and pressures of everyday life. You might find them relaxing on the porch, sipping a glass of icy lemonade, and watching the fireflies dance. They work hard, but they know how to play, too. They get together for a Trivial Pursuit tournament, followed up by some homemade ice cream—or they pack a picnic lunch and ride their bicycles to the park.

Members of healthy families recognize their "breaking point"—the point at which stress has become too much. At that point they step back, cancel their scheduled activities, and get together for some good, spirited fun. They diffuse stress with laughter and play, and the members of healthy families share a great sense of humor.

## Positive and Equal Interaction

In healthy families, the family is important; it's a priority to each of the members. Family members take time from work and other activities and give it to each other—and if one member of the family has an emergency or deadline pressure, other members rally around in support. They try hard not to bring work home at night or on the weekends, and they plan carefully so there is plenty of time for family activities. Those family times reflect equality and sharing between family members. No one member dominates; there are no cliques or coalitions. Family members perform sometimes-complicated juggling acts to give a fair share to each other.

## Leisure Times

Healthy families have a balanced amount of leisure time—spending some of it in pursuit of their own activities and some of it together as a family. Healthy families usually say that the most enjoyed activities are the ones that are the least structured: playing touch football in the leaves on the front lawn, shopping for a new television set, deciding to sleep outside on a warm summer night. And although it's important to spend leisure time together as a family, members of healthy families usually spend time, too, with just one other family member: A husband and wife get away together for the evening, two sisters go horseback riding together, or a father takes his six-year-old daughter out to lunch. The leisure time that families spend together isn't just "leftover" time; it's a priority that is definitely planned.

## Shared Responsibility

Parents in healthy families delight in the chance to give their children responsibility—and then they follow through by helping their children fulfill their responsibility. Family members realize that they need each other, and everyone pitches in to make sure the family keeps running smoothly. Everyone shares in the running of the household; one person does not exist to "serve" the others. Members of healthy families share responsibility for more than just chores; they also take responsibility for creating a great home atmosphere, for boosting each other up, and for providing support. Children who take responsibility are praised, recognized, and commended for their efforts.

## A Sense of Right and Wrong

Although values are a very personal thing and vary from family to family, values in healthy families clearly include the differences between right and wrong. Those differences are taught to all family members. The husband and wife agree on basic values, and give their children clear, specific guidelines about what is right and wrong.

## Traditions

Healthy families share traditions. Some involve special occasions (the kids always put out a plate of cookies for Santa Claus, and there's always a big Easter egg hunt the morning before Easter). But some "traditions" are part of the everyday fabric of life, too (every Sunday afternoon Grandma comes over for dinner, and Mom makes the rounds every night to tuck everyone in bed).

Healthy families treasure their stories and the things family members have left behind—a yellowed diary kept by an early farmer, a collection of letters from a young immigrant to his parents in the homeland, a patchwork quilt pieced from a thousand tiny scraps of fabric and stitched by hand in front of a stone fireplace.

Rituals are an important part of healthy families; some are very simple (a child gets to choose the dinner menu on her birthday). Families are eager to accept all their members, new babies and elderly grandparents alike, and the door is always open for visits, even when no invitation has been extended.

## Religion

Healthy families seem to share a strong religious core that brings them faith, a set of moral values, and a system of beliefs as a guideline. Parents make it a priority to pass religious faith on to their children by example and to help their children understand various tenets of the faith. Even when parents are not of the same religious faith, they tend to take the strong aspects of each religion and use them as strengths in the family. Healthy parents do not force a child to accept a religion, but encourage it by example.

## Respect for Privacy

Although healthy families enjoy each other and do plenty of things as a group, they also recognize the need to nurture each person as an individual. In a healthy family, parents recognize that each person is a private being who has the right to be alone—physically or emotionally—sometimes. The right to be private is the right to be different, the right to change gradually over the years, the right to mature, and the right to eventually leave home as a mature, functioning adult.

Respecting privacy means knocking on a child's closed door before entering the room; it also means allowing a child to make some of his or her own decisions and respecting confidences.

## Service

Healthy families stress the importance of service to others—not only within the family circle, but outside it as well. Parents encourage their children to participate in volunteer activities, and they set an example by doing it themselves. In addition, family members are hospitable and make others feel comfortable in their home.

## Solving Problems

The healthy family is not a problem-free family, but it is a family that works toward solving problems. Members admit problems, face them head-on, and do whatever is needed to solve the problems. If necessary, they seek outside help. They expect problems—because they know that problems are a part of everyday life, so they develop their own problem-solving abilities to work things out.

# The Health Benefits of Strong Families

*The family is our refuge and springboard;*
*nourished on it, we can advance*
*to new horizons. In every*
*conceivable manner, the family is*
*the link to our past, bridge to our future.*

—Alex Haley

As with all basic relationships, the family determines to a large extent how healthy its members are. Those who belong to a healthy family find that their stress levels are lower, they suffer significantly less illness, and they recover from illness and disease much more rapidly. Their coping mechanisms are better, and they are able to function at a higher level. Those from healthy families, overall, are healthier people.

In a special Gallup Poll commissioned by *American Health* magazine, Americans credit much of their health—and most of their positive health changes—to the influence of the family. In the poll, 87 percent of those surveyed reported making positive health changes during the past few years; they included quitting smoking, drinking less alcohol, controlling job stress, exercising more, losing weight, and eating healthier foods.

The family, not the physician, was responsible for those changes, poll results show. The editor of the magazine reported the poll results with the comment: "Family and loved ones shape our health habits more than doctors do. . . . The computer showed that marriage and family played an even deeper role than we realized."

Social support has been proved to be an important factor in protecting good health and long life. And if you belong to a strong, healthy family, you've got "an unconditional charter membership in an emotional support group wherever you roam."[46] No one is in a better position to help than your family; no one knows you better. Members of your family can be counted on to provide practical and concrete aid in times of crisis. One family counselor summed it up this way: "The person from a really supportive family doesn't have to go it alone. That person is part of something bigger—a family that cares enough to let him or her know he or she is okay."[47]

The strongest social ties we have are our family—our parents, spouse, siblings, and children. Research has shown that of all the different kinds of social support available, that provided by the family is the most critical and the strongest.[48] And the family unit itself is a source of the joy that brings good health. In a variety of studies, parents have expressed that children provide love and companionship, give a sense of self-fulfillment, and bring joy and pleasure as parents watch children develop and grow.

If it is true that stress causes disease, which has been proven beyond doubt through years of scientific studies, it is also true that a strong family helps an individual cope better with stress—thus reducing the risk of illness and disease. As one researcher put it, "During periods of crisis, as doubts arise and confidence flags, families offer reassurance and bolster the individual in his resolution. This is particularly important during periods of loss, desertion, or other crises."[49] Studies of people during particularly stressful periods—such as the Depression and World War II—showed that family integration, family adaptability, and marital adjustment were the factors most enabling people to adjust to crisis.

Studies of other stressful situations illustrate the buffering effect of strong families. The American farm crisis provides an example.[50] During the 1970s, farmers faced incredible odds: The cost of production skyrocketed, but they couldn't command a high enough price for farm commodities. Many farmers faced staggering debt; some underwent foreclosure. A number of family farms were destroyed in the process.

As many as half the farmers in some states were bankrupted. Those who weren't teetered on the edge, not knowing from one month to the next whether they would survive financially—or whether it would be their farm on the next auction block. In one small Iowa community of only 8,000, three farmers committed suicide in an eighteen-month period because of the prospect of losing their farms.

Consider the stress created by this kind of scenario. The family faced not only economic distress, but also a feeling of personal failure. Some of the farms had been run by families for many generations; the failure or loss of a farm was an embarrassment and disgrace not only for the farmer, but also for dozens of members of the extended family. The economic and emotional load for the head of the family would be unbearable—and the children, who had nothing to do with the source of the problem and little control over its solution, undoubtedly stood to pay much of the price in the form of stress.

Some of these farm families undoubtedly suffered tremendously. But many, according to research, rallied. They fought off the effects of stress. They did not fall prey to illness or disease as a result. They were families. The strength of the family—its interactions, communication patterns, and problem-solving abilities—enabled it to weather the storm.

The unique social support provided by families comes from several different functions in the family. A family endows a person with the feeling that he or she is loved and cared for. It gives a person a sense of being valued and esteemed. And it gives a person a sense of belonging to a group—a group in which he or she has responsibilities and obligations. All of that translates into a buffer for the stress we all experience in daily living—and it helps prevent disease and illness.

Evidence of that buffering effect abounds.[51] Children experience less stress from hospital procedures when parents are present—so many hospitals are now allowing parents to stay in the room with sick infants and children. People with strong families recover more quickly from surgery, tend to follow medical instructions, maintain treatment recommendations, take prescribed medications, and get better more quickly with fewer complications.

People with strong families also tend to manage chronic illness better. Wendy Auslander, a medical social worker at Washington University, studied children with diabetes; she found that the most significant factor influencing children's metabolic stability was family stress. Her findings are important nationally: Diabetes affects more than 1 million children in the United States. Auslander and her colleagues discovered that children with the healthiest families were best able to control their disease. It's not just diabetes, either, says Auslander. The strength or weakness of the family and the findings of her study can be generalized "to other diseases, like cystic fibrosis, asthma, renal disease, and leukemia."[52]

People with strong families are more likely to survive a heart attack. And people with strong families are less likely to develop heart disease—even when standard risk factors are present.

People with strong families are able to weather the storm of unemployment—and in a situation that often causes illness, they are often buffered from getting sick. People with strong families do better after the death of a loved one. They do better, in fact, in almost any stressful situation.

Research shows that a strong family can even mitigate the stresses usually experienced by single-parent families. Generally, single-parent families are seen as problematic, and the experience of losing a parent through separation, divorce, or death has been shown to lead to health problems in children. However, the strength of the remaining parent and his or her ability to create a cohesive family unit helps overcome some of those problems—indicating that it is the strength of the family, not the number of parents, that has the greatest impact. In one Canadian study of 138 two-parent families and single-parent families headed by women, researchers looked at how the health of the children was impacted by family cohesiveness.[53] They especially looked at family cohesion, family pride, general self-efficiency, network support, community support, family income, the mother's educational level, internal locus of control, and the mother's nontraditional sex role orientation. They found that strong families—even those headed by a single parent—promote the health of their members because of their ability to focus on healthy behavior and to make and act upon informed choices about healthy living.

Finally, people in strong families tend to live longer than people in weak families or people without children. People who are married do best; compared to married people, those who were previously married have higher death rates regardless of whether they live alone, live with their older children, or live with others. In fact, previously married people who live with relatives other than their parents or their children are more than 50 percent more likely to die.[54] Researchers believe that part of the protective power of strong families comes from the quality of social support felt by their members.

People with strong families are twice as likely to be alive at any given age, and studies have shown that members of strong families even *expect* to live longer.[55] Family therapists and researchers Nick Stinnett and John DeFrain summed it up this way:

> *Strong families are pleasant, positive places to live because members have learned some beneficial ways of treating each other. Family members can count on each other for support, love, and loyalty. They can talk to each other, and they enjoy each other.*
>
> *Members of strong families feel good about themselves as a family unit or team; they have a sense of belonging with each other—a sense of "we." At the same time, no individual gets lost or smothered; each family member is encouraged to develop his or her potential.*

*Finally, strong families can best be defined as places where we enter for comfort, development, and regeneration and places from which we go forth renewed and charged with power for positive living.*[56]

## Family Reunions: More than a Good Time

Family reunions are more than just fun. They apparently provide some health benefits, too. Researchers were first prompted to study the health benefits of family reunions after watching what happens in the wild: Elephants have a practice of gathering around a sick beast, offering help and support. Also, the oldest healing form in tribal medicine involved bringing the whole family—the entire clan—together and working things through for a few days.

Harold Wise, M.D., who has studied family reunions, believes that they can have tremendous healing power, even for conditions as serious as cancer.

As a result of the research of Wise and others, some physicians have begun encouraging "therapeutic" family reunions. Extended families are brought together to rally around a sick member. Family members are encouraged to tune in to each other. One person is encouraged to speak for the others. Wise says it's "a very primal feeling, a sense that you have stepped out of time. And once the family is into that level, no one will leave."

Wise says that, although he doesn't understand exactly how the reunions work, he does know that they work. He has experienced only one reunion in which the family member did not improve in health. "It's a very moving event," he says. "And to my astonishment, there have been some remissions of the disease in the dying person."

Wise believes that the reunions—in which family members are urged to bring up problems, discuss feelings, and forgive each other—help people feel more "connected," which brings tremendous health benefits. According to Wise:

*I have a lot of notions about what's happening, but I don't have a theory that satisfies me. All I know is that the reunions are very healthful for the family. And as the ill person is a part of the family, it's also critical to that person.*

*You can clear out everything that prevents families from getting together, the unresolved grief, the unexpressed anger, and get to what lies underneath— a tremendous amount of love. If people feel supported and loved, they seem to heal better. The immune system seems to work better. But whether there's a remission of the disease or not, I know that this work is important for the healing of the family itself.*[57]

Having a family reunion is only one way to boost the strength of your family. Try developing other family traditions or customs, too, that have special meaning for every member of your family. You might come up with certain rituals you always remember on birthdays, anniversaries, or other holidays. Or your customs might be as simple as gathering the family for prayer before everyone leaves in the morning, reading a few pages of a classic novel together at bedtime, or going on a family walk around the block just before dinner. You might try a "penny parade"—each time you reach a corner, flip a penny. Heads, you go left—tails, you go right.

Another good idea is to take on a volunteer effort as a family. Involve the entire family from the beginning. Work together to decide on a project, to plan for what each family member will do, and to carry out all your plans. If you're creative, you'll be able to find ways to involve even young children.

Or try working together on a project that benefits everyone in the family. Try a family garden—work together to plan what you'll plant, read up on how to plant, prepare the soil, place the seeds, and stake off the area. Take turns watering and weeding, and work together to harvest. You might even set up a family "assembly line" to preserve your harvest by freezing, canning, or drying it.

Finally, you might consider setting aside a regular, structured block of time for "family night" or family councils. Use a certain night each week or each month to make plans, compare schedules, discuss problems, set goals, or work on a special project. Make sure you add some fun time—a romp in the leaves, a swim at the local pool, or a round of banana splits for everyone!

## ENDNOTES

1. Leonard A. Sagan, *The Health of Nations* (New York: Basic Books, 1987).
2. Phillip L. Rice, *Stress and Health: Principles and Practice for Coping and Wellness* (Monterey, Calif.: Brooks/Cole Publishing Company, 1987), 122.
3. Jerrold K. Footlick, "What Happened to the Family?" *Newsweek* (Special Issue), winter/spring 1990, 16.
4. Footlick, "What Happened to the Family?" 17.
5. J. Higley et al., "A Nonhuman Primate Model of Excessive Alcohol Intake: Personality and Neurobiological Parallels of Type I- and Type II-Like Alcoholism," in M. Galanter, ed., *Recent Developments in Alcoholism, Vol. 13: Alcoholism and Violence* (New York: Plenum Press, 1997); and J. Higley, et al., "Low Central Nervous System Serotonergic Activity Is Traitlike and Correlates with Impulsive Behavior," *Annals of the New York Academy of Sciences* 836 (December 29, 1997): 39–56.
6. B. McEwen et al., "Corticosteroids, the Aging Brain and Cognition," *Trends in Endrocrinology and Metabolism* 10, no. 3 (1999): 92–96.
7. T. Comery et al., "Rapid Communication: Differential Rearing Alters Spine Density on Medium-Sized Spiny Neurons in the Rat Corpus Striatum: Evidence for Association of Morphological Plasticity with Early Response Gene Expression," *Neurobiology of Learning and Memory* 63 (1995): 217–19.
8. D. Liu et al., "Maternal Care, Hippocampal Glucocorticoid Receptors, and Hypothalamic-Pituitary-Adrenal Activity," *Science* 277 (September 12, 1997): 1659–62.

9. M. Gunnar, "Early Adversity and the Development of Stress Reactivity and Regulation," in C. A. Nelson, ed., *The Effects of Adversity on Neurobehavioral Development, Minnesota Symposia on Child Psychology* 31 (New Jersey: Lawrence Erlbaum Associates, 2000).

10. Stephen Suomi, "Attachment in Rhesus Monkeys," in J. Cassidy and P. Shaver, eds., *Handbook of Attachment: Theory, Research, and Clinical Applications* (New York: Guilford Press, 1999).

11. James J. Lynch, *The Broken Heart: The Medical Consequences of Loneliness* (New York: Basic Books, 1977).

12. Lynch, *The Broken Heart.*

13. Ibid.

14. Ibid.

15. Ibid.

16. Ibid.

17. Ibid.

18. Ibid.

19. B. Bower, "Teenagers Reap Broad Benefits from 'Authoritative' Parents," *Science News* 136 (1989): 117–18.

20. Bower, "Teenagers."

21. John Pekkanen, "Keys to a Longer, Healthier Life," *Reader's Digest,* March 1983, 25–32.

22. Sagan, *The Health of Nations.*

23. A. E. Jorm, K. B. G. Dear, B. Rodgers, and H. Christensen, "Interaction Between Mother's and Father's Affection as a Risk Factor for Anxiety and Depressive Symptoms: Evidence for Increased Risk in Adults Who Rate Their Father as Having Been More Affectionate Than Their Mother," *Soc Psychiatry Psychiatr Epidemiol* 38 (2003): 173–79.

24. H. Stephen Glenn and Jane Nelsen, *Raising Children for Success* (Fair Oaks, Calif.: Sunrise Press, 1987).

25. Glenn and Nelsen, *Raising Children for Success.*

26. Dolores Curran, *Stress and the Healthy Family* (Minneapolis, Minn.: Winston Press, 1985).

27. Harriet B. Braiker, *Lethal Lovers and Poisonous People* (New York: Pocket Books, 1992).

28. N. E. Mahon, A. Yarcheski, and T. J. Yarcheski, "Anger, Anxiety, and Depression in Early Adolescents from Intact and Divorced Families," *Journal of Pediatric Nursing* 18, no. 4 (2003): 267–73.

29. Kevin Fiscella and Thomas L. Campbell, "Association of Perceived Family Criticism with Health Behaviors," *Journal of Family Practice* 48, no. 2: 128–34.

30. "Pain: Is It All in Your Family?" *Executive Fitness,* May 1987, 7.

31. "Pain: Is It All in Your Family?"

32. Arthur J. Barsky, *Worried Sick: Our Troubled Quest for Wellness* (Boston: Little, Brown, 1988).

33. Blair Justice, *Who Gets Sick: Thinking and Health* (Houston, Texas: Peak Press, 1987), 37–38.

34. Justice, *Who Gets Sick.*

35. Steven Locke and Douglas Colligan, *The Healer Within: The New Medicine of Mind and Body* (New York: E. P. Dutton, 1986), 141.

36. Locke and Colligan, *The Healer Within,* 145.

37. S. I. McMillen, *None of These Diseases,* rev. ed. (Old Tappan, N. J.: Fleming H. Revell Company, 1984).

38. Locke and Colligan, *The Healer Within,* 118–19.

39. Ibid.

40. Ibid.

41. Sagan, *The Health of Nations.*

42. Dennis Drotar, "Relating Parent and Family Functioning to the Psychological Adjustment of Children with Chronic Health Conditions: What Have We Learned? What Do We Need to Know?" *Journal of Pediatric Psychology* 22, no. 2: 149–65.

43. Barbara Powell, *Good Relationships Are Good Medicine* (Emmaus, Pa.: Rodale Press, 1987).

44. G. R. Parkerson, Jr., J. L. Michener, L. R. Wu et al., "Associations Among Family Support, Family Stress, and Personal Functional Health Status," *Journal of Clinical Epidemiology* 42, no. 3: 217–29.

45. From Dolores Curran, *Traits of a Healthy Family* (Minneapolis, Minn.: Winston Press, 1983).

46. Sharon Faelten, David Diamond, and the editors of *Prevention* magazine, *Take Control of Your Life: A Complete Guide to Stress Relief* (Emmaus, Pa.: Rodale Press, 1988), 273.

47. Faelten et al., *Take Control of Your Life.*

48. C. E. Ross and J. Mirowsky, "Family Relationships, Social Support and Subjective Life Expectancy," *J Health Soc. Behav.* 43, no. 4 (December 2002): 469–89.

49. Sagan, *The Health of Nations.*

50. Rice, *Stress and Health,* 140.

51. Nick Stinnett and John DeFrain, *Secrets of Strong Families* (New York: Berkley Books, 1985).

52. "Cutting Family Stress Aids in Controlling Child's Illness," *Deseret News,* July 16, 1989, 11A.

53. Marilyn Ford-Gilboe, "Family Strengths, Motivation, and Resources as Predictors of Health Promotion Behavior in Single-Parent and Two-Parent Families," *Research in Nursing & Health* 20, no. 3: 205–17.

54. Richard G. Rogers, "The Effects of Family Composition, Health, and Social Support Linkages on Mortality," *Journal of Health and Social Behavior* 37, no. 4: 326–38.

55. Ross and Mirowsky, "Family Relationships."

56. Stinnett and DeFrain, *Secrets of Strong Families.*

57. Source unknown.

# CHAPTER 13

# Grief, Bereavement, and Health

*Every man has his secret sorrows which the world knows not;*
*and oftentimes we call a man cold when he is only sad.*

—Henry Wadsworth Longfellow

## Learning Objectives

- Understand the relationship between loss and grief.
- Define grief and bereavement.
- Explain the health consequences of bereavement.
- Explain how grief and bereavement impact mortality.
- List ways of helping to reduce the risk of grief on health.

For more than 2,000 years, people have recognized that grief—the overwhelming sorrow that follows a loss—can make people sick; even longer ago, philosophers and physicians knew that grief alone could kill. An early epitaph by Sir Henry Wootton crisply summarizes the effect that grief and bereavement can have on those who mourn:

*He first deceased; she for a little tried*
*To live without him; liked it not, and died.*[1]

Clearly, we've made considerable advancements in medical technology during the past 2,000 years. But something else is just as clear: Grief still makes people sick. And, unfortunately, it even kills them. Although some come through the experience of loss and the grief that follows it with relative ease, many are not so fortunate. Grief-related disorders can range all the way from mild distress and depression to major illness and death.

Our understanding of the grief and bereavement process is made all the more important by several emerging trends:[2]

- Most deaths in the United States occur in health care settings, such as hospitals and long-term care facilities; an estimated 60 percent happen in hospitals or medical clinics, and an additional 16 percent occur in nursing homes or hospice facilities. Staff in these health care settings have an increased role in caring for survivors and helping through the initial grief process.

- Research on grief and study of the care that is given to survivors have increased dramatically in both scope and frequency in the last twenty years.

- Biomedical research advances made during the past twenty years have the potential of substantially improving our understanding of the biological changes that occur as part of the grief and bereavement process.

- There are likely to be greater demands on the nation's health care systems—including the demand for end-of-life services—as the sizable "baby boomer" generation ages and faces death.

## The Loss That Leads to Grief

Researchers and physicians have long recognized a specific pattern relating to human loss: Loss is often followed by depression and disease. Early physicians recognized it. Some chronicled that entire kingdoms and villages in England were "daunted" by the death of a national hero.[3]

Today loss is still recognized as a precursor to distress, depression, and disease. Loss has even been implicated as a factor in premature death. Dr. Arthur Schmale studied forty-two consecutive patients admitted to the Rochester Memorial Hospital; their medical problems ranged from cardiovascular problems to respiratory, digestive, and skin diseases. Hoping to find some common thread among them, he interviewed patients and their families regarding the events that led up to the illness. Schmale did indeed find a common thread: loss. Thirty-one of the patients—approximately 75 percent—developed their disease within one week of the loss of a loved one. The loss led to feelings of helplessness or hopelessness, and illness followed.[4] Researchers believe that the illness and death that so often follow loss is no coincidence: Researcher Steven Schleifer of New York's Mount Sinai Hospital estimates that 20 percent of all people who die within a year of losing a spouse die as a direct result of the loss.[5]

Loss has been shown to be a factor in a variety of illnesses, but it seems to have particular influence in some—notably, cancer. Renowned general and pediatric surgeon Bernie Siegel, who has become well known for his work with cancer patients, said, "One of the most common precursors of cancer is a traumatic loss or a feeling of emptiness in one's life. When a salamander loses a limb, it grows a new one. In an analogous way, when a human being suffers an emotional loss that is not properly dealt with, the body often responds by developing a new growth. It appears that if we can react to loss with personal growth, we can prevent growth gone wrong within us."[6]

The loss that precedes illness doesn't always have to be the loss of a person or a relationship. Illness might also follow the loss of a job, the loss of self-respect, the loss of feelings of usefulness, the loss of security, or the loss of an important possession. In fact, grief and illness do not always necessarily follow a loss that involves death or separation from a loved one. One study yielded the "unexpected finding" that other losses had greater impact on health than did bereavement.[7]

Possessions may be especially important to elderly people, and the loss of a cherished possession may place them at particular risk for illness. According to researchers, possessions for the elderly seem to explain where they fit in and how they are related to the bigger scheme of things. When the elderly "see their possessions as extensions of themselves or as a personal record of their memories and experiences, then depriving older people of objects they care about may be the equivalent of destroying their identity."[8]

For children, another kind of loss—the loss of a parent—can be particularly devastating. In research performed twenty-five years ago, Dr. Rene Spitz was the first to describe "marasmus," the physical wasting away of infants who suddenly lost their mothers. These infants refused to eat and eventually died, even when they were force-fed.[9] (Marasmus is discussed in greater detail in Chapter 12.)

In an attempt to determine the impact of parental loss on children, Spitz and Katherine Wolf carefully observed ninety-one infants who were reared in foundling homes in the United States and Canada (see Chapter 12). All of the infants were physically well cared for, but they didn't gain weight or grow as rapidly as other infants. In fact, some of them even lost weight. Despite excellent physical care, the infants seemed anxious and depressed. Of the ninety-one infants in the study, thirty-four—or more than one-third—died despite what researchers say was "good food and meticulous medical care."[10] Even among those who survived, almost all showed varying signs of emotional and physical retardation. The last trimester of an infant's first year of life seems to be of particular significance. Most of the deaths in the study occurred during this period.

Parental loss—the loss of a parent through death, separation, or divorce—has been shown in a wide variety of studies to lead to later health problems. Unfortunately, the likelihood of losing a parent has remained almost constant since 1900. Even though mortality rates have dipped—making it less likely that a parent will die—the divorce rates have increased, making it more likely that divorce or separation will affect the family.[11]

From what researchers can determine, early loss of a parent leads to both physical and psychological illness. In an expansion of his earlier study, Schmale and other members of the Rochester Medical School research group studied adult patients who had been admitted to the hospital with physical complaints. A significant number of the men and women had lost one or both parents early in life. Now, as adults, they had suffered some new loss—or had merely been threatened with such a loss—and they reacted with physical illness, including cardiac disorders.[12]

Philadelphia researchers studied records of cardiac patients obtained through the Middlesex County Heart Study and the Midtown Manhattan Mental Health Study. A significant number of the coronary disease patients had lost their fathers—most of them between the time they were five years old and seventeen years old.[13]

The psychological problems that follow the loss of a parent can be devastating, too. Delinquency, accidents, psychosis, and suicide are all more pronounced among children who lost a parent early in life. The risk of suicide is seven times greater among children who have lost both parents than for those raised in an intact family.[14]

Eager to find out how much influence parental loss had over thoughts of suicide, researchers decided to study college students. They examined students who had come from intact families; they also studied students who had been separated from at least one parent during childhood. The differences between the two groups of students were vast: Only 10 percent of the students from intact families had ever had serious thoughts about suicide. In sharp contrast, almost half of the students who had lost a parent had seriously contemplated ending their own lives.[15]

## Grief: The Natural Effect of Loss

According to one psychologist, grief is the natural and predictable process of healing from the pain of loss. Grief has been called the "quintessential mind-body problem," providing rich evidence of how an emotional experience translates into very real biological results. Psychiatrist Paul Pearsall calls grief a completely natural emotion—as natural, in fact, as joy—and concludes that his patients who grieve the most intensely are also those who experience the greatest joy.

Because it is a process of healing, grief is necessary. Those who don't grieve, says Professor of Psychiatry Glen Davidson, become chronically disoriented. An entire array of studies shows that incomplete or abnormal grief can cause serious physical and psychological problems.

For grief to progress "normally," most experts agree, a person needs to pass through the stages of grief made famous by Dr. Elisabeth Kübler-Ross:

- Denial—a disbelief that the loss has actually occurred.

- Anger over the loss.

- Bargaining—a person typically "bargains" with him or herself or with God, desperately attempting to reverse the loss by offering something in exchange.

- Depression—feeling intense sorrow over the loss.

- Acceptance of the loss.

- Hope for the future.

Even though grief is normal and natural and necessary, it can cause illness because it involves intense emotions, and because it is so inseparably connected to loss. The best health protection against the consequences of grief is to allow enough time to grieve—enough time for the healing process to take place—and to affirm and acknowledge feelings about the loss. Psychiatrist Glen Davidson, chief of thanatology at Southern Illinois University School of Medicine, emphasizes that a wide range of emotions is apt to accompany grief. In his in-depth work with mourners, he has found that emotions like sorrow, guilt, anger, depression, fear, shame, anxiety, and loneliness are all normal.[16]

As the old saying goes, "Time heals all wounds." Nothing could be more appropriate in describing what's needed to heal grief. Research now shows that trying to stifle grief, trying to "keep a stiff upper lip," is actually more stressful on the body than allowing yourself to grieve. "Formal psychiatry suggests that 'uncomplicated bereavement' should be over and done with in two months. That's ridiculous," says Gerald Koocher, an expert on grief and chief psychologist at Children's Hospital in Boston. "A person can grieve continuously for a loved one for as long as two years, and intermittently for many years after." There is nothing wrong or unhealthy about it.[17]

Other researchers in the area of grief agree with Koocher's assessment. Stephen Goldston, a psychologist who has done comprehensive research on grief, says we have adopted a cultural attitude that

*A person who isn't "back to normal" four to six weeks after a loss is somehow sick or wallowing in self-pity. This places a burden on grieving people, who then think they should "snap out of it" after a few weeks. But people just can't recover from a major loss that quickly. And when they don't, they are made to feel abnormal or guilty about experiencing normal, understandable emotions.*

> *In fact, it takes most people a full year to resume life after bereavement, and it can take as long as three. They find ways to cope with a loss themselves, at their own pace. In fact, that is really the only way to handle grief.*[18]

Although Davidson's research shows that the average recovery time from a major loss is between eighteen and twenty-four months, that time can vary greatly—and can even be much longer under some circumstances—without being considered prolonged or abnormal.

A number of things can help ease the grieving process and can reduce the risk of ensuing illness. Among them are regular exercise, a balanced diet, a healthy fluid intake, and plenty of rest. Critical to the eventual healthy outcome is a nurturing social network. Mourners who have good support from family and friends (even if it's just a few close friends) do better than those who don't have such support. And, researchers say, as important as all the other factors is attitude—courage to face the loss and willingness to fully rejoin life.

## The Health Consequences of Bereavement

*Bereavement*—the loss of a loved one through death—is a special kind of *grief* (the distress that results from bereavement). A universal experience, it has been described as the process of disbanding from someone who played an important role in one's life—someone who is now gone. Bereavement has been defined by some researchers as a "broad term that encompasses the entire experience of family members and friends in the anticipation, death, and subsequent adjustment to living following the death of a loved one."[19] That definition would include external circumstances and changes—such as a change in living conditions—as well as the internal, physiological changes and the expressions and experiences of grief.

Grief, on the other hand, has been defined as "a complex set of cognitive, emotional and social difficulties that follow the death of a loved one."[20] Researchers who use that definition point out that people vary enormously in the kind of grief they experience, its duration and intensity, and their way of expressing it.

Because much of the research does not differentiate between grief and bereavement, the studies cited throughout the rest of this chapter may use both or either term to describe the same general phenomenon.

The intense and prolonged grief involved in bereavement have been shown to have significant health risks, ranging all the way from immune system disorders to suicides, sudden deaths, and increased death rates from all causes. According to research, how you grieve determines to a large extent how healthy you stay.[21]

According to the National Institute of Mental Health, the likelihood of suffering through bereavement at some time in your life is great. Each year, an estimated 8 million Americans suffer the death of an immediate family member. There are approximately 800,000 new widows and widowers each year in this country. Suicide occurs in at least 27,000 families each year (and probably in many more, since suicide is heavily underreported). Approximately 400,000 children and young adults under the age of twenty-five die each year in the United States.[22]

Because of the tremendous increase in grief research over the past two decades, we know much more about bereavement and its effects on the body:

- *Everyone experiences loss, but not everyone reacts to that experience in the same way—and there is no one clearly defined way to grieve.* There are many factors that can influence the way a person grieves—among them gender, age, stage of development, familial relationships, religion, culture, existing social networks, history of loss, previous trauma, the type of loss (anticipated, violent, or traumatic), the quality of the relationship with the deceased person, and the presence of any depressive or other psychiatric disorder. Most people cope well with loss—but because we haven't fully identified all the "normal" responses to loss, it's sometimes difficult to determine when someone has a problematic reaction to grief.[23]

- *We have made progress in distinguishing "normal" reactions to grief from complicated grief and in determining the risks that complicated grief entails.* A small, but significant, percentage of the population experiences complicated—sometimes called "pathological"—grief. We have made progress in defining what that means, and we also know that those are the people who are most likely to suffer adverse physical reactions to their grief.[24]

- *Maintaining continuing emotional or psychological bonds with the deceased is not necessarily a sign of pathological grief.* We used to think that "breaking bonds" with the deceased was a critical part of normal, healthy grief.[25] Recent research,[26] however, indicates that people who maintain emotional and psychological ties to the deceased can often have a very positive adaptation to bereavement.

- *Positive emotions are possible following loss.*[27] In fact, the loss of a loved one might change a person in very positive ways. Researchers have found numerous accounts of people who have been transformed for the better as a result of struggling with the loss of a loved one.[28]

- *Some people do not experience what we understand as distress or grief following the loss of a loved one.*[29] In the past, we considered someone who didn't experience distress or grief as having an abnormal or pathological reaction, both of which indicated problems. However, researchers now realize that the death of a loved one may actually signal the end of a very difficult situation, relief from a terminal illness, or even the end of an abusive relationship,[30] which would obviously not cause distress. Even when negative circumstances did not exist, the loss of a loved one may result in important personal growth.[31]

- *Research shows that grief counseling may not help people who are going through "normal" grief—and, in fact, it might even be detrimental.*[32]

- *Significant advancements have been made in identifying, measuring, and understanding the biological effects of grief.*[33] These advances can help us more clearly understand how pathological grief may lead to negative health effects and will help us determine how to help those who are grieving.

In describing the events that are likely to occur as part of bereavement, National Institute of Mental Health researchers say that "the bereaved are very likely to be susceptible to serious illness and even death. At a minimum, bereaved people may report pain; gastrointestinal, sleep, and appetite disturbances; and other vegetative symptoms that may signal the onset of a depression. Especially in the elderly, these symptoms may be misdiagnosed as organic. However, some studies suggest a link between bereavement and specific diseases such as cancer, heart disease, and ulcers."[34]

A special type of bereavement occurs when a woman involuntarily loses her baby during pregnancy. Research shows that women tend to experience greater symptoms of grief than do their male partners. In one study involving 109 Australian women who lost their babies either during pregnancy or at birth,[35] 91 percent of the women saw the death as the worst thing that had ever happened to them, and 77 percent said the death of the baby led to a marked decline in their ability to function. Most reported that their social environment did not give them "permission" to grieve. However, 68 percent said they were eventually able to attribute something positive to the experience.

In another study of seventy-four African American women,[36] almost all the women said they considered the loss to be of the *baby*, not the pregnancy. Contemplating memories of the baby helped these women, as did reliance on spiritual and religious practices and beliefs and the effort to connect with other people.

Another special type of bereavement occurs in parents who lose a child—a type of loss that is regarded as more intense than the loss of a spouse or parent.[37] Parents who lose a child are more likely to suffer from increased anxiety and other types of distress;[38] conflict and anger, breakdown in communication, differences in grief intensity, and lowered expression of intimacy between parents;[39] and complicated grief.[40] In one study of 204 families who lost a child by accident, homicide, or suicide, parents indicated it took three or four years to put the child's death into perspective; those whose children died by homicide suffered the highest rate of posttraumatic stress disorder, and marital satisfaction decreased over time for all parents, regardless of how the child died.[41]

A decade ago a prominent psychologist maintained that every death has at least two victims—and that it is the surviving "victim" who hurts the most deeply. The surviving victim, the one who is left behind, is at significantly higher risk for a number of health problems.

A survivor's health is at least partly dependent on how much he or she thinks about or talks about the death. To study that effect, researchers obtained coroner's records of everyone who had died in a large metropolitan area within a single year and singled out the people who had committed suicide or died in a car accident.[42] To further narrow the study, any deaths used as part of the study had to meet three criteria. The deceased person had to have (a) been married, (b) been between the ages of twenty-five and forty-five, and (c) died within twenty-four hours of the suicide attempt or accident.

Researchers then sent questionnaires to the surviving spouses approximately one year after the death; 62 percent of those who received them returned the questionnaires. The questionnaires tried to determine three things:

1. What kind of illnesses the survivors had in the year following the death.
2. How much the survivors had talked to others about their spouse's death.
3. How much they thought about their spouse's death.

Three interesting findings emerged. First, the more people talked about a spouse's death, the fewer health problems they had during the year following the death. Second, the more they talked about the death, the less they thought about it. Finally, the more they thought about the death, the more health problems they had.

The spouses of car accident victims had more health problems than the spouses of suicide victims. Those whose spouses died in car accidents tended to talk about the accident less and think about it more; those whose spouses died as a result of suicide seemed more eager to seek out a "listening ear" and to talk about the death.

Apparently the health effects of widowhood depend in part on how old the person is when he or she is widowed. Although divorce takes a greater toll at older ages, the harmful health effects of widowhood are greater at younger ages. The younger a person is when a spouse dies, the greater the likelihood that health problems or premature death will follow.[43]

The health effects of widowhood also depend on how swiftly the spouse dies—and, even then, there are differences in the ways men and women react. A study led by researchers from Yale looked at whether bereavement led to different health outcomes in men and women, depending on gender.[44] The study involved almost 100 women and more than 50 men, who were first interviewed when their terminally ill spouses were admitted to the hospital and who were followed for more than two years. The study looked for all kinds of physical and behavioral problems known to be associated with grief and bereavement, including heart attack, heart disease, stroke, smoking, alcohol abuse, sleep problems, and depression. They noted any hospitalization and also recorded how the men and women rated their own health at periodic follow-up intervals.

The researchers found that both men and women suffered three distinct symptom "clusters"—traumatic grief, depression, and anxiety. Both men and women experienced easing of these symptoms over a similar period of time; neither the men nor the women were able to ease their emotional stress more rapidly than the other group. But the way these symptoms impacted health was different for men and women, depending on gender.

At approximately the one-year anniversary of their wives' death, the men in the study who suffered a high level of grief had an increased rate of accidents, hospitalization, and "physical events" (being told by a physician that they had cancer, stroke, or heart attack). The women in the study who had significant grief had a high rate of sleep changes. Men who suffered depression had higher rates of hospitalization and accidents; women who were depressed had higher rates of arthritis, thoughts of suicide, and poor self-rated health. High levels of anxiety tended to produce poor self-rated health among both men and women.[45]

At approximately two years after the spouse's death, high levels of grief caused high blood pressure among the men; it caused heart problems, "physical events," and changes in eating habits among the women. Significant depression caused high blood pressure, poor self-rated health, and changes in sleep habits for men; high depression caused higher levels of traumatic grief among the women. And high levels of anxiety caused thoughts of suicide among the men, but heart attack and stomach problems among the women.[46]

Research conducted at the University of Utah in Salt Lake City and sponsored by the National Institute on Aging led to findings that women fare better than men when a spouse dies suddenly, and that men do better than women after a spouse dies of a chronic illness.[47] According to the research, men whose wives die suddenly are at 52 percent greater risk of dying soon than are men of similar age and background whose wives are still alive. If the wife dies of chronic illness, her husband's risk of premature death drops to 13 percent—still elevated above normal, but one-fourth the risk of those whose wives die suddenly.

The risks appear to be reversed for women. Sociologist Ken R. Smith, who spearheaded the study, says that a woman whose husband dies of a chronic illness faces 49 percent higher risk of premature death than other women her age whose husbands are still alive. If the husband dies suddenly, her risk of premature death plummets to 1 percent.

Smith speculates that the difference between men and women has to do with the woman's role as caregiver. Men whose wives died suddenly aren't prepared for the loss of the one who nurtured them; if the wife dies of a chronic illness, the man has probably had a chance to "prepare" by finding someone to take care of his needs. A woman, on the other hand, faces the burden of giving care to a chronically ill husband and the financial loss that follows his death.[48]

Those who are caregivers—especially the elderly—may suffer particular effects of grief once the patient dies,[49] depending on how much strain was involved in the caregiving. In a study of 129 people between the ages of sixty-six and ninety-six (three-fourths of whom were women, and 90 percent of whom were Caucasian), researchers divided the group into caregivers who were strained, caregivers who were not strained, and people who were not caregivers.

The strained caregivers suffered greater symptoms of depression and had worse health practices—they didn't take time to go to the physician when they were sick, didn't get enough rest, had trouble slowing down, didn't take time to exercise, and forgot to take medications. The people who were not caregivers had higher levels of depression, increased use of antidepressants, and suffered weight loss. The nonstrained caregivers fell somewhere in the middle, experiencing only minor increases in depression. However, researchers indicate that the death of a spouse may not necessarily increase the levels of distress for strained caregivers, who may interpret the death as the relief of a significant burden.

Widowhood seems to have a profound effect especially on the well-being of men.[50] It has been theorized that the effects may be greatest on women because "relationships are more important to women" and because "women measure their importance by how well they attract men. Thus, without a man a widow becomes a lesser creature."[51] Research shows, however, that men may be even harder hit than women. And recent research shows that the effects become greater with age: The older the man, the more health is affected by the loss of a spouse, adult child, parent, sibling, or friend.[52]

Dr. Anne Peplau, a psychologist at the University of California, Los Angeles, says:

> One of the myths we have been debunking is that the people you really need to worry about are lonely old ladies, that men somehow do better. The evidence comes out overwhelmingly opposite—women seem to be better able to adjust to

*old age and widowhood than men do, especially if the men are not married. Through most of men's lives, marriage seems to provide a social buffer for them. If their wives die before they do, men are in trouble in terms of their physical health and their mental health.*[53]

Studies bear out Peplau's contention that men are less able to make full adjustments. In one large-scale study, researchers observed bereaved men and women beginning in the second year after the spouse's death and continued the study through the tenth year. They found a slight but significant increase in illness and death among the men when compared with the rates of illness and premature death among the women—especially among men who did not remarry.[54]

Adjustment following the death of a spouse depends on a number of factors, including age, the quality of the relationship, self-blame, and self-assessment of initial grief symptoms. Findings from one study of relatively young widowed people (between the ages of twenty-one and fifty-five) found the following:[55]

- The people who adjusted the best tended to focus on "what they did" rather than the broader aspect of "who they were" in looking at the valued parts of their lives, and they depicted their lives as mostly good with only a limited number of setbacks.

- Those who felt greater satisfaction in their relationship with their spouse tended to maintain continuing bonds with the spouse—and had higher levels of grief-specific symptoms five years later. The greatest factor seemed to be the extent to which the bereaved person used continuing bonds, rather than the type of expression involved.

- People who blamed themselves for the death or some aspect of the death were much more likely to suffer complicated grief—with adverse effects on long-term adjustment to the loss.

- Those who underestimated their initial grief symptoms tended to improve relatively more over time. Those who overestimated their initial grief symptoms were less likely to improve over time.

- People who showed facial expressions of negative emotions within six months of the death were more likely to have physical complaints and signs of depression five years later. And those who had higher levels of emotional processing at six months tended to have higher than expected levels of grief symptoms five years later.

In general, an entire host of symptoms and illnesses strike with greater frequency among the bereaved. One mail survey evaluated the health of a group of widows in the Boston area; all were under the age of sixty, and each had been widowed thirteen months earlier. Researchers then found a group of 199 other women who were used as a matched control group; they were extremely similar to the widows in age, profession, and other circumstances, except that members of the control group were married.[56] Researchers looked at (a) what kinds of physical symptoms each of the groups had, (b) which group had the most physical symptoms, and (c) which group had the greatest "deterioration in health" during the previous thirteen months.

Findings of the study confirmed the health problems associated with bereavement. Members of the widowed group had a significantly higher number of physical symptoms, ranging from sleeplessness to serious disease conditions, such as asthma. The most common symptoms generally associated with bereavement were headaches, dizziness, fainting spells, skin rashes, excessive sweating, indigestion, difficulty in swallowing, and chest pain.[57]

The second part of the study continued to confirm that the bereaved have more health problems: 28 percent of the bereaved reported that they had experienced a significant deterioration in health, whereas only about 4.5 percent of the control group had experienced such a decline.[58]

A study of the survivors of more than 200 deaths showed a significant correlation between bereavement and morbidity. Those who lose a loved one (through death, divorce, or separation) are much more likely to become ill than those who suffer no such loss. Studies further show that if the death occurs as a result of chronic illness, the survivors will have an increase in minor illnesses, but if the death is sudden, the survivors will have an increased risk for serious illnesses.[59]

As a result of the many studies that have been completed, we know that bereavement—the process of "disbonding" that follows the loss of a spouse or other significant person in our lives—leads to a significant number of problems, including heart disease, immune system dysfunction, suicides, and sudden deaths.

The ability of a person to make sense of a death may depend in large part on religious faith. In one study,[60] researchers studied 205 adults who had suffered the loss of a spouse/partner, parent, child, sibling, other relative, or friend; they asked participants whether they had been able to make sense of the death or had been able to find anything positive in the experience. The researchers found that people who were able to understand the death in terms of their existing worldviews were generally able to make sense of the death without much problem; those with fewer problems were also the ones who had religious or spiritual beliefs about death that helped them make sense of the situation.

Those who were able to make sense of the death within the first six months were much less likely to suffer emotional distress—and those who couldn't make sense of the death within the first six months were also unlikely to be able to make sense of it later. Most reported that they had perceived something positive from the experience—most often growth in character, strengthening of relationships, and changes in perspective. Importantly, making sense of the death and finding something positive in the death are not related.

Another study,[61] of relatives and friends of dying patients in a London care center, found that those with strong spiritual beliefs had the strongest pattern of recovery over the nine months following the death. Those with low levels of spiritual belief showed little change by nine months following the death, but then tended to recover quickly from then on. Those with no spiritual beliefs actually showed a decline at nine months that intensified at fourteen months following the death. Authors of the study suggest that the strength of spiritual beliefs may play a role in the timing and resolution of grief following the death of a loved one.

## Heart Disease

We've all heard about people who "died of a broken heart." According to research, there may be much more fact than fiction to that notion. As an example, the heart attack rate of widows between the ages of twenty-five and thirty-four is five times that of married women in the same age group.[62] In an attempt to determine the rate of premature death among widowed people, researchers studied nearly 4,500 people aged fifty-five years and older. During the first six months after a spouse's death, the rate of premature death was startling: Nearly 40 percent of the survivors died during the first six months. The mortality rates gradually decreased over the next few years until it had become the same as control groups by the end of five years. Almost half of all the deaths during the first six months were due to heart problems. As a result, researchers dubbed it the "broken heart" study—and announced that the bereaved can, indeed, die of a broken heart.[63]

Subsequent studies have confirmed the findings, although the exact percentages vary slightly. One study concluded that widowers are significantly more likely to die than men the same age who have not lost their wives; the increased risk for the men persists for at least six years unless the man remarries. The study results, they say, bear out the notion of "dying from a broken heart."[64]

A handful of critics have eyed bereavement studies with suspicion, saying that marriage and remarriage may not have that great an influence after all. The people involved in these studies, the critics say, were probably too sick to get remarried—and that's not only why they failed to remarry, but it's probably why they died, too. But the results of a number of studies directly refute that line of thinking. The most persuasive was a study in which a high number of surviving spouses died during the first six months of bereavement. The study finding "clearly implies that the increase in mortality in widows and widowers is not due to the fact that these individual are simply too sick to remarry. Most of the increase in sudden deaths occurs before there would have been sufficient time to remarry in any event."[65] The "broken heart" syndrome might again have influence: Three-fourths of the bereaved people who died fell prey to either arteriosclerosis or coronary thrombosis.

In another study, the "broken heart" notion held true, but those who died had a different kind of bereavement. Dr. William Greene and his colleagues carefully studied the circumstances surrounding twenty-six Eastman Kodak Company employees who died of sudden coronary deaths. To gather their information, they studied medical records and also interviewed the next of kin, usually the wife. Most of the twenty-six men who had died suddenly from coronary heart problems were grieving—not the loss of a spouse, but a child. More than half were depressed over "the departure of the last or only child in the family for college or marriage." Greene and his colleagues also noticed during the course of the study that a large number of patients who had a heart attack but who survived to reach the hospital mentioned that a child had recently left home.[66]

## Immune System Function

Researchers say there's a logical reason why the bereaved have greater health problems than usual: The process of bereavement compromises the immune system. Researchers first discovered a link between bereavement and impaired immune system function in 1977. Four Australian researchers decided to study immune system response in twenty-six people who had lost their spouses. The researchers conducted blood tests two weeks after the spouses died and again six weeks later. They then compared the test results with people whose spouses were still living. The results demonstrated for the first time that bereavement had real, physical effects. In both sets of blood tests—the test two weeks after the deaths and the test six weeks later—there were significant drops in both T and B cell activity.[67]

Numerous follow-up studies have shown the same result. Physicians from Florida's Veterans Administration Medical Center and the University of Miami School of Medicine studied a group of sixty men; the average age was fifty-four. Each man had experienced serious illness or death of a close family member during the previous six months. In each case, the men had a reduced activity level of lymphocytes, cells vital to the functioning of the immune system.[68]

A team of researchers at Mount Sinai Hospital in New York City headed by psychiatrists Steven Schleifer and Marvin Stein and immunologist

Steven Keller studied a group of men whose wives had died from breast cancer. To test how well the widowers' immune systems were functioning, researchers injected the men with a mitogen, a chemical that kicks the immune system into gear and triggers lymphocyte activity. For two months following the wives' deaths, the widowers' immune activity (measured by the response of T cells and B cells) was "significantly suppressed." For a year longer, the men's immune systems didn't completely bound back; throughout the year, the immune system lymphocytes showed only an "intermediate level" of activity. In assessing the results of the study, Schleifer and his colleagues summarized that the increased death rate among bereaved widowers is due to the changes in the immune system.[69]

Test results are similar for women who are bereaved. Dr. Michael Irwin and his colleagues at the University of California, San Diego, measured natural killer-cell activity in women whose husbands had recently died. The role of natural killer cells is a vital one: They appear to protect the body against viral disease and against tumor growth; natural killer cells become immediately activated against virus and tumor cells, even when they have never been exposed to those cells previously. The researchers compared natural killer-cell activity among widows to natural killer-cell activity among women whose husbands were healthy.

The results showed that the women whose husbands were healthy had normal levels of natural killer-cell activity. Those who were bereaved—whose husbands had died—had "significantly reduced" natural killer-cell activity.[70]

Part of the effect of bereavement may have to do with perception and attitude—how we think and, specifically, our thoughts regarding the loss. Some scientists have theorized that it is the brain (the center of thought) that governs how we react to bereavement.

That theory is supported by a study conducted at Norway's University of Bergen. Thirty-nine Norwegian women were studied approximately one month after the death of their husbands, and again a year later. Researchers found that immunity was strongest among women who had good "coping"— defined as a positive expectation about the outcome of the experience.[71]

Results of a study involving women who had undergone abortion also demonstrate that the theory may have credence. Research scientists from Israel's Weizmann Institute of Science and Jerusalem's Kaplan Hospital studied women who had lost their unborn children.[72] Some of the women had experienced spontaneous abortion (miscarriage); others had requested medically induced abortions. Researchers were interested in finding out what factor influenced the immune system. Was it the type of abortion, or was it how the women perceived the abortions?

To test the women, psychiatrists divided them into two groups. In the first group were those who did not accept the abortion, regardless of the way it happened. In the second group were the women who were more accepting, less anxious, and less upset. Blood samples were then taken and compared with each other as well as with samples from women of similar ages who had not suffered the loss of an unborn child. The women who were having trouble coping and adjusting to the loss of the child suffered "a definite shift" in immune system activity; they had "more feeble T cell strength" than the women who had adjusted better to the loss. The woman's thinking seemed to be the critical factor; whether the abortion was accidental and unplanned or medically requested didn't seem to make a difference.[73] As one researcher said, "The heart cannot decide that a loved one's death in a train wreck is too much to bear; the liver does not feel the shame of embarrassment; the immune system does not know whether its client is employed or not, divorced or happily married. It is the brain that knows and feels."[74]

One reason for immune system shifts during bereavement could be due to a simple hormone. During periods of active mourning, separation, depression, and high levels of uncertainty, the levels of the hormones called corticosteroids are vastly increased. In the bloodstream, corticosteroids put a damper on the immune system's antibody response. They prevent the immune system from completely kicking into gear, they lower immune response, and they make the body susceptible to all kinds of illness.[75] Recent research at Norway's University of Bergen shows that immune system function improves significantly after one year of bereavement.[76]

## Sudden Deaths

Those who are mourning a loss have a higher than expected rate of sudden death. We already discussed the sudden deaths among Eastman Kodak employees in Rochester; at least half of the sudden deaths were preceded by "the departure of the last or only child in the family for college or marriage."[77] Throughout most of medical history, physicians have documented cases in which a person died suddenly and unexpectedly following a loss; in fact, "grief" used to be listed as a cause of death on death certificates.[78] As medicine became more sophisticated and technology became more advanced, however, physicians began searching instead for signs of disease or illness; the factor of "grief" as a cause of death became mere speculation among friends and family members.

In any event, a number of researchers have shown that loss, grief, mourning, and bereavement can and do result in sudden death. One of the most notable researchers in the field, Dr. George Engle, studied 170 sudden deaths in 1971. Engle, who is affiliated with the Rochester University Medical School in New York, studied 170 newspaper reports (many from the Rochester press) of sudden death during a six-year period. Engle used the

170 deaths in his study because he could rule out suicide as a factor and because he could reconstruct the circumstances surrounding the deaths. The following are examples of the cases:

- During a physical examination, a fifty-two-year-old man passed an electrocardiogram with "flying colors"; the test showed no evidence of coronary disease. Six months later, his wife died of lung cancer. The day after her funeral, the man died suddenly of a massive myocardial infarction (heart attack).

- When an eighty-eight-year-old man was told of the sudden death of his daughter, he began wringing his hands and asking, "Why has this happened to me?" Even though he had no known heart disease, he developed acute pulmonary edema while talking on the phone to his son; he died just as a physician reached his house.

- A seventy-one-year-old woman rode in the ambulance with her sixty-one-year-old sister, who was pronounced dead on arrival at the hospital. The instant she received the news that her sister was dead, the older woman "collapsed." Physicians did an electrocardiogram, which showed she had sustained damage to her heart; within a few minutes, she developed ventricular fibrillation (disruption of the heart's rhythm) and died.

- A thirty-one-year-old woman had been having headaches, nausea, and eye problems when her close friend and neighbor—also thirty-one—died suddenly of an abdominal hemorrhage. She herself died two days later of a brain tumor.

- A twenty-two-year-old woman had malignant paraganglioma, a cancer of the sympathetic nervous system, but she was still able to go on automobile rides with her mother. On one such ride, the mother was in an accident, thrown from the car, and killed. Even though the daughter was not injured, within a few hours she lapsed into a coma and died. Results of the autopsy revealed widespread cancer but proved that she had not been injured in the accident.

- A fourteen-year-old girl suddenly "dropped dead" when told that her seventeen-year-old brother had died unexpectedly.

- An eighteen-year-old girl died suddenly and unexpectedly when told that her grandfather, who had helped rear her, was dead.[79]

In more than half of the sudden deaths he investigated, Engle was able to document that the death was immediately preceded by some kind of interpersonal loss. In both men and women, most of the deaths occurred after the collapse or death of a loved one, during acute grief (within sixteen days of the loss), or during the threat of loss of a loved one.[80]

As in the last two cases, the kinds of sudden death that occur as a result of grief or bereavement don't just happen to the elderly or to people who are already ill. Engle points out that they often occur in young, apparently healthy people. When they suddenly and unexpectedly lose someone close, they apparently become convinced that life is "unbearable." In many ways, says Engle, they simply "will their own death."

Other researchers have noted the same phenomenon. In Engle's hometown of Rochester, two cousins provided a classic example—although they were not part of Engle's study. The cousins, Pete and "Re-Pete," were the same age, had married sisters, and had lived within two blocks of each other throughout their lives. At the age of sixty-nine, Pete died of liver cancer. Less than twelve hours later, Re-Pete suffered a heart attack and died at the same hospital.[81]

Researchers Ian Wilson and John Reece reported on the case of inseparable twin sisters in North Carolina. Neither married or stayed away from the other for any prolonged period. When they were twenty-one, both of the young women started showing signs of schizophrenia; within ten years, both had to be hospitalized. During the next year, they were in and out of the hospital several times; with each readmission they became worse, until finally they both refused to eat. Hospital authorities theorized that they reinforced each other's behavior and refusal to accept food, so the twins were separated and placed on separate floors of the hospital. Early one morning, one of the twins was found dead. Within minutes her twin sister went to the window, looked up at her sister's room a floor above, and—without even knowing that her sister was dead—slumped to the floor. She, too, was dead.[82]

The phenomenon isn't isolated to people. Based on his years of research, Engle says that animals, too, seem to give up and die suddenly if a lifelong companion dies. Based on his studies, he tells the following story of Charlie and Josephine, who had been inseparable for thirteen years:

> In a senseless act of violence, Charlie, in full view of Josephine, was shot and killed in a melee with the police. Josephine first stood motionless, then slowly approached his prostrate form, sank to her knees, and silently rested her head on the dead and bloody body. Concerned persons attempted to help her away, but she refused to move. Hoping she would soon surmount her overwhelming grief, they let her be. But she never rose again; in fifteen minutes, she was dead.
>
> The remarkable part of the story is that Charlie and Josephine were llamas in the zoo! They had escaped from their pen during a snowstorm and Charlie, a mean animal to begin with, was shot when he proved unmanageable. I was able to establish from the zookeeper that to all intents and purposes Josephine had been normally frisky and healthy right up to the moment of the tragic event.[83]

Another phenomenon related to the sudden death among the bereaved has been dubbed the "anniversary" death: A bereaved person may die suddenly and unexpectedly on the anniversary of a loved one's death. Sometimes these deaths occur on actual anniversaries; at other times, they occur as the result of a powerful reminder of the dead person. For example, the widow of Louis "Satchmo" Armstrong suffered a fatal heart attack as she played the final chord of "St. Louis Blues" at a memorial concert for her husband.[84]

## Suicides

Suicide rates increase among the bereaved as well. In an early study, researchers examined the incidence of suicide among the widowed in Massachusetts between 1948 and 1952. Consistent with earlier studies, researchers Brian MacMahon and Thomas Pugh found that the bereaved did have a higher incidence of suicide. The rate of suicide among the bereaved was the highest during the first year after a loved one's death. During that first year, the suicide rate was two and a half times higher than expected. During the second through fourth years of bereavement, the suicide rate dropped, but was still higher than normal—about one and a half times higher.[85]

In a review of death records in Finland for the years 1972 to 1976, more than 95,000 widowed persons were studied. The suicide rate was 242 percent higher than expected among men and women who had lost a spouse. The most profound increase was during the first month of bereavement: Suicides rose 17 times among the men who had lost a spouse and 4.5 times among the women who had been widowed. According to the researchers, the rates gradually dropped after the first month, but still remained "substantially" higher than normal.[86]

## General Mortality Rates

When all causes of death are considered, the bereaved have a much higher death rate than people of the same age whose spouses are living. Although the exact statistics vary according to the specific study, the results are the same: People who are widowed are more likely to die early.

In the study conducted in Finland, the rate of death from all causes was 6.5 percent higher than expected for their age and gender. The increase was sharpest during the first months; during the first week alone, mortality rates doubled for both men and women. Women seemed to recover more rapidly than men to the emotional rigors of being widowed: Their death rates from natural causes returned to average by the end of the first month. In men older than sixty-five, the death rates returned to average by the end of six months. Men younger than sixty-five fared the worst: After being widowed, their death rates were still 50 percent higher than expected after three years.[87]

Studies done in England confirmed that men are affected more gravely. In those studies, 4,486 bereaved men older than sixty-four were studied. During the first six months of bereavement, their death rates increased more than 40 percent over what would have been expected for men of their age. After six months, the mortality rates started to gradually decline until they reached the death rates for married men of the same age.[88] Because almost half the deaths in the study involved heart disease, it became known as "the broken heart study."[89] According to one researcher, the death rate from cardiovascular disease was 67 percent higher among the men in the study than would have been expected among the widowers.[90]

Widows are affected as well. They die at rates three to thirteen times as high as those of married women for every known major cause of death.[91] For both men and women, the effects of bereavement increase the risk of premature death. In fact, men and women who lose their mates are among the highest-risk groups for premature death. As mentioned earlier, studies conducted at New York's Mount Sinai School of Medicine indicate that about 35,000 bereaved partners die each year—and that one in five can be directly attributed to the loss of their mate.[92]

Results of a study by the National Institute on Aging show that death rates are indeed higher during the first two years after the death of a mate—but widowed persons who survive the two years resume the likelihood of living a normal life expectancy. The study, which involved 14,000 adults in the United States and West Germany, half of whom were widowed, was conducted from 1970 to 1981. During the first two years after the death of their spouses, the widowed had a "consistently higher death rate" than those of the same age who were married. The newly widowed were more likely to die as a result of disease or accidents and also more likely to commit suicide. But, data reveal, "after the two-year mark, the mortality rate slowed significantly, and the researchers could see no differences in the health and well-being of the long-term widowed and married people of the same age."[93]

Findings of the U.S./West German study may not hold true across the board, say other researchers. The results of other studies show that the risk of premature death stays high for widowers for at least six years after they lose their wife, unless they remarry. For women, the risk is not as great during the first year, but becomes greatly increased during the second year.[94]

Studies conducted in a rural community in Wales showed that the death rate among the bereaved was considerably higher during the first year. Researchers studied 903 close relatives of almost 400 residents who died during a five-year period. Nearly 5 percent of the relatives died within the first year after being bereaved; only 0.7 percent of the nonbereaved people of the same age who lived in the same community died during the year.[95] Study results showed a sevenfold increase in the death rate for surviving close relatives—spouses, children, parents, or siblings. The place of death was also significant: If the person died in the hospital, the relative's risk of death during the first year was two times higher. If the person died elsewhere, the relative's risk jumped to five times higher.

Although death rates are higher overall for bereaved people, studies consistently show that there are unusually high death rates for certain conditions—and that those differ between men and women, and even somewhat with age. According to statistics, bereaved women tend to die more often than expected from cancer, heart disease, tuberculosis, cirrhosis, and alcoholism. Bereaved men have a higher risk of dying from heart disease, tuberculosis, influenza, pneumonia, cirrhosis, alcoholism, accidents, and suicide.[96] Results of the study in gender differences conducted at Yale, however, urge caution in separating the genders when considering the impact of bereavement. According to the Yale researchers, further studies are needed, especially surrounding the ways gender influences the mental and physical impact of the death of a spouse.[97]

Regarding mortality rates, one researcher who did an extensive review of the literature[98] cautions that a number of issues complicate the interpretation of published findings about the relationship of bereavement and increased mortality. He argues that these findings should be considered tentative, and that the prospective data on grief, depression, immune function, and neuroendocrine function are needed before it will be possible for researchers to substantiate claims that bereavement either weakens the immune system or causes premature death.

# Cutting the Risk

The best thing bereaved people can do to protect themselves, researchers say, is to surround themselves with people who are supportive. If they perceive that their social support is strong, they will reap the protective health benefits.

Researchers studied a group of women thirteen months after the death of their husbands. The group was divided into those who perceived their social support to be adequate and those who did not. Only about one in five of those who felt their social support was good had poor health; in stark contrast, almost nine of ten of the women with inadequate social support had poor health.[99]

Researchers then took the women who felt their support was inadequate and put them in a program of supportive counseling; the women were able to gain tremendous social support from the counselors and the group. As a result, the percentage with poor health went from a staggering 86 percent to only 13 percent. In summing up the findings, researchers said that "adverse health effects associated with bereavement are absent or at least reduced when the individual maintains close supportive relationships."[100]

In a similar study, 200 widows were assessed during the first few weeks following the husband's death. Researchers judged that 64 of them were at high risk for developing disease because of weak support from family and friends, an ambiguous relationship with the husband, and additional life crises at the time of the study. Researchers took the 64 widows considered to be at high risk and divided the group in half. Half of the group received no support; the other half received support and counseling. At thirteen months following the bereavement, the group that had received social support and counseling did the best; only about a third showed increased health problems. Both mental and physical symptoms increased in more than half of the unsupported group.[101]

In the final analysis, support may be the most crucial factor. A study led by Itzhak Levav of the University of Hebrew and Hadassah School of Public Health and Community Medicine looked at the effect of support on bereavement. Researchers examined 3,600 Israeli parents who had lost adult sons either in the Yom Kippur War of 1973 or through accidents occurring between 1971 and 1975. The bereaved parents were compared with the general populace, and researchers compared not only illness and disease but death rates as well. The widowed and divorced mothers of the deceased sons did have increased mortality—but the married parents demonstrated "no consistent evidence of an elevated risk of death." Researchers conducting the study concluded that marriage—and the social support it provides—protects against the potential health and mortality dangers of bereavement.[102]

How can you best help the bereaved? According to research, traits that help protect a person in the event of loss include social support, strong religious belief, rituals, and belief that one can control the bereavement.[103] One writer suggests the following:

- Be there.
- Listen.
- Avoid clichés.
- Keep in touch.
- Send a note.
- Be patient.
- Accentuate the positive.

And, the writer says, don't forget to touch—a hug or a squeeze of the hand can do wonders.[104]

## ENDNOTES

1. Wolfgang Stroebe and Margaret S. Stroebe, *Bereavement and Health* (Cambridge, Mass.: Cambridge University Press, 1987), 1.

2. Center for the Advancement of Health, *Report on Bereavement and Grief Research* (New York: BrunnerRoutledge, 2004), 495.

3. Stroebe and Stroebe, *Bereavement*, 2.

4. James J. Lynch, *The Broken Heart: The Medical Consequences of Loneliness* (New York: Basic Books, 1977).

5. Larry Dossey, *Meaning and Medicine: A Doctor's Tales of Breakthrough and Healing* (New York: Bantam Books, 1991), 90.

6. Bemie S. Siegel, *Love, Medicine, and Miracles* (New York: Harper & Row, 1986).

7. S. A. Murreil, S. Himmelfarb, and J. F. Phifer, "Effects of Bereavement/Loss and Pre-event Status on Subsequent Physical Health in Older Adults," *International Journal of Aging/Human Development* 27, no. 2 (1988) 89–107.

8. Ann McCracken, "Emotional Impact of Possession Loss," *Journal of Gerontological Nursing* 13, no. 2: 14–19.

9. Lynch, *The Broken Heart*.

10. Ibid.

11. Leonard A. Sagan, *The Health of Nations* (New York: Basic Books, 1987).

12. Lynch, *The Broken Heart*.

13. Ibid.

14. Sagan, *The Health of Nations*.

15. Ibid.

16. Brent Q. Hafen and Kathryn J. Frandsen, *People Who Need People: The Importance of Relationships to Health and Wellness* (Evergreen, Colo.: Cordillera Press, 1987), 37.

17. Sharon Faelten, David Diamond, and the editors of *Prevention* magazine, *Take Control of Your Life: A Complete Guide to Stress Relief* (Emmaus, Pa.: Rodale Press, 1988), 134.

18. Faelten et al., *Take Control*.

19. G. Christ, G. Bonanno, R. Malkinson, and S. Rubin, "Bereavement Experiences After the Death of a Child," in Institute of Medicine, M. Field, and R. Behrman, eds., *When Children Die: Improving Palliative and End-of-Life Care for Children and Their Families* (Washington, D.C.: National Academy Press, 2003), 554.

20. Christ et al., "Bereavement Experiences," 555.

21. J. Amold, "Rethinking Grief: Nursing Implications for Health Promotion," *Home Health Nurse* 14, no. 10 (September 1997): 777–83.

22. "NIMH Issues Guides to Bereavement," *Behavior Today*, November 7, 1988, 2.

23. Center for Advancement of Health, *Report on Phase I of the Grief Research Gaps, Needs, and Action Project* (Washington, D.C.: Center for Advancement of Health, 2003).

24. H. Prigerson and S. Jacobs, "Traumatic Grief as a Distinct Disorder: A Rationale, Consensus Criteria, and a Preliminary Empirical Test," in M. Stroebe et al., eds., *Handbook of Bereavement: Consequences, Coping, and Care* (Washington, D.C.: American Psychological Association, 2001).

25. M. Stroebe, "Bereavement Research and Theory: Retrospective and Prospective," *American Behavioral Scientist* 44 (2001): 854–65.

26. M. Stroebe, D. Klass, and T. Walter, "Process of Grieving: How Bonds Are

Continued," in M. Stroebe et al., eds., *Handbook of Bereavement: Consequences, Coping, and Care* (Washington, D.C.: American Psychological Association, 2001).

27.  G. Bonanno, "Introduction: New Directions in Bereavement Research and Theory," *American Behavioral Scientist* 44 (2001): 718–25.

28.  L. Calhoun and R. Tedeschi, "The Positive Lessons of Loss," in R. Neimeyer, ed., *Meaning Reconstruction and the Experience of Loss* (Washington, D.C.: American Psychological Association, 2001), 157–72.

29.  G. Bonanno, "Grief and Emotion: A Social-Functional Perspective," in M. Stroebe et al., eds., *Handbook of Bereavement: Consequences, Coping, and Care* (Washington, D.C.: American Psychological Association, 2001).

30.  C. Wortman and R. Silver, "The Myths of Coping with Loss Revisited," in M. Stroebe et al., eds., *Handbook of Bereavement: Consequences, Coping, and Care* (Washington, D.C.: American Psychological Association, 2001).

31.  Calhoun and Tedeschi, "The Positive Lessons."

32.  J. Jordan and R. Neimeyer, "Does Grief Counseling Work?" *Death Studies* 27 (2003): 765–86; and H. Schut, M. Stroebe, J. van den Bout, and M. Terheggen, "The Efficacy of Bereavement Interventions: Determining Who Benefits," in M. Stroebe et al., eds., *Handbook of Bereavement: Consequences, Coping, and Care* (Washington, D.C.: American Psychological Association, 2001).

33.  K. Goodkin, T. Baldewicz, N. Blaney, D. Asthana, M. Kumar, P. Shapshak, B. Leeds, J. Burkhalter, D. Rigg, M. Tyll, J. Cohen, and W. Zheng, "Physiological Effects of Bereavement and Bereavement Support Group Intervention," in M. Stroebe et al., eds., *Handbook of Bereavement: Consequences, Coping, and Care* (Washington, D.C.: American Psychological Association, 2001); and M. Hall and M. Irwin, "Physiological Indices of Functioning in Bereavement," in M. Stroebe et al., eds., *Handbook of Bereavement: Consequences, Coping, and Care* (Washington, D.C.: American Psychological Association, 2001).

34.  "NIMH Issues Guides to Bereavement," 3.

35.  T. Uren and C. Wastell, "Attachment and Meaning Making in Perinatal Bereavement," *Death Studies* 26 (2002): 279–306.

36.  P. Van and A. Meleis, "Coping with Grief after Involuntary Pregnancy Loss: Perspective of African American Women," *Journal of Obstetrics, Gynecology, and Neonatal Nursing* 32, no. 1 (2003): 28–39.

37.  Christ et al., "Bereavement Experiences," 554.

38.  S. Rubin and R. Malkinson, "Parental Response to Child Loss Across the Life Cycle: Clinical and Research Perspectives," in M. Stroebe et al., eds., *Handbook of Bereavement: Consequences, Coping, and Care* (Washington, D.C.: American Psychological Association, 2001).

39.  Christ et al., "Bereavement Experiences."

40.  Ibid.

41.  S. Murphy, L. Johnson, L. Wu, J. Fan, and J. Lohan, "Bereaved Parents' Outcomes 1 to 60 Months After Their Children's Deaths by Accident, Suicide, or Homicide: A Comparative Study Demonstrating Differences," *Death Studies* 27, no. 1 (2003): 39–61.

42.  J. H. Chen, A. J. Bierhals, H. G. Prigerson, S. V. Kasl, C. M. Mazure, and S. Jacobs, "Gender Differences in the Effects of Bereavement-Related Psychological Distress in Health Outcomes," *Psychological Medicine* 29, no. 2 (1999): 367–80.

43.  Chen et al., "Gender Differences."

44.  Ibid.

45.  James J. Pennebaker and Joan R. Susman, "Disclosure of Traumas and Psychosomatic Processes," *Social Science Medicine* 26, no. 3 (1988): 327–32.

46. Sheldon Cohen and S. Leonard Syme, *Social Support and Health* (Orlando, Fla.: Academic Press, 1985).

47. "Swiftness of Spouse's Death Affects Mate's Mortality Risk," *Medical World News,* September 11, 1989, 27.

48. "When Death Does Us Part: The Difference Between Widows and Widowers," *Psychology Today,* November 1989, 14.

49. R. Schulz, S. Beach, B. Lind, L. Martire, B. Zdaniuk, C. Hirsch, S. Jackson, and L. Burton, "Involvement in Caregiving and Adjustment to Death of a Spouse: Findings from the Caregiver Health Effects Study," *Journal of the American Medical Association* 285 (2001): 3123–29.

50. Cohen and Syme, *Social Support.*

51. Genevieve Davis Ginsburg, "Coping with Widowhood: 'Who Am I Without My Mate'?" *50 Plus,* June 1987, 44–53.

52. T. R. Fitzpatrick, "Bereaved Events Among Elderly Men: The Effects of Stress and Health," *Journal of Applied Gerontology* 17, no. 2 (October 1996): 204–28.

53. Louise Bemikow, *Alone in America* (New York: Harper and Row, 1986).

54. "On the Health Consequences of Bereavement," *New England Journal of Medicine* 319, no. 8 (1988): 510–11.

55. J. Bauer and G. Bonanno, "Doing and Being Well (for the Most Part): Adaptive Patterns of Narrative and Self-Evaluation During Bereavement," *Journal of Personality* 69 (2001): 451–82; G. Bonanno and N. Field, "Examining the Delayed Grief Hypothesis Across 5 Years of Bereavement," *American Behavioral Scientist* 44 (2001): 798–816; N. Field and G. Bonanno, "The Role of Blame in Adaptation in the First 5 Years Following the Death of a Spouse," *American Behavioral Scientist* 44 (2001): 764–81; N. Field, E. Gal-Oz, and G. Bonanno, "Continuing Bonds and Adjustments at 5 Years After the Death of a Spouse," *Journal of Consulting and Clinical Psychology* 71 (2003): 110–17; and M. Safer, G. Bonanno, and N. Field, "'It Was Never That Bad': Biased Recall of Grief and Long-Term Adjustment to the Death of a Spouse," *Memory* 9, no. 3 (2001): 195–204.

56. Stroebe and Stroebe, *Bereavement,* 143.

57. Ibid.

58. Ibid., 145.

59. J. Van Eijk, A. Smits, F. Huygen, and H. van der Hoogen, "Effect of Bereavement on the Health of the Remaining Family Members," *Family Practitioner* 5, no. 4 (1988): 278–82.

60. C. Davis and S. Nolen-Hoeksema, "Loss and Meaning: How Do People Make Sense of Loss," *American Behavioral Scientist* 44 (2001): 726–41.

61. K. Walsh, M. King, L. Jones, A. Tookman, and R. Blizard, "Spiritual Beliefs May Affect Outcome of Bereavement: Prospective Study," *British Medical Journal* 324 (2002): 1–5.

62. Lynch, *The Broken Heart.*

63. Cohen and Syme, *Social Support.*

64. 'NIMH Issues Guides," 3.

65. Lynch, *The Broken Heart.*

66. Ibid.

67. Blair Justice, *Who Gets Sick: Thinking and Health* (Houston, Tex.: Peak Press, 1987), 188.

68. Justice, *Who Gets Sick,* 189.

69. Signe Hammer, "The Mind As Healer," *Science Digest,* April 1984, 47–49, 100.

70. "Bereavement: An Immune Reaction," *Mind/Body Health Digest* 1, no. 2 (1987): 2.

71. Torill Christine Lindstrom, "Immunity and Health After Bereavement in

Relation to Coping," *Scandinavian Journal of Psychology* 38, no. 3 (September 1997): 253–59.

72. Steven Locke and Douglas Colligan, *The Healer Within: The New Medicine of Mind and Body* (New York: E.P. Dutton, 1986), 72.
73. Locke and Colligan, *The Healer Within.*
74. Robert Ornstein and David Sobel, "The Healing Brain," *Psychology Today,* March 1987, 48–52.
75. Marc Pilisuk and Susan Hillier Parks, *The Healing Web* (Hanover, N. H.: University of New England Press, 1986).
76. Torill Christine Lindstrom, "Immunity and Somatic Health in Bereavement: A Prospective Study of 39 Norwegian Widows," *Omega: Journal of Death and Dying* 35, no. 2 (1997): 231–41.
77. Lynch, *The Broken Heart.*
78. Justice, *Who Gets Sick,* 192.
79. Ibid., 192–93.
80. Lynch, *The Broken Heart.*
81. Justice, *Who Gets Sick,* 194.
82. Ibid.
83. Ibid., 194–95.
84. Ibid., 196.
85. Lynch, *The Broken Heart.*
86. Jaakko Kaprio, Markku Koskenvuo, and Heli Rita, "Mortality After Bereavement: A Prospective Study of 95,647 Widowed Persons," *American Journal of Public Health* 77 (1987): 293–87.
87. Kaprio et al., "Mortality."
88. Lynch, *The Broken Heart.*
89. Cohen and Syme, *Social Support.*
90. Peter Reich, "How Much Does Stress Contribute to Cardiovascular Disease?" *Journal of Cardiological Medicine,* July 1983, 825–31.
91. Claudia Wallis, "Stress: Can We Cope?" *Time,* June 6, 1983, 48–54.
92. Brent Q. Hafen and Kathryn J. Frandsen, *People Who Need People* (Provo, Utah: Behavioral Health Associates).
93. "If Surviving Spouse Endures 2 Years, Normalcy Returns," *Deseret News* and United Press International.
94. "NIMH Issues Guides," 3.
95. Lynch, *The Broken Heart.*
96. Hafen and Frandsen, *People Who Need People.*
97. Chen et al., "Gender Differences."
98. P. R. Duberstein, "Death Cannot Keep Us Apart: Mortality Following Bereavement," in P. R. Duberstein and J. M. Musling, eds., *Psychodynamic Perspectives on Sickness and Health* (Washington, D.C.: American Psychological Association, 2000), 250–331.
99. Pilisuk and Parks, *The Healing Web.*
100. Ibid.
101. Robert Ornstein and David Sobel, *The Healing Brain: Breakthrough Discoveries About How the Brain Keeps Us Healthy* (New York: Simon & Schuster: 1987), 195.
102. R. Weiss, "Risk of Death from Grief May Be Low," *Science News* (2001): 184, 135.
103. Gass, "The Health of Conjugally Bereaved Older Widows: The Role of Appraisal, Coping, and Resources," *Research in Nursing and Health* 10 (1987): 39–47.
104. Victor M. Parachin, "Eight Ways to Say I Care," *Complete Woman,* April 1991.

# Part IV

# Spirituality and Health

This section of the book defines spirituality and the spiritual concepts of altruism, faith, hope, and optimism. The healing components of spirituality are introduced, and the current research that supports those healing concepts is discussed. The chapters and topics presented in this section are:

**Chapter 14**   *The Healing Power of Spirituality*

**Chapter 15**   *The Healing Power of Altruism*

**Chapter 16**   *The Healing Power of Faith and Religion*

**Chapter 17**   *The Healing Power of Optimism*

CHAPTER 14

# The Healing Power of Spirituality

*It is difficult to make a man miserable while he feels he is worthy of himself and claims kindred to the great God who made him.*

—Abraham Lincoln

## Learning Objectives

- Be able to define spirituality, religion, and healing.
- Identify the effects of spiritual well-being on physical and mental health.
- Describe the effects of spiritual and religious practices on health.
- Clarify the essence of spiritual well-being, particularly as defined by health outcomes.

"Everyone who is seriously involved in the pursuit of science becomes convinced that a Spirit is manifest in the Laws of the Universe," reflected Albert Einstein—"a Spirit vastly superior to that of man, and one in the face of which we, with our modest powers, must feel humble."

A Harris Poll asked 1,254 people about their aches and pains. The results were rather surprising. First of all, what age group do you suppose has the most pain? The answer was: young adults! And the pains were highly associated with the "hassles of life." (Compare the discussion of pain and anxiety in Chapter 5.) But then the next surprise: Where do you suppose they got their best relief? Physicians provided relief 73 percent of the time. Other practitioners were 65–70 percent helpful. But the most helpful of all were their *spiritual counselors*—at 85 percent. What would spiritual counseling have to do with physical pain? Could it be by reducing the stress of life's hassles?

Here's a similar example: Most people with a chronic muscle pain condition called fibromyalgia seek "alternative care," that is, help beyond the usual medical system. A survey of these chronic pain patients asked what had been helpful to them, and, on a scale of 1 to 10, how helpful to them. Here are the results:[1]

| Therapy | Percentage Using | Satisfaction (0–10) |
|---|---|---|
| ▪ Over-the-counter items | 70 | 5 |
| ▪ Dietary modifications | 26 | 5 |
| ▪ Practitioners | 40 | 8 |
| ▪ Spiritual Practices | 48 | 9 |
| ▪ Prayers | 41 | |
| ▪ Meditation | 38 | |
| ▪ Relaxation | 10 | |
| ▪ Self-help | 6 | |
| ▪ Spiritual healing | 5 | |

Note that the spiritual practices listed were regarded as even more helpful than the practitioners consulted. How would spiritual health improve pain management?

Before we assign any definition to spiritual health, consider history: Spirituality and medicine were intertwined from the beginning of time. The earliest doctors of which we have record were the religious figures in tribes and groups—the priests and the medicine men and women. Cardiologist Bruno Cortis points out that disease was originally considered to be supernatural, and those who dealt with disease were the ones considered to have power over the spirits. Not until Hippocrates, says Cortis, was medicine separated from religion.

For millennia before the late 1800s, medicine, hospitals, and beliefs about health were intimately tied to religion and the need for divine help in healing. After the scientific revolution, medicine went in the opposite direction (perhaps to an extreme), thinking of healing processes along purely biological and psychological lines. "Germs" and other offenders caused disease, and the way to treat or prevent disease was to kill or avoid the causative agent. But then, as we became more aware, it was obvious that some people exposed to disease causing agents got sick, and some didn't. The concept of "host resistance" evolved. As described through many chapters in this book, many factors play into that resistance: not only organic problems, but also social factors and such things as coping ability. All of these modulate the homeostasis and immune responses that make up the disease-resistant person. So now the pendulum is swinging back toward rediscovering the role that spiritual issues play in the well-being (health) equation. Almost three-quarters of Americans say that their coping and overall approach to life are centrally grounded in their religious beliefs.[2] In a Gallup Poll (1990), 85 percent of Americans considered spirituality to be important in their daily lives, and 61 percent believe that spirituality or religion can answer most of life's perplexing problems. Surveys suggest that a very large majority (86 percent) believes that God, prayer, and spiritual practices are very important to them in healing at a time of serious illness.[3] And several reviews of medical literature (involving hundreds of studies) show that both spiritual and religious factors play a significant role in both the prevention of illness and in health outcomes when people are recovering from physical or mental illness.[4] The scientific studies are quite consistent in demonstrating a significant beneficial effect of spiritual issues on health outcomes. These benefits cross different religions, nationalities, ages, genders, and types of medical practice.[5] So maybe the ancients knew something important about spirituality and healing after all.

The ancients were not alone in their discovery of the importance of spirituality to health. Evidence suggests that increasing numbers of physicians today are taking the spirituality of their patients into account as part of patient care.[6] These physicians are forming a "therapeutic alliance" with their patients that affirms the importance of their spirituality. Indeed, says one writer, "As physicians respectfully explore patient spirituality, a reciprocal enhancement in patient regard for physicians and a deepening of the alliance between patients and their physicians becomes possible, potentially resulting in more effective treatment."[7]

The same type of spiritual involvement is being incorporated into mental health treatment and has been recognized as "a crucially important dimension" in acute mental care.[8] Unfortunately, a patient's religious beliefs and values may be difficult to discern and respond to in the context of acute mental illness, which poses a significant challenge and requires extra effort. Many organizations are taking steps toward recognizing the importance of spirituality in mental health treatment; in the United Kingdom, the Code of Professional Conduct requires that mental health nurses "recognize and respect the uniqueness and dignity of each patient, including their religious beliefs."[9]

As physicians have sought support and training in dealing with their patients on a spiritual level, rapidly increasing numbers of medical schools and other training programs have responded favorably. Funds have also been dedicated to the spiritual education of physicians. For example, the John Templeton Foundation recently established start-up grants for medical schools to initiate courses in spirituality and medicine as a regular part of physician education.

Research shows that patients, too, are supportive of a patient/physician relationship that takes spirituality into account. A number of studies show that patients long for their physicians to be more involved with them on a spiritual level. In a survey of the American public, 74 percent of sick patients feel a physician should:

- introduce a discussion about an ill patient's spiritual needs,
- refer a patient to a spiritual advisor (rabbi, priest, minister, chaplain), or
- suggest prayer.

At the end of life, the number hoping for their physician to include spiritual considerations increases to 90 percent (but this is done only 24 percent of the time). A Gallup Poll indicates that 60 percent of patients would like their physicians to pray with them.[10] At the very least, new guidelines suggest that physicians should ask patients about their spiritual beliefs, practices, and values as a routine part of assessment, and should incorporate those into the patient's ongoing care.[11] When the local culture of a community is taken into consideration, activities such as prayer, anointing, testimonials, and other worship practices can be explored as potential health resources.[12] When this type of medicine is practiced, a patient is much more likely to enjoy both physical and spiritual health.

In discussing the tremendous freedom spiritual health can bring, Dr. Bernie Siegel uses the example of people who, through no choice, are in less than desirable conditions (such as ghettos or the poverty-stricken areas of Third World countries):

> You always have a choice about how you feel. Listen to Jesse Jackson say that you may not have chosen to be down, but you have a choice as to whether you want to try to get up. . . . Listen to Mahatma Gandhi, who said, "Let us not kill our enemies but kill their desire to kill." And so you have a choice about how you behave, whether you are in prison, whether you are in a concentration camp, or whether you are sick. You have a choice.[13]

## What Is Spirituality and Spiritual Health?

Before discussing spiritual health, let's look at the terms *religion, spirituality,* and *healing.* The word *religion* derives from the Latin root *religio,* which signifies a bond between humanity and some greater-than-human power. In ancient times, the experience of interacting with that power, and the rituals involved, were central to religion. More recently, religion has seemed to become less a personal experience with that power and, in some cases, more identified with a fixed system (denominations, theologies, etc.).[14] Religion and its beliefs provide ways to interpret the deeper purposes of life, to give life and its events meaning and structure, and to organize one's actions in keeping with those precepts. Religious communities provide a means to explore and share spiritual ideals and experience, and potentially to receive caring support. At times, however, there is also potential for being judged and excluded for violating the society's norms.

Motivations used in religious groups to encourage "proper" behavior can vary: either using unconditional love and support, or else perhaps motivating with conditional guilt, shame, and fear. The health and well-being effects of religion can thus vary with which approach is taken. In some of the studies cited,[15] *intrinsic* religious experience improved health, but *extrinsic* religious commitment showed little benefit.[16] Intrinsic religion refers to being motivated by core, internalized beliefs that reflect deeply who a person is and that for which he or she most hopes. Intrinsic religion is deeply God-centered and not subjected as much to social pressures and conformity. Extrinsic religious commitment, on the other hand, usually involves using religion for other ends, such as security, social acceptance, or self-justification. Extrinsic religion is often driven by social pressures and conformity, and tends to be more self-centered. As we shall see, intrinsic religion is healthy, but extrinsic religiosity is not.

The word *spirituality* derives from the Latin *spiritus,* meaning breath or life. In the Jewish and Christian traditions, biblical words translated "spirit" (Hebrew *ruach* and Greek *pneuma)* to also mean breath (and the source of life). And much like Eastern religions today, ancient biblical people used breathing meditative techniques to "breathe in" and thus experience spiritual power. Shamanic healing ceremonies among native Americans and Polynesians invoke similar rituals of drawing healing spiritual power within one who needs it. The experience of oneness with the sources of spiritual power and life seems central to spirituality. Those same energies are sensed as sources of healing. In recent years, the rise of secularism and the yearning for such experience with the transcendent has led to many nonreligious approaches to seeking spirituality, such as the New Age Movement and nonreligious meditation.

In recent health research, religion usually is associated with the institutional and ritual-practice elements, while spirituality refers more to personal experience with the transcendent. But what exactly is spiritual well-being? Interestingly, we may be able to help define the answer to that important question by scientific analysis of which spiritual elements powerfully affect mental and physical well-being (health). From this data, the mind/body connection appears increasingly to be a mind/body/spirit triad.

Defining *healing* reveals some fascinating overlap between medical and spiritual terminology. Drawing once again on ancient wisdom, the words *heal* and *health* originally referred to being made *whole,* and are associated with "holy." The biblical Greek word *sozo* is translated as both "to heal" and also "to save." The biblical Greek word *soteria* is translated as either "health" or "salvation." Thus, to ancient religious people, salvation, the end goal of religious and spiritual practice, meant total well-being (health): spiritual, mental, physical, and social. That insight is worthy of our consideration today.

To heal also has to do with bringing separated things back together, as in skin that has been cut, or a broken relationship. It thus has to do with *creating oneness:* not only reestablishing homeostasis of physical systems, but also mentally and socially becoming "at one"—no longer torn or alienated from oneself, from others, or from the sources of one's spiritual strength. As we shall see, when people heal social and spiritual relationships, they tend to heal physically as well. We tend to artificially separate these things, but the larger brain, mind, and soul do not.

Healing tends to make people feel more fully alive and more grateful for life. Indeed, gratitude for all that life is may be one of the best markers for spiritual well-being. This usually means more than simply a return to the former condition. It involves enlarging the circle of our being to include more that is loved and understood.

Dr. Bernie Siegel tells the story of a woman who had been reared in an alcoholic family where everyone committed suicide. She wrote that she felt she "didn't have a choice" regarding the family she was born into, and that she felt like she was a prisoner. But, she wrote to Siegel, "When I let love into my prison, it healed all the things in my life." She still has her illness, but she is at peace. "We don't have choices about who our parents are and how they treated us," Siegel says, "but we have a choice about whether we forgive our parents and heal ourselves."[17]

Spirituality is not the same as organized religion, although spiritual experience is the cornerstone of religion. And spiritual health is not the same thing as physical health: A person can enjoy optimum spiritual health while battling the ravages of terminal cancer.

Indeed, healing does not always "result in a physical cure," points out *Psychology Today* editor Marc Barasch. "But the quest for wholeness is never in vain, no matter what the outcome. To find it, we may have to forsake, once and for all, that misapprehension that sees Good in what aggrandizes us, Beauty in what is unblemished, Wholeness only in what is intact. For those who can summon the courage to tread a path with heart, illness's dark passage may provide a glimpse not only of what it is like to become whole, but what it means to be fully human."[18]

"I believe that the power of the mind goes far beyond what I first imagined," wrote renowned radiation oncologist O. Carl Simonton, following years of research on the connection between the mind and the body. "In addition, I believe that, beyond the body and mind, there is another aspect of healing that needs to be addressed: the spiritual aspect. . . . The dictionary defines spirit as the life principle, especially in humans, and the feelings and motivating part of our lives. . . . Our work with patients has demonstrated that health involves body, mind, and spirit. And while the mind alone can be used to influence the physical state, it is used most effectively when it is aware of spirit."[19]

One researcher, R. Banks, attempted to arrive at a definition of spirituality by questioning health professionals, health educators, health students, and others who worked within the health and medical fields. Her characterization eventually merged many of the ideas of people involved in health. Her definition of the spiritual dimension involved eight different ideas:[20]

1. Something that gives meaning or purpose to life

2. A set of principles or ethics to live by

3. The sense of selflessness and a feeling for others—a willingness to do more for others than for yourself

4. Commitment to God, and an ultimate concern

5. Perception of what causes the universe to work the way it does

6. Something for which there is no rational explanation—recognition of powers beyond the natural and rational

7. Something perceived as being known or hazily known—something for which there is no easy explanation, and so it becomes a matter of faith

8. The most pleasure-producing quality of humans

Combining all of these ideas and others she collected, Banks identified what she believed to be the four aspects of spiritual health:

1. The spiritual dimension of health acts as a unifying force that integrates the other dimensions of health: physical, mental, emotional, and social. The spiritual dimension unites the other dimensions of health, bringing them into a whole.

2. The spiritual dimension of health creates or brings into focus a meaning in life. The exact components of that meaning vary from one individual to another. For one, it may be centered on family relationships, whereas for another it may be focused on humanitarian efforts or the result of professional effort. Regardless of the source of the meaning, it can serve as a powerful inner drive for personal accomplishment. And regardless of its source, it is vital. Without some meaning in life, the will to live is lost.

3. Because the spiritual dimension of health transcends the individual, it has the capacity to be a common bond between individuals. It rises above the individual and goes beyond the limits of the individual. With this common bond, we are enabled to share love, warmth, and compassion with other people—and we are able to do unselfish and compassionate

things for others, things that go beyond ourselves. We are able to put someone else's life, safety, security, and interest before our own. This common bond also enables us to follow a set of ethical principles—and to make a commitment to God (or some other source of spiritual power).

4. The spiritual dimension of health is based on individual perceptions and faith. We acknowledge that there is some power at work, a power other than the natural and the rational. We acknowledge and perceive that such a power is the cause behind the natural workings of the universe. Our perceptions and our faith bring us pleasure and convince us of our ability to survive.[21]

In *The Path of Transformation*, Shakti Gawain writes that "contact with our spiritual self gives us an expanded perspective on our lives, both as individuals and as part of humanity. Rather than just being caught up in the daily frustrations and struggles of our personality, we are able to see things from the perspective of the soul. We're able to look at the bigger picture of life on earth, which helps us to understand a lot more about why we're here and what we're doing. It helps to make our daily problems seem not quite so huge, and makes our lives feel more meaningful."[22]

Indications of spirituality include prayer, a sense of meaning in life, reading and contemplation, a sense of closeness to a higher being, interactions with others, and other experiences that reflect spiritual interaction or awareness.[23] The scope of decisions influenced by spirituality is vast; the wide range of decisions that have spiritual overtones include the degree of sexual intimacy engaged in, the decision to donate organs, the movies seen, the literature read, the music sung or listened to, smoking, drinking alcohol, taking drugs, and many more.[24]

Still another researcher, using many of the same basic components, developed a slightly different definition of spiritual health. Optimum spiritual health, he says, is the ability to develop our spiritual nature to its fullest potential. Part and parcel of that is the ability to discover and articulate our own basic purpose in life. It's the ability to learn how to experience love, joy, peace, and fulfillment. And it's the experience of helping ourselves and others achieve full potential.[25]

One of the keys to spirituality and spiritual health lies in our relationship with others and the experiences we share. Those experiences are of prime importance. According to researchers who spoke at Harvard Medical School's Conference on Advances in Behavioral Medicine, the greatest benefits of spirituality are rooted in experience, not just belief. Apparently, those who "believe" but do not experience miss out on the psychological and physical benefits of spirituality. (Speakers were quick to point out that many people probably have spiritual experiences all the time, but do not recognize them as such.)

The notion of spirituality itself implies that we are able to give as well as to receive[26]—that we can receive love and joy and peace and fulfillment, but that, through our experiences, we can give those things as well. We can give peace to another by offering words of encouragement or forgiveness. We can give joy by giving someone else a deeply desired gift. We can share love by countless acts of sacrifice, by considering someone else first. Spirituality can be manifested by listening to a friend's heartaches, by walking with a child, by leaving a box of groceries on the porch of a young family whose husband lost his job. Spirituality can be enhanced by sitting at the edge of a meadow studded with wildflowers, befriending someone who is lonely, listening to a symphony.

Through the spiritual dimension, we emphasize our "connectedness" to other members of the human family. Because of that connectedness, say some, we have a responsibility to help others experience spiritual growth—to help others find joy, peace, fulfillment, and a purpose in life. When we do so, we find that the experience is reciprocal; as we affect the spirituality of others, we receive help and support as well.[27]

An important distinction has to be made: In this results-oriented society in which we live, we need to realize that spirituality and spiritual health are a process or a journey, not an end point. It is a lifestyle, not a prescribed set of activities to accomplish on a onetime basis. There is no standard recipe to follow to achieve spirituality or spiritual health; spirituality and spiritual health involve intentional choices made over an entire lifetime. They involve living a series of experiences that define and fulfill our purpose in life and lead us to feelings of joy, peace, and love.

According to Joan Borysenko:

> *Wholeness has to do with the acceptance of both darkness and light, so that the work of healing and transformation can begin. Healing is a state of authenticity that allows freedom of creativity and is marked by peace, joy, compassion, and acceptance of the wide range of emotions that carry the information required to continue learning. It is a splendid coincidence that healing is often associated with better physical functioning, but the person who is truly evolving toward healing realizes that illness is a part of a Sacred Mystery that can never be reduced solely to the physical, emotional, behavioral, or spiritual (in the limited perspective we have as human beings). In the words of Stephen Leaven, we must evolve toward becoming responsible to our illness (and all life-crises), rather than getting stuck in feeling responsible for it.[28]*

## Influences on Health

Spirituality and the cultivation of spiritual health can have an influence on physical, mental, and emotional health—sometimes in very dramatic ways. The impact of spirituality on health may be due in part to the fact that "attitudes, of faith, hope, and commitment imply an internal locus of control, and following an ethical path that involves fulfillment, purpose, and meaning may lead to enhanced self-esteem and a sense of connectedness with self and others."[29]

How could such things as a sense of control or purpose, of love or hope, cause better physical health? Looking at it naturalistically, let's take the example of pain, or of depression with its damage to health. In Chapters 5 and 6, we described the neurochemistry of how depression or anxiety causes more disease and pain (through deficiencies of neurotransmitters such as serotonin, norepinephrine, GABA, or dopamine), and how enhancing the function of these neurotransmitters reduces pain or depression. Earlier we cited studies of how spiritual practices reduce pain. Interestingly, in studies at the University of California, Los Angeles, a personal sense of control was shown to significantly increase serotonin function (much like an antidepressant medication would). And deeply loving relationships and vivid spiritual experience raise dopamine levels. Also, getting "turned on" with purpose to a project that is believed in can raise central norepinephrine levels. Meditation can raise GABA function, a neurotransmitter that calms the overresponsive nervous system characteristic of many common illnesses such as headache, irritable bowel, or chronic pain. Each of these neurochemical effects improves nervous system suppression of pain. So all this may explain somewhat how a person with pain who falls in love and experiences joy will at times find his or her pain subsiding. And perhaps also how interventions that quiet hostility and improve relationships can reduce heart attacks.

Cardiologist Bruno Cortis asks, "How can health be without spirituality? Can the body live without the soul that makes it? The spiritual powers within far surpass any others; transcendent, they lift all of humanity."[30] Experienced clinician and educator Paul Pearsall, who founded and directs the Problems of Daily Living Clinic in the Department of Psychiatry at Sinai Hospital in Detroit, remembers a woman who exemplified spiritual health:

> *I will never forget her. As she laughed, her hand went to her forehead to brush her hair from her eyes. Purple numbers were tattooed on her wrist. She called them her death marks but said that they had strangely protected and renewed her life during her suffering. She had been tortured, seen her own parents and almost all of her relatives killed, and had lived in the agony, squalor, and starvation of a prison camp for most of the young years of her life. She had every reason to be weak, bitter, sick, and depressed. Instead, she was one of the most joyful, hardy women I have ever met.[31]*

Pearsall attributes her health, strength, and resilience to a deep sense of spiritual strength. She was a person whose spirituality enabled her to find meaning and purpose in life—even in the midst of crisis.

Similarly, Victor Frankl, himself a Jewish survivor of a Nazi prison camp and an astute observer of what allowed some to bear it well, eloquently describes the key to such resilience as a sense of purpose and meaning. In his classic book, *Man's Search for Meaning,* Frankl describes how resilient people find meaning in all the vicissitudes of life, even in such a tragedy as the camp.

Researchers are beginning to view spirituality with new interest, especially as it relates to physical health. One who is pioneering such research is Kenneth Pelletier who, with his colleagues at the Corporate Health Promotion Project at the University of California, San Francisco, is investigating the link between spirituality and health. Pelletier started his research by investigating the lives of top business executives and other prominent people who have achieved what most consider to be "success."

He found, first, that most of the professionally successful men and women participating in the study had strong spiritual values and beliefs. Further, virtually all of them had suffered a major psychological or physical trauma early in life. Despite these traumas—or maybe because of them, Pelletier surmises—these people now have a more effective style of coping with life crises.[32] (As discussed in the Harvard Medical School conference, spiritual people weather crises better—partially because they are able to find purpose and meaning in life despite the crisis and even from the crisis.)

Preliminary findings from the study found the correlation between good spiritual health and good physical health to be "striking." People with a deep sense of spirituality reported less use of medical services, less minor illness, and more complete recovery from minor illness than the national average. Similar findings were reported from a study of 300 terminally ill and nonterminally ill hospitalized adults. Those with the greatest spirituality, even though their illnesses were terminal, showed resilient emotional health. Spirituality was significantly related to "low death fear, low discomfort, decreased loneliness, emotional adjustment, and positive death perspectives among terminal cancer and other seriously ill patients."[33]

In another study of more than 100 geriatric patients at a clinic, researchers measured each patient's "religious activity" by determining the amount of each one's religious community activity, private devotional activity (such as prayer), and intrinsic religious orientation. They found that those who had little religious activity had much higher rates of cancer, chronic anxiety, depression, cigarette smoking, and alcohol use. On the other hand, patients with high levels of religious activity enjoyed better overall physical and mental health.[34]

Some of the improvement in overall health may well relate to the benefits of spiritual practice on mental health and reduction of feeling stressed. In his text on the subject, Pargament concluded that the evidence showed that spirituality can reduce anxiety, foster better intimacy, enhance a sense of purpose and meaning for life, and foster personal growth and control.[35] A panel of experts carefully reviewed many studies in the medical literature,[36] and concluded that spirituality and religiousness were in particular related to greater

- subjective well-being,
- life satisfaction, and
- marital satisfaction,

and less

- depression symptoms,
- delinquency, and
- drug and alcohol abuse.

For dealing with stressful events, some aspects of religious coping (e.g., seeking reassurance from God and seeking support within one's religious community) were more helpful than others (e.g., praying for a miracle). On the other hand, some forms of religiousness had deleterious mental effects (e.g., beliefs in a punitive God, extrinsic religiosity, conflict with or feeling judged by clergy, and hyperrigid religiousness).

Mindful meditative practice reduces anxiety in the long term.[37] This has been shown to reduce physical problems considerably, as do other treatments for anxiety.[38] For example, transcendental meditation, by reducing stress hormones, can lead to regression of carotid artery thickening[39] (compared to progressive thickening in control groups) and improved coronary disease outcomes.[40]

Psychiatrist and psychosomatic physician Gerald Epstein has focused almost two decades of research on the spiritual components of health by analyzing what is found in the biblical Ten Commandments.[41] Rather than relate the Ten Commandments to any specific religion or religious belief, Epstein analyzed their content and teachings in the context of spirituality and spiritual health in general. He found that the Ten Commandments are a "prescription for healthful living. . . . The first five outline the proper relationship of human beings to God, the last five the proper relationship of human beings to human society; all of them are finely and intricately related to each other."

And the teachings in the Ten Commandments give us information for our own spirituality, he notes. One message is that we should not place our faith in the authority of a doctor as an ultimate healer. Pearsall states, "Determination on the part of the patient, not the physician, is what makes healing and joy possible."[42] Or, as Buddha summarized, "It is you who must make the effort. The masters only point the way." Pearsall remarks that contemporary psychologists call this combination of faith and determination a "sense of trust"—"a trust in the spirit of God within each of us as the source of all joy."

Epstein points out that spirituality "also means that in understanding illness, one should regard agents such as disease-bearing organisms as simply one component of a process involving God and human beings, human beings and ethics, human beings in relationship to each other."[43] Those relationships are an essential part of spirituality and spiritual health—and, Epstein says, this aspect of spirituality emphasizes what is positive about relationships. Those in truly great relationships know the joy that comes in desiring the good of the beloved. In this, a person comes to feel more fully alive.

Similarly, says Pearsall, choosing to care well for oneself is another aspect of spirituality. This requires a good sense of self-acceptance:

> We seem to be alienated from our own affection for ourselves. We believe that once we lose weight, make more money, or learn some new skill, we will then become more acceptable to ourselves. This sequence is backward. We must begin with a celebration of self, not a diagnosis of our flaws. If you can't say something good about yourself, maybe you shouldn't be saying anything at all until you look a little closer at just how special you really are. . . . To love oneself is only possible by first learning to love others and by developing a tolerance, acceptance, and empathy that are necessary if we are ever going to get closer to one another than we have been until now.[44]

## Crisis as a Growth Experience

People with a deep sense of spirituality see life differently. They have a purpose, they enjoy a sense of meaning in life, and they have a broader perspective. Spirituality buffers stress; people with a deep sense of spirituality are not defeated by crisis. They are able to relax their minds, elicit the relaxation response, and heal more quickly and completely.

At a deep level, how important is growth to you, that is, being better today than you were five years ago, and being wiser and stronger tomorrow than you are today? To most of us, that seems very important. Yet we often try to avoid the very parts of life that best bring that maturation. Much of what life is about seems to be related to that growing process: becoming wiser and more loving. Praying for no difficulties is probably a prayer that is unlikely to be answered. And those who acknowledge life's purposes, and even enjoy rising to the challenge, become more resilient.[45]

Spirituality helps people interpret crisis in a growth-producing way, and, as a result, they are able to use illness as a means of spiritual growth. Even when a disease takes a life, spirituality can make the experience one of positive growth. In talking about how spirituality can influence attitude, Bernie Siegel remarks, "I simply try to heal the life. I hate to have somebody die with an unhealed life. I hate to have somebody die who says, 'I have never lived; I have never experienced love; I have always felt worthless.' Through the disease, I try to bring something to their lives, so the disease can be a gift."[46]

In the effort to "heal a life," Siegel says, we need to figure out "what is the self trying to get me as a patient to learn about myself?" . . . "If you turn toward what threatens you and say, 'Why are you here? Why do you want to kill me? What can I learn from you?' then you help heal your life and find out who you are."[47] He further says that when "you take on life's afflictions and challenges, you are a winner." He adds that he hopes people can

> understand that there can be a gift in the disease and you can help heal everyone around you. Hemingway said that the world breaks everyone and some of us are strong at the broken places. I am talking about people who are strong at the broken places: the quadriplegics can have healed lives; people who aren't cured of cancer can be incredibly inspiring and teach all of us; people with multiple sclerosis can teach us.[48]

Not everyone will attain a cure. At some time or another, everyone will die. But people who are busy living, who are trying to make changes in their lives, experience great growth even in the face of serious illness. People who face disease with that attitude, Siegel says,

> define their disease as a gift, a challenge, a wake-up call, a new beginning, and a beauty mark. And they are not necessarily saying, "I am cured." The exceptional people accept their mortality. They have heard they're going to die, but they don't take it as a sentence. So they don't go home and die. They take it as an opportunity to live until they die.[49]

In discussing the entire issue of spirituality and the growth that can come from illness or other adversity, Siegel talks about what he calls "a spiritual flat tire":

> I simply say that sometimes adversity and affliction direct you into the proper place so that when you have a flat tire that makes you miss a plane that later crashes, you embrace the tire, bronze it, and hang it over your fireplace as the spiritual flat tire that saved your life. But while you are fixing the tire you are screaming and yelling and getting dirty and mad that you are going to miss your plane. There are many things in life that redirect our lives. So I don't judge things as good, bad, right or wrong. Just sit back and say, "We'll see."[50]

In using illness as an opportunity for spiritual growth, Siegel says that we need to accept the illness (which is far different from becoming resigned to it), view it as a source of growth, and view it as a positive redirection in life. Perhaps most important, says Siegel, is to infuse your situation with spirituality and love:

> *The only way you can live forever is to love somebody: then you can really leave a gift behind. And when you live that way, as I have seen happen with people who have physical illnesses, it is even possible to decide when you die. You can say, "Thank you, I've used my body to its limit. I have loved as much as I possibly can, and I'm leaving at two o'clock today." And you go. Then maybe you spend half an hour dying and the rest of your day living. But when these things are not done, you may spend a lot of your life dying, and only a little living.*[51]

Spiritual healing, says one researcher, "is not a complicated system of diagnoses and remedies but seems to work on the level of unselfish love and compassion. Not an emotional love which is bound up with one's own needs, but a caring, unconditional, detached love with no beginning and no end."[52]

The Reverend Michael Harper pointed out the importance of spirituality to health when he said, "We need to see that we cannot escape from either the spiritual or the physical. We cannot be wholly saved by drugs or medical treatment, nor can we detach our bodies from our spiritual lives. Biblical language and understanding makes it obligatory for us to have a healing ministry which relates the spiritual to the physical and the physical to the spiritual. By ignoring the one we are doing a disservice to the other and are ignoring human and divine realities."[53]

## The Power of Prayer on Health

A seventy-six-year-old Spanish-speaking man who lives in a small village north of Santa Fe, New Mexico, described the essential rhythms of his life in this way:

> *For us the day begins with a prayer of thanks to God, for giving us another day here. And in the evening, when we go to bed, we stop and say thank you, dear Lord, for the gift of another day with our children and grandchildren. It is only a few moments any of us is here, we know—because life goes on and on and on, and we're but one stalk of corn, and many stalks are planted and grow and are harvested, season after season. But the one who puts us here and then gathers us up—He is the one who should hear from us with a please, a thank you, a wave, a smile. If we cry, He'd like to know why. If we're happy, He'd like to know why. It's not right to think you're the lord and master of this place. He is the one who has His eyes on us and wants the best for us.*
>
> *True, we have to build our lives for ourselves; He has let us do that. But He's not beyond giving us a boost now and then—if we ask! When we get sick, we don't go right down to Santa Fe or Albuquerque right away. No sir, we stop*

*and try to figure out what has happened; and we call the priest; and we get down on our hands and knees and call Him to us, the Lord, and tell Him what's up. When we do that—well, you hear what you've said, and believe me, there are times when just listening to your own prayers makes you feel better!*[54]

The elderly villager is right: Your own prayers can make you feel better. Prayer signals a commitment to a set of moral and ethical values. It is a signpost of our spirituality and is at the core of most spiritual experiences. According to a recent Gallup Poll, 87 percent of all Americans pray to God. When we pray, we are in a state of relaxed alertness, peace, joy, contentment, and emotional release. During prayer, we empty the mind, yet we receive some inner direction. Part of the magnetism of prayer comes from our own belief, our own faith—the powerful suggestion that prayer will work, that something will happen.[55]

A study of nearly 4,000 mostly Christian people over age sixty-five found that those who never or rarely prayed ran about a 50 percent greater risk of dying over a period of six years.[56] The authors postulate that the relaxation and meditative effects of prayer may play a role in the protection it provides. From a naturalistic perspective, one might also think that the 64 percent of people who pray for their health,[57] and trust in prayer's efficacy, tap into the power of hope and expectation that improves outcomes (see Chapter 16).

It's the subtle peace and quiet effect of prayer that may be the most effective. In one study of spontaneous remission of cancer conducted at Kyushu University School of Medicine in Japan, researchers found that prayer preceded the cure in every case. But, say the researchers, it wasn't "robust, aggressive prayer for specific outcomes, including eradication of the cancer" that did the trick, but "a prayerful, prayerlike attitude of devotion and acceptance."[58]

Dr. Larry Dossey, an internist who has pioneered prayer research, writes, "I would describe prayer as any psychological activity—conscious or unconscious—that places us in closer contact with the transcendent. This can involve words, but it can also be subconscious or unconscious. Prayer can even occur during sleep. The state of mind that I call prayerfulness seems to involve certain fairly specific qualities, in particular, empathy. The most successful prayer experiments have always linked outcome to the empathy, love, and sense of involvement felt by the people doing the praying."[59]

## The Relaxation Response

Prayer has powerful physiological effects on the body as well. Of 131 controlled experiments on prayer-based healing, more than half showed statistically significant benefits.[60] Dr. Herbert Benson, associate professor of medicine at the Harvard Medical School and chief of the Section on Behavioral Medicine at the New England Deaconess Hospital, has focused the last two decades of his clinical work on what he has come to call the "relaxation response." The relaxation response is the body's ability to enter a "scientifically definable state" of relaxation. During the relaxation response, changes occur in the body. Metabolism slows down, blood pressure drops, breathing slows, heart rate lowers, and even the brain waves are less active.[61]

According to Benson, the relaxation response, "with all its physiological benefits, has most often and effectively been elicited through forms of prayer."[62] In his own practice, as he has struggled to teach patients the relaxation response, he has watched the great physical results of prayer. He has written extensively of those results; in one woman, crippling angina was resolved. In another, life-threatening high blood pressure was dropped.

The relaxation response gives us a clue as to one reason why prayer improves health: It helps us meditate, relieving stress. Prayer may be the most common kind of meditation in the Western world. When patients pray, they're focusing on their deepest values and drawing on spiritual power that develops a sense of connectedness and also develops hope. And that has been known to affect medical outcomes. The mind has the ability to heal when those elements are elicited.

Apparently, most of the benefits from prayer come from what researchers call "meditative" prayer—being still, knowing that God is God. According to University of Akron Sociologist Margaret Poloma, research suggests that people who use only active prayer but don't get into meditative prayer "aren't as likely to find peace and serenity" through their prayers.[63]

Poloma and her colleague, Brian Pendleton, found that different types of prayers affected people in different ways. Happiness, they say, seems to be predicted not by the frequency of prayer, but by its quality. In a study of 560 Akron-area residents, Poloma and Pendleton identified four main types of prayer that are performed away from church:

1. Meditative (feeling or quietly thinking about God)

2. Colloquial (asking for guidance or forgiveness)

3. Petitional (asking for explicit favors)

4. Ritual (reading specific prayers)[64]

According to Poloma and Pendleton, meditative prayer was closely associated with "existential well-being" and religious satisfaction, whereas colloquial prayer was related to overall happiness.

When we ourselves pray, we reap tremendous physical, emotional, and spiritual benefits. And if current research is correct, we may also reap the benefits from the prayers of others on our behalf.

### The Effects on Other People

According to some research, prayer can have a powerful impact on people, even though they don't know prayers are being offered in their behalf.

Arthur Kennel, assistant professor of medicine at Mayo Medical School in Rochester, Minnesota, says, "I pray for my own patients, and I feel my prayers benefit them."

Dr. Kennel is not alone. In a nationwide poll asking doctors whether they believe patients benefit from prayer and whether they themselves pray for patients, the results favored prayer. Half of the doctors questioned said that they believe prayer helps patients; two-thirds of the doctors responding said that they pray for their patients.[65]

In a highly publicized scientific study of prayer in a medical setting, R. B. Byrd, over ten months, randomly divided 393 patients of a coronary care unit to either be prayed for or not.[66] Neither the patients nor the physicians knew who was in each group. Those praying knew specific names and diagnoses. Those prayed for did significantly better on standard measures of outcome such as time in the hospital, complication rates, medications needed, and new symptoms. A similar study at the Mayo Clinic, however, was unable to replicate this effect when patients were unaware of the prayer.[67]

A number of physicians pointed out that prayer, as an expression of spirituality, can work in concert with medical treatment to bring about physiological changes and recoveries. Francis MacNutt, director of the Christian Healing Ministries, echoed that sentiment: "In no way do I conceive prayer for healing as a negation of the need for doctors, nurses, counselors, psychiatrists, or pharmacists. God works in all these ways to heal the sick; the ideal is a team effort to get the sick well through every possible means."[68]

## The Healing Power of Forgiveness

Essential to a spiritual nature is forgiveness—the ability to release from the mind all the past hurts and failures, all sense of guilt and loss. Counselor Suzanne Simon defines forgiveness as a "process of healing." What some have also called "the first step on the pathway to healing," forgiveness enables one to banish resentment. It is, as Dr. Joan Borysenko put it, "accepting the core of every human being as the same as yourself and giving them the gift of not judging them."[69]

According to psychotherapist Robin Casarjian, founder and director of the Lionheart Foundation, forgiveness is "a relationship with life that frees the forgiver from the psychological bondage of chronic fear, hostility, anger, and unhealthy guilt."[70] Forgiveness, she says, is an attitude that implies that you are willing to accept responsibility for your perceptions, realizing that "your perceptions are a choice and not an objective fact."

We forgive others, and we must forgive ourselves. According to one researcher, forgiveness "removes whatever has blocked your creative mind from operating positively for you and for your good."[71]

Forgiveness isn't easy; in fact, most people who responded to one poll said they had great difficulty in forgiving others. Apparently, forgiveness is the most difficult when we are called upon to forgive ourselves. Psychologists estimate that at least seven of every ten people carry throughout life a sense of guilt—a feeling of having committed a sin or mistake for which they have never been forgiven.[72]

Forgiveness is not condoning negative, inappropriate behavior, whether your own or someone else's, says Casarjian. It is also not "pretending everything is just fine when you feel it isn't, or assuming an attitude of superiority or self-righteousness." Instead, she says, it is a "decision to see beyond the limits of another's personality . . . and to gradually transform yourself from being a helpless victim of your circumstances to being a powerful and loving co-creator of your reality."[73]

Our own chosen thoughts about what the offender has done are far more powerful in creating our reaction than is their act itself. For example, when Ingrid saw her physician for abdominal pains and headaches, she spoke very angrily and in condemning terms about her teenage daughter's sassy, rebellious attitude the day before. "Cally makes me so angry! I hate her when she acts that way!" To Ingrid, Cally's acts seemed to reach inside her to make Ingrid bitterly angry and hateful, causing her to lash out at Cally with putdowns in retaliation.

Afterward, however, Ingrid felt some remorse, even guilt, about the way she had put her daughter down. "I don't want to be that kind of mother," Ingrid admitted. "Cally is going through a lot, and trying to let go of being dependent and controlled by me. I don't deserve to be treated that way, but neither does she. When I try to put myself in her shoes, and see the world through her eyes, I can feel my heart softening and the anger melts away."

Ingrid was beginning to understand an essential key to reclaiming one's life, to feeling the sense of personal control that has been so consistently linked to better health and medical outcomes. That key is called forgiveness. Forgiveness can at first seem difficult, like giving a magnanimous gift to some jerk who doesn't deserve it, or like letting them off the hook of deserved consequences and retribution. However, with a bit of reflection, the real meaning of forgiveness begins to emerge. Forgiveness is refusing any longer to blame someone else, or circumstances, for *making* one feel or act in ways they would not want. Forgiveness is taking back control of one's life, behavior, and personal actions. This recovery of a sense of personal control is essential to wholeness and well-being (health). A low sense of personal control leads to all the negative emotions: anger, guilt, fear, anxiety, and frustration (with all of their adverse health implications). On the other hand, a high sense of personal control (of one's self, not of the world out there) leads to all the positive emotions: confidence, inner peace, hope, and loving kindness (even for a rebellious daughter).

The foremost way to get a high personal sense of control is to fully accept personal responsibility for how one chooses to think about and respond to the acts of others (or of fate). Blaming makes it feel like the other has taken control of you—making you act and feel ways you would not want. But the fact is they don't have that kind of control over you. Only you do. So call your control back by refusing to blame any longer what they have done for making you be other than what you want to be— by forgiving. Such a choice may well require help beyond your own. Forgiveness is taking back control of your life, and if possible, as Ingrid did, seeing the pain or insecurity that drives the other's behavior. This may even lead to compassion.

To determine the physical effects of forgiveness, it is first necessary to determine what happens to us physically when we don't forgive. The resulting hatred drives all the mechanisms causing poor health described in the chapters on stress (Chapter 2) and anger (Chapter 4). With forgiveness, the anger and resentment dissolve. The body stops pouring high-voltage chemicals into the bloodstream. The healing begins.

One of the greatest examples of the healing power of forgiveness can be found in nature. As one author put it:

> *Nature always forgives. Nature is the great giver and the great forgiver. Should you cut your hand with a sharp knife, the forces of nature set about immediately to repair the damage. It was a mistake to cut your hand, but nature does not withhold the repairing of the wound. Nature immediately forgives and starts at once to make repairs. If you eat food that does not agree with you and you have indigestion, nature immediately starts to repair the damage. Although it was a mistake to eat the wrong food, you do not need to go through the rest of your life with indigestion. Nature even repairs the ravages of the battlefield by covering it with grass and flowers. [No one] can go forward if he is tied to the past. No one can think straight and efficiently if his mind is cluttered up with thoughts of hate or memories of hurts and mistakes; hence the necessity of forgiving so that we can love ourselves, our neighbor, and God.[74]*

To bring a greater sense of forgiveness into your own life, try following what Dwight Wolter presented as the "tools of forgiveness."

- Begin by letting go of your unforgiving stance.
- Admit that the events and feelings you are struggling with really happened.

- Admit that the past cannot be undone. After all, there is really no hope for a better yesterday.

- Recognize that you no longer need to depend on others, including your parents, for approval. When you realize your independence, you assume your rightful power and you learn to be who you want to be regardless of the actions of others.

- Don't expect others to respond to your efforts to forgive.

- Release any unrealistic expectations of yourself.

- Accept others for who they are rather than who you want them to be.

- Be flexible about rules of conduct for yourself and others.

- Talk about issues as they come up.[75] Refuse any longer to blame.

In addition to those suggestions, Robin Casarjian suggests fostering a forgiving attitude by praying, meditating, expressing gratitude (to people or to a higher power), spending time in nature and allowing yourself to experience its wonder, serving others selflessly, and creating through any art form.[76]

## Church Affiliation and Health

Religion, basically, is a science in how to know God—and research has shown that people with active religious faith and people who are strongly affiliated with a particular church generally enjoy better health. Religion is "the personal beliefs, values, and activities pertinent to that which is supernatural, mysterious, and awesome, which transcends immediate situations, and which pertains to questions of final causes and ultimate ends of man and the universe."[77]

There are two basic orientations of religion:

1. **Personal.** Religion involves a person's values, beliefs, and attitudes. Spiritual experience is the cornerstone of religion; if spiritual experience is in one's belief system, it becomes the only way to God. The personal orientation of religion can be either intrinsic or extrinsic. Those with an intrinsic sense of religion participate in their chosen religion for spiritual reasons; to them, the religion comes first and is a dominating force in their lives. Those with an extrinsic sense of religion do not share the "zeal" or commitment of those with an intrinsic orientation; religion for them is secondary and does not represent a primary need. They "belong," but they do not "live" their religion.[78]

2. **Institutional.** Individuals adopt a church or religion because of group-related benefits: They enjoy attending church, participating in group activities or rituals, and receiving community support.

Studies indicate that religion may enhance health and well-being in at least four ways:[79] first, through social integration and support; second, through the establishment of a personal relationship with a divine other; third, through the provision of systems of meaning and existential coherence; and fourth, through the promotion of specific patterns of a more healthy personal lifestyle.

Regardless of how it works, evidence exists that religion does enhance health. Numerous studies conducted over the past decade provide evidence that, on average, high levels of religious involvement are associated with better health. These studies have involved both men and women, numerous racial and ethnic groups, people from diverse social and economic backgrounds, people of all ages, and members of a wide variety of different churches. While some studies focus on particular religions (such as Mormons or Adventists) as being protective of health, others show that factors such as frequency of attendance and religious belief are also important in protecting health.[80]

Studies that examined the rate of heart disease, high blood pressure, stroke, cancer, digestive disease, physical disability, self-rated health, and self-reported symptoms showed a strong relationship between religious participation and good health.[81] A study by the National Institute on Aging found that elderly people living at home who attended church regularly were less depressed and physically healthier than those who did not attend church.[82] New studies show that:

- Those patients who undergo open-heart surgery have a much greater chance of surviving if they gain comfort and strength from religious faith.[83]

- Those who enjoy regular religious affiliation live longer, probably in part because regular church attendance promotes social support.[84]

- The elderly who regularly attend church have significantly better physical and mental health and lower death rates[85] (one study, in fact, showed that some elderly people in New Haven, Connecticut, actually postponed the timing of their death until the conclusion of major religious holidays, such as Easter or Christmas).[86]

In one study of 850 male hospital patients, researchers at a North Carolina Veterans' Administration hospital found that religion was an important coping factor for the men. One in five said religion is "the most important thing that keeps me going." Nearly half of the patients rated religion as very helpful to them in coping with the situation of being hospitalized. According to the men in the study, they derived a feeling of peace and comfort from prayer, Bible study, faith in God, and the emotional support of a pastor or other church members. Those who were religious had high levels of social support, low levels of alcohol use, and significantly less clinical depression.

A detailed review of all such studies[87] revealed that high religious commitment is associated with the following:

**Better physical health outcomes**

- 212 studies: 75 percent positive; 17 percent mixed; and 7 percent negative (including heart disease, cancer, survival, hypertension, general health, and overall functioning)

**Better mental health outcomes**

- 18/19 studies: better adjustment and coping
- 15/15 studies: less drug abuse
- 20/24 studies: less alcohol abuse
- 15/18 studies: less psychiatric illness
- 13/19 studies: less depression

**Better quality of life**

- 18/19 studies: better life satisfaction
- 10/10 studies: better marriage adjustment
- 20/22 studies: better overall well-being
- 14/21 studies: less death anxiety

Let's discuss some specifics of these studies. For example, Harold Koenig and David Larson studied 542 people aged over sixty, finding that over a year, those who attended church at least weekly were hospitalized 56 percent less (43 percent less after controlling for illness, age, and depression). Also, when hospitalized, those affiliated with any religion stayed less than half as long as those who claimed no religion.

"Many people—especially those with fewer health, social, and financial resources—turn to religion for solace in the face of situations over which they have no control," said the researchers, commenting on the study. "Their religious beliefs and involvement may counteract feelings of helplessness, provide meaning and order to challenging life experiences, and restore a sense of control."[88]

Researchers at Duke University, confirming these positive effects of religion on health, theorized that the relationship had to do with the comfort religion provides in time of difficulty or crisis.[89]

Patients themselves tend to confirm those theories. An Internet study recruited 157 people to describe their "alternative" practices in mental health.[90] Most of those surveyed had bipolar mood disorders, depression, or schizophrenia. The methods most commonly used were:

- Spiritual/religious practices    50 percent
- Meditation    43 percent
- Massage    31 percent
- Yoga    20 percent
- Imagery    17 percent
- Herbs    16 percent
- Dietary supplements    13 percent

Eighty-six percent were also taking medication. Adding the above practices provided the following enhanced benefits (each reported by more than 20 percent of the group):

- Increased calmness and stability
- Better cognitive function
- Improved relationships
- Greater sense of purpose
- Feeling spiritually nurtured
- Improved general functioning

In a study of elderly people who were depressed, Bosworth found that the significantly better improvement in those who were religious came from much more than simply social support.[91]

## Attendance and Affiliation

According to nationwide surveys, more than 90 percent of all Americans profess a belief in God; a recent Gallup Poll puts that number as high as 95 percent. According to the Gallup Poll, almost three-fourths of all Americans hold basic Christian beliefs; two-thirds believe that the Bible is "inspired . . . of God." More than half believe in life after death.[92] According to the *New York Times*, almost 90 percent of all Americans report some religious affiliation.

Despite their belief in God, Christ, and the Bible, many American Christians are not active in church affiliations. While 85 percent of Americans consider religion "very important or fairly important" in their lives,[93] their church attendance does not always reflect that attitude. According to a Gallup Poll, only about 40 percent of all Americans attend a place of worship weekly, and about 60 percent attend monthly.[94]

Even churchgoers have a growing dissatisfaction with organized religion. Of those surveyed, 59 percent think churches spend too much time on organization issues; 32 percent believe organized religion is too restrictive in its moral teachings. And almost one in four of the respondents to the Gallup Poll say they turned away from their church in search of "deeper spiritual meaning."[95]

Even so, extensive research indicates that active participation in a church or synagogue boosts health,[96] acts as a buffer against stress, and may even prolong life. Researchers at Southern California College found that elderly people who are religiously active tend to be more optimistic and better able to cope with illness than people who are less religious. University of Portland Sociologist Robert W. Duff said the research is consistent with other studies, including one of his own that showed that religiously active older persons had relatively high life satisfaction ratings.

Religious faith and involvement may be even more life-enhancing than was previously believed, especially for the elderly, according to research by Yale Psychologist Stanislav Kasl and Rutgers University Psychologist Ellen Idler. The pair studied the health and well-being of almost 3,000 retirement-aged residents of New Haven, Connecticut. They found that religious involvement did enhance the well-being of the seniors. According to Idler, "There actually may be a common-sense connection here. It seems reasonable that those people who say they get a great deal of strength and comfort from religion are often those who need it the most—those who are ill."[97]

Religious affiliation appears to protect health at the other end of the age spectrum as well. A study of 19,000 high school seniors conducted at the University of Michigan explains one reason why religious affiliation appears to protect the health of adolescents: Those who have a strong religious affiliation are less likely to behave in ways that compromise their health, such as getting into fights, carrying weapons, smoking cigarettes, using marijuana, and driving under the influence of alcohol. They are also *more* likely to behave in ways that enhance their health, such as eating well, getting proper nutrition, getting regular exercise, and getting plenty of rest.[98] Research shows that religious beliefs and behaviors are fairly widespread among American teens. Among those aged thirteen to seventeen, 95 percent report being affiliated with a religious group or denomination, and 40 percent say they try very hard to follow the teachings of their religion. Of youth in that age group:[99]

- 95 percent believe in God or a universal spirit.
- 93 percent believe that God loves them.
- 91 percent believe in heaven.
- 76 percent believe that God observes their actions and rewards or punishes them.

Interestingly, an adolescent's health may even be protected by the fact that his or her *mother* regularly attends church. A study of 143 teenagers in the Baltimore area looked at the significant risks for psychiatric disorders and examined adolescents who were considered a high risk. Researchers found that those whose mothers attended religious services at least once a week had greater overall satisfaction with their lives, had more involvement with their families, felt greater support from friends, and had better skills in solving health-related problems. The only factor that had a greater influence in the study was family income.[100]

People who attend church or synagogue on a regular basis have a much lower rate of diseases than those who attend less frequently or do not attend at all. Churchgoers have especially low rates of heart disease, lung disease, cirrhosis of the liver, and some kinds of cancer.[101] For example, men who attend church infrequently or not at all are at almost twice the risk of dying of arteriosclerotic heart disease—and that's even when other risk factors (such as smoking and social status) are taken into consideration. They are more than four times more likely to die of cirrhosis of the liver. And women are more than three times as likely to die of cancer of the cervix if they aren't frequent churchgoers.[102]

One review of 200 epidemiological studies found that religion improved health in eight different areas: cancer of the uterus and cervix, all other cancers, colitis and enteritis, cardiovascular disease, hypertension and stroke, general health, general longevity, and disease and death among the clergy.[103]

## Relationship to Church Teachings

In addition to the above probable reasons for a religion's protective nature, many churches prescribe behavior that prevents illness or assists in the treatment of illness. Some religions actively promote healthier lifestyles, such as eating less meat, drinking less alcohol, avoiding caffeine-containing foods and drinks, and not smoking.[104] Other examples of religious prescriptions for healthy behavior include encouragement to eat a diet of healthy, nutritious foods; promotion of proper rest, life balance, and exercise; encouragement of family and social patterns of helping and caring; and proper utilization of available health care systems.

Church teachings often encourage support in times of need, and they cultivate attitudes that may give individuals a helpful perspective with which to face stressful life situations (a belief in life after death, for example, makes it much less stressful to face the terminal illness of a loved one).[105]

Many churches also discourage behavior that is harmful to health, often counseling against harmful drugs, immoral activities (including promiscuous sex), and activities that have a high probability of injuring the body.[106]

Researchers point out, however, that not all religions act to preserve life and promote health. Some religions include the use of contaminated substances in rituals, burials, and other practices; placing the dead in rivers; ritual suicide; religious wars; tortures and executions in the name of religion; and endogamous marriage customs that may engender and perpetuate genetic disorders. Some, too, prohibit members from seeking modern medical treatment or from practicing modern health principles—although churches with these policies are in the distinct minority.[107]

Still another way that churches protect health may lie in attitude. According to researcher Ellen Idler at Rutgers University, the religious teachings of many churches help foster a more positive approach to illness, pain, or disability.[108]

A prominent theory regarding how churches protect the health of their members rests with the well-known fact that social support boosts and protects health. People who are active in a church are not as likely to be lonely. Members of a church affiliation are much like members of an extended family; they provide comfort, companionship, and even material assistance when needed. Ministers and other church leaders visit the ill, marry couples, provide comfort when a family member dies, speak at the funeral, and give counsel in difficult circumstances. Churches offer tradition and social support that are lacking in many communities.[109]

Leonard Sagan says that lifestyle prescriptions are probably at least partly responsible for the better health of active church members—but he is convinced that "support provided by the social network" may be the more important force in boosting the health of active church members. "For one thing," he points out, "membership in other organizations, such as the military services, is also associated with a reduction in mortality."[110]

It's not only physical health that is benefited, but mental and emotional health as well. Famed psychotherapist Carl Jung commented:

> *During the past thirty years, people from all the civilized countries of the earth have consulted me. I have treated many hundreds of patients. . . . Among all my patients in the second half of life—that is to say, over thirty-five—there has not been one whose problem in the last resort was not that of finding a religious outlook on life. . . . It seems to me that, side by side with the decline of religious life, the neuroses grow noticeably more frequent.[111]*

As previously noted, religious commitment has been shown to enhance overall mental health. Maryland psychologist John Gartner reviewed 200 studies on religious commitment and mental health. Those studies showed that the religiously faithful have lower suicide rates, lower drug use and abuse, less juvenile delinquency, lower divorce rates, higher marital happiness, better overall well-being, and better recovery from mental illness.

"Religious belief gives life a context and restrains many self-destructive impulses," explains Gartner. "For many people it appears to be a solid floor for mental health."[112]

Regardless of why religion works to boost health, regular participation seems to be a key. It is associated with increased life span and decreased mortality, even after controlling for age, sex, and various other risk factors.[113]

## Specific Illnesses

Regular church attendance apparently has an impact on a number of specific diseases as well. One is cardiovascular disease. Researchers have found that the more active a person is in a religion, the less chance he or she has of incurring myocardial infarction. The same holds true with people born of a religiously homogeneous marriage.[114] In addition, people who attend church regularly are at lower risk for myocardial degeneration, chronic endocarditis, arteriosclerotic heart disease, and degenerative heart disease.

In addition to benefiting the cardiovascular system, twenty-two out of twenty-seven studies found that the frequency of religious attendance is "significantly associated" with good health. People who go to church frequently, the studies say, have fewer incidences of hypertension, positive pap smears, cervical cancer, neonatal mortality, emphysema, cirrhosis of the liver, suicide, colorectal cancer, cancer-related pain, and physical symptoms in general.[115]

In summary, spiritual practices and attitudes that have been proven to be associated with enhanced physical health include the following:

- Hope
- Forgiveness
- Giving up hostility
- Altruism
- Loving, supportive relationships—community
- Prayer
- Meditation
- Feeling close to God

# The Essence of Spirituality and Spiritual Well-Being

What, then, is the essence of spiritual well-being, the state toward which spiritual and religious practices are best directed? Perhaps, from a scientific perspective, we might discover the answer in those spiritual elements that most powerfully impact mental and physical well-being.

*Health* has been defined by the World Health Organization as total well-being (physical, mental, social, and spiritual), not just the absence of disease. Others have defined health as the quality of existence in which one is at peace within oneself (physically, mentally, and spiritually) and in good concord with the environment. Health science requires the measurements of studies. We can measure physical health very well and mental health quite well, but how do we measure spiritual health?

As one looks at the hundreds of studies in this book for the mental (mind) elements that most powerfully affect physical health (body), at least four become very obvious:

- **A sense of empowerment and personal control**—not necessarily over the environment, but rather over one's self and responses in that environment. This involves being and acting in accord with one's deepest values in any situation—a type of spiritual integrity to deep wisdom.

- **A sense of connectedness**—to one's deeper self, to others, to the sources of one's empowerment, and even to the earth and universe, and all regarded as good.

- **A sense of purpose and meaning**—giving of one's self for a purpose of value and something believed in, thus having an altruistic sense of mission about one's life. And also sensing purpose in the present here-and-now circumstances—whether difficult or joyful—honoring growth and having a vision of one's potential.

- **Hope**—not necessarily for a specific outcome, but for the wisdom and capability to deal well with whatever comes, and for something of value to come of it.

Notice that these "mental" elements (proven to improve physical and mental health) are at their core also very spiritual elements. We propose that they thus define some of the most important principles of spiritual well-being.[116] Directing one's spiritual practices and religious motivations toward these principles has been shown to improve total health. Violating these principles, even with the best of intentions, is likely to cause problems.

For example, a parent or religious leader who has very good intentions for a person, may use guilt or shame to motivate better behavior. Does that empower the person, or make him or her feel less capable? Does throwing guilt connect us or disconnect us? Does shaming create hope, or imply that one is unworthy? On the other hand, motivating improvement instead with love that accepts people right where they are in their process, conveying a belief and trust in them to rise to their own greater wisdom, might enhance each of the above four principles of spiritual well-being. Thus, knowing what we are going toward might guide one's approach to both religion and spirituality. It seems important not to confuse means and ends. Religion is a means to an end of spiritual well-being. Done well, religion can be a very powerful means to that end. But, losing sight of those end principles, religion not done so well could cause difficulty.

Physician Rachel Naomi Remen, medical director of the Commonweal Cancer Help Program and a member of the Scientific Advisory Board for the Inner Mechanisms of the Healing Response Program for the Institute of Noetic Sciences, says it may be easiest to define the spiritual by defining what it isn't. The spiritual, she says, is not the moral. Nor is it the ethical. The spiritual is also not the psychic, nor is it the religious.

The spiritual, she says, "is inclusive. It is the deepest sense of belonging and participation. We all participate in the spiritual at all times, whether we know it or not. There's no place to go to be separated from the spiritual. . . . The most important thing in defining spirit is the recognition that spirit is an essential need of human nature. There is something in all of us that seeks the spiritual. This yearning varies in strength from person to person but it is always there in everyone. And so healing becomes possible."[117]

Our relationship to spirit, says allergist William L. Mundy, defines our very being:

> *The wonderful organism that we are, comprised of billions of parts, many working together on a similar project within a confine we call an organ, or hundreds of millions of cells all performing a similar function, all working together to make us tick as a human being, can hardly be brought down to a simplistic (or profoundly complicated) system of chemical reactions. We need more than science to explain such divine miracles.*[118]

## ENDNOTES

1. Pioro-Boisset, *Arthritis Care Res* 1996; 9: 15.
2. A. E. Bergin and J. P. Jensen, "Religiosity of psychotherapists: A national survey," *Psychotherapy* 27:(1990) 3–7.
3. CBS News Poll 1998 and Yankelovich Partners U.S. Survey. Reported in C. Wallis, "Faith and Healing," *Time* 6/24/96, 62.
4. D. B. Larson, *The Faith Factor, Volume II: An Annotated Bibliography of Systematic Review and Clinical Research on Spiritual Subjects* (Rockville, MD: National Institute for Healthcare Research, 1993); D. B. Larson and S. S. Larsen, *The Forgotten Factor in Physical and Mental Health, What Does the Research Show?* (Rockville, MD: National Institute for Healthcare Research, 1994); D. A. Matthews and D. B. Larson, *The Faith Factor, Volume III: Enhancing Life Satisfaction* (Rockville, MD: National Institute for Healthcare Research, 1995); A. E. Bergin, "Psychotherapy and Religious Values," *Jl of Consulting and Clin. Psychother* 48:(1980) 95–105; and I. R. Payne, et al., "Review of Religion and Mental Health: Prevention and Enhancement of Psychosocial Functioning." *Prevention in Human Services* 9:(1991) 11–40.
5. J. S. Levin, "How Religion Influences Morbidity and Health: Reflections on Natural History, Salutogenesis and Host Resistance," *Soc Sci Med* 43:(1996) 849–64.
6. "MD's Discover Prayer is Good Medicine," *Alternative Therapies in Clinical Practice* 4, no. 2, 59, 1997.

7. David G. Hamilton, "Believing in Patients' Beliefs: Physician Attunement to the Spiritual Dimension as a Positive Factor in Patient Healing and Health," *American Journal of Hospice and Palliative Care* 15, no. 5, 276–9, September/October 1998.

8. P-J. Charters, "The Religious and Spiritual Needs of Mental Health Clients," *Nursing Standard* 13, no. 26, 34–36, October 1999.

9. United Kingdom Central Council for Nursing, Midwifery, and Health Visiting, *Code of Professional Conduct* (London: UKCC, 1992).

10. George Gallup, quoted at the Harvard Mind/Body Institute Symposium: Spirituality and Healing in Medicine II, December 1996.

11. Hamilton; W. L. Larimore, M. Parker, and M. Crowther, "Should Clinicians Incorporate Positive Spirituality into Their Practices? What Does the Evidence Say?" *Ann Behav Med* 24:(2002) 69–73; and P. S. Mueller, D. J. Plevac, and T. A. Rummans, "Religious Involvement, Spirituality, and Medicine: Implications for Clinical Practice," *Mayo Clin Proc* 76:(2001) 1225–35".

12. Mary Rado Simpson and Marilyn Givens King, "'God Brought All These Churches Together': Issues in Developing Religion-Health Partnerships in an Appalachian Community," *Public Health Nursing* 16, no. 1, 41–49, February 1999.

13. Graves, "The High Priest of Healing."

14. D. B. Larson, J. P. Swyers, and M. E. McCullough, *Scientific Research on Spirituality and Health.* The John Templeton Foundation.

15. Matthews and Larson, *The Faith Factor, Volume III.*

16. M. J. Donahue, "Intrinsic and Extrinsic Religiousness: Review and Meta-analysis," *Jl Personality and Social Psychology* 48:(1985) 400–19.

17. Bernie Siegel, *"How to Live Between Office Visits"* (New York: HarperCollins Publisher, 1993) 13.

18. Marc. I. Barasch, "The Healing Path: A Soul Approach to Illness," *The Psychology of Health, Immunity, and Disease,* vol. B, 10, in Proceedings of the Sixth International Conference of the National Institute for the Clinical Application of Behavioral Medicine.

19. O. Carl Simonton and Reid Henson, *The Healing Journey* (New York: Bantam Books, 1992), 13.

20. R. Banks, "Health and the Spiritual Dimensions: Relationships and Implications for Professional Preparation Programs," *Journal of School Health* 50: 1980, 195–202.

21. Banks.

22. Shakti Gawain, *The Path of Transformation* (Mill Valley, Calif.: Nataraj Publishing, 1993), 77.

23. Pamela G. Reed, "Spirituality and Well-Being in Terminally Ill Hospitalized Adults," *Research in Nursing and Health* 10: 1987, 335–44.

24. Glenn E. Richardson and Melody Powers Noland, "Treating the Spiritual Dimension Through Educational Imagery," *Health Values* 8(6): 1984, 28.

25. Larry S. Chapman, "Developing a Useful Perspective on Spiritual Health: Love, Joy, Peace, and Fulfillment," *American Journal of Health Promotion* (Fall 1987): 12.

26. Chapman, 13.

27. Chapman, 13.

28. Joan Borysenko, "Exploring the Heart of Healing: New Findings on Body-mind and Soul," *The Psychology of Health, Immunity, and Disease,* vol. B, 33, in Proceedings of the Sixth International Conference of the National Institute for the Clinical Application of Behavioral Medicine.

29. Phillip J. Waite, Steven R. Hawks, and Julie A. Gast, "The Correlation Between Spiritual Well-Being and Health Behaviors," *American Journal of Health Promotion* 13, no. 3, 159–62, January/February 1999.

30. Dr. Bruno Cortis, "Spirituality and Medicine," in *Proceedings of the Fourth National Conference on the Psychology of Health, Immunity, and Disease,* published by the National Institute for the Clinical Application of Behavioral Medicine.

31. Paul Pearsall, *Super Joy* (New York: Doubleday, 1988), 1.

32. From "The Spirit of Health," *Advances: Journal of the Institute for the Advancement of Health* 5(4): 1988, 4.

33. Reed.

34. H. G. Koenig, D. O. Moberg, and J. N. Kvale, "Religious Activity and Attitudes of Older Adults in a Geriatric Assessment Clinic," *Journal of the American Geriatric Society* 36(4): 1988, 362–74.

35. K. I. Pargament, *The Psychology of Religion and Coping: Theory, Research and Practice* (New York: Guilford Press, 1997).

36. Larson, Swyers, and McCullough, *Scientific Research,* 59–61.

37. J. Kabat-Zinn, et al., "Effectiveness of a Meditation-based Stress Reduction Program in the Treatment of Anxiety Disorders," *Am J Psychiatry* 149:(1992) 936–43.

38. J. J. Miller, K. Fletcher, and J. Kabat-Zinn, "Three-year Follow-up and Clinical Implications of a Mindfulness-based Stress Reduction Intervention in the Treatment of Anxiety Disorders," *Gen Hosp Psychiatry* 17:(1995) 192–200.

39. A. Castillo-Richmond, *Stroke* 2000; 31(3): 568–73.

40. J. W. Zamarra, et al., "Usefulness of the Transcendental Meditation Program in the Treatment of Patients with Coronary Artery Disease," *Am J Cardiology* 77:(1996) 867–70.

41. Gerald Epstein, "Hebraic Medicine," *Advances: Journal of the Institute of Advancement of Health* 4(1): 1987, 56–66.

42. Pearsall, 215.

43. Epstein, 58.

44. Pearsall, 54.

45. S. O. Kobasa, "How Much Stress Can You Survive?" *American Health* Sept., 1984, 67.

46. Siegel, 130.

47. Siegel, 130.

48. Siegel, 130.

49. Siegel.

50. Siegel.

51. Rick Fields, Rex Weyler, Rick Ingrasci, and Peggy Taylor, *Chop Wood, Carry Water* (Los Angeles, Calif.: Jeremy P. Tarcher, 1984).

52. A. Taylor, *I Fly Out with Bright Feathers: The Quest of a Novice Healer* (London, Fontana/Collins, 1987).

53. Elissa F. Patterson, "The Philosophy and Physics of Holistic Health Care: Spiritual Healing as a Workable Interpretation," *Journal of Advanced Nursing* 27, no. 2, 287–93, 1998.

54. Robert Coles, "The Power of Prayer," *50 Plus* (December 1987): 44.

55. Blair Justice, *Who Gets Sick: Thinking and Health* (Houston, Tex.: Peak Press, 1987), 275.

56. H. G. Koenig, et al., *Jl Gerontology* June 2000.

57. CBS News Poll 1998.

58. Larry Dossey, *Healing Words* (San Francisco: HarperSan Francisco, 1993), 31.

59. Larry Dossey; "Evidence of Prayer's Healing Power," *Brain/Mind* (December 1993): 4–5.
60. Rupert Sheldrake, "Prayer: A Challenge for Science," *Noetic Sciences Review* (Summer 1994): 5.
61. Herbert Benson, *Your Maximum Mind* (New York: Times Books/Random House, 1987), 6.
62. Benson, 46.
63. Gurney Williams III, "Holy-istic Healing," *Longevity* (March 1994): 28.
64. *Journal of Psychology and Theology* 19: 71–73.
65. "Does Prayer Help Patients?" 35.
66. R. B. Byrd, "Positive Therapeutic Effects of Intercessory Prayer in a Coronary Care Unit Population," *Southern Med Jl* 81:(1988) 826–29.
67. J. M. Aviles, et al., "Intercessory Prayer and Cardiovascular Progression in a Coronary Care Unit Population: A Randomized Controlled Trial," *Mayo Clin Proc* 76:(2001) 1192–98
68. A. M. McCaffrey, et al., "Prayer for Health Concerns: Results at a National Survey on Prevalence and Patterns of Use," *Arch. Int. Med* 164:(2004) 858–62.
69. Joan Borysenko, *Minding the Body, Mending the Mind* (Reading, Mass.: Addison-Wesley Publishing Company, 1987), 176.
70. Robin Casarjian, "Forgiveness: An Essential Component in Health and Healing," in *Proceedings of the Fourth National Conference on the Psychology of Health, Immunity, and Disease,* published by the National Institute for the Clinical Application of Behavioral Medicine.
71. Dan Custer, *The Miracle of Mind Power* (Englewood Cliffs, N.J.: Prentice Hall, 1960).
72. Custer.
73. Casarjian.
74. Custer.
75. Dwight Lee Wolter, *Lotus* (Spring 1994): 53.
76. Robin Casarjian, *Forgiveness: A Bold Choice for a Peaceful Heart* (New York: Bantam Books, 1992), 232–33.
77. Harold G. Koenig, James N. Kvale, and Carolyn Ferrel, "Religion and Well-Being in Later Life," *The Gerontologist* 28(1): 1988, 18–27.
78. Harvard Medical School and New England Deaconess Hospital, Proceedings of "Advances in Behavioral Medicine: Clinical Practices and Research," February 28–March 3, 1989.
79. Christopher G. Ellison, "Religious Involvement and Subjective Well-Being," *Journal of Health and Social Behavior* 32:(1991) 80–99.
80. Christopher G. Ellison and Jeffrey S. Levin, "The Religion-Health Connection: Evidence, Theory, and Future Directions," *Health Education and Behavior* 25, no. 6, 700–20, December 1998.
81. J. S. Levin and P. L. Schiller, "Is There a Religious Factor in Health?" *Journal of Religion and Health* 26, 9–36, 1987.
82. William W. Parmley, "Separation of Church and State (of Health)," *Journal of American College of Cardiology* 28, no. 4, 1047–48, October 1996.
83. Parmley.
84. W. J. Strawbridge, R. D. Cohen, S. J. Shema, and G. A. Kaplan, "Frequent Attendance at Religious Services and Mortality over 28 Years," *American Journal of Public Health* 87, 957–61, 1997.
85. Neal Krause, "Religion, Aging, and Health: Current Status and Future Prospects," *Journal of Gerontology* 52B, no. 6, S291–S293, 1997.

86. E. L. Idler and S. V. Kasl, "Religion, Disability, Depression, and the Timing of Death," *American Journal of Sociology* 97, 1052–79, 1992.

87. Matthews and Larson, *The Faith Factor, Volume III.*

88. H. G. Koenig and D. B. Larson, "Use of Hospital Services, Religious Attendance and Religious Affiliation."

89. "Religion Aids Coping with Illness," *Mental Medicine Update* (Spring 1993): 2.

90. "Religion as a Variable in Psychiatric Studies," *Behavior Today,* February 27, 1989, 6.

91. H. B. Bosworth, et al., "The Impact of Religious Practice and Religious Coping on Geriatric Depression," *Int Jl Geriatr Psychiatry* 18:(2003) 905–14.

92. "The Empty Church Syndrome," *Psychology Today,* November 1988.

93. Andrew J. Weaver, Laura T. Flannelly, Kevin J. Flannelly, Harold G. Koenig, and David B. Larson, "An Analysis of Research on Religious and Spiritual Variables in Three Major Mental Health Nursing Journals, 1991–1995," *Issues in Mental Health Nursing* 19, no. 3, 263–76, May–June 1998.

94. G. H. Gallup, *Religion in America: 1992–1993* (Princeton, N.J.: Gallup Organization, 1993).

95. "The Empty Church Syndrome."

96. Leonard A. Sagan, *The Health of Nations* (New York: Basic Books, 1987), 137.

97. "Faith Vital to Seniors' Well-Being," *Brain/Mind and Common Sense, American Journal of Sociology,* 97: 1052–79.

98. John M. Wallace, Jr. and Tyrone A. Forman, "Religion's Role in Promoting Health and Reducing Risk Among American Youth," *Health Education and Behavior* 25, no. 6, 721–41, December 1998.

99. G. H. Gallup, Jr. and R. Bezilla, *The Religious Life of Young Americans* (Princeton, N.J.: George H. Gallup International Institute, 1992).

100. Stuart R. Varon and Anne W. Riley, "Relationship Between Maternal Church Attendance and Adolescent Mental Health and Social Functioning," *Psychiatric Services* 50, 799–805, 1999.

101. Michael Argyle, *The Psychology of Happiness* (London: Methuen and Company, 1987), 196.

102. Argyle.

103. Laurel Arthur Burton and Jarad D. Kass, "How to Make the Best Use of a Patient's Spirituality," in *Proceedings of the Fourth National Conference on the Psychology of Health, Immunity, and Disease,* published by the National Institute for the Clinical Application of a Behavioral Medicine.

104. Mark Bricklin, Mark Golin, Deborah Grandinetti, and Alexis Lieberman, *Positive Living and Health* (Emmaus, Pa.: Rodale Press, 1990).

105. George K. Jarvis and Herbert C. Northcott, "Religion and Differences in Morbidity and Mortality," *Social Science Medicine* 25(7): 1987, 813–24.

106. Jarvis and Northcott.

107. Jarvis and Northcott.

108. Bricklin et al.

109. Brent Q. Hafen and Kathryn J. Frandsen, *People Need People: The Importance of Relationships to Health and Wellness* (Evergreen, Colo.: Cordillera Press, 1987) 25.

110. Sagan, 137–38.

111. S. I. McMillen, *None of These Diseases* (Old Tappan, N.J.: Fleming H. Revell Company, 1984), 208.

112. John Gartner, Dave Larson, and George Allen, *Journal of Psychology and Theology,* 19: 6–25.

113.  Jeffrey S. Levin and Preston L. Schiller, "Is There a Religious Factor in Health?" *Journal of Religion and Health* 26(1): 1987.

114.  Levin and Schiller.

115.  Jeffrey S. Levin and Harold Y. Vanderpool, "Is Frequent Religious Attendance Really Conducive to Better Health?: Toward an Epidemiology of Religion," *Social Science Medicine* 24(7): 1987, 589–600.

116.  N. L. Smith, "Healing as the Masters Healed," *Jl Collegium Aesculapium* 1988 (Winter):17–27; presented at the Harvard Conference on Spirituality in Medicine, March 14, 2002, and also at the Psychiatry Grand Rounds University of Maine, September 23, 2003, and University of Utah, November 6, 2002.

117.  Rachel Naomi Remen, "On Defining Spirit," *Noetic Sciences Review* (Autumn 1988): 7.

118.  William L. Mundy, "Curing Allergy with Visual Imagery," *The Psychology of Health, Immunity, and Disease*, vol. A, 437, in *Proceedings of the Sixth International Conference of the National Institute for the Clinical Application of Behavioral Medicine*.

CHAPTER *15*

# *The Healing Power of Altruism*

*I don't know what your destiny will be, but one thing I know:
the only ones among you who will be truly happy are those
who will have sought and found how to serve.*

—Albert Schweitzer

## Learning Objectives

- Define altruism and identify the aspect of altruism that may help protect health.
- Discuss how altruism boosts health.
- Identify the characteristics of the altruistic personality.
- Discuss the health benefits of volunteerism and the characteristics of volunteer work that are most beneficial to health.
- Understand how love contributes to well-being and longevity.

**P**hysician and philosopher Albert Schweitzer proclaimed during a selfless career what he believed to be the prescription for happiness. True happiness, he said, is to be found only by serving others. New clinical research has verified that service not only is a prescription for happiness but is a prescription for improved health as well. As German-born physicist and Nobel Prize winner Albert Einstein said, "Only a life lived for others is worth living."

Altruism—the act of giving of oneself out of a genuine concern for other people—has been called one of the healthiest of human attributes. Albert Einstein said, "Many times a day I realize how much my own outer and inner life is built upon the labors of my fellow men, both living and dead, and how earnestly I must exert myself in order to give in return as much as I have received."

A recent Gallup Poll shows that Americans contribute more than $104 billion per year to good causes. The value of our volunteer time equates to an additional $150 billion each year. According to studies, altruism is one of the biggest sources of revenue for the U.S. gross national product.[1]

The ability to "connect" by regarding another's needs as above one's own appears to contribute to a longer and healthier life. Scientists are beginning to conclude that doing good for others is good for a person—especially for the nervous system and the immune system. The effects of genuine altruism may be so powerful that even thinking about altruistic action may give your immune system a boost.[2]

Harvard psychologists who wanted to find out how altruistic thoughts impact us conducted a precise experiment on a group of volunteers; the accurate measure was the amount of germ-fighting substance in the saliva of the volunteers. The amount of the substance provides a clear indication of how well the immune system is working. Psychologists measured the saliva of the volunteers both before and after they watched each of three films. The first was a gentle film on gardening, the second was a Nazi war documentary, and the third was a documentary about Mother Teresa, the Nobel Prize–winning nun who has dedicated charitable works to the poor, the lepers, and the orphans in India's most poverty-stricken regions.

Measurements of saliva showed no change during the first two films. After reviewing the third film, the amount of immune agent in the volunteers' saliva rose sharply, even among those who said they dislike Mother Teresa. Volunteers who merely watched altruistic service experienced an actual physical change—one that could possibly help them stay healthier.[3]

Altruism may actually be one of our earliest skills. Bowling Green State University psychologist Jaak Panksepp believes that helping had an integral part in our biological evolution because it's necessary for reproduction and the survival of certain species. In the evolution of the human species, cooperative efforts may have been not only helpful to survival but also, says Panksepp, a key factor in the development and expansion of the human brain. "Intrinsic helping tendencies may thus, like dominance urges, be embedded in the human brain structure," he theorizes, or "may even be part of what we think of as human nature itself."[4]

## How Altruism Boosts Health

While researchers know that altruism promotes health, they are just beginning to find out how and why. In addition to the direct link to the immune system, it may counteract stress. Canadian physician Hans Selye, one of the world's authorities on the physiological effects of stress, concluded that altruism can help combat the effects of stress by preventing nervous system "overload." By doing good deeds for others, Selye believed, a person wins their affection and gratitude—and the resulting "warmth" helps protect the person from stress.[5]

There may even be a physiological reason for that "warmth": Varied research has shown that altruistic action stimulates the brain to release endorphins, powerful natural painkillers that literally make us feel better. Those endorphins may also be a key to relieving the effects of stress.

Allan Luks, executive director of the Institute for the Advancement of Health in New York City, shares the view that altruistic deeds help relieve stress. He says that "people who help others frequently report better health than people who don't help. They relate an improved sense of well-being, and decreased problems with stress-related health conditions."[6]

We know that the cumulative effects of stress are negative. Kenneth R. Pelletier, associate clinical professor at the University of California School of Medicine, says, "Under conditions of extreme stress, the immune system is depressed. The number and activity of white cells falls. The activity of the natural killer cells is reduced. There are changes in the ratio of helper cells to suppressor cells of the immune system."[7]

New evidence shows that the cumulative effects of altruism, of giving a helping hand and reaching out to others, are positive. Although stress can compromise the immune system, positive emotions related to altruism—emotions like love and compassion—help stabilize the immune system against the normal immunosuppressing effects of stress. That effect may go so far, Pelletier believes, that altruism may even help slow down the inevitable deterioration of the immune system as a person ages.[8] And, because of the social contact and sense of purpose associated with altruism, good deeds may help prevent some stress to begin with.

In his landmark book, *The Broken Heart: The Medical Consequences of Loneliness,* University of Maryland School of Medicine researcher James Lynch says, "The mandate to 'Love your neighbor as you love yourself' is not just a moral mandate. It's a physiological mandate. Caring is biological. One thing you get from caring for others is you're not lonely. And the more connected you are to life, the healthier you are."[9]

Some specialists believe that altruism actually helps to preserve life—and a few believe that it is even part of the survival instinct. When University of California, Los Angeles, sociologist Linda Nilson studied data from more than 100 disasters, she found that those who survived and did the best were those who reached out to help others. The "tribal cohesiveness" that stemmed from the helping process, says Nilson, is what enabled many to survive even tremendous odds.

Epidemiologist James House and his colleagues at the University of Michigan's Survey Research Center carried out a landmark study of 2,700 people in Tecumseh, Michigan. The study period spanned more than a decade as House and his coworkers followed the volunteers carefully to determine what impact their social relationships had on their health. What

House discovered was a powerful testimony for altruism. Among the people studied in Michigan, those who did regular volunteer work had better health and longer lives. House concluded that doing volunteer work, more than any other activity, dramatically increased life expectancy—and probably health as well.[10] Among the Michigan residents studied, the men who did no volunteer work were two and a half times as likely to die during the study as men who volunteered at least once a week.

Other studies confirm House's findings. Psychiatrist George Vaillant followed Harvard graduates for four decades. He found that altruism was one of the major qualities that helped the graduates cope with the stresses of life. The absence of altruism apparently has the opposite effect. After an in-depth study, social psychologist Larry Scherwitz of San Francisco's Medical Research Institute concluded that people who are self-centered are more likely to develop coronary heart disease, even when other risk factors are taken into account.

The factor of self-centered thoughts and behavior can in itself contribute to the stress that may lead to disease. Dean Ornish, director of California's Preventive Medicine Research Institute, says, "When a person has a sense of isolation, often what comes with that are feelings of not having enough or not being enough. The person says, 'if only I had more'—more power, more money, more love, whatever—'then I'd be happy.' Once that view of the world is set up, it's ultimately self-defeating because if people don't get more of it, whatever it is, they feel stress. And even when they do, it's never enough."[11]

Altruism and its associated good deeds, says Ornish, help free us from "the stress cycle" by turning our focus away from self-involvement and toward those we are helping.[12] Once our involvement is focused on others, we begin to show the qualities consistent with altruism: a high degree of optimism, a strong sense of purpose and spirituality, and a continued involvement with other people.

Even the way we talk reflects how we feel about others—and possibly how healthy we are. In interviews, people with the least evidence of altruism were those who referred to themselves with the pronouns *I, me,* and *my* most often—and they were also the ones most likely to develop coronary artery disease.

A group of studies done on altruism found that people who care for others are physically, emotionally, and mentally healthier than those who concentrate more on their own needs. It can even boost the ability to learn. College students who volunteered in a Head Start–based Family Literacy Project in Connecticut were studied to determine the impact of their volunteerism. Researchers found that those students who engaged in regular volunteer work had greater self-knowledge, had greater social awareness, and performed better in academics. They also did better in the areas of personal growth, self-esteem, and personal efficacy. The students themselves reported finding more meaning in what was learned in the classroom, increased awareness of important social issues, greater appreciation for diversity, and decreased negative stereotypes.[13]

Many researchers believe that altruism is an inborn characteristic intended to help boost health and longevity. One of them, bioethics researcher Willard Gaylin, says, "We are born with a natural caring tendency. I don't think it's so rare. We take care of infants who certainly do nothing to deserve it. They're not attractive. They wake you in the middle of the night. They urinate on you. They vomit on you. And yet we love them and care for them."

People who care for others also tend to have an important health-preserving quality: optimism. Psychologist Martin Seligman, author of *Learned Optimism,* says that altruism is an activity "that presupposes a belief that things can change for the better." Optimists, he maintains, "have better health, better immune systems, and so live longer. Indirect evidence would then indicate that altruists might live longer."[14] For more on optimism and health, see Chapter 17.

One of the most profound examples of the health and longevity benefits of altruism comes from the life of philanthropist John D. Rockefeller, Sr.[15] Rockefeller entered the business world with gusto and drove himself so hard that by age thirty-three he had earned his first million dollars. Ten years later he owned and controlled the world's largest business. By the time he was fifty-three, he was the world's first billionaire.

Meanwhile, the people he had crushed in this pursuit of wealth hated him; workers in Pennsylvania's oil fields hanged him in effigy, and he was guarded day and night by bodyguards pledged to protect his life. He had developed alopecia, a condition in which hair falls out; his digestion was so poor that all he could eat was crackers and milk. He was plagued by insomnia. The doctors who struggled to help him agreed that he wouldn't live another year.

Then something happened to John D. Rockefeller. He began to think of—and care about—others more than he did himself. He decided to use his billions of dollars for the benefit of others. Hospitals, universities, missions, and private citizens were the beneficiaries of the hundreds of millions of dollars he gave through the Rockefeller Foundation. His generosity aided in the discovery of penicillin. His contributions to medicine enabled researchers to find cures for tuberculosis, malaria, diphtheria, and many other diseases that had robbed so many of life. His contributions helped rid the U.S. South of its greatest physical and economic plague, the hookworm.

When Rockefeller began using his riches to help other people, he helped himself. For the first time in years, he was able to eat normally. He felt renewed. He slept soundly. He defied the odds and lived to see his fifty-fourth birthday—and many birthdays after that. He kept on giving and caring for others, in fact, until he died at the age of ninety-eight.

## The Altruistic Personality

What makes a person altruistic? Some believe it's instinct, stemming from the time when people lived in small groups of hunters and gatherers. According to Stanford anthropologist John Tooby, those early hunters/gatherers depended highly on each other, not only for food and shelter, but also for survival.[16]

In a supporting point of view, New York psychologist Linda R. Caporall cites a series of experiments conducted over ten years and reported in *Behavioral and Brain Sciences*. The studies show that human nature is basically social, not selfish—and she agrees that altruism probably stems back to hunter/gatherer times.[17]

A growing number of researchers believe that altruism is a capacity shared by everyone to some extent or another. Altruism can be learned, say the researchers, depending on social and cultural background, the stage of moral or self-development, previous opportunities to learn altruism, the sense of responsibility and empathy, and the particular situation in which one is called upon to help.[18]

Other researchers believe in a certain "personality"—that altruistic people seem to have a set of personality traits enabling them to reach out to others. In a classic study of altruism, Samuel P. Oliner and Pearl M. Oliner studied the "rescuers" who provided help to the Jews during Hitler's reign of terror. These rescuers were altruistic—so much so that they often risked their own lives and safety to help others. According to Oliner, altruism is fueled by "empathy, allegiance to their group or institutional norms, or commitment to principle."[19] University of California, Irvine, Professor Kristen Monroe says that research shows altruists tend to view themselves as one with all of humanity rather than acting only in their own behalf.[20]

The Oliners say altruistic people never regard others as inferiors; they have a firm conviction that all people have universal similarities.[21] One rescuer summarized the attitude by remarking that "Jews were just people. We neither looked down on them nor did we look up to them. We never felt they were any different."

The altruistic people the Oliners studied valued human relationships more than money, and focused on others rather than on themselves. They believed that ethical values were to be applied universally—that people are worthy of tolerance and respect regardless of their race, religion, or class. They emphasized the values of helpfulness, hospitality, concern, and love, and they sensed a universal obligation to be of help to others. Their commitment to caring for others extended well beyond their friends and loved ones.

The "rescuers" believed in the right of innocent people to be free from persecution—and most were moved by the pain of others. They also had a tendency to believe in a victim's innocence, to believe that people are victimized by external circumstances and not by inherent character flaws. With deep empathy for the sadness and helplessness of others, these rescuers felt a personal responsibility for helping to relieve others' pain and sadness.

That empathy may have been one of their most important emotions. Considerable evidence, both anecdotal and that based on scientific experiments, suggests that empathy somehow connects people. It forms a literal bond, acting almost as a "glue" between living things. We know it works between people, and even between people and animals. Now researchers at Princeton University's Engineering Anomalies Research Laboratory have proved that it even works to connect people and machines. According to Larry Dossey, studies show that "the effects of empathic bonding transcend space and time."[22]

These altruistic people had a healthy perspective about themselves. They did not suffer from self-interest or self-preoccupation, both of which reduce the ability to care for others. They did not think too highly of themselves (people with too much self-esteem believe they should be the recipients, not the bestowers, of attention and care). Nor did they think too poorly of themselves (people with too little self-esteem become so absorbed by their own distress that they can't worry about other people's needs). Most were highly independent of the opinions and evaluations of others; they tended to act on their own and did not seek or need external reinforcement for their activities. Actually, most were embarrassed by the thanks or appreciation they received.

The altruistic people the Oliners studied were very "connected" to others, especially to diverse people and groups. They enjoyed close family relationships and had a strong sense of belonging to the community. Their attachment to others began early in life and extended beyond family to embrace friends, acquaintances, and even strangers. The rescuers had a tendency to befriend people who were different from themselves. They perceived their relationships with their family of origin as being very close.

Their commitment to caring was profound—and their internal compulsion was so strong that they often made the decision to help almost instantaneously. They felt a strong sense of inner control, but did not feel the need to control others; although they believed they could control events and shape their own destiny, they were also willing to risk failure. When something didn't go as planned, they spent little time mourning those failures.

Most important, they believed they could succeed when others were convinced of failure.

To these rescuers, caring was not a spectator sport—it compelled action. They assumed personal responsibility not because others required it, but because they would have been unhappy if they had failed to act. Although they placed a value on hard work and economic prudence, they never expected a monetary reward for their altruistic actions. They performed those deeds without ulterior motives. The Oliners summed up the rescuers in their study as "not saints, but ordinary people who nonetheless were capable of overcoming their human frailties by virtue of their caring capacities."

The personality traits the Oliners observed among the rescuers are not peculiar to that group of people; the traits, researchers believe, are common among most altruistic people. Nor does altruism necessarily stem from a church or a religious belief; repeated research shows that church members are no more altruistic as a group than are other people.[23] University of Massachusetts psychologist Ervin Staub believes that altruistic people share three general traits:

1. They have a positive view of people in general.

2. They are concerned about others' welfare.

3. They take personal responsibility for how other people are doing.[24]

The tendency toward altruism is a trait that is established early in life, according to a number of researchers. Psychologist Alfie Kohn noted that altruism may be as dramatic as donating a kidney, or as "mundane as letting another shopper ahead of you in line. But most of us do it frequently and started doing it very early in life. . . . Caring about others is as much a part of human nature as caring about ourselves."[25]

In studying outstanding altruists, researcher Christie Kiefer found that background and family values help determine the altruistic personality. The altruists she studied "came from families that were warm and nurturing. The emotional self-acceptance they developed in that environment liberated them to be generative, creative, playful, and relaxed." In addition, says Kiefer, they learned a sense of social responsibility from their parents or from another prominent person in their early lives—a sense that "committed them to action on behalf of others or their community."[26]

In their book, *The Altruistic Personality*, the Oliners cited the important lesson all of us can learn from the "rescuers":

> *Rescuers point the way. They were and are "ordinary" people. They were farmers and teachers, entrepreneurs and factory workers, rich and poor, parents and single people, Protestants and Catholics. Most had done nothing extraordinary*

*before the war nor have they done much that is extraordinary since. Most were marked neither by exceptional leadership qualities nor by unconventional behavior. They were not heroes cast in larger-than-life molds. What most distinguished them were their connections with others in relationships of commitment and care. It is out of such relationships that they became aware of what was occurring around them and mustered their human and material sources to relieve the pain. Their involvements with Jews grew out of the ways in which they ordinarily related to other people. . . .*

*They remind us that such courage is not the providence of the independent and the intellectually superior thinkers but that it is available to all through the virtues of connectedness, commitment, and the quality of relationships developed in ordinary human interactions.*[27]

## The Health Benefits of Volunteerism

A recent Gallup survey revealed that 52 percent of all American adults and 53 percent of all American teenagers are involved in some kind of volunteer work. Many do it without organizational support. On their own, they figure out ways to help those who need it or those who are less fortunate. When asked why, two-thirds say it is because they want to "help people." That instinct to help occurs early in life; as early as the second year of life, a child will respond to someone in distress by reaching out with a comforting touch, offering a favorite toy, or bringing a parent to help.

People who volunteer, help, and care for others benefit more than the recipients of the help. The acts of volunteering, helping, and serving appear to bring important health benefits to the volunteer. Examples abound. Consider the Retired Senior Volunteer Program, which places a quarter of a million elderly people in community volunteer jobs each year. National Director Alfred N. Larson recognizes the health benefits those seniors have, saying, "Doctors tell us that elderly people who engage in volunteer work are a lot better off, visit the doctor less often, and have fewer complaints."[28] A study of 2,700 residents of Tecumseh, Michigan, showed that men who volunteer for community organizations are two and a half times less likely to die from all causes of disease than those who don't get involved in volunteer work.[29]

One elderly volunteer in Baltimore explained, "Involvement makes you keep well so you can keep giving. It makes you take care of your health. It's a blessing to ward off old age."

The health benefits aren't restricted to consciously taking better care of health, however. Yale University Professor of Public Health Lowell Levin points out that "when you're a helper, your self-concept improves. You are somebody. You are worthwhile. And there's nothing more exhilarating than that. That can influence your health." Consider these examples:

- Kay Arnold joined SENSE, a group of Connecticut entertainers who perform for the elderly and disabled. Her audiences benefit—and Kay herself says her volunteer work gives her "a sense of worth I never had before." And when she performs, her arthritis pain disappears.

- Vince Ward is advertising and public relations director for one of the nation's largest telecommunications firms. His job is considered one of the highest-stress positions imaginable, yet he does not have high blood pressure. How has he been able to overcome one of the most common physiological effects of stress? The key could lie in the way he spends his spare time. Vince Ward is busy away from the office, too, raising money for a children's home, working with parolees from Kansas State Penitentiary, and donating blood to the Community Blood Bank of Greater Kansas City.

- In one study, the experiences of more than 1,700 women who regularly volunteered to help others were analyzed at the Institute for the Advancement of Health in New York City. The women who helped experienced relief of actual physical ailments, including headaches, loss of voice, pain due to lupus and multiple sclerosis, and depression. Approximately 90 percent of the women in the survey rated their health as better than or as good as others their age.[30]

Women in two major studies about volunteerism described a "helper's high," similar in nature to the "runner's high" experienced during exercising.[31] Research at Carnegie Mellon University shows that volunteerism helps improve mood and gives a "high." Scientists studying the phenomenon believe the act of volunteering, of serving and helping others, may cause the release of endorphins. One researcher who has been studying the effects of altruism in animal studies concludes that it is "just about proven that it is our own natural opiates, the endorphins, that produce the good feelings" associated with reaching out to help others.[32]

Deeper insight about the "high" experienced by volunteers stemmed in part from a study conducted by Allan Luks, then at the Institute for the Advancement of Health, and psychologist Howard Andrews, a senior research scientist with the New York State Psychiatric Institute. What did they learn? After collecting surveys from more than 3,000 volunteers, they found twofold health benefits from volunteer work. The "healthy-helper syndrome," as they call it, starts with a physical high—a "rush" of good feeling that is characterized by increased energy, sudden warmth, and a sense of euphoria. The physical sensations associated with the "helper's high"—

which 95 percent of the people surveyed experienced—suggest that the brain releases endorphins in response to the act of helping.

The second stage of the healthy-helper syndrome—which more than half of the volunteers reported—is a longer lasting sense of calm and heightened emotional well-being. Together, say Luks and Andrews, the "high" associated with volunteering is a powerful antidote to stress, a key to happiness and optimism (see Chapter 17), and a way to combat feelings of helplessness and depression.[33]

A national survey that led to the definition of the healthy-helper syndrome definitely delineated the two distinct phases—one an "immediate physical feel-good sensation," the second a sense of calmness and relaxation. According to Luks, the survey showed that those who volunteer have better perceived health, and that the more often they volunteer, the greater the health benefits. Luks says those who volunteered once a week reported ten times better health and had specific improvements in health that ranged from less pain and fewer colds to overall well-being.[34]

Famed Harvard cardiologist Herbert Benson, well-known for his research on the effects of relaxation, feels that helping others works much the same way as yoga, spirituality, and meditation to help people "forget oneself, to experience decreased metabolic rates and blood pressure, heart rate, and other health benefits."[35] Volunteer service can result in a condition sometimes described as "helper's calm" or helper's high. Under stress, the heart pumps faster, the adrenal glands release corticosteroids (the "stress hormones"), organ functions are disrupted, and breathing speeds up. As a result, the person is more sensitive to pain, and the stress hormones that start coursing through the veins raise the level of blood cholesterol, elevate blood sugar, and reduce functioning of the immune system.

Apparently volunteer service works in the opposite way, reducing the effects of stress.[36] It works so well, in fact, that people in various studies have reported "treating" their stress-induced illnesses by engaging in altruistic volunteer work.

According to Luks and Howard, the volunteers who experienced the healthy-helper syndrome noticed an improvement in their own physical ills, including fewer arthritis pains, lupus symptoms, asthma attacks, migraine headaches, colds, and bouts of flu. The researchers believe that volunteerism, or altruism, can also alleviate the stress and other physiological conditions that lead to heart attacks.

Luks and Howard credit a combination of factors for the improved health of volunteers: "the strengthening of immune system activity; the diminishing of both the intensity and awareness of physical pain; the activation of emotions vital to the maintenance of good health; the reduction of the incidence of attitudes, such as chronic hostility, that negatively arouse and damage the body; and the multiple benefits to the body's systems provided by stress relief."[37]

## One-on-One Contact

The benefits of volunteer work depend on several factors. According to Allan Luks and Peggy Payne, the most health benefits from volunteering occur when you make personal contact, do it frequently (two or more hours a week), help a stranger, find a shared problem, work with an organization, use your skills, and "let go" of results.[38]

Of those, one of the most important is one-on-one contact—that the helper actually connect with people. The health benefits of volunteer work don't seem as pronounced when the volunteer simply donates money (no matter how important the cause) or spends volunteer time doing things isolated from close physical contact.[39] The physical contact seems to be a key. It is vital to good health and longevity.

In their book *The Healing Brain*, physician David Sobel and psychologist Robert Ornstein argue that the brain's major function is not logical thought, but protection of the body from illness. And, they say, the brain "cannot do its job of protecting the body without contact with other people. It draws vital nourishment from our friends, lovers, relatives, lodge brothers and sisters, even perhaps our coworkers and the members of our weekly bowling team."[40]

The direct contact involved in volunteer work seems to provide some of its value, but the direct contact apparently doesn't have to be physical, as long as it's one-on-one. In various studies, people who have done one-on-one crisis counseling or intervention by telephone have experienced and reported helper's high, whereas those doing nonpeople tasks, such as stuffing envelopes, don't experience the "high."

And helper's high results most from helping people we don't know: The greatest chance of experiencing helper's high in several experiments was correlated with giving service to strangers.[41]

## Desire to Volunteer

In addition to actual contact with the people one is helping, another important factor in achieving the health benefits of volunteer work seems to hinge on the word *volunteer:* A person has to want to do it. Forcing a person to be of help doesn't reap the health benefits of the helping service. In fact, some researchers now believe that one reason why altruism benefits health is that it gives one a sense of control—but only by being able to choose the circumstances of the altruistic deeds.

That sense of control may even be crucial. A number of studies have shown that a lack of control can undermine health (as discussed elsewhere in this book). One landmark project carried out in a housing project for the elderly in San Francisco underscores the health benefits that follow the sense of control that volunteer work brings.

Meredith Minkler, cofounder of the project and a professor at the University of California's School of Public Health, reports that isolated elderly people living in single-room-occupancy hotels were brought together as volunteers to improve the neighborhoods where they were living. Together, they established minimarkets in the hotels in which they lived, brought down the crime rate, and brought about a number of other improvements. Meanwhile, their health improved. Their sense of well-being increased. Some even recovered from serious illnesses, and one ignored a doctor's "death sentence," living several years longer than had been predicted.[42]

## Liking the Work

Another factor in reaping health benefits from volunteer work is to choose work a person likes to do—something that is suitable, brings pleasure, and is a joy to do. If volunteer work does not bring happiness or even make a person feel slightly exhilarated, he or she should probably consider switching to another project or type of work.

## Consistency

Consistency seems important, too. Although an occasional good deed is certainly appreciated by the recipient, it doesn't seem to carry the same health benefits to the bestower as regular altruistic acts or consistent volunteer work. In studies of altruism and volunteerism, the greatest health benefits have been reaped by those who do consistent, regular volunteer work—at least once a week.[43]

## Motive

Will you get the good-health benefits of volunteer work if you embark on a project out of selfish motives to improve your own health? Some say you can. Luks, who has been involved in studying the benefits of altruism, points out that "people help for all sorts of reasons: empathy for the homeless; peer pressure from a neighbor; guilt over some problem; or pressure from church or community. But it doesn't seem to matter. If they continue with the helping, most likely, they'll get the feel-good sensation."[44]

Research shows that people may not fare as well if they expect repayment for their altruism or if they expect something in return. If repayment is expected but withheld, the helper does not gain the emotional benefits from helping, says Carnegie Mellon University researcher Gail Williamson.[45]

The "repayment" expected by some volunteers varies tremendously, too; some expect monetary reward, whereas others hope for payment in terms of increased status.[46]

Volunteer work has several unique aspects that could make the health benefits even greater. First, good feelings—and, almost certainly, health benefits—last far beyond the altruistic act itself. People in one study described more than one positive benefit associated with helping; 95 percent felt good while helping, and almost 80 percent said that the good feelings kept recurring long after the helping activity had ended.[47]

Participants in studies say they can recapture the helper's high, although sometimes not as intensely, by merely remembering or thinking about their charitable acts. For those participants, the health benefits of helping—fewer aches and pains, relief of depression, strength, energy, and increased self-worth—kept returning when they remembered the altruistic deeds. In fact, more than 80 percent could recapture the physical benefits just by thinking about their volunteer work.[48]

For the best health benefits from volunteering, researchers advise avoiding "unhelpful helping"—a style of volunteerism that causes the person being helped to actually become progressively more helpless and to eventually lose skills. To avoid that kind of helping, David Sobel offers these suggestions:

- Try to empower the person you're helping; you need to help that person gain as much control over his or her own life as possible.

- Encourage independence.

- As much as you can, allow the other person to make decisions.

- Give the other person clear responsibilities whenever possible—even for things you know you could do better or faster.

- Break down complicated tasks into small, easy steps.

- Allow mistakes and reward efforts, even if the results fall short of what you expected or what you know is possible.

- Limit your availability; the person you are helping should be increasingly independent. If you are always there, you stifle independence instead.

- Don't shield the person from all bad news or all problems; allow the person to appropriately express disappointment, anger, or sadness.[49]

And, because volunteering can become very demanding, Sobel advises that you avoid burnout by doing the following:

- First, monitor yourself and watch for the signs of burnout. You're probably getting burned out if you feel overwhelmed, helpless, out of control, resentful, guilty, or stressed.

- Pay attention to your own needs; if your own bucket is empty, you won't have anything to share with someone else.

- Recognize your limits. It would be nice to help at the homeless shelter every night, but that's just not realistic for most people. Or you might have a difficult time volunteering at a center for abused children if you were abused and have not dealt with those issues in your own life.

- Get help if you need it.

- Pace yourself; go only as fast as you comfortably can. Take what you can handle, and pass on what will overwhelm you.

- Don't get discouraged; if things don't work out with a certain situation, find another helping situation that's better for you. You might feel overwhelmed in a situation where you're expected to help a gang member rehabilitate—try helping an elderly person learn to read instead.

- Cancel any guilt trips you're considering.

- Finally, give yourself a pat on the back. You deserve it![50]

## Love: The Emotion Behind It

In essence, the health benefits of altruism and volunteer service may depend on the driving emotion behind it all—love, a projection of one's own good feelings onto other people. True love for others is a reflection of love of oneself,[51] a willingness to project warmth and affectionate concern. The love that brings health benefits goes beyond romantic love and kinship ties to include feelings of friendship, compassion, respect, admiration, and gratitude for others. True love, too, is a verb—an action word that calls on us to demonstrate and apply our good feelings through specific actions or deeds.

After a careful analysis of thousands of his patients, psychiatrist Alfred Adler wrote, "The most important task imposed by religion has always been, 'Love thy neighbor. . . .' It is the individual who is not interested in his fellow man who has the greatest difficulties in life and provides the greatest injury to others. It is from such individuals that all human failures spring."[52]

According to researchers who have studied the effects of love, a truly loving relationship—one of acceptance and safety—is earmarked by freedom from expectations and demands. And when that kind of relationship exists, they say, love and health go hand in hand.

Some even believe that love is an important key in the healing process. People who become more loving and less fearful, who replace negative thoughts with the emotion of love, are often able to achieve physical healing.

Most of us are familiar with the emotional effects of love, the way love makes us feel inside. But it doesn't stop there. True love—a love that is patient, trusting, protecting, optimistic, and kind—has actual physical effects on the body, too.

Bernie S. Siegel, prominent Yale surgeon and oncologist, claims that love and support, whether from an individual or a group, is an important facet of all healing. Its importance is so marked that even outsiders who observe the loving process can see clear evidence of its healing effects. Based on his own observations over the years, Siegel says, support and love from a physician can even result in noticeable improvement in a patient's condition.[53] Reflecting on his own practice, which has spanned more than three decades, Siegel concludes, "Someday we will understand the physiological and psychological workings of love well enough to turn on its full force more reliably. Once it is scientific, it will be accepted."[54]

Although we are not yet at that ideal level of understanding, there is much we do know and understand about the physiological effects of love. One of the most important effects of love is a boost of immune system function. Based on his studies, Harvard psychologist David McClelland concludes that love aids lymphocytes and improves immune functions—even though he is not sure how.[55]

Tests conducted at the Menninger Clinic in Topeka, Kansas, seem to confirm the effect of love on the immune system. At the clinic it was found that people who were romantically in love had white cells that were significantly more active in fighting infection. As a result, they suffered fewer colds. They also had lower levels of lactic acid in their blood, which means they were less likely to get tired, and they had higher levels of endorphins in their blood, which may contribute to a sense of euphoria and may help reduce pain.[56]

People with personality traits that enable them to love others and to enjoy intimate relationships tend to fare better overall in immune system function. In a group of studies, those who loved and cared most for others had the best immune system balance: a high ratio of helper/suppressor T cells and low levels of the stress hormone norepinephrine.[57] Those who scored highest on the ability to have an intimate relationship also had the highest levels of immunoglobulin A, an important immune agent that enables people to resist disease.[58]

Scores of other studies point out the importance of love to good health.[59] In one, people who were isolated had a twofold to threefold increased risk of death from heart disease and all other causes. In another, people who felt loved and supported developed much less atherosclerosis of the coronary arteries (a major risk factor for heart disease). In another, elderly adults who felt loved and supported had lower cholesterol levels and better immune function.

Writing in the journal *Science,* Dr. James House summed up the notion that it's the "10 to 20 percent of people who say they have nobody with whom they can share their private feelings, or who have close contact with others less than once a week, who are at most risk."[60]

## Love and Animals

The power of love has even been profoundly demonstrated in experiments with animals. Love and the handling that goes along with it have been shown to influence a baby animal's weight gain, emotional reactions, ability to respond to stress, and learning behaviors.[61] Studies have shown that animals raised without love (and the handling that goes along with it) have weakened immune systems.

Animals deprived of love also have a greater tendency to develop disease, whereas those exposed to love and handling seem better able to resist disease. In one experiment, two groups of laboratory rabbits were each fed a diet high in fat. One group of rabbits was treated routinely in the laboratory. The other group was shown "love"; these rabbits were talked to, handled gently, and petted often. The rabbits that were shown affection developed significantly less atherosclerosis than the rabbits treated routinely.[62]

## Love and Children

Although an absence of love seems to weaken the immune system in animals, it has also been shown to reduce an animal's ability to deal with stress. The same appears to be true of humans. And the earlier people have the benefit of a strong, loving relationship, the better they seem to be able to resist the deleterious effects of stress.

In the book *Vulnerable but Invincible*, the effects of an early loving relationship become apparent. To determine in part what helps us resist stress, researchers studied 650 children reared in poverty on the island of Kauai in the Hawaiian Islands. Their families had a multitude of problems. Many of the children were reared by single-parent mothers who were themselves troubled by depression and schizophrenia in addition to the rigors of extreme poverty.

Researchers first did an extensive follow-up on the children when they turned ten years old. Half of them were already in serious trouble. Many had serious physical problems and problems in school, among other difficulties. Eight years later, researchers did another follow-up on the children, now eighteen years old. One-fourth of them had developed "very serious" physical and psychological problems. By the time they became adults, more than three-fourths showed the effects of their impoverished environment. Many had profound psychological and behavioral problems; even more were in poor physical health.

Of greatest interest to researchers, however, were the 15 to 20 percent who remained resilient. Despite their impoverished and difficult existence, these children were able to successfully resist the stress of that environment. Study findings give us a powerful insight into the effect of love. The children who remained resilient and well had a warm and loving relationship with another person during their first year of life. The children who developed serious psychological and physical problems did not.

Psychotherapist Harmon Bro, a former professor at Syracuse University, emphasizes the importance of early, affirming love. People who have "never developed the capacity for loving find lovelessness reflected in their bodies"—in poor health, muscular tension, shallow breathing, and other physical "ills" that reflect in a very real way an illness of the spirit.

## ENDNOTES

1. Alfie Kohn, "Do Religious People Help More? Not So You'd Notice," *Psychology Today,* December 1989, 66.
2. Eileen Rockefeller Growald and Allan Luks, "Beyond Self," *American Health,* March 1988, 51–53.
3. Growald and Luks, "Beyond Self."
4. Allan Luks and Peggy Payne, *The Healing Power of Doing Good* (New York: Fawcett Columbine, 1992).
5. Growald and Luks, "Beyond Self."
6. Sarah Lang, "Extend Your Hand, Extend Your Life," *Longevity,* March 1989, 18.
7. Lang, "Extend Your Hand," 19.
8. Ibid.
9. James, Lynch, *The Broken Heart: The Medical Consequences of Loneliness* (New York: Basic Books, 1977).
10. Growald and Luks, "Beyond Self," 51–53.
11. Lang, "Extend Your Hand," 19.
12. Ibid., 19.
13. J. Primavera, "The Unintended Consequences of Volunteerism: Positive Outcomes for Those Who Serve," *Journal of Prevention and Intervention in the Community* 18 (1999): 1–2.
14. Lang.
15. S. I. McMillen, *None of These Diseases,* rev. ed. (Old Tappan, N. J.: Fleming H. Revell, 1984), 188–89.
16. Geoffrey Cowley, "A Disaster Brings Out the Best in People. Why?" *Newsweek,* November 6, 1989, 40, 44.
17. Bruce Bower, "Getting Out from Number One," *Science News* 137 (1990): 266–67.
18. Tom Hurley, "Another Look at Altruism: Notes on an International Conference," *Noetic Sciences Building,* August/September 1989, 3.
19. Samuel P. Oliner and Pearl M. Oliner, *The Altruistic Personality: Rescuers of Jews in Nazi Europe* (New York: Macmillan/Free Press, 1988).
20. "Dr. Frederick Franck: An Artist, Physician, and Author Searches for What It Means to Be Human," *Your Personal Best,* November 1989, 14–15.
21. Oliner and Oliner, *The Altruistic Personality.*
22. Larry Dossey, *Healing Words* (San Francisco: Harper San Francisco, 1993), 110–13.
23. Kohn, "Do Religious People Help More?"
24. Alfie Kohn, "Beyond Selfishness," *Psychology Today,* October 1988, 38.
25. "Research: Altruism and Transformation," *Noetic Sciences Review,* autumn 1990, 33.

26. "Research: Altruism and Transformation."

27. Oliner and Oliner, *The Altruistic Personality.*

28. Allan Luks with Peggy Payne, "Helper's High," *New Age Journal,* September/October 1991, 49, 121; from Allan Luks with Peggy Payne, *The Healing Power of Doing Good: The Health and Spiritual Benefits of Helping Others* (New York: Ballantine Books, 1991).

29. David Sobel, "Rx: Helping Others," *Mental Medicine Update,* winter 1993, 6.

30. Allan Luks, "Helper's High," *Psychology Today,* October 1988, 39–42.

31. Luks, "Helper's High," 39.

32. "The Return of Generosity," *Health,* August 1989, 13.

33. Luks and Payne, "Helper's High."

34. Ibid.

35. Luks, "Helper's High," 42.

36. Ibid.

37. Luks and Payne, "Helper's High," 121.

38. Ibid.

39. Luks, "Helper's High."

40. Growald and Luks, "Beyond Self," 52.

41. Luks and Payne, "Helper's High."

42. Lang, "Extend Your Hand," 19.

43. Ibid.

44. Ibid.

45. "The Return of Generosity," *Health,* August 1989, 13.

46. Cowley, "A Disaster."

47. Howard F. Andrews, "Helping and Health: The Relationship Between Volunteer Activity and Health-Related Outcomes," *Advances* 7, no. 1 (1990): 25–34.

48. Luks, "Helper's High," 42.

49. Sobel, "Rx: Helping Others."

50. Ibid.

51. Arnold Fox and Barry Fox, *Wake Up! You're Alive* (Deerfield Beach, Fl.: Health Communications, 1988) 75.

52. McMillen, *None of These Diseases,* 124.

53. Mary Carpenter, "Modern-Day Faith Healing: Why Doctors Are Listening, Not Laughing," *Self,* September 1987, 202–5.

54. Blair Justice, "Think Yourself Healthy," *Prevention,* June 1988, 31–32, 105–8.

55. Justice, "Think Yourself Healthy."

56. Ibid.

57. Blair Justice, *Who Gets Sick: Thinking and Health* (Houston, Tex.: Peak Press, 1987), 257.

58. Justice, "Think Yourself Healthy."

59. Studies summarized from Dean Ornish, "The Healing Power of Love," *Prevention,* February 1991, 60–66, 135–41; from Dean Ornish, *Dr. Dean Ornish's Program for Reversing Heart Disease* (New York: Random House, 1990).

60. Ornish, "The Healing Power of Love."

61. Fox and Fox, *Wake Up!* 85.

62. Justice, *Who Gets Sick,* 258.

# CHAPTER 16

# The Healing Power of Faith and Religion

*We act in faith, and miracles occur.*

—Dag Hammerskjold

## Learning Objectives

- Understand how spirituality, religion, and faith differ.
- Understand what faith is, and its impact.
- Discuss the influence of spirituality, religion, and faith on health.
- Understand how faith has been used as a healing agent.
- Define the placebo effect, understand how it is related to faith, and discuss the myths associated with placebos.
- Discuss how placebos work and how the expectations of a physician can impact health.

French novelist George Sand penned the sentiment that faith "is an excitement and an enthusiasm: it is a condition of intellectual magnificence to which we must cling as to a treasure, and not squander in the small coin of empty words." If the results of recent studies are correct, faith—along with spirituality and religion—are treasures, not only in the spiritual sense but also as a potent factor in both good health and healing influence.

As discussed in Chapter 14, spirituality and religion are similar in many ways—and, in fact, overlap in some ways. *Spirituality* involves an integrative energy that "encompasses all aspects of human being and is a means of experiencing life."[1] It is often based on experience, not intellect, and can be manifested in experiences and interconnectedness not only with a divine being but also with self, the earth, the environment, the cosmos, nature, animals, or relationships with others. Spirituality comes from the Latin term *spiritus*, which means "the breath," or that which is most vital to life.

Generally, it is part of every aspect of life and provides purpose, meaning, strength, and guidance in shaping the journey of life.[2]

*Religion* is generally recognized as the way in which people practice or express their spirituality; it is the organized practice of a person's beliefs. Some describe religion as a "search for significance in ways related to the sacred."[3] Religion is a personal way of expressing spirituality through rites and rituals based on creeds and communal practices.[4] It is from the Latin term *religare,* meaning to bind together. Religion can also affect every aspect of life, including family life, sexual activity, human development, economic status, political beliefs, social organizations, criminal behavior, and even personality characteristics.

While spirituality and religion are similar in many ways, they do have some important distinctions:[5]

- Spirituality focuses on individual growth, while religion focuses on creating community.

- Religion is much more formal in worship, systematic in doctrine, and authoritarian in direction, and involves more formally prescribed behaviors than does spirituality.

- Spirituality is much more difficult to identify and objectively measure than is religion.

- Spirituality is emotion-based and focuses on inner experiences; religion is behavior-based and focuses on outward, observable practices.

- Spirituality is universal and emphasizes unity with others; religion is particular and segregates one group from another.

So, where does the concept of *faith* enter in?

American philosopher Ralph Waldo Emerson wrote extensively of faith, and penned in his later years the sentiment that "all he had seen and experienced caused him to have faith in that which he could not see. Whoever reasons only according to what the five bodily senses reveal or believes that the only means of knowing is through seeing, hearing, tasting, smelling, and feeling is controlled by appearances."[6]

Indeed, faith must "rise above what our five senses tell us, for they only report the appearance of the physical world."[7] Or, as one behavioral health scientist put it, "I see miracles as the playing out of natural or divine law with which we were not formerly acquainted. For example, though some considered the fact that Columbus did not fall off the edge of a 'flat' earth to be a miracle, the real miracle was the opening of the layer of consciousness that allowed Columbus to perceive the earth as being round before he set sail."[8]

That scientist, Deirdre Davis Bingham, said she sometimes thinks of us "as being in the center of nesting Russian eggs. Our reality is limited by the wooden shell of the particular egg in which we find ourselves. As we drill conceptual holes in the immediate shell and glimpse a new layer of possibilities, that shell begins to crack and we have a new realm of reality." It is in the nature of scientific inquiry (and human consciousness) that major advances come from people who look at things in a different way—who break through the shell of their immediate nesting egg.[9]

Medical and scientific research conducted over the past two decades have demonstrated clearly that what exists is not as important as what we believe exists. Personal belief gives us an unseen power that enables us to do the impossible, to perform miracles—even to heal ourselves. It has been found that patients who exhibit faith become less concerned about their symptoms, have less severe symptoms, and have less frequent symptoms with longer periods of relief between them than patients who lack faith.

That is not to say that faith should replace modern medicine. Instead, it should be used in conjunction with modern medicine—used to enhance the effects of medicine and to strengthen its impact. Even staunch medical practitioners recognize that faith plays a vital part in the healing process. As early as the sixteenth century, the great surgeon Ambrose Pare noted in one surgical report, "I dressed the wound, and God healed it."

An increasing number of physicians guide their patients toward faith as an integral part of the healing process. The latest research shows that, according to a nationwide survey, 80 percent of family physicians have recommended that their patients seek religious counsel and exercise faith as part of treatment for everything from substance abuse and mood disorders to terminal illness. The study's lead author, Dr. Timothy P. Daaleman of the University of Kansas Medical Center in Kansas City, says that more and more doctors are acknowledging the important role of faith and spirituality in health.[10]

The growing interest in spirituality, religion, and faith as they relate to health is creating compelling research as well as compelling questions—some of which still have not been completely answered. How does religious faith influence health? Do spiritual or religious people enjoy better physical or mental health throughout their entire lives? How are spirituality, religion, and faith related to a sense of well-being? Can spirituality, religion, or faith influence—and possibly change—the way people adapt to chronic illness and impending death? Are some religious practices associated with lower disease rates and longer life?

Religion and healing have always been closely tied, but research into religion and health is not always as clear as it may seem. There are important biological, cultural, social, and psychological influences on health that can be difficult to isolate from religious influences—especially in people for whom religious practice is an integral part of life. And some are distressed by the attempt to scientifically explain spirituality—which, by its very nature, is intensely personal and experiential and cannot really be reduced to a test tube or a laboratory.[11] Others are disturbed by the attempt to study religion as it impacts health because such a study may give the message that religion is only valuable if it "works." Interesting questions are also being raised about the impact of faith on health.

Because of these questions and areas that still lack clarity, it's important to determine what role spirituality, religion, and faith may have in health and longevity. Spirituality, as a personal and inner reflection, may have profound influence—and religious orientation may have a broad array of influences that impact health, moderate risk, and help people cope better with all kinds of experiences in life. During those times in life when people are faced with the most difficult experiences, they may call on the deepest and most profound aspects of spirituality, religion, and faith. As such, there are compelling reasons to understand the impact these factors can have.[12]

The growing appreciation of faith among members of the medical community is characterized in the comments of Dr. Joan Borysenko, a former instructor at Harvard Medical School:

> Two thousand years ago a woman who had suffered prolonged uterine bleeding approached Jesus of Nazareth. Coming up to him in a crowd, she touched the hem of his garment and was instantly healed. Jesus turned to her and explained that it was her faith that had made her whole. After centuries of slow progress toward rational explanations of the physical world, even scientists can at least begin to appreciate the truth of His assessment. We are entering a new level in the scientific understanding of mechanisms by which faith, belief, and imagination can actually unlock the mysteries of healing.[13]

The medical community is smart to take a broader interest in spirituality and religion—because Americans in general are a spiritual and religious people. According to recent research:[14]

- 95 percent of all Americans believe in God or a higher power.
- 75 percent of Americans say that their religious faith forms the foundation for their approach to life.
- 73 percent of Americans say that prayer is an important part of their daily life, and 33 percent of all Americans use prayer to heal their medical conditions.
- 74 percent of all Americans associate the word *spirituality* with positive feelings.

- 65 percent of Americans associate religion with positive associations.

- 59 percent of all Americans describe themselves as both spiritual and religious.

- More than 40 percent of Americans attend weekly religious services.

## The Impact of Faith

An excellent example of the impact of faith—and the detriment of its absence—occurred in the Philippines during World War II.[15] American soldiers who had been bathing in contaminated streams had been infected with schistosomiasis, a parasitic worm infection. The soldiers had been treated with a complete regimen, but remained hospitalized four months after they were first diagnosed. They should have been healed, but they felt vaguely ill; they complained of symptoms ranging from abdominal cramps to headaches to vague weakness and fatigue. Attending physicians were puzzled. The soldiers were well fed. They were being housed in comfortable accommodations. They had benefited from the best available medical care for the condition. Yet none had healed.

Johns Hopkins School of Medicine psychiatrist Jerome D. Frank, then an Army doctor, was asked to investigate the situation and offer some clues as to why the men were not responding to treatment. After exhaustive interviews and examinations, he found that faith had a great deal to do with the soldiers and their prolonged illness.

The soldiers were confused and frightened about their prognosis and about what would happen to them. They were getting a mixed message about their illness. Their doctors were telling them that schistosomiasis was not a serious malady and that they would regain their health. At the same time, radios in the background were broadcasting "scare stories" about the disease in an effort to keep the American soldiers from bathing in the contaminated streams. The soldiers didn't know who to believe—the doctors who tried to soothe them or the radio announcers who detailed a grisly fate. Then there was confusion about what would happen. The Army was incredibly inconsistent about how the soldiers were treated. Some were shipped home. Some were detained in the Army hospital. Still others were sent back into combat.

Making the situation even worse were the doctors and nurses themselves. Carrying overwhelming caseloads, they did not have the time to devote undying attention to the soldiers stricken with schistosomiasis; as time went on, they were faced with the frustration that none of the soldiers was recovering. Before long, doctors and nurses were treating the soldiers with abrupt detachment—a sign to the soldiers that something was seriously wrong. The soldiers lacked faith, not because of some fault of their own, but because the confusing situation did not allow the opportunity to develop faith. The soldiers did not expect a cure, so none came.

The evidence says that faith can heal—or that it can be a very powerful element in the healing process. When combined with conventional treatment and optimism, faith can make the difference.

## The Influence of Spirituality, Religion, and Faith on Health

Many peoples and cultures in the world believe that spirituality and health are intimately connected; according to Dr. Deepak Chopra, "Spirituality is not meant to be separate from the body. . . . Sickness and aging represent the body's inability to reach its natural goal, which is to join the mind in perfection and fulfillment."[16] And since religion is the organized expression of spirituality, it, too, is closely related to health.

Many studies have demonstrated a powerful connection between spirituality, religion, and health. For example, research has shown that those who attend religious services one or more times a week have dramatically lower death rates—especially from coronary artery disease (50 percent less), emphysema (56 percent less), cirrhosis of the liver (74 percent less), and suicide (53 percent less).[17] Other research on the connection between religion and health has shown the following:[18]

- There is a positive relationship between religion and both physical and mental health.

- Many depend on spirituality and religion as their main method of coping with physical health problems and the stress of surgery.

- Most older people say that spirituality and religion help them cope with or adapt to personal losses or difficulties.

- People who attend religious services at least once a week are half as likely to be depressed.

- Those who both attend religious services at least once a week and read religious scriptures at least daily are much less likely to have high blood pressure.

- Those who attend religious services at least once a week and who pray or read religious scriptures at least daily are almost 90 percent less likely to smoke cigarettes.

- High levels of religious involvement are associated with the practice of positive health behaviors, including self-care.

- Religious involvement may help boost immune function, facilitate healing and recovery, and prevent postsurgical infection.

- Religious involvement is associated with reduced levels of pain in cancer patients; improved physical functioning, medical regime compliance, and self-esteem; and lower anxiety and health-related worry a year after surgery among heart transplant patients.[19]

- Religious involvement can change the perception of people with disabilities so that they perceive themselves as less disabled and more capable.

- Spirituality and religious involvement have been associated with longer life, better health, more hopefulness, healthier lifestyle choices, less cardiovascular disease, decreased incidence of cancer, longer marriages, less depression, and an expanded social network.

All the effects of religion may not be positive, however—when taken to an extreme, religion can actually have negative effects on health. For example, extremely devout religiosity can cause inflexibility, narrow-mindedness, unusually high expectations, and excessive guilt—which can result in neuroses, anxiety, isolation, alienation, or depression. In addition, some religions discourage appropriate mental and physical health care or encourage their followers to discontinue traditional medical treatment. Finally, religious cults can alienate people from their support networks (including family and friends); some have even encouraged suicide.[20] It's important to remember that these are *extremes*, however, and that the general impact of spirituality and religion, when appropriate, promotes health and well-being.

Religious advocates have always believed in the power of faith to influence health and healing. Now, growing scientific evidence is convincing the medical and scientific community about the power of faith on the human body. One of the strongest proponents of the impact of faith on health is psychiatrist Harold Koenig, director of Duke University's Center for the Study of Religion/Spirituality and Health. For more than a decade, his studies on the role of faith in many medical conditions have shown a definite relationship between the two. Thanks to his work and that of other prominent researchers, material that was once considered only "anecdotal" has been accepted as solid scientific evidence.[21]

The power of faith over health begins in the mind. Cardiologist Herbert Benson makes a convincing case for the power of the mind with the example of the classic film, *Lawrence of Arabia*. While watching this epic, even people in air-conditioned theaters became extremely hot and thirsty; during intermissions, the concession stands were inundated with people demanding ice-cold drinks. It was, as Benson terms it, an "epidemic of thirst." The moral of the story, Benson says, is that "the influential and even life-changing forces we encounter are often not those things that are externally real. In the case of the film, of course, people weren't really deprived of water, but they identified with those waterless conditions so thoroughly that their bodies became 'convinced' they were on the Arabian dunes."[22]

According to Benson, medical and scientific research "are demonstrating ever more clearly that the things we can touch, taste, and measure frequently have to take a back seat to what we perceive or believe to be real." If the mind is that powerful, then what the mind believes can, in fact, have tremendous influence over the body. Belief or faith, says Benson—whether it's deep in the mind or heart or focused on some outside object, like a physician—can play a key role in generating a response in the body. Apparently, he says, "just having a strong belief is enough to cause things to happen in our physiology, but this is a very ticklish point. It does seem that just the state of belief, which can emanate from a variety of personal, philosophical, or religious orientations, is itself a powerful force."[23]

In his book *Super Immunity*, psychologist Paul Pearsall sums up research conducted at Michigan State University that proves that a single cell can be controlled by how we think. In describing the study results, Pearsall says that "the mind alters every cell in the body."[24]

A dramatic example of that power was provided by a sixteen-year-old boy with congenital ichthyosiform erythrodermia, a serious skin disease that causes a hardening and blackening of the skin. There is no known cure for the disease. The boy's condition had deteriorated to such a degree that his skin was harder than fingernails, and bacterial infection had set in. To demonstrate the power of the mind over the body, a hypnotist challenged the boy to "see" his skin as becoming normal. Within five days of the hypnosis, the boy's hard, damaged skin fell off; it was replaced with reddened, but more normal-looking, skin. Within ten days, the boy's skin had returned to normal—a phenomenon verified by three independent medical researchers.[25]

According to Benson, faith has been shown in countless studies to have a powerful influence over the body. So great is its power, in fact, that faith has been used to successfully relieve headaches, reduce angina pains, control hypertension, overcome insomnia, prevent hyperventilation attacks, help alleviate backaches, enhance cancer treatment, control panic attacks, reduce cholesterol levels, reduce overall stress, and alleviate the symptoms of anxiety—which include nausea, vomiting, diarrhea, constipation, short temper, and inability to get along with others.[26]

A review of studies measuring faith shows some impressive results and helps confirm the power of faith over physiological processes.[27] In one study, people showed a powerful ability to inhibit the growth of fungus cultures by concentrating on them for fifteen minutes from a distance of several feet. In another, people were able to significantly stimulate or inhibit the growth of bacteria. In a study conducted by the Mind Science Foundation, people were able to decrease the destruction of red blood cells. In still other studies, people even exerted influence over plants and animals. In one study conducted at the Mind Science Foundation, volunteers had a potent effect over people several rooms away.

A good example of faith's power over physiological processes is its influence over blood pressure. According to researchers Jeffrey S. Levin of Eastern Virginia Medical School and Hearold Y. Vanderpool of Galveston's University of Texas, devoutly faithful groups of people tend to have lower blood pressure than comparison groups of people.[28] Faith is so powerful, say researchers, that it has been shown to be effective against diseases like cancer, believed incurable in many cases. Harvard's Joan Borysenko studied cancer patients who were considered to be long-term survivors; she found that the attribute they had in common was strong faith.[29]

Faith also apparently increases the ability to resist stress and strengthens the body against the physical changes that can accompany stress. In one study, two psychiatrists, an endocrinologist, and a cancer specialist in New York City teamed up to determine which hormones were released under the stress of a truly life-threatening situation. For their "life-threatening situation," they chose women who were undergoing breast biopsies to determine whether they had cancer. To ascertain how much distress each woman was suffering, the researchers took daily measurements of hydrocortisone (a hormone secreted by the adrenal glands in response to stress) for three days before the women underwent the biopsy.[30]

They found that the amount of distress a woman suffered was not dependent on the crisis of probably having cancer. Instead, researchers determined that the amount of stress suffered was determined by the woman's psychological defenses—her outlook and her beliefs in general. The woman who suffered the least amount of stress (and whose adrenal hormones were the lowest) reported that she regularly used faith and prayer to cope with life's stressful events.

"People with a strong faith, whether from religious beliefs or just good experience with trust, are the ones who stick it out in the worst circumstances," reports psychologist Shlomo Breznitz, visiting scientist with the National Institute of Mental Health. "The best example is a mining disaster," Breznitz points out. "Miners are taught that if they should become trapped in a cave-in, there are certain things they should do and not do to stay alive. There is only limited oxygen, so they have to conserve their energy. It's futile to spend it trying to dig their way out. It's the miners who are able to maintain hope that they will be rescued, even when there's nothing else they can do, who have the best chances of surviving."[31]

# The Healing Power of Faith

The power of faith is probably more apparent in the healing process than in any other aspect of medicine. And, according to researchers who have studied the effects of faith, the stronger the faith, the more certain the healing power. As one researcher put it, "The faith that heals, that 'removes mountains,' must be a certainty about something which cannot be seen and cannot now be proved."[32]

Researcher Daniel Goleman maintains that belief "is the hidden ingredient in Western medicine and every traditional system of 'healing' I know about. In the West, doctors have long been aware of its curative power. A large number of illnesses can be treated more successfully if the patient believes in a particular cure."[33]

Psychiatrist Jerome Frank ascribes even greater powers to faith. He says faith is the element in even modern medicine that brings about a recovery. "The physician's main function is to use his medical skills to stimulate the patient's mechanisms of repair," Frank explains. "Nonmedical healers, whether African witch doctors or religious faith healers in Western countries, intuitively understand this. Their rituals and laying on of hands are designed to release or strengthen the patient's inner healing powers."[34]

"Faith" is not the property of a certain religion, nor does it owe its effectiveness to a certain shrine or ritual. All religions have members who have experienced seemingly magical, spontaneous cures from life-threatening or incurable diseases. Miracles have occurred at shrines scattered throughout the world, and patients who seemed stripped of any possibility of a cure have responded to a broad spectrum of rituals (such as laying on of hands). The key to these experiences is not the religion or the shrine or the ritual itself, but the faith of the person who is healed.

"There is no denying that religious shrines unleash powerful healing emotions of hope in the pilgrim," maintains Frank. "One cannot attribute this to any particular religious faith or object of worship, since all religions can cite instances of these seemingly magical cures. The more likely explanation is that the cure results from the individual's state of mind—his expectant faith."[35]

## Healing and the Religious Shrine

One obvious example is that of probably the best-known healing shrine, Lourdes, France. Since the visions of Marie Bernarde Soubirous and the discovery of the healing spring in the middle of the nineteenth century, there have been countless documented cases of people who went to the spring with faith and who were cured of severe illness. Lame people have left Lourdes with the ability to walk; the deaf have been blessed with the gift of sound, and sight has been restored to the blind. Many of the cures have been dramatic.

Today, more than 2 million people visit Lourdes each year in hope of being healed; they come from all corners of the world, and many have been told there is no cure for their condition. For most people, Lourdes is a last resort. Many make the pilgrimage only after years of drugs and therapies that have not yielded results.

The reputation of Lourdes as a "healing" shrine is well deserved. People are healed, sometimes of lifelong conditions. Are those healings due to some magical property of the springs themselves? Or to a special healing power possessed by the priests, nurses, and orderlies? Probably the healing is due to the expectant faith of the pilgrim who comes to Lourdes to be healed. As one eyewitness describes the scene at the shrine each afternoon, "The sick line up in two rows. . . . Every few feet, in front of them, kneeling priests with arms outstretched praying earnestly, leading the responses. Nurses and orderlies on their knees, praying too. . . . The Sacred Host is raised above each sick one. The great crowd falls to its knees. All arms are outstretched in one vast cry to Heaven. As far as one can see in any direction, people are on their knees, praying."[36]

The stirring services, the sense of support, and the outpouring of emotion at Lourdes and shrines like it "can only serve to reinforce the expectant faith that pilgrims bring with them," explains Frank. This faith, he adds, explains "the spontaneous remissions of disease and improved bodily functions experienced by some, as well as the increased sense of hope and improved morale that even the uncured take home with them."[37]

## Other Examples of Faith and Healing

Lourdes (and other shrines like it) is only one example of how faith works to heal the sick. There are many other examples, and a number of scientific studies have even been able to document the healing power of faith. In one study, researchers studied a group of patients who were about to undergo surgery for detached retina. The researchers gave each patient a "score" that reflected his or her expectations about the surgery. After the surgery, the surgeon—who did not know the patient's "score"—gauged the speed of recovery and noted any complications. Those who had faith in the surgeon and faith in their own ability to cope with the surgery did the best. The researchers concluded that the body's own healing ability is actually stimulated "by a patient's faith in the healer and his methods, an optimistic outlook toward the treatment, and other psychological variables that, taken together, may be called an attitude of expectant faith."

In one stunning experiment, Harvard psychologist David McClelland took fourteen Harvard undergraduates with common colds to a psychic healer within twenty-four hours of the time their symptoms first appeared. The therapy was simple: The healer said, "You're healed."

But were they?

McClelland had listed thirty-two cold symptoms and had asked the students to rate their symptoms both before and after the visit to the psychic healer. All but five students said their symptoms were better. But here's the best part: The nine students who felt better also had higher levels of immunoglobulin A (IgA) in their saliva. IgA is an immune antibody that battles upper respiratory infections. In other words, their immune systems had been activated.[38]

A separate study provides a graphic description of how powerful faith can be in the healing process—even when the faith is not justified. A hospital-based physician was frustrated with three patients who, despite his best efforts, had not been helped by medical treatment. All three were women in their sixties. One suffered from chronic inflammation of the gall bladder. One was wasting away after failing to recuperate from surgery for pancreatitis. And one had inoperable cancer of the uterus; to complicate matters, she also had tremendous swelling of the legs and anemia.

The doctor called in a faith healer but did not tell any of the women about him. He practiced his rituals on an absentee basis, without any of the three patients knowing anything about it. After twelve healing sessions, there was no change in any of the patients' conditions. The physician dismissed the faith healer.

Then the physician went to the three patients, described the faith healer in enthusiastic and glowing terms, and told the women that they were extremely lucky: The faith healer would be working on their behalf each morning for three days. Of course, this wasn't true; the doctor had dismissed the faith healer. But as far as the women were concerned, they believed that the faith healer was working for them.

What the doctor saw was both dramatic and almost unbelievable: All three patients were relieved of their symptoms. All three were able to leave the hospital within a week. The patient with pancreatitis, who had been literally wasting away, got out of bed after what she believed to be the first "healing session." She rapidly gained thirty pounds—a feat medical science had been unable to help her accomplish. And she remained well, without any relapse of her condition. Most amazing was the cancer patient. The swelling in her legs disappeared. Her red blood cell level rose, reversing her anemia.

Five days after the "healing sessions" began, she returned home—where she was able to function normally until her death several months later.

Some, eager to dismiss the phenomenon of faith healing, overlook the impact of faith on health. By doing so, say many researchers, they risk overlooking a potentially powerful source of healing for many patients. Responding to criticism in his field about the prospect of faith healing, one professor of nursing wrote:

> It may be that some force is activated that we do not yet understand (although [scientists] offer us perfectly rational explanations), but . . . we risk putting an incredibly useful idea outside scientific and rational enquiry, thereby keeping it out of the mainstream of health care—exactly where it is needed. A bit of humility, clear thinking, and free speech in the face of the awesome mystery of healing would not come amiss from very many of our "healers."[39]

Beyond the work of faith healers and other practitioners, faith itself can not only stimulate the body's own healing mechanisms, but also apparently influence the way drugs work in the body. Mary Baker Eddy, the founder of Christian Science, pronounced before the turn of the twentieth century that "when the sick recover by the use of drugs, it is the law of a general belief, culminating in individual faith, which heals."[40] And cardiologist Herbert Benson makes much the same argument in our day when he maintains that "a new drug given by a doctor who believes in it enthusiastically is far more potent than the same drug given by a skeptical doctor. The doctor marshals his patient's belief and power to help himself. But a patient may be able to get better without a doctor, simply calling on his belief in some outside force."[41]

One of the most striking and profound examples of how faith influences even the course of medication is the well-known story of a patient treated by Dr. Bruno Klopfer in the late 1950s. The patient was suffering from a widespread lymphoma—a serious cancer of the immune system—that was in its late stages. At the time, a drug called Krebiozen was being touted as a cure for cancer. The patient demanded that Klopfer administer Krebiozen, and the doctor agreed. Within two days of receiving the Krebiozen, the patient experienced a remarkable turnaround. As one account described it, the large tumors that covered his body began "melting like snowballs." After ten days of treatment with Krebiozen, the patient was released from the hospital, apparently free of disease. Klopfer believed that a medical miracle had occurred.

A medical miracle had occurred—but it was due to the patient's faith in the Krebiozen, not due to the drug itself. As fate would have it, that faith was short-lived. A few months after the patient was released from the hospital, newspapers around the country announced that Krebiozen was worthless. The patient's tumors promptly reappeared.

Klopfer was fascinated by this turn of events. Based on the patient's history, he strongly suspected that it had been the patient's belief that had cured him and that the drug had nothing to do with it. Klopfer became convinced that he could once again harness the man's faith if the conditions were right. He called his patient in, reassured him, and told him the newspaper accounts were inaccurate and an extra-strength, improved, refined form of the drug had just been released to physicians. Klopfer offered this "refined" form of the drug to his eager patient. But Klopfer didn't actually have any improved Krebiozen. What he gave his patient was actually distilled water.

With distilled water coursing through his veins, the patient who believed that he had a new super Krebiozen staged another remarkable recovery. Within days, his tumors again disappeared. He was released from the hospital a second time, again apparently disease-free.

Unfortunately, it didn't last. Three months after his recovery, the patient read a newspaper report published by the American Medical Association. Definitive tests had proven beyond a doubt, the report said, that Krebiozen was worthless. Top-ranking officials in the American Medical Association proclaimed the drug as useless in the fight against cancer. The patient, who had left the hospital three months earlier free of tumors, read the report. His faith was shattered. His tumors ballooned. Two days after he read the newspaper report, he literally laid down and died.

## Transfer of Energy Theory

One way in which faith healers have attempted to harness faith and bring about healing is through "laying on of hands," a ritual that dates to ancient times. "Spiritual healing by the laying on of hands has been practiced for as long as recorded history," notes psychiatrist Daniel Benor. "The Bible is replete with tales of unusual cures by the prophets, Christ, and the Apostles. Virtually every known culture has included healers among its healthcare professionals."[42]

An eighteenth-century physician who practiced the laying on of hands expressed his hope that a physicist would someday be able to substantiate scientifically what went on during these rituals: Why should not the proximity of the human body, which can restore the brilliance of a faded pearl, exert upon a neighboring body, by means of an aura or radiation, an influence that stimulates or tranquilizes the other's nerves? Surely there may be attraction and revulsion, sympathy and antipathy, between individual and individual.[43]

Today's faith healers, says psychiatrist Jerome Frank, explain their power in different ways: Some believe they serve as a conduit for supernatural healing energy or that they transmit healing power generated by other members of the group; others believe that the healing force comes from within them. Patients who have undergone healing by laying on of hands often report a sensation of intense heat, although this does not register on a thermometer. Nevertheless, the evidence suggests that laying on of hands often does accelerate wound healing, and there have been cases in which patients who have been in wheelchairs for years suddenly rise and walk during the ritual.[44]

The "transfer of energy" theory has received widespread support among faith healers who practice the laying on of hands. Dolores Kreiger, a professor of nursing at New York University, teaches a version of laying on of hands to her students and claims that the ritual "redistributes the patient's energy."[45]

Another practitioner who claims to be using the laying on of hands for "some kind of an energy exchange" is University of South Carolina Nursing Researcher Janet Quinn. The U.S. Department of Health and Human Services has awarded Quinn grant money to prove her hypothesis and to determine whether the practice might benefit heart surgery patients.[46]

One Connecticut hospital has decided to offer laying on of hands as a service to patients who want it—not, some are eager to point out, as a "potential cure for any ailment," but to "provide emotional and religious support to the community." Acting under the expert advice of the National Institute of Healthcare Research in Maryland, hospital administrators are careful not to promise results to anyone, but those results have come for many. One, a fifty-four-year-old former IBM executive on leave from her job, enjoyed remarkable remission from multiple sclerosis, which had confined her to a wheelchair for eighteen months. Those who participate in the laying on of hands at the hospital point out that therapeutic touch changes the energy field that emanates from the body, making it possible to heal illness and injury.[47]

In fact, many who practice the laying on of hands say they have a specific task related to energy fields, according to Toni Tripp-Reimer, associate professor of nursing and adjunct professor of anthropology at the University of Iowa. The practitioner first identifies, then brings back into equilibrium, disrupted energy fields that surround the patient's body. "In theory, the therapist has a balanced energy field," Tripp-Reimer explains. "Being stronger, the therapist's field helps to bring the patient's back into proper balance."[48]

Indeed, a technique called Kirlian photography may give some credence to the "energy exchange" theory. Kirlian photography is a special kind of photography that reveals the spectacular color corona that surrounds the body. The corona of a healthy person is sharp and bright; a sick person has a blurry or cloudy corona composed of duller colors. Researchers who have photographed a practitioner's hands before and after "laying on of hands" show that the coronas surrounding the fingers and hands are brighter and more colorful after the ritual than before.

Other interesting research has studied the effects of "therapeutic touch," which doesn't involve physical contact. Instead, the healer's hands are held a short distance away from the skin as the healer performs the technique.

In one landmark study, researcher David P. Wirth used forty-four patients who had full-skin-thickness surgical wounds on their arms. The patients were asked to stick their arms through holes in a wall for five minutes a day; researchers told the patients that physicians were measuring "biopotentials" from the surgical site.

In actuality, however, something else was happening. For twenty-one of the patients, the room on the other side was vacant. For twenty-three of the patients, a therapeutic practitioner did noncontact therapeutic touch each day. Every few days, physicians who had no knowledge at all of the therapeutic touch measured the wounds of all forty-four patients.

What happened? By the eighth day, wounds of the patients who received therapeutic touch were significantly smaller and showed much less variation than those of the other patients. By the sixteenth day, thirteen of the twenty-three patients who had therapeutic touch were completely healed. None of the patients who had stuck their arms through holes into a vacant room was healed.

Wirth points out that the therapeutic touch itself was the reason for the healing. Because the patients didn't know they were receiving the touch, they weren't influenced by the placebo effect, suggestion, expectation, or belief.[49]

## Faith and the Placebo Effect

One of the most striking demonstrations of faith in action is the placebo effect: the physical change that occurs as a result of what we think a pill or a procedure will do. According to Yale oncologist and surgeon Bernie Siegel, "What the placebo suggests to us is that we may be able to change what takes place in our bodies by changing our state of mind."[50]

A remarkable example of the placebo effect stands out in the memory of Dr. Stephen Strauss, chief of the Laboratory of Clinical Investigation at the National Institute of Allergy and Infectious Diseases. He tells of a woman in her thirties who was "very significantly impaired" by chronic fatigue syndrome. She had no energy, was unable to work, and spent most of her time at home. During a study to determine the effectiveness of a new chronic fatigue drug, however, her strength was restored and she underwent a full recovery.

"She and her parents were so thrilled with her recovery that they were blessing me and my colleagues," remembers Strauss, the principal investigator in the study. Here's the amazing part: The woman was one of the study participants who received not the chronic fatigue drug, but a placebo—a pill that *looked* like the chronic fatigue drug but that contained no active ingredients. It was her *belief* in the treatment, not the treatment itself, that effected her recovery.[51]

## What Is a Placebo?

A placebo has been defined as "any effect attributable to a pill, potion, or procedure, but not to its pharmacodynamic or specific properties."[52] Another general definition of placebos is "substances or procedures without specific activity against the condition being evaluated."[53] If a person deeply believes that a pill is going to work in a certain way, chances are it will—even if the pill is fashioned of nothing more than table sugar, distilled water, or saline solution.[54] The healer is actually faith, not pharmacology.

The word *placebo* comes from the Latin word meaning "placate" or the phrase meaning "I will please." In fact, one of the earliest medical definitions of placebo—penned in the early 1800s—described it as "an epithet given to any medication adopted more to please than to benefit the patient."[55] Placebos have been used by physicians since the time of Hippocrates.

We know a placebo to be "a pill that is given with the intention of treating a medical disease, but which has no specific biological or chemical activity against the condition."[56] But a placebo doesn't necessarily have to be a pill; it can be a potion, a surgical procedure, or any other medical procedure. A physician can even be a placebo. And, according to researchers, the effects of a placebo are not imaginary but can be physically measured with physiological tests. Experts tell us also that the effects of a placebo are often more potent than those of the actual medication or procedure.[57]

One dramatic example of the placebo effect occurred in a New York hospital in 1950. In the experiment, Dr. Stewart Wolf treated women who were suffering severe nausea and vomiting from pregnancy. Wolf told the women he was going to give them a drug known to alleviate nausea and vomiting. In reality, however, Wolf gave the women syrup of ipecac—a drug used to induce vomiting.

What happened? The patients' nausea and vomiting disappeared after taking the syrup of ipecac. According to researchers, the women's belief in the drug's powers was so potent that it actually counteracted the pharmaco-logic actions of the drug.[58]

A more recent example of the placebo effect stemmed from a large, multicenter study called the Beta Blocker Heart Attack Trial. As reported in the British medical journal *Lancet,* Dr. R. Horowitz and his colleagues gave heart attack patients either a beta blocker or a placebo. The researchers then compared the rates of death among patients who did or did not take their medication.

Even after taking into account factors like family history, cigarette smoking, or psychological characteristics, the researchers found that those who didn't take the beta blocker as prescribed were 2.6 times more likely to die than those who did take the beta blocker. The surprise occurred with the placebo group: Those who did not take the placebo also had an increased rate of death when compared with those who did take the placebo—even though it contained no medication at all.[59]

Norman Cousins defined a placebo as

> *not so much a pill as a process, beginning with the patient's confidence in the doctor and extending through the full functioning of his own immunological system. The process works not because of any magic in the tablets but because the human body is its own best apothecary and because the most successful pre-scriptions are those that are filled by the body itself.*[60]

Placebos have everything to do with faith: A patient believes that the pill or procedure will work, so it does. The key is the meaning of the experi-ence for the person. Placebos work on a wide range of medical disorders, and they work an astounding percentage of the time—an estimated one-third to one-half of the time. Officials also estimate that almost half of all the prescriptions written today are for placebos—drugs that have no actual effect on the condition for which they are prescribed, but that may bolster a patient's belief (and therefore the patient's own healing mechanisms). A perfect example is when a doctor prescribes antibiotics for the flu. Antibi-otics are not effective against viruses, such as the influenza virus. But patients who faithfully take antibiotics in the belief that these will make them better usually recover faster.

According to a review published in the *Journal of the American Medical Association,* placebos can be effective in a variety of disorders—and can affect practically any organ system in the body. A host of studies has shown that placebos are effective against angina pectoris, rheumatoid arthritis, pain, hay fever, headache, cough, peptic ulcer, and high blood pressure. Studies cited in the *Journal of the American Medical Association* article also show that placebos can be effective when used against psychiatric disorders, such as depression, anxiety, and schizophrenia.[61]

## How Do Placebos Work?

"Expectation is a powerful thing," says Dr. Robert DeLap, head of one of the Food and Drug Administration's Offices of Drug Evaluation. "The more you *believe* you're going to benefit from a treatment, the more likely it is that you *will* experience a benefit."[62]

No one is absolutely certain how placebos work, but there are several theories. A number of studies show that the answer might be endorphins. Absolute belief in a pill, a treatment, or even a practitioner seems to stimulate the brain to release endorphins, which relieve pain and may speed healing.[63]

Another theory revolves around research conducted by a Finnish physiologist in which actual physiological changes were triggered by the patient's imagination. According to the study, powerful influences on the placebo effect include the patient's observation of his own physical reactions, the patient's observation of the physician's behavior, and information from other sources that may verify the effects of the placebo.[64]

Expectations may actually cause physical reactions. In one Canadian study, more than half of the men who got placebo pills reported significant relief from symptoms of benign enlargement of the prostate gland, including faster urine flow. Researcher J. Curtis Nickel, who participated in the study, theorized that the men's positive *expectations* of the experimental drug's benefits may have actually eased nerve activity and caused smooth muscles in the bladder, prostate, and urethra to relax.[65]

Another theory is that placebos may be explained by people's differing sensitivity to bodily symptoms. There are two general types:

1. **Reducers.** These people are slow to perceive symptoms consciously. Even when they do perceive symptoms, they tend to deny them or ignore them until they get quite severe. In general, reducers do not get worried or alarmed about bodily symptoms—and are not as vulnerable to the effect of placebos.[66] Being a reducer isn't good in all situations, however. Studies have found that the absence of sensory input and stimulation can be very disturbing. Researchers have even noted that prisoners who are reducers and who are incarcerated get so starved for sensation that they deliberately hurt or mutilate themselves.

2. **Amplifiers.** These people amplify sensations that other people would be unaware of. They are even made uncomfortable by situations that most people would find to be neutral. According to researchers, these people seem "hard-wired" into their brains from the time they are born.

Somewhere in between the reducers and the amplifiers are the rest of us. How vulnerable a person is to the effects of a placebo depends on how aware he or she is of body symptoms. Researchers have found that seven characteristics determine whether you feel more symptomatic than the average person:

1. **Age.** Generally, the older the person, the more symptoms he or she feels and reports to a physician.

2. **Gender.** Women consistently report more bodily symptoms than do men. In fact, many studies indicate that women are more sensitive to changes in their bodies, feel less healthy, take more medications, and think of themselves as prone to illness more than do men in general.

3. **Social class.** People who have higher incomes and who are better educated generally believe themselves to be in better health. In general, as social class declines, the prevalence of medical symptoms and ill health increases.

4. **Ethnic background.** Studies show that Jews and Italian Americans exhibit an emotional and expressive response to pain. Anglo Americans, on the other hand, are more stoic and less likely to become as overwrought about illness. At the extreme end of the scale are the Irish Americans, who tend to completely deny pain.

5. **Marital status.** Single people over the age of thirty are more troubled by symptoms than are their married counterparts.

6. **Degree of self-consciousness.** People who are extremely self-conscious are more aware of bodily symptoms and more likely to report symptoms of illness.

7. **Control.** People who feel dependent on others and who feel less able to control what happens to them in life report more frequent and more severe symptoms.[67]

## Myths About Placebos

To understand how powerful faith is, it's important to understand how powerful the placebo effect can be—and important to debunk the most common myths about placebos:[68]

1. *Any symptoms that respond to placebos must be imaginary.* Nothing could be further from the truth. Research conducted at Harvard Medical School shows that placebos have been effective in relieving the very real symptoms of colds, headaches, seasickness, angina, anxiety, and post-operative pain.[69]

   Placebos have been shown to relieve symptoms that can be scientifically monitored. An excellent example of this was a woman who was complaining of severe nausea and vomiting. Nothing her doctors had been able to do for her seemed to help. Laboratory instruments were used to measure her stomach contractions; the pattern of contractions she exhibited was proof that she was indeed suffering from the nausea that she reported. Her symptoms were very real.

Her doctors finally offered her what they called an "extremely powerful" new wonder drug that would, without a doubt, relieve her nausea. Sure enough, within twenty minutes of taking the new drug, the woman's nausea disappeared. Not only did the nausea disappear, but the stomach contractions she was having also returned to normal.

The drug the woman had been given was syrup of ipecac, a standard remedy to induce vomiting. The woman's faith was so strong—and the placebo effect, as a result, was so powerful—that the drug actually had an opposite effect in relieving her nausea and vomiting.[70]

In other studies, placebos were powerful enough to stop symptoms that could not have been imaginable because they are easy to observe: coughs, nasal discharge, and skin rashes, for example. They have also been effective against symptoms that are easy to measure, such as fever and high blood pressure.

2. *Response to a placebo is a sign of mental illness.* As shown in the previous example of the woman who was nauseated and vomiting, placebos have an actual effect. It's faith, not mental illness, that is at work.

3. *Placebos cannot influence objective physiologic processes.* Just the opposite is true. Placebos have been found to have a profound influence over physiologic processes. One dramatic example was the story cited earlier about the lymphoma patient whose tumors "melted like snowballs" when he was given distilled water that he believed was a wonder drug. Placebos have been shown in scientific studies to affect the rate of stomach secretions, white blood cell counts, fever, blood cholesterol, dilation and constrictions of the pupils of the eye, and the stages of sleep.

In a classic experiment at a medical school, a pharmacology professor lectured to the students about the differences between stimulants and sedative medication. He went into great detail, describing the effects that each has on the body. He also described the side effects that each might have. He then told the students that he wanted them to take the medications and measure each other's responses. Half the class was given a pink pill ("stimulant") and the other half was given a blue pill ("sedative") to take. The students then measured and recorded each other's symptoms, blood pressure, and heart rate. Even though the pills were not real, the students experienced physiological reactions. About half had specific sedative-related physiological reactions that could be measured with laboratory equipment—such as decreased blood pressure, slowed heart rate, or increased pulse and blood pressure. They also experienced characteristic effects of the "stimulants," such as dizziness, watery eyes, and abdominal pain.

The researchers concluded that the color of the pills, coupled with the students' expectant faith, brought on literal physiological changes when they took the placebos.[71]

4. *Placebos can do no harm since they cannot cause any real side effects.* In the case just described, half of the medical students who took the pink or blue pills experienced not only appropriate physiological changes, but also the side effects generally associated with stimulants and sedatives. See the "Negative Effects" section later in this chapter for more examples.

In a variety of studies, placebos have been shown to cause very real side effects including nausea, skin irritation, hearing loss, diarrhea, constipation, headache, erratic heartbeat, pain, dizziness, insomnia, and even addiction. One researcher described a total of thirty-eight toxic effects directly attributable to placebos. The most common was drowsiness; others included headaches, nausea, and vomiting. Some of the effects were serious, such as impairment of liver function. Some side effects of placebos are so serious that patients have required hospitalization.[72] These negative effects are referred to as the "nocebo" effect.

In the Canadian study on benign prostate enlargement, men who took the placebo experienced the negative side effects generally ascribed to prostate medications—including impotence and reduced sex drive, nausea, diarrhea, and constipation.[73] In a separate study, researchers tested the effects of a drug called mephenesin on anxiety. Half of the patients in the study were given the drug, and half were given a placebo. The drug and the placebo produced almost identical side effects in the patients. Study participants complained of dizziness, nausea, and sleep disturbances as side effects. But these side effects were incurred by both the people who took the medication and the people who took the placebos.

One of the subjects had a severe reaction that mimicked shock: fainting, reduced blood pressure, and clammy white skin. That patient displayed the exact same reaction whether he took the drug or the placebo.[74]

## Physicians' Expectations

Many studies have indicated that a drug—real or placebo—is much more effective when the physician who administers it has strong faith in it. In fact, studies cited by Dr. Alfred Berg of the University of Missouri show that a physician's expectations of a drug's effectiveness can alter the "outcome of therapy by about 25 to 30 percent in either direction."[75] Studies have repeatedly shown, he says, that a drug works best when a physician's hopes for it are at their highest.

Researcher Jerry Solfvin extensively examined the power of the physician's underlying beliefs. Solfvin did three separate double-blind studies of the use of vitamin E in treating angina pectoris, the chest pain caused by coronary artery disease. Two of the studies were conducted by skeptics who did not believe vitamin E had any effect; sure enough, it didn't have any effect for the patients involved in the study. But the third study was conducted by an enthusiastic doctor who did believe that vitamin E would work. And, sure enough, it did.[76]

A similar, but earlier, experiment took place during the 1950s, when controversy surrounded the new drug meprobamate (one of the earliest tranquilizers). The doctors who believed in it consistently found that it worked; the skeptics thought it was no better than a placebo.

Researchers designed a double-blind study and involved two physicians— one who had an "enthusiastic, therapeutic" approach, and the other who had a "skeptical, experimental" approach toward the drug. Here's the catch: The doctors didn't know which pills were the placebos and which were the meprobamate. Neither did the patients. In fact, they didn't even know they were being involved in an experiment.

What happened? The meprobamate proved to be much more powerful than the placebo—but only for the physician who believed in it. The patients treated by the skeptical physician enjoyed no drug benefit at all from either pill.[77]

Dr. J. Mostyn Davis, a family practitioner at Pennsylvania's Geisinger Medical Center, remembers the time he prescribed what he believed to be a long-acting appetite suppressant. His patients, he relates, had great success with the drug. When he found out that the drug was, in fact, only a short-term appetite suppressant, he continued to use the drug in the same way, without telling the patients. But, he remembers, "now it worked for only a few hours! Was I unconsciously giving cues to my patients?" The mystery remains to this day.[78]

The physician, in fact, may be one of the most powerful placebos. One writer commented that the placebo effect "demonstrates that the physician functions as a healer. Because the medical profession relies so heavily on science and thus concentrates on diseases rather than illness, deals with cases rather than patients, and seeks to cure rather than provide care, physicians have lost faith in themselves as therapeutic instruments. Medicine has long been accused of being the silent profession, and it must be recognized that a physician is not merely a conduit of pills and procedures. Throughout history, rhetoric has moved people; and if people can be so moved to march, vote, or go to battle, certain words can have a tremendous effect on how someone feels."[79]

## Negative Effects

While the placebo effect can be positive and can bring on relief of symptoms as well as overall cures, the placebo effect can also be negative. People who believe that they are going to get sick actually can—and do. Cardiologist Herbert Benson, who has studied the placebo effect in depth, maintains that there are "dozens of examples throughout history of the scourge of negative placebo effects. Some even mimic terrible contagious diseases and can spread through large populations."[80]

An example of a negative placebo effect from history is the dancing manias that occurred during the Middle Ages. People who believed that they were "possessed" jerked and danced around uncontrollably in the streets. According to Benson, the sight of one person would arouse others until there were sometimes groups of more than a hundred jamming the streets. After hours of this dancing, Benson says, the victims would fall to the ground, exhausted. Some—who were actually healthy but believed that something was wrong with them—"dashed their brains out by running against walls and corners of buildings or rushed headlong into rapid rivers."[81]

Two examples from our own day show the power of faith and what can happen when it is misdirected. During the morning shift at a midwestern electronics plant, one worker suddenly became faint. Just moments later, a coworker who had helped the first victim also dropped to the floor. Within three hours, twenty of the factory workers had been taken to the hospital by ambulance complaining of the same set of symptoms: dizziness, headache, nausea, and difficulty breathing. Before the "plague" was over, at least ninety-three of the factory workers were afflicted with the strange sickness, which the victims attributed to a sickening odor wafting through the factory. These sicknesses persisted, even though the plant was closed three times while the maintenance engineers conducted detailed inspections and found no possible source for an odor.

In another example, a cargo ship damaged at sea was forced to dock in New Zealand. When it docked, unlabeled containers of an unknown chemical split open, spreading terrible-smelling fumes throughout the entire area. Local officials, alarmed by the fumes, immediately evacuated the area. People's belief that the horrible-smelling fumes were toxic was fueled by the quick reaction of local officials in evacuating the area. Panic spread like wildfire; hundreds of people were rushed to local hospitals, supposedly sick from inhaling the toxic fumes. When calmer heads prevailed and the chemical was finally identified, it was thoroughly tested. Even though it smelled bad, it was totally harmless.

## The Power of the Placebo

How powerful is the placebo effect? In recent tests, the placebo has "reduced attacks in angina patients by 82 to 93 percent; eased the suffering of almost two-thirds of migraine patients by 50 percent or more; given significant relief to about a third of patients with severe pain (without being addictive or interfering with mental function); led to improvement in up to half of patients with ulcerative colitis; resulted in healing of duodenal ulcers in 50 to 60 percent of patients; and significantly reduced tenderness of the joints in 22 percent of rheumatoid arthritis sufferers."[82]

There are many medical examples of the placebo effect—and examples of how it has worked, whether in medical form or in the form of surgery. In one study, the Coronary Drug Project Research Group compared five-year mortality rates among patients who were given the cholesterol-lowering drug clofibrate (Atromid-S) or a placebo.[83] Researchers observed each patient in the study to determine how faithful each was in taking the prescribed medication. The patients who took the clofibrate every day lived longer than the patients who frequently missed doses. The patients who took placebos every day also lived longer than the patients who frequently missed doses of placebos. There was no difference in mortality between the patients who regularly took clofibrate and the ones who regularly took placebos.

In another study, researchers tested the drug Stellazine on patients with chronic psychiatric illness. Half of the patients in the study received Stellazine, and half received a placebo. Neither the doctors who administered the medications nor the patients knew who were receiving active drugs and who were receiving placebos.[84]

To double-check their results, the researchers ran the test twice, using different sets of patients and different doses of both the drug and the placebo. In the first experiment, the patients who took Stellazine showed an improvement rate of 32 percent. The patients taking the placebo did even better, showing an improvement rate of 35 percent. In the second experiment, researchers doubled the dose of both the drug and the placebo. The patients experienced even greater improvement this time: The ones who took the Stellazine enjoyed an improvement rate of 67 percent. But, again, the ones taking the placebo did even better: Their improvement rate was 72 percent.

In summing up the results of the experiment, researchers say that "in many cases, particularly in those involving a person's state of mind, the effect of medication is influenced by the hope of cure, coupled with a belief in the physician, who in some unknown way conveys his sense of the strength and effectiveness of the drug."[85]

The placebo can even work in cases of "faith healing." New York psychologist Lawrence LeShan, an avid experimenter and authority in faith healing, relates an incident that he calls "the most dramatic single result" in his long experience. According to LeShan, a man he knew asked LeShan to do a long-distance healing for an extremely painful condition that required immediate and intensive therapy. As LeShan tells it, "I promised to do the healing that night, and the next morning when he awoke a 'miraculous cure' had occurred. The medical specialist was astounded, and offered to send me pre- and posthealing x-rays and to sponsor publication in a scientific journal. It would have been the psychic healing case of the century except for one small detail. In the press of overwork, I had forgotten to do the healing!" The patient who believed that he had meditated in his behalf had been healed anyway.[86]

The power of the placebo also extends to surgery. Alan Roberts, director of medical psychology at Scripps Clinic and Research Foundation, and his colleagues studied almost 7,000 patients who once had one of a number of treatments that were later thoroughly discredited, such as a surgical procedure for intractable asthma or the use of special dyes and fluorescent light on herpes sores. Even though the treatments were later found to be useless, 40 percent had reported "excellent" improvement, and another 30 percent had reported "good" results. In summing up his findings, Roberts said, "I think physicians have always been embarrassed by the notion that people get better when they're given dummy pills or dummy treatments."[87]

Some of the most convincing evidence regarding the placebo effect stems from surgical procedures in which incisions are made while the patient is under anesthesia, but no operation is performed.[88] One of the most classic examples of this hails from the mid-1950s. At that time, a new surgical procedure was introduced to help relieve the chest pains from coronary heart disease. The surgery, called an "internal mammary artery ligation," involved tying off an artery in the chest, with the result that more blood was available to the heart.

Initial response to the surgery was overwhelming. Almost half of the patients reported an improvement in chest pain—and two-thirds of them said that the improvement was considerable. Surgeons who pioneered the operation said that the patients also did better on an electrocardiogram after the surgery, and their exercise tolerance also improved. Thousands of patients requested the surgery, and the operation gained in popularity.[89]

But all of the surgeons who looked into the operation were not equally enthusiastic about it. In fact, two groups of surgeons were extremely skeptical and decided to test the procedure against a placebo. (Note: This kind of a test would not be allowed under today's rules of medical ethics.) For their test, the skeptical surgeons randomly divided patients slotted for surgery into one of two groups. The first group would receive the internal mammary artery ligation, as planned. The second group, without knowing it, would be put under general anesthesia, an incision would be made in the chest, the incision would be closed, yet no surgical procedure would have been performed on any artery.

The results were almost identical, whether the patients had arteries tied or not. Many of the patients in both groups experienced less anginal pain, increased tolerance for exercise, improvements on the electrocardiogram, and a reduced need for nitroglycerin. The studies demonstrated that "ligation of the internal mammary artery was no better than a skin incision, and that such an incision could lead to a dramatic, sustained placebo effect."[90]

After more than 10,000 patients underwent surgery, the surgery was abandoned. It was replaced by coronary artery bypass surgery, an operation that is still performed today. In coronary artery bypass surgery, diseased sections of the arteries that feed the heart are replaced by a new vein created from sections of veins removed from the patient's legs. At first glance, the surgery seems to be a resounding success: More than 90 percent of the patients who receive it report that their symptoms are relieved. Three-fourths of the patients who undergo surgery also perform better on an exercise stress test than they did before undergoing surgery.

But the placebo is at work again. All the patients actually receive the surgery, but of those who say they feel better, only about one in five—20 percent—show actual improvement of heart function when they are tested. Approximately 60 percent show no improvement at all; they are the same as they were before the surgery. And the other 20 percent are actually worse than they were before the surgery.[91] The percentages bear strong testimony to the power of faith: Patients who receive bypass surgery believe it will help them. And it does "help" more than 90 percent of them to feel better, even though only a small fraction actually improve.

The placebo effect has been shown to influence even the immune system. A number of animal studies have shown that the immune system can literally be "conditioned" by placebos, and a human study conducted at the University of Arkansas proved that expectations can determine the outcome of immune function.[92]

The researchers in the study told nine people who were positive for the tuberculosis skin test that they would be given a skin test on each arm once a month for the next six months to determine if they were still positive for the bacteria. Each month the subjects were tested. For the first five months, the right arm of each person was injected with a tuberculin solution. The left arm of each person, without the patient's knowledge, was injected with a simple saline solution. Naturally, the skin reaction appeared on the right arm of each person, but not the left arm. For the test during the sixth month, the researchers reversed the procedure: Saline was injected into the right arm, and the tuberculin solution was injected into the left arm. Nobody expected a reaction to occur on the left arm, so it did not. Only traces of a reaction occurred on any of the volunteers, even though all were still positive for the bacteria.[93]

Medically speaking, faith can move mountains. What we believe and what we expect are often more powerful than even the most potent pill or the most skilled surgeon's knife. Our task, then, is to unleash that powerful faith in a positive way, a way that will enhance our own healing.

One of the most diligent physicians of all time recognized the power and value of our faith and our beliefs. When he was asked to explain the secret of African witch doctors, humanitarian Albert Schweitzer replied with a simplicity that carries a message for all of us:

*The witch doctor succeeds for the same reason all the rest of us succeed. Each patient carries his own doctor inside him. We are at our best when we give the doctor within each patient a chance to go to work.*[94]

## ENDNOTES

1. N. Goddard, "A Response to Dawson's Critical Analysis of 'Spirituality as "Integrative Energy,"'" *Journal of Advanced Nursing* 31, no. 4 (2000): 968–79.
2. Caroline Young and Cyndie Koopsen, *Spirituality, Health, and Healing* (Thorofare, N.J.: Slack Incorporated, 2005), 59.
3. Thomas G. Plante and Allen C. Sherman, *Faith and Health: Psychological Perspectives* (New York: Guilford Press, 2001).
4. Young and Koopsen, *Spirituality,* 60.
5. Ibid., 60.
6. Dan Custer, *The Miracle of Mind Power* (Englewood Cliffs, N.J.: Prentice Hall, 1960).
7. Custer, *The Miracle.*
8. Deirdre Davis Brigham, "Shifting Consciousness, Creating Epiphanies, and Enabling Miracles," *The Psychology of Health, Immunity, and Disease,* vol. B, 49, in *Proceedings of the Sixth International Conference of the National Institute for the Clinical Application of Behavioral Medicine.*
9. Brigham, "Shifting Consciousness."
10. Linda Liu, "Faith Cures (Even Doctors Believe It!)," *McCall's* 126, 92, July 1999.
11. Thomas G. Plante and Allen G. Sherman, "Research on Faith and Health: New Approaches to Old Questions," in Plante and Sherman, *Faith and Health.*
12. Plante and Sherman, "Research."
13. Joan Borysenko, *Minding the Body, Mending the Mind* (Reading, Mass.:

Addison-Wesley Publishing Company, 1987), 10.

14. D. B. Larsen and H. G. Koenig, "Is God Good for Your Health? The Role of Spirituality in Medical Care," *Cleveland Clinic Journal of Medicine* 67, no. 2 (2000): 80–84; D. A. Matthews, "Prayer and Spirituality," *Rheumatic Diseases Clinics of North America* 26, no. 1 (2000): 177–87; and R. O. Scott, "A Look in the Mirror: Finding Our Way in This New Spiritual Landscape," *Spirituality and Aging* 4, no. 1 (2001): p. 26.

15. Examples of servicemen are from Jerome D. Frank, "Emotional Reactions of American Soldiers to an Unfamiliar Disease," *American Journal of Psychiatry* 102: 1946, 631–40, as reported in "The Medical Power of Faith," *Human Nature* (August 1978): 40–47.

16. Young and Koopsen, *Spirituality*, 61.

17. Ibid.

18. Ibid.

19. Carl E. Thoresen, Alex H. S. Harris, and Doug Oman, "Spirituality, Religion, and Health: Evidence, Issues, and Concerns," in Plante and Sherman, *Faith and Health*.

20. Young and Koopsen, *Spirituality*, 61.

21. Harold Koenig, *The Healing Power of Faith: Science Explores Medicine's Last Great Frontier* (New York: Simon & Schuster, 1999).

22. Herbert Benson, *Beyond the Relaxation Response* (New York: Times Books, 1984).

23. Benson, *Beyond*.

24. Paul Pearsall, *Super Immunity* (New York: McGraw-Hill, 1987).

25. Pearsall, *Super Immunity*.

26. Benson, *Beyond*.

27. Studies summarized from "Review Confirms 'Healing' Effects," *New Sense Bulletin* 16(8): 1991, 1.

28. Christina V. Miller, "Mental Powers: Divine Power over Blood Pressure," *Longevity*, September 1989, 78.

29. Borysenko, *Minding the Body*.

30. Blair Justice, "Those Who Stay Healthy," *New Realities*, July/August 1988, 35–39, 69–71.

31. Daniel Goleman, "Denial and Hope," *American Health*, December 1984, 54–61.

32. Custer, *The Miracle*.

33. Daniel Goleman, "The Faith Factor," *American Health*, May 1984, 48–53.

34. Frank, "Emotional Reactions."

35. Ibid.

36. Ibid.

37. The study descriptions are from ibid.

38. Larry Dossey, *Meaning and Medicine: A Doctor's Tales of Breakthrough and Healing* (New York: Bantam Books, 1991), 158–59.

39. Steve Wright, "Speaking Out," *Nursing Times* 95, no. 10, 19, March 10–16, 1999.

40. Mary Baker Eddy, *Science and Health* (New York: Harper & Row, 1875).

41. Goleman, "The Faith Factor."

42. "Review Confirms 'Healing Effects.'"

43. Leonard A. Sagan, *The Health of Nations* (New York: Basic Books, 1987).

44. Frank, "Emotional Reactions."

45. "Healing or Hoping?" *American Health*, January/February: 1987, 55.

46. "Healing or Hoping?"

47. Associated Press, "Hospital Tries Out Laying on of Hands," *Modern Healthcare* 28, no. 19, 50, May 11, 1998.
48. Bernhardt J. Hurwood, "Healing and Believing," *Health,* June 1984, 15–21.
49. Larry Dossey, *Healing Words,* 48.
50. Bernie Siegel, *Peace, Love, and Healing* (New York: Harper & Row, 1989), 21.
51. Tamar Nordenberg, "The Healing Power of Placebos," *FDA Consumer,* January/February 2000, 14–17.
52. Stewart Wolf, "The Pharmacology of Placebos," *Pharmacological Reviews* II: 1959, 689–704.
53. "Success of Placebos May Be Connected to Imagery," *Brain/Mind Bulletin* 14(10): 1989, 1, 8.
54. Nordenberg, "The Healing Power."
55. O. H. P. Pepper, "A Note on the Placebo," *American Journal of Pharmacy* 117: 1945, 409–12.
56. Arthur J. Barsky, *Worried Sick: Our Troubled Quest for Wellness* (Boston: Little, Brown, 1988).
57. Stewart Wolf, "Effects of Suggestion and Conditioning on the Action of Chemical Agents in Human Subjects: The Pharmacology of Placebos," *Journal of Clinical Investigation* 29: 1950, 100–9.
58. Herbert Benson and Eileen M. Stuart, *The Wellness Book* (New York: Birch Lane Press, 1992), 9.
59. Benson and Stuart, *The Wellness Book.*
60. Robert Ornstein and David Sobel, *The Healing Brain* (New York: Simon & Schuster, 1987), 37.
61. Herbert Benson and Mark D. Epstein, "The Placebo Effect: A Neglected Asset in the Care of Patients," *Journal of the American Medical Association* 232: 1975, 1225–26.
62. Nordenberg, "The Healing Power."
63. Morton Hunt, "Faith, Hope, and Placebos," *Longevity,* May 1991, 74.
64. "Success of Placebos May Be Connected to Imagery."
65. Nordenberg, "The Healing Power."
66. Information on "reducers" and "amplifiers" is from Barsky, *Worried Sick.*
67. Ibid.
68. Howard Brody, "The Placebo Response," *Drug Therapy,* July 1986, 106, 115–31.
69. Hurwood, "Healing and Believing."
70. Robert Ornstein and David Sobel, *Healthy Pleasures* (Reading, Mass.: Addison-Wesley Publishing Company, 1989), 29.
71. Ornstein and Sobel, *The Healing Brain,* 79–80.
72. J. Mostyn Davis, "Don't Let Placebos Fool You," *Postgraduate Medicine* 88(4): 1990, 22.
73. Nordenberg, "The Healing Power."
74. Wolf, "The Pharmacology of Placebos."
75. "Success of Placebos."
76. Dossey, *Healing Words,* 135.
77. Ibid., 135–36.
78. Davis, "Don't Let Placebos Fool You."
79. Howard M. Spiro, "Are Placebos Legitimate Therapy?" *Patient Care,* May 15, 1991, 69.
80. Benson, *Beyond.*
81. The three examples are from ibid.

82.  Hunt, "Faith," 68.
83.  Brody, "The Placebo Response."
84.  Frank, "Emotional Reactions."
85.  Ibid.
86.  Larry Dossey, *Healing Words* (San Francisco: HarperSanFrancisco, 1993), 78.
87.  Rita Rubin, "Placebos' Healing Power," *U.S. News and World Report,*
     November 22, 1993, 78.
88.  Herbert Benson and D. P. McCallie, "Angina Pectoris and the Placebo Effect,"
     *New England Journal of Medicine* 300(25): 1979, 1424–29.
89.  E. G. Diamond, C. F. Kittle, and J. E. Crockett, "Evaluation of Internal Mam-
     mary Artery Ligation and Sham Procedure in Angina Pectoris," *Circulation* 18:
     1958, 712–13; and L. A. Cobb, G. I. Thomas, D. H. Dillard, K. A. Merendino,
     and R. A. Bruce, "An Evaluation of Internal-Mammary-Artery Ligation by a
     Double-Blind Technic," *New England Journal of Medicine* 260(2): 1959, 1115–18.
90.  Benson and McCallie, "Angina Pectoris."
91.  Ornstein and Sobel, *The Healing Brain,* 81.
92.  G. R. Smith and S. M. McDaniel, "Psychologically Mediated Effect on the
     Delayed Hypersensitivity Reaction to Tuberculin in Humans," *Psychosomatic
     Medicine* 45(1): 1983, 65–70.
93.  Smith and McDaniel, "Psychologically Mediated Effect."
94.  Source unknown.

# CHAPTER 17

# The Healing Power of Optimism

*Every good thought you think is contributing its share
to the ultimate result of your life.*

—Grenville Kleiser

## Learning Objectives

- Define optimism.
- Discuss the characteristics of optimists.
- Understand how optimism influences health.
- Discuss the impact of optimism on immune function and healing.
- Understand the influence of optimism on mental health and performance.

According to Webster's dictionary, optimism is "an inclination to anticipate the best possible outcome." To redefine it psychologically, according to Ornstein and Sobel, optimism is "the tendency to seek out, remember, and expect pleasurable experiences. It is an active priority of the person, not merely a reflex that prompts us to 'look on the sunny side.'"[1]

A growing body of evidence indicates that optimists live longer and they probably enjoy better health along the way as well. Scientific evidence suggests that optimism, the habit of positive thinking, has a specific effect on the physiological functioning of the body. In a real, physical sense, optimists are healthier. Their immune systems are stronger. And as a group, they do live longer.

## Who Are Optimists?

Optimists are people who generally believe that good, rather than bad, things will happen to them. They believe that the future will work out well; they approach the world in an active, productive way. They take reality into account, but they do everything possible with the reality they find. Optimism has a lot to do with other positive qualities as well, such as happiness, self-efficacy, and hardiness.

The readers of *Psychology Today* were asked what happiness means to them. More than 52,000 responded. Compiling their answers, the authors of the survey concluded that happiness "comes from tending one's own garden instead of coveting one's neighbor's. . . . Happiness, in short, turns out to be more a matter of how you regard your circumstances than of what the circumstances are."[2]

Research shows that an optimistic bias is far more common than was once considered. The community of psychotherapy is realizing that normal, healthy individuals do downplay their faults and the negative things that happen to them—and that the people who lean toward optimism are the most healthy, both physically and mentally.

Psychologists Shelley Taylor of UCLA and Jonathon Brown of Southern Methodist University in Dallas say that research shows that most people view themselves in an optimistic light. "They judge themselves to be nicer, smarter, more charming, and prettier than even their closest admirers judge them to be," the psychologists assert. "Normal, healthy people see themselves more kindly than does the cold eye of the camera or even the caring eyes of family and friends. They think they're more talented and able than they are."[3]

Even aside from improving health, optimism is a positive force. "Optimism galvanizes people," says University of Michigan Psychologist Christopher Peterson. "It sets you in motion. To be optimistic in the true sense is not to wear a smile button, but to be a problem-solver."[4]

The "experts" used to believe that it was important to have a cold, hard perception of reality. Psychologist Robert Ornstein and physician David Sobel point out that psychologist Sidney Jourard once wrote, "The ability to perceive reality as it 'really is' is fundamental to effective functioning. It is considered one of the two preconditions to the development of health." Ornstein and Sobel continue that modern psychology and clinical research contradicts this—and that healthy people are not accurate perceivers of reality. "Expecting to be pleased, healthy people cultivate a set of illusions. They inflate their own importance and have an exaggerated belief in their ability to control their destiny."[5]

While a significant amount of research has been done on optimism, there are still four unresolved issues in regard to the influence of optimism on health:[6]

1. Should optimism and pessimism be considered as polar ends of a single dimension—attitude—or should they be considered as two separate dimensions?

2. How important is optimism in promoting health? What *unique* effects does it have, as considered separately from all other influences?

3. How are the effects of optimism related to health?

4. Can specific health behaviors change or mediate the relationship between optimism and health?

## Characteristics of Optimists

Seven-year-old Kealan Jewell is positive about everything. She unabashedly declares she's one of the most popular girls in her class. When asked what she wants to be when she grows up, she doesn't think twice. "I'm going to be an artist," she says. "I'd like to write a book, but I can't find the time."[7]

Kealan is an optimist, as are most other children her age. So was American philosopher Henry Thoreau, who used to lie in bed for a few minutes every morning to think positive thoughts. He would remind himself that he was healthy, that his mind was alert, that his work was interesting, that the future looked bright, and that many people trusted him. When he got out of bed, he entered a world filled with the kind of positive, good people and opportunities that he expected—a kind of "self-fulfilling prophecy."

It usually is easy to tell the difference between an optimist and a pessimist. The optimist has an entirely different explanation for things. The optimistic driver acknowledges (or "blames") the reduced visibility, the slick and snow-packed streets, and other adverse conditions for his accident. Then he realizes he hasn't had much experience on snowy roads and tells himself that he'll have to be more careful until he gets more experience. The pessimistic driver, on the other hand, blames himself. His internal reasoning goes something like this: "I'm such a poor driver. I'll never learn to drive safely. Every time I try something new, I screw it up."[8]

Optimists have a number of qualities in common. Probably the most common is that they see the good in situations and they truly expect things to go their way. According to Michael Scheier, professor of psychology at Pittsburgh's Carnegie Mellon University, researchers are finding that "anticipating a favorable outcome leads an optimist to do things that actually determine the final outcome. Optimists expect things to turn out well, but they also do things that can change the course of events."[9]

In addition, optimists see events in their lives as controllable—an apt attitude because, says Scheier, optimism comes from the Latin word *ops*, meaning power. When something bad does happen, optimists are not defeated. Instead, they make a plan of action, follow it, and work quickly before the situation gets out of hand. They expect that they will be able to handle anything that comes along (and they are usually right).

Optimists don't give up; they are known for their perseverance. Optimists have a knack for staying focused on the positive and are able to keep going when others might quit.

When something bad happens, optimists view it as an isolated occurrence—not as part of a general trend or life pattern. In day-to-day events, in fact, optimists dismiss the bad and instead internalize the good. They interpret events and circumstances in their favor, a trait that helps them stay positive even when confronted by situations they truly cannot control (such as the death of a loved one).

Optimists tend to see the future through "rose-colored glasses." They believe that they will have a happy life filled with adventure and good health. When they marry, they believe that the marriage will succeed and be fulfilling; they don't consider or dwell on the possibility of divorce. When they have children, they believe that their children will be happy and healthy and well-behaved. In essence, they don't think about the bad things that could happen. But underlying their attitude is a firm belief that if something bad does somehow occur, they'll be able to "fix it" with no problem.

All this cheerfulness is not to say that optimists can't face reality or see when they're "in over their heads"; optimists express acceptance or resignation when needed. University of Miami Psychologist Charles Carver says that researchers "don't want to imply that people should put on a happy face and go around being mindlessly cheerful all the time. Even optimists have occasional doubts or fail sometimes. By resignation, we mean the ability to say, 'I'm not going to pretend this isn't happening, but if I have to put up with it, I will.'"[10] Scheier maintains that they have the instinct to know when to charge forward or when to back off—and their optimistic attitude helps them cope far more effectively when situations come up.

In his book *You Can't Afford the Luxury of a Negative Thought*, popular author Peter McWilliams and his coauthor John-Roger summarize optimism with this challenge:

> *It's as though there were two attorneys in your mind, one gathering evidence for "Life is Awful" and the other gathering evidence for "Life is Wonderful." You're the judge and can rule out any evidence you want. Your decision is final. Which judicial ruling do you suppose would lead to more joy, happiness, peace, and ease?*[11]

## How Optimism Influences Health

When diagnosed with ankylosing spondylitis, a devastating degenerative disease, former *Saturday Review* editor Norman Cousins refused to give up. He fought back, using a number of factors (such as enhanced nutrition, optimism, and laughter) to overcome his disease. When news of his amazing recovery surfaced, much of the attention focused on the factor of laughter—which, although it was important, was not the only thing that Cousins believes led to his recovery.

"I didn't say that I was cured through laughter, but it made for interesting and catchy newspaper treatment," Cousins says, referring to the accounts of his fight against the illness. "Laughter played a part, of course, but laughter was a metaphor for the full range of positive emotions—hope, faith, love, determination, confidence—all the things that are part of the ability of the human mind to get the most out of whatever is possible."[12]

A growing body of evidence gives increasing credibility to the idea that optimism and positive emotions promote health. Even positive denial can be health-promoting. Psychologist Richard Lazarus believes that a sense of "positive denial"—a refusal to believe in something negative, as long as it is not carried to the extreme—helps keep hopes up, sustains morale, improves health, and reduces anxiety.[13] But researchers who have conducted studies on attitude and beliefs agree with one basic principle: A positive attitude and belief in the body's own healing abilities can certainly supplement medical treatment, but should never replace it. Cousins, Yale oncologist and surgeon Bernie Siegel, and others who are at the "battle front," stress the idea that the best possible outcome results when optimism and positive thinking work hand-in-hand with the medical treatment offered by competent physicians.

Exactly what role can optimism play, then? For one thing, it appears that an optimistic attitude can actually protect a person from getting sick in the first place. For the study conducted by Petersen and Vaillant on a group of armed services veterans who had graduated from Harvard University, Seligman and his colleagues recently reviewed the original comments, questionnaires, health records, and other data for ninety-nine of the Harvard graduates who participated in the study. The researchers found that the men who were the most optimistic in their original writings had the best health forty years later. Their own perception of their experiences was significantly associated with later physical and mental illness; those with an optimistic outlook were healthy, and those with a gloomy outlook were ill (or dead).[14]

In writing down their experiences during the war, the pessimists, who were in worse health at the end of the study, penned remarks like, "Giving orders was sometimes very hard, if not impossible, because I always had this problem of dealing with men under me, even later in the war when I had the appropriate rank."

The healthy optimists, on the other hand, recorded sentiments such as, "During the war I was occasionally bored, because anyone who's ever been on a ship is bored to tears." The optimist, even though he had a bad experience, didn't blame it on his own shortcomings. He was bored, but isn't everyone bored on a ship?

In summing up the study, Seligman and his colleagues wrote, "If you always go around thinking, 'It's my fault, it's going to last forever, and it's going to undermine everything I do,' then when you do run into further bad events, you become at risk for poor health."[15]

Optimism has been shown to have an impact on all kinds of disease conditions, including those as serious as cardiovascular disease. With cardiovascular disease being the most prevalent cause of death in the United States—affecting one in four people every year—researchers have tried to identify not only the causes of heart disease, but also what makes successful patients able to make the health changes they need.

A huge role in changing cardiovascular health behaviors is what researchers call "dispositional optimism,"[16] the belief that one's outcomes will be positive instead of negative. Optimists, say the researchers, are more likely than pessimists to believe that good outcomes are attainable and bad outcomes are avoidable, so the optimists put forth greater effort to attain the desired outcome.[17]

Various studies have provided "compelling evidence"[18] that dispositional optimism contributes to greater success among cardiac patients. In a study conducted at the University of Massachusetts Medical Center, patients in a cardiac rehabilitation program were studied to determine which ones were most successful in making the behavioral changes needed to protect their cardiac health. Those who were most optimistic at the beginning of the program had the greatest success in reducing levels of saturated fat, increasing aerobic exercise capacity, reducing body fat, and generally lowering their cardiac risk.[19]

Optimism and pessimism can even play a role in maladies as simple as the common cold. Carnegie Mellon University Psychologist Sheldon Cohen worked with other researchers at the Common Cold Unit in England to determine what factors were at play in susceptibility to colds. Their findings point the finger at optimism and pessimism, and "suggest the possibility that there is a relationship between psychological factors and susceptibility to colds."[20]

In three separate studies constructed in much the same way, researchers tested undergraduate college students to see which had optimistic outlooks and which had pessimistic outlooks; they then tracked the students for various periods to see which got sick, had adverse symptoms, or had to visit the doctor.

Psychologist Christopher Peterson studied students at Virginia Tech in Blacksburg, Virginia. He reported that pessimistic students were ill twice as many days and had four times as many doctor visits over the course of a year compared with optimistic students. Peterson expressed particular interest in the fact that 95 percent of all the ill students had infectious diseases—the common cold, sore throats, flu, pneumonia, ear infections, venereal diseases, and mononucleosis. Apparently the pessimistic students were less able to fight infection. "This suggests that how we view things may directly affect our immune system," he says.[21] The pessimists, he points out, may have been more likely to get colds and other illnesses in part because they were less apt to seek medical advice or take simple medical precautions.

Peterson was able to confirm his theories with results from several other studies. In one study,[22] he and his colleagues studied summer school students at the University of Michigan. Again, he assessed general style to determine whether each student was pessimistic or optimistic. Then researchers carefully followed the health of each student, asking for an assessment on a daily basis. Again, the pessimists were the most ill—and 95 percent of the reported symptoms were from colds or the flu, suggesting a breakdown in the ability to resist infectious diseases.

In a similar study, in which Carnegie Mellon researchers found that optimistic students reported fewer ills, researchers wrote, "Pessimists, as a rule, care less about their health. In addition, pessimists blame themselves for their failures but then do little to further improve their lot. Optimists, on the other hand, view failures as problems that can be fixed. They meet their problems head on, form a plan of action, and achieve results."[23]

The impact of optimism on health may be due to the tendency of optimists to take control, proactively engage in improving their conditions, attend to health threats, and engage in health-promoting behaviors. Researchers point out that optimism influences health-promoting behavior because optimists focus on problems and work to solve them rather than avoiding those problems. When they think something is attainable, optimists will continue to strive toward their goal, even when progress is difficult or slow.[24]

Studies have shown that those who are most optimistic in their outlook also pay the greatest attention to health risks and threats. Research at the University of Maryland showed that people who are optimistic about their health and their future in general are much more likely to pay attention to information about health risks or threats to health and to act positively on that information.[25]

Some believe that optimists are unrealistic in their outlook, ignoring or avoiding the very real negative factors that surround them. The results of several fascinating studies show, however, that optimists are generally very realistic about their situations. But instead of reacting with a negative outlook, they proactively work to cope with difficult situations and bring about positive change. In one, researchers collected information from 3,000 people living in high-rise public housing in more than two dozen neighborhoods.

According to Michael Greenberg, professor and codirector of the New Jersey Graduate Program in Public Health at Rutgers University:

> *Network television, newspapers, public policy documents, and scholarly studies tell Americans that high-rise, public housing projects in Chicago, Detroit, New York City, and other cities are places where nightmares are born and lived. Residents are characterized as terrorized by gangs, unable to move around within their buildings because of unlit hallways and malfunctioning elevators, afraid that their children will become victims of illegal drugs and stray bullets, unfairly treated by police and the judicial system, and subjected to numerous other indignities and risks that cumulatively cause hopelessness.*[26]

Greenberg realized that these conditions challenge dispositional optimism—the "expectation that people will work for a positive outcome even under difficult conditions."[27] Greenberg's study, which canvassed more than two dozen neighborhoods, was part of an ongoing project aimed at understanding how residents of decaying, crime-ridden neighborhoods characterize their environment. Specifically, Greenberg and his colleagues designed their study to

- Determine the degree to which optimism (and the health-related behaviors associated with it) existed in high-rise public housing.

- Determine whether optimists realized the severity of the problems that existed in their housing.

- Determine whether optimists were more likely to engage in behavior that would protect their own health and the health of others in the housing.

Before he began his formal study, Greenberg spanned a period of three years during which he had informal conversations with more than four dozen people who

> *lived adjacent to a massive rat-infested trash pile or an unremediated hazardous waste site, or across the street from houses that were stripped of their aluminum siding and copper pipes and then burned by drug-addicted arsonists. Rather than cringing in fear at their difficult neighborhood conditions, some residents felt they could control their local environment. They welcomed the challenge of improving the neighborhood, spoke about activities . . . to improve the neighborhood, and expected, or at least hoped, for a positive outcome. . . . These kind of responses are associated with dispositional optimism.*[28]

These informal conversations—using people "who were interviewed because they were standing outside when the author was in the neighborhood rather than being scientifically selected"—led Greenberg to wonder how dispositional optimism impacted the residents of these projects. For his formal study, Greenberg chose a controversial high-rise public housing project in central New Jersey. At the time of the study, the project had been threatened with demolition for about a decade; more than 200 of the units were occupied, and the project was surrounded by a bridge, a heavily used highway, and a group of low-rise housing units occupied primarily by lower-middle-income blacks and Hispanics. As a foundation for his survey, Greenberg relied on questions in the U.S. Department of Commerce's biannual *American Housing Survey for the United States*. Survey respondents were asked first to indicate whether certain potentially harmful situations existed in the project (such as crime or decaying conditions). Then they were asked whether they were willing or able to take action on their own behalf or on behalf of the neighborhood. A standard test was used to determine whether each survey respondent was an optimist or a pessimist.

Here's what Greenberg found: Optimists and pessimists identified about the same number and types of problems and amenities in the neighborhood. Their rating of neighborhood quality was almost identical, too. In other words, the optimists didn't minimize the serious problems that existed in their housing project. However, the optimists were *much* more likely to attend a public meeting, participate in a church or civic function, and in other ways engage in neighborhood activities that helped them cope with extremely difficult conditions. They were also more likely to proactively engage in trying to solve the problems than to withdraw, as did the pessimists.[29]

## Optimism and Healing

Not only can optimism help keep a person healthy, but it can also boost the body's own mechanisms to speed the healing process. Anxious to see exactly how much power the mind has over the body, researchers decided to look at the example of warts. Warts are caused by a virus, and they are controlled by the immune system. When the immune system does not work to control the virus, warts appear. Researchers at Boston's Massachusetts General Hospital hypnotized patients with intractable warts and told them, under hypnosis, that the body would heal itself. In almost all the cases, the body did just that; the warts disappeared.

Psychologist and avid skier Lonnie Barbach pulled the ligaments in her left knee and spent a painful six weeks on crutches. Two years later, she injured her right knee in the same way—skiing—and to the same extent. This time she pulled all her optimism to the fore and used mental training to imagine that her ligaments were tightening and that the pain, soreness, and swelling were diminishing. Without using crutches, she was completely healed in fewer than three weeks.[30]

Optimism can make a big difference in surgical outcomes, too. In a study conducted by Dr. Charles S. Carver of the University of Miami and

Dr. Michael F. Scheier of Carnegie Mellon University, coronary bypass surgery patients were questioned the day before surgery and again one week after surgery. Based on the results of the first interview, researchers categorized each patient as being an optimist or a pessimist. While their mental attitudes were different, their physical conditions were similar and the outlook for their recovery was the same.[31]

Not everyone had the same results after surgery, however. The optimists were busy making plans for the time when they would be released from the hospital; after surgery, they sought information about what they could do to improve their recovery. The pessimists, on the other hand, took an "observer" stance and were much less involved in helping themselves. Although the outlook was the same for all patients, the optimists had a much speedier recovery, marred by fewer complications. In summing up the study, Carver concluded that "optimists may experience more success because they deal with their problems earlier than pessimists do, and in a more direct, goal-oriented way. . . . They use a strategy for coping that is most adaptive and least dysfunctional."[32]

Optimism may make such a difference to recovery that some hospitals have begun using aids to boost it—such as an "artificial window" that provides a peaceful scene as well as simulating the change between day and night. Stanford was the first medical facility in the country to use the window, a four-by-five-foot computer-controlled light box behind a blowup of a slide shot by California nature photographer Joey Fischer. Fischer saw the need for the "window" when his own father had a heart attack and spent many hours counting holes in the hospital ceiling tiles because there was nothing else to look at. In the window is a peaceful pasture topped by billowing clouds; an electronic digital timer produces 650 separate light changes every twenty-four hours, mimicking dawn to twilight.[33]

Optimism can even make a difference in illnesses as grave as cancer. A University of California, Los Angeles, research team launched a national survey of cancer specialists in an attempt to find out which psychosocial factors were most important in helping patients overcome the disease. A total of 649 oncologists responded to the survey, and reported on their experiences in treating more than 100,000 cancer patients. More than 90 percent of the physicians who responded to the survey said that the most significant factor in effective treatment was the attitude of hope and optimism.[34]

A number of studies confirm that point of view. In one, Sandra Levy and her colleagues at the University of Pittsburgh School of Medicine studied middle-aged women who had breast cancer. They put special emphasis on the psychological factors that seemed related to survival, especially the differences between optimism and pessimism. They carefully interviewed each of the thirty-six women at the beginning of the study and then observed them for four years. Although optimism was not the strongest predictor (the number of initial cancer sites was the strongest predictor), Levy was able to fairly accurately predict who would still be alive at the end of four years based on their outlook. The optimists won out.[35]

Dr. G. Frank Lawlis and Jeanne Achterberg, a husband-wife team at the University of Texas Health Science Center in Dallas, conducted a series of studies that showed that people become and stay healthy in response to optimism and positive attitude—and that optimism has an impact even on cancer. In their studies, Lawlis and Achterberg studied the personalities of 200 terminal cancer patients; they found that certain personality traits were common to those who lived much longer than they had been expected to live: The survivors utterly refused to give up. They were open to new ideas. They rejected their role as invalids. They refused to accept the limits of their illness. And, most important, they were optimistic. They believed in themselves, in their ability to beat the cancer.

Thirty years of cancer research by Dr. Lawrence LeShan has shown that those who do best are those who remain optimistic. Norman Cousins, a longtime believer in the impact of emotions, says that "emotions play a profound part in bringing on disease and in helping to combat it. What you think, what you believe, and how you react to experiences can impair or aid the workings of the body's immune system."

Indeed, a positive attitude and a belief that you can overcome illness go a long way in boosting immunity and conquering disease, according to significant evidence obtained from clinical practice and carefully controlled studies. Many examples have been reported of patients whose positive attitudes helped them conquer their supposedly terminal conditions—especially cancer.

One study in England helps substantiate that philosophy. Dr. Steven Greer and his colleagues followed the progress of women who underwent mastectomies for early-stage breast cancer; he evaluated the psychological condition of each patient and her attitude toward her disease. Five years later he noticed a common thread among those who had overcome the disease: They reacted with either strong denial or a fighting spirit, buoyed by the optimism that the cancer would not defeat them.[36]

## Imaging

A positive personality and mindset can do even more. Researchers now believe that a positive practice called *imaging* may mobilize the body's physical resources. Positive imaging—the ability to concentrate on images that represent the body's fight against disease—is a newly recognized and little-understood phenomenon that has begun to attract considerable attention in the medical profession. It was first used as a therapy to treat illness by Dr. O. Carl Simonton, with the Cancer Counseling and Research Center in Fort

Worth, Texas. Although scientists and researchers don't understand its effects on the immune system, one thing is obvious: It can sometimes help, even when the odds for recovery seem bleak. As we understand it, positive imaging seems to be an example of the power of the mind over the body.

Impressed by Simonton's results and curious about the effect of imaging on the immune systems of cancer victims, George Washington University Biochemist Nicholas Hall began teaching the system of positive imaging to his patients. One of Hall's patients was a man with prostate cancer that had metastasized to the bone marrow. Hall taught his patient imaging, and the patient was tested one to two times a week while he was practicing it. While the patient was practicing imaging, his white blood cell count was up and his body produced greater amounts of thymosin, a thymic hormone that might help regulate the immune response. When instructed to stop imaging, the patient's white blood cell count dropped severely and thymosin was almost undetectable in his body. Research has found that imagery can help reduce pain and stress, alter the course of disease, and improve patients' outlook on their illness.[37]

Psychologist Patricia Norris, clinical director of the Biofeedback and Psychophysiology Center at the Menninger Foundation, relates a remarkable story about positive imaging. Anna, who had a malignant tumor growing rapidly at the back of her neck, had been given only three months to live. The cancer had virtually crippled her: She was hunched over, her head was forced painfully to one side, and her right arm was paralyzed and contracted. Her doctor had instructed her to do the sensible thing: Go home and make the necessary arrangements for the futures of her young children.

Norris instructed Anna in positive imaging. Anna began to visualize her tumor as a dragon on her back; she imagined her white blood cells to be knights that were attacking the tumor with swords.

A year later, Norris saw Anna again. A remarkable change had taken place: Her arm was fully mobile, and the tumor had shrunk. The next time the two met, Anna was in total remission. (Note: Although imaging may be helpful in some circumstances, it should never replace appropriate and proven medical treatment.)

## Other Methods of Using Optimism to Heal

One oncologist in Houston utilizes optimism to its fullest: Before he ever treats a patient for cancer, he introduces the patient to another patient who has survived and conquered the same condition. This method has met with some success.

Another factor that can't be ignored is the simple fact that optimists tend to do more toward prevention and respond more actively if they do become ill.[38] They tend to exercise better health behaviors. And if they get sick, they respond in a more positive way by getting more sleep, decreasing work loads, visiting the physician, and following the physician's orders.

## Optimism: A Boost to Immunity

Experts in the field of psychoneuroimmunology have learned that there is a complex relationship between the brain and the immune system. Tucked beneath the breastbone in the chest is the thymus gland, the organ that produces T cells (immune blood cells). Psychologists Karen Bulloch, Denis Darko, and Michael Irwin found that an intricate network of nerve fibers connects the thymus gland with other parts of the immune system—the spleen, lymph nodes, and bone marrow—as well as to the cells of the body and the brain itself.

Research also indicates that there are hormonal and chemical links between the brain and the immune system.[39] According to experiments by immunologist Ed Blalock at the University of Alabama at Birmingham, "The immune cells communicate with the brain in the same way the brain and glands talk to them—through hormones." Blalock found that "the immune cells can produce hormones, such as growth hormone, thyroid-stimulating hormone, and reproductive hormones."[40]

While at the National Institute of Mental Health, Candace Pert and her colleague, Michael Ruff, announced that monocytes—the immune cells that help heal wounds, ingest bacteria, and repair tissue—are sensitive to chemicals produced in the brain. These chemicals, called neuropeptides, are concentrated in the brain's limbic system, the center that controls emotions.[41]

Emotions, then, can have impact on the immune system—and optimism is one of the emotions that seems to have the strongest ties. In his work over several decades, psychologist Seligman found real physiological differences between pessimists and optimists. In one study, he and his colleagues measured the disease-fighting cells in the blood of 300 people whose average age was seventy-one. The optimists had the healthier immune systems.[42]

In another study measuring optimism and the immune system, Leslie Kamen and her colleagues at the University of Pennsylvania studied mostly healthy middle-aged and elderly adults. Each was interviewed, and blood samples taken from each were measured to determine robustness of the immune system. Adults who were optimistic were found to have the strongest immune response; those who were pessimistic had the weakest.[43]

Other studies have yielded similar results. At the Medical Illness Counseling Center in suburban Maryland, ten cancer patients added guided imagery to their conventional chemotherapy treatment in an attempt to mobilize their own defenses against their cancers. After a year, all ten were still alive. And blood tests showed that their white blood cells had multiplied to fight the cancer cells.[44]

In a study at Michigan State University, patients used a combination of imagery and relaxation coupled with the optimistic belief that their treatment would work. Among those in the study, patients were able to cause an average of 60 percent of their white blood cells to leave the bloodstream and enter the surrounding tissue.[45]

In a study at Harvard, a group of people imagined that their T cells were attacking cold and flu viruses. That imagery—boosted by optimism—caused both T cell counts and immunoglobulin A counts to increase, multiplying the strength of the immune system.[46]

The ability of optimism to boost the immune system may hold benefits for victims of acquired immune deficiency syndrome (AIDS), which ordinarily knocks out the body's immune system. New York psychologist Lewis Katoff maintains that positive thinking plays "an important role" in helping AIDS victims survive longer. Katoff, reporting on the first-ever study of the attitudes of AIDS victims who have survived three years or longer, said of the victims that they "are not depressed. They refuse to give up."[47]

## Optimism's Effect on Mental Health and Performance

In addition to better physical health, optimists score better on performance and mental health—especially in resisting the effects of stress. Writing about some of the greatest entrepreneurs of our day, *Success* editor Scott DeGarmo penned the sentiment that "learning how to rebound with optimism is part of adapting to a world of constant change." Optimism, he says, is one of the key characteristics of the men and women who change the shape of the nation through their entrepreneurial ventures. He quotes Ralph Waldo Emerson in saying that these optimists display "a wild courage, a stoicism not of the schools but of the blood."[48]

Seligman, who has studied optimism extensively, says that the "link between optimism and performance is basically persistence. Optimists keep at it; pessimists give up and fail, even if they have equal talent. And because optimists are always hopeful about the outcome, they tend to take more risks and try more new things."[49]

Seligman has shown that optimists are more successful and perform better than pessimists in almost all fields, including education, business, sports, and politics. He successfully predicted that Bush would face Dukakis in the 1988 presidential campaign long before the crowded field of contenders was narrowed, and he made his prediction based solely on optimistic characteristics. "Forget about the deficit and prayer in schools," one researcher summed. "A leading determinant for political wins is the level of optimism candidates convey. Dukakis and Bush came out on top, based on careful analysis of their stump speeches. Alexander Haig, on the other hand, was at the bottom of Seligman's list of optimistic traits (as was Gary Hart), and the first to withdraw."[50]

Seligman has long been convinced that optimists perform so much better than pessimists in almost every way that optimism should be taken into account when hiring personnel. He was able to convince insurance giant Metropolitan Life that his theory was right—and he developed a twenty-minute written examination to screen applicants for the trait of optimism. Metropolitan Life then administered the test to 15,000 recruits, many of whom had failed the industry examination the first time. The examination separated the optimists from the rest of the pack, and Metropolitan Life hired a new sales force based on optimism.

The new hiring strategy was an unfailing success. By the end of the first year, the optimists were outselling the others by 20 percent. By the end of the following year, they were outselling the others by 50 percent.[51]

Optimism is also one of the best-known buffers against the deleterious effects of stress. Studies have shown that people who meet stress head-on with a sense of optimism and control don't get ill as often as those who meet stress with pessimism. Or, as one writer so aptly put it, "Winners are healthier than whiners."[52]

Researchers at Ohio State University studied more than 200 adults who had been categorized as optimists or pessimists based on scientifically accepted questionnaires. They found that those who were optimists had far less stress, less anxiety, and fewer health problems a year after they were initially categorized. Even more important than being optimistic, says study lead author Susan Robinson-Whelan, it may be crucial to *not* be pessimistic.[53]

Optimists do better under stress because they're less likely to believe that the source of stress is all-encompassing or overwhelming. They're less likely to turn to drugs or alcohol in an attempt to escape from stress. They're more likely to make recommended changes when ill—and more likely to follow prescriptions by a physician. They're more likely to take better care of themselves—a boon no matter what the source of stress.

Another reason why optimists fare better under stress than pessimists is the trait called dispositional optimism, which we discussed earlier. According to researchers from Carnegie Mellon University, optimists view the world more positively

> for the simple reason that they take more positive actions to improve it. They were found to deal with stressful situations by focusing directly on the problem at hand. They tended to "positively reinterpret" a difficult situation, focusing on what they could learn from it or the discovery of some new truth about life.

*Pessimists, by contrast, tended to deal with stress by attempting either to disengage from it, to deny it, or simply to complain about it—techniques poorly suited for achieving positive results.*[54]

## Optimists and Longevity

There's a real physiological reason why optimists live longer, and researchers believe that it lies in a complex set of "messages" that the mind sends to the body. As a result of his work with thousands of critically ill patients, Yale surgeon Bernie Siegel believes the following:

> *The body responds to the mind's messages, whether conscious or unconscious. In general, these may be either "live" or "die" messages. I am convinced we not only have survival mechanisms, such as the fight-or-flight response, but also a "die" mechanism that actively stops our defenses, slowing our body's functions and bringing us toward death when we feel our life is not worth living.*[55]

Optimists, it seems, give consistent "live" messages to the body—and, as a result, live longer. Results of a number of studies have confirmed the theory that people with a cheerful outlook on life generally get to enjoy life longer.

In one study, researchers pored through the pages of the *New York Times* and the *Philadelphia Inquirer* analyzing the quotes of all the Baseball Hall of Fame players who played major league baseball between the years 1900 and 1950. Based on the players' comments about the game, researchers were able to tag which were optimists and which were pessimists. The pessimists—those who ascribed their success as being short-lived or due to luck—lived significantly shorter lives than the optimists.[56]

How you perceive your health to be—whether your perception is or is not accurate—also seems to have a significant bearing on how long you will live. People who believe that they are in bad health—even if they are, in reality, in good or excellent health—have an increased mortality risk. And those who believe that their health is good are literally at a reduced risk of dying, even if "objective" measures (such as medical examinations and laboratory tests) show that they are actually in poor health.

Researchers in one study tracked 6,298 adults in Alameda County, California, for nine years. Men who were "health pessimists" (believed they were in poor health) had two times the mortality risk of men who were "health optimists." The mortality risk among women was a striking five times higher for those pessimistic about their health.[57]

Optimism, then, can be a powerful factor in life. It can, according to results flooding in from the vast number of studies being conducted, be a potent determinant in how healthy we are and how long we live. An increasing number of physicians who are "in the trenches" with patients every day continue to express the firm belief that optimism, more than almost any other attitude, can open the way to health and healing.

Interested in becoming more optimistic? Researchers suggest the following ways to boost your optimism:

- Realize you may need to make a lifestyle change.
- Start small by choosing one area of your life in which to become more optimistic, then become aware of the way you think in relation to that area.
- Take a good, hard, critical look at your beliefs about yourself and about that area of your life: How realistic are they?
- Set goals that are small enough to achieve quickly, then reward yourself when you meet those goals. It's important to reward yourself when you reach even the most modest goal.
- Seek out optimistic people; seek a good friend.
- "Play" at being optimistic; stay flexible.[58]

In the book *Mind/Body Medicine: How to Use Your Mind for Better Health,* editors Daniel Goleman and Joel Gurin suggest the following ways to raise an optimistic child:

- Be consistent, positive, and responsive.
- To the extent that you can, "program" the child's world to be consistent, positive, and responsive.
- Give the child responsibility; encourage independence and involve the child in a variety of age-appropriate activities.
- Set realistic goals and encourage problem solving.
- Teach the child not to generalize from specific failures; instead, help the child see failure as a challenge to do better next time.
- Encourage humor as a way of coping.
- If the child expresses pessimistic views, challenge them.
- As best you can, screen the child's peers and teachers for pessimistic tendencies.
- And, finally, be a role model yourself of realistic optimism.[59]

Norman Cousins, whose own experiences formed the foundation for his remarkable work with others, says:

> Yes, I know that my optimism can be carried too far—but I also know that no one is smart enough to fix its limits; and that it is far better to pursue a remote and even unlikely goal than to deprive oneself of the forward motion that goals provide. My life has been an education in these essentials, and I could no more turn away from them than I could deny my own existence. . . . Some people

*may interpret the effort as overwrought do-goodism; but the risk is worth taking nonetheless, for every once in a while it happens that hope can rekindle one's spirits, create remarkable new energies, and set a stage for genuine growth. At least nothing I have learned is less theoretical than the way the entire world seems to open up when courage and determination are connected to truly important aims.*[60]

# ENDNOTES

1. Robert Ornstein and David Sobel, *Healthy Pleasures* (Reading, Mass.: Addison-Wesley Publishing Company, 1989), 149.
2. P. Shaver and J. Freedman, "Your Pursuit of Happiness," *Psychology Today,* August 26, 1976, 29.
3. Ann Ranard, "The World Through Rose-Colored Glasses," *Health,* August 1989, 58.
4. Carolyn Jabs, "New Reasons to Be an Optimist," *Self,* September 1987, 170–73.
5. Ornstein and Sobel, *Healthy Pleasures,* 169.
6. Joel E. Milam, Jean L. Richardson, Gary Marks, Carol A. Kemper, and Allen J. McCutchan, "The Roles of Dispositional Optimism and Pessimism in HIV Disease Progression," *Psychology and Health* 19, no. 2 (April 2004): 167–81.
7. Example is from Ranard, "The World," 58.
8. Joan Borysenko, *Minding the Body, Mending the Mind* (Reading, Mass.: Addison-Wesley Publishing Company, 1987), 120.
9. Sharon Faelten, David Diamond, and the editors of *Prevention* Magazine, *Take Control of Your Life: A Complete Guide to Stress Relief* (Emmaus, Pa.: Rodale Press, 1988), 306.
10. Faelten et al., *Take Control,* 308.
11. Peter McWilliams and John Roger, *You Can't Afford the Luxury of a Negative Thought* (Los Angeles, Calif.: Prelude Press, 1989), 133.
12. "Hope: That Sustainer of Man," *Executive Health,* sec. II, 20(30): 1983, 1–4.
13. T. P. Hackett and N. H. Cassem, "Development of a Quantitative Rating Scale to Assess Denial," *Journal of Psychosomatic Research* 18: 1974, 93–100.
14. Bruce Bower, *Science News,* July 23, 1988.
15. From Ornstein and Sobel, *Healthy Pleasures,* 167.
16. James A. Shepperd, JoAnn J. Maroto, and Lori A. Pbert, "Dispositional Optimism as a Predictor of Health Changes Among Cardiac Patients," *Journal of Research in Personality* 30: 517–34, 1996.
17. M. F. Scheier and C. S. Carver, "A Model of Behavioral Self-Regulation: Translating Intention into Action," in Louise Berkowitz, ed., *Advances in Experimental Social Psychology,* vol. 21, 303–46 (New York: Academic Press, 1988).
18. Shepperd, Maroto, and Pbert, "Dispositional Optimism," 1996.
19. Ibid.
20. Daniel Goleman, *New York Times,* April 20, 1989.
21. Jabs, "New Reasons," 171.
22. Christopher Peterson and Lisa M. Bossio, *Health and Optimism* (New York: Free Press), 1991, 34.
23. Devera Pine, "Cruising Attitude," *Health,* August 1987, 20.
24. Karina Davidson and Kenneth Prkachin, "Optimism and Unrealistic Optimism Have an Interacting Impact on Health-Promoting Behavior and Knowledge Changes," *Personality and Social Psychology Bulletin* 23(6): 617–25, June 1997.
25. Lisa G. Aspinwall and Susanne M. Brunhart, "Distinguishing Optimism from Denial: Optimistic Beliefs Predict Attention to Health Threats," *Personality and*

*Social Psychology Bulletin* 22(10): 993–1003, October 1996.

26. Michael Greenberg, "High-Rise Public Housing, Optimism, and Personal and Environmental Health Behaviors," *American Journal of Health Behavior* 21(5): 388–98, September–October 1997.
27. Greenberg, "High-Rise Public Housing," 1997.
28. Ibid.
29. Ibid.
30. Bernie Zilbergeld and Arnold A. Lazarus, "Use Your Head," *Shape,* June 1988, 115, 146–52.
31. Clive Wood, "Optimism and Health: Expecting the Best," *Mind/Body/Health Digest,* 1(3): 3.
32. Wood, "Optimism."
33. Jean Seligman and Linda Buckley, "A Sickroom with a View," *Newsweek,* March 26, 1990, 61.
34. Norman Cousins, *Head First: The Biology of Hope* (New York: E. P. Dutton, 1989), 217.
35. Peterson and Bossio, *Health and Optimism,* 35–36.
36. Henry Dreher, "Cancer and the Mind: Current Concepts in Psycho-Oncology," *Advances,* Institute for Advancement of Health, 4(3): 27–43.
37. Rebecca Stephens, "Imagery: A Strategic Intervention to Empower Clients," *Clinical Nurse Specialist* 7(4): 1993, 170–71.
38. Peterson and Bossio, *Health and Optimism,* 124–26.
39. Steven Locke and Douglas Colligan, *The Healer Within* (New York: E. P. Dutton, 1986).
40. Armand Tanny, "The Healthy Optimist," *Men's Fitness,* February 1989, 112.
41. Daniel Goleman, *New York Times Magazine,* September 27, 1987.
42. Ranard, "The World," 59.
43. Peterson and Bossio, *Health and Optimism,* 36–37.
44. Will Stapp, "Imagine Yourself Well," *Medical Self-Care,* January/February 1988, 27–30.
45. Stapp, "Imagine Yourself Well."
46. Ibid.
47. "Expert Hopeful About AIDS Therapy," *Deseret News,* June 20, 1991, A8.
48. Scott DeGarmo, "Optimism: The Secret Weapon," *Success,* July/August 1987, 4.
49. Eric Olsen, "Why Optimists Win," *Success,* December 1988, 32.
50. Olsen, "Why Optimists Win."
51. Jill Neimark, "The Power of Positive Thinking," *Success,* September 1987, 38–47.
52. Faelten et al., *Take Control,* 309.
53. Julia Van Tine, "Become an Optimist," *Prevention* 50(6): 32, June 1998.
54. "Squelching Stress with Optimism," *Men's Health,* September 1987: 3, summarizing information from the *Journal of Personality and Psychology* 51(6): 1987.
55. Editors of *Prevention* Magazine Health Books, *The Complete Book of Cancer Prevention* (Emmaus, Pa.: Rodale Press), 495.
56. Ornstein and Sobel, *Healthy Pleasures,* 168.
57. Blair Justice, "Think Yourself Healthy," *Prevention,* June 1988, 31–32, 105–8.
58. David Burns, *Feeling Good* (New York: Avon Books–HarperCollins, 1999).
59. Daniel Goleman and Joel Gurin, eds., *Mind/Body Medicine: How to Use Your Mind for Better Health* (New York: Consumer Reports Books, 1993), 364.
60. Cousins, *Head First,* 68–69.

# Part V

# Perception and Health

This section focuses on perception, or how we see the world, and its effect upon health. Explanatory style discusses the health impact of how people perceive the events in their lives. This, in turn, affects their internal or external locus of control, their positive or negative self-esteem, and the positive power of humor and laughter. The chapters and topics presented in this section are:

**Chapter 18**    *Explanatory Style and Health*

**Chapter 19**    *Locus of Control and Health*

**Chapter 20**    *Self-Esteem and Health*

**Chapter 21**    *The Healing Power of Humor and Laughter*

# Explanatory Style and Health

*An optimist may see a light where there is none, but why must
the pessimist always run to blow it out?*

—Michel de Saint-Pierre

## Learning Objectives

- Define explanatory style.
- Describe the effects of explanatory style.
- Understand the effects of explanatory style on physical and mental health.
- Discuss the effects of explanatory style on immune function.

I t's the first baseball game of the summer, but the sultry afternoon is unusually hot for June. The sun hangs lazily above the western horizon and you absentmindedly wipe the moisture from your forehead with the back of your hand. In an effort to get some relief from the heat, you lift your frosty soft drink to your lips. Take a look at it. Is it half empty? Or is it half full? Your answer reveals what researchers call your explanatory style—and it can help determine your physical and mental health.

## What Is Explanatory Style?

Explanatory style is the way in which people perceive the events in their lives. It's the habitual way in which people explain the bad things that happen to them. In reality, it's a habit; it's a way of thinking that people use when all other factors are equal and when there are no clear-cut right and wrong answers.

According to Martin E. P. Seligman, "Explanatory style is much more specific and scientifically testable than mood. It focuses on three dimensions of our accounting for the good and bad events in our lives. Pessimists attribute bad events, such as the loss of a job, the breakup of a marriage, or a falling-out with a friend, to causes that are long-lasting or permanent, that are pervasive and affect everything they do, and that are their own fault. Optimists see the causes of such events as temporary, limited to the present case and the result of circumstances, bad luck, or other people's actions. A pessimist sees success at work, in love, or in friendship as due to luck; an optimist, as due to his or her own efforts and skill."[1]

Imagine that a driver skids into a school bus on a snowy day. The person with the pessimistic explanatory style moans, "I am the world's worst driver! It is beyond my ability to drive safely. I always foul things up!" The person with the optimistic explanatory style thinks, "I'm just a beginner, and beginners have to expect a banged fender once in a while. I'll have to be extra careful until I'm a little more practiced. Besides, these roads sure are slick! And the snow made it so it was difficult to see exactly where I was and how far I had to stop."[2]

The person with the pessimistic explanatory style interprets one negative event as an "omen," a sign as to how the rest of his or her life will turn out. The person with the optimistic explanatory style sees an isolated bad event as just that: isolated.

People with a pessimistic explanatory style can be identified by three thought patterns that give clues about what they're thinking in their conversation.

1. *Pessimists assume the problem is stable, or never-ending.* They are sure "it will never go away" instead of "it's a one-time thing." The pessimistic snowy-day driver, for example, believes that "I'll never learn to drive safely" in the snow.

2. *Pessimists believe the problem is global,* that it affects a broad spectrum of activities instead of an isolated incident.[3] The snowy-day driver opines, "Every time I try something new, I screw it up." A pessimist believes that a bad event "is going to ruin my whole life" instead of seeing a bad event as something with a specific cause that "has no bearing on the rest of my life."

3. *Pessimists internalize everything.* They believe everything is "my fault." The snowy-day driver is convinced that the accident happened because "I'm a bad driver." In contrast, the person with an optimistic explanatory style ascribes the accident to slick roads, poor visibility, some other adverse weather conditions, or merely a spot of bad luck—being in the wrong place at the wrong time.

To sum it up, pessimists tend to attribute their problems to permanent personal inadequacies that undermine everything they do. Optimists usually view a setback as a one-time thing attributable to bad luck, some external factor, or at least to a specific cause that can be remedied.[4]

University of Pennsylvania Psychologist Martin Seligman describes it neatly: "Explanatory style is a theory about your past, your future, and your place in the world."[5] Once you've formulated your theory, he adds, you tend to find evidence for it in any situation that comes along.

Paul Rosch, president of the American Institute of Stress, used the example of a roller-coaster ride to illustrate the difference between someone with an optimistic and a pessimistic explanatory style: "Look at how two people might experience a roller-coaster ride. One has his back stiffened, his knuckles are white, his eyes shut, jaws clenched, just waiting for it to be over. The wide-eyed thrill seeker relishes every plunge, can't wait to do it again."[6]

## How Permanent Is Explanatory Style?

Once you've developed an explanatory style, are you stuck with it forever? This question evokes considerable controversy among the nation's leading researchers. Many believe that we stick to one explanatory style throughout our lives. Some evidence does exist to support that notion.

The University of Pennsylvania, psychologist Martin Seligman, doesn't think that explanatory style—of even bad events—has to stay the same. Seligman, a pioneer in psychoneuroimmunology research, is convinced that explanatory style—which is basically a belief system—can be changed. Results of his work demonstrate that people can be trained to change their outlook.[7]

## What Are the Effects of Explanatory Style?

Regardless of whether researchers believe that a basic explanatory style can be changed, they do agree on one thing: Explanatory style has an extremely powerful influence on health and wellness. According to research found in *Health and Optimism*, certain kinds of thoughts are more powerful in predicting health and wellness:

- Manifest thoughts and beliefs
- Explanations for setbacks and disappointments
- What someone thinks about the real world—its events, their causes, and their aftermath
- Thoughts that are responsive to other people
- Beliefs that lead to action[8]

Explanatory style, says Seligman, works like a self-fulfilling prophecy. The way a person "explains events in his life can predict and determine his future," Seligman explains. "Those who believe they are the masters of their fate are more likely to succeed than those who attribute events to forces beyond their control."[9]

Yale oncologist and surgeon Dr. Bernie Siegel agrees, and points out that a negative explanatory style can halt the healing process and put a damper on the immune system. From his work with cancer patients, he points out, "If I said to patients, you have two choices if you want to get well—you can change your lifestyle or have an operation—the majority would say, 'Operate. It hurts less.'"[10] Siegel says that patients who get well when they're not supposed to are "not having accidents or miracles or spontaneous remissions. They're experiencing self-induced healing."[11]

Siegel, who works with patients to help them change their explanatory style and to resolve stress and conflict in their lives, tells of remarkable changes in the course of disease as a result. "As I saw people learning to live with their illnesses, I saw them gaining incredible control over their wellness," he says. "I saw people dealing with conflict in their lives and then, suddenly, having their cancer shrink or disappear. These were things I had never seen before. I was astonished. And as a physician, I felt uncomfortable with it. They were getting better and I hadn't lifted a finger."[12]

A woman named Roz had cancer so advanced that her physicians sent her to a nursing home to die. But Roz hated the nursing home, and she had the kind of explanatory style that enabled her to take hold of the situation. Instead of "passively accepting her situation," Siegel says, "she stood up and led a revolution in the nursing home. She returned home and her cancer went away."[13]

In referring to explanatory style, William Wilbanks, professor of criminal justice at Florida International University, refers to "the New Obscenity. It's not a four-letter word, but an oft-repeated statement that strikes at the very core of our humanity. The four words are: 'I can't help myself.'"[14] This kind of explanatory style, says Wilbanks, "sees man as an organism being acted upon by biological and social forces, rather than as an agent with a free will. It views offenders not as sinful or criminal but as 'sick.' By ignoring the idea that people face temptations that can—and should—be resisted, it denies the very quality that separates us from the animals."

## The Influence of Explanatory Style on Health

Siegel maintains that a negative explanatory style is harmful to the body. On the other hand, he says, an optimistic explanatory style and the positive emotions it embraces—such as love, acceptance, and forgiveness—stimulate the immune system and kick the body's own healing systems into gear. An optimistic explanatory style sends "live" messages to your body and helps promote the healing process.[15]

Although it's essential to have an optimistic explanatory style, says Siegel, it's also crucial to use that explanatory style to deal with the realities in life:

> *Learning to let go of negative emotions is the key. The person who smiles on the outside and is hurting on the inside is not dealing with himself or his life. All his "live" mechanisms are told to stop working. Doctors see examples of this every day. You are making rounds at the hospital and you ask a patient how she's doing and she says "Fine." But you know she's not doing fine. Her husband ran off with another woman. Her son is on drugs. And she has cancer. But still she says, "Fine." When I find a person who answers, "Lousy," I say, "That's wonderful! You want to get better so you're dealing with the truth. If your mind and body are feeling lousy and you're relating to that, you'll ask for help."*[16]

## Impact on Mental Health

According to the most recent research, explanatory style can have a tremendous impact on mental health—and the explanatory style that is considered "normal" is probably much more optimistic than what researchers once believed it was. According to researchers writing in the *Psychological Bulletin*, it was once considered "normal" for people to have accurate perceptions of themselves, the world, and their future; this was a quality considered essential for good mental health. Recent research, however, indicates that "overly positive" evaluations of self, "exaggerated" perceptions of control, and "unrealistic optimism" are characteristic of normal human thought.[17] (See Chapter 17 for a further discussion of this.)

The kind of optimistic explanatory style that researchers describe helps promote other aspects of mental health—the ability to care about others, the ability to be happy or contented, and the ability to engage in productive or creative work—because it "distorts" incoming information in a positive direction and dilutes negative input until it is no longer threatening. All in all, say researchers, an optimistic explanatory style helps people adapt in a healthy way when something negative or stressful happens.

A pessimistic explanatory style, on the other hand, can lead to depression. Princeton University Psychologists Susan Nolen-Hoeksema and Joan Girgus showed in their study that explanatory style was a much more important factor in depression than was mood—and that explanatory style is much more permanent than mood. In their study, Nolen-Hoeksema and Girgus repeatedly tested third, fourth, and fifth graders on both mood and explanatory style. The kids who started out in a momentarily happy mood but who had a pessimistic explanatory style were depressed within three months of the time the study began. The ones who had an optimistic explanatory style but who were depressed for some reason in the month the study began tended to bounce back and feel upbeat and happy three months later.[18]

According to researchers, a pessimistic explanatory style can lead to anxiety, eating disorders, and a number of emotional problems. It also leads to what researchers call *dysphoria*—a variety of negative emotional states that cause you to "just feel bad." That dysphoria can take the form of depression, anxiety, guilt, anger, or hostility.[19]

## Impact on Physical Health

A growing body of evidence suggests that explanatory style can be a potent predictor of physical health. According to research, a pessimistic explanatory style can depress immunity. Scientists from the University of Pennsylvania, Yale University, and Sydney's Prince of Wales Hospital involved elderly men and women in a study designed to determine the effect of explanatory style on immunity. According to researchers, those with a pessimistic explanatory style had a lower ratio of T-helper cells to T-suppressor cells and had a poorer T-lymphocyte response when their immune system was challenged.[20]

Explanatory style can even affect the way the body reacts to surgery. After years of medical practice, one surgeon vowed that he would never operate on a patient who believed he (or she) would die, because that's what always happened.

In one study designed to measure the impact of explanatory style on surgical outcomes, researchers asked patients six to twelve months before their surgery was to take place to rate their expectations of surgery and the problems associated with surgery.[21] Researchers then gave the patients questionnaires just before surgery and four more times over the next two years. The patients' attitudes and expectations about the surgery (their explanatory style) turned out to be powerful predictors. The patients who expected fewer problems had better outcomes. The ones who expected more problems got exactly that. Two years later they had physical problems, dissatisfaction with the surgery, and mood disturbances.

Apparently, how people feel about their own health can actually determine how good their health is. Yale Medical School Researcher Stanislav Kasl and Rutgers University Sociologist Ellen Idler studied more than 2,800 men and women aged sixty-five years and older. What they discovered is that our own opinion about the state of our health is an even better predictor of health than objective factors—such as what a physician can determine through laboratory tests. It's even a better predictor than behaviors, such as cigarette smoking. For example, people in the study who smoked cigarettes were twice as likely to die during the next twelve years as people who did not smoke. But people who thought they were in "poor" health were seven times as likely to die as those who thought they were in "excellent" health.[22]

People with pessimistic explanatory styles have a tendency to blame themselves for anything bad that happens to them. That tendency can interfere with health, recovery, and healing. In one study, researchers analyzed the hospital reports of people who were hospitalized for the treatment of acute burns. People with pessimistic explanatory styles tended to blame themselves for the burn—and also had more pain, greater depression, and less compliance with the instructions of nurses and physical therapists.[23]

Researchers who have studied explanatory style and its impact on health have found that it can influence healing time and the course of the illness in several major diseases, such as cancer and coronary disease. In one pilot study of cancer patients who had advanced melanoma, University of Rochester Researcher Sandra Levy reported that "an optimistic explanatory style was the number one psychological predictor of who would live the longest."[24]

One study conducted by Martin Seligman and his colleagues at the University of Pennsylvania involved thirteen patients with malignant melanoma. They found that the best predictor of a patient's survival time was the "absence of a helpless explanatory style." The absence of a helpless style, in fact, was an even more potent predictor than the activity of the patient's natural killer cells.[25]

In another study—this one of women who had recurring breast cancer—Levy and her colleagues studied the common links among women who had the longest cancer-free period between episodes of the disease. The most common denominator among women whose cancer was slow to return was an optimistic explanatory style.[26]

Siegel maintains that one of the most important keys to cancer survival is attitude, and, based on his work with cancer patients, explanatory style contributes a great deal to the ability of people to fight their cancer. He says that the majority of cancer patients are willing to take on the role of "observer," sitting back and letting a physician direct the treatment. About one in five are happy to die because "their lives are in shambles." The rest—about 15 to 20 percent—have explanatory styles that make them "truly exceptional survivors."[27]

Interestingly, the results of one study show that cancer patients who have a *moderate* explanatory style actually do better: While positive attitude was important, those who were positive for the present actually had better outcomes than those who were extremely positive for the future. Optimism for the day, as opposed to heavy expectations for the future, helped cancer patients do better in a variety of ways; those who were focused on the future tended to do less well and faced greater disappointment in many cases.[28]

University of Georgia Researcher James Dabbs studied a group of male college students to determine the effects of explanatory style on health. He found that the optimists in the group had a higher level of the male hormone testosterone, which, he says, provides evidence that optimism and explanatory style influence our secretion of hormones.[29]

Attitude and explanatory style can even impact the circulatory system and the outlook for people with coronary heart disease. Sophisticated instruments and testing procedures have enabled researchers to watch the brain in action. Blood flow in the brain literally changes as thoughts, feelings, and attitudes change. The results of a variety of studies show that people with pessimistic explanatory styles are at increased risk of atherosclerosis, blockage of coronary arteries, and heart attack.

Study results reported to the Society of Behavioral Medicine by Dr. Daniel Mark, a Duke University heart specialist, followed up on 1,719 men and women who had undergone heart catheterization, a common procedure to check for clogging of the arteries. All of the people in the study had heart disease. Those with pessimistic explanatory style—the ones who doubted they would recover—fared much more poorly than those with an optimistic style. Of the pessimists, 12 percent were dead within a year—more than twice as many as the 5 percent of the optimists. In summing up the study, Mark emphasized that "the mind is a tremendous tool or weapon, depending on your point of view."

In another study, researchers found that those with an optimistic explanatory style also had much better results following coronary bypass surgery. One of the most dangerous complications following coronary bypass surgery is high blood pressure. In this study, people with optimistic explanatory styles had better attitudes about the surgery, had more favorable pulse rates after surgery, and had less hypertension after surgery. High blood pressure following surgery was reduced from 75 percent to less than 45 percent among those with healthy attitudes. An optimistic explanatory style also strongly affects the pace of recuperation, the incidence of complications, and the overall outcome of the surgery.[30]

Explanatory style may even enable researchers to predict which people will get sick. In one study, Martin Seligman and his colleagues at the University of Pennsylvania rated 172 undergraduate students on what kind of explanatory style they had. The researchers then predicted which ones would get sick. After a month, they found their predictions were right on. A year later, their predictions still held true.[31]

People with an optimistic explanatory style have better health for reasons that are described in more detail in the chapters that follow. Some of those factors include stronger immunity, good social support, and a willingness to continue better health habits.[32] Another reason, say researchers, is that people with a pessimistic explanatory style generally react to illness with helplessness and a lack of fighting spirit—factors that have in themselves been linked to poor health.[33]

## A Healthy Style, a Healthy Immune System

One of the reasons an optimistic explanatory style leads to better health may be that an optimistic style tends to increase the strength of the immune system. Robert Good, former president and director of the Memorial Sloan-Kettering Cancer Hospital in New York, maintains that an optimistic explanatory style and the positive attitude it fosters can actually alter our ability to resist "infections, allergies, autoimmunities, or even cancer."[34]

According to researchers, the hypothalamus control center of the brain—the part that is involved in attitudes and outlook—is directly "wired" to the immune system. If a portion of the hypothalamus is electrically stimulated, antibodies increase; if it is cut, immune activity is depressed. The same thing happens in response to thoughts, beliefs, and imaginations—things that are "not ephemeral abstractions, but electrochemical events with physiological consequences."[35] Siegel mirrors that belief and points out that positive emotions and attitudes actually stimulate the immune system.

Michael A. Lerner, the founder of Commonweal, a cancer hospice in southern California, and a MacArthur Foundation Genius Award winner, says the attitudes linked to an optimistic explanatory style can even boost the immune system enough to defeat cancer: "Attitudes themselves have a very potent effect on the immune system. You become different than the person who developed the cancer. Becoming a different personality may change the environment the cancer grew in; it may become so inhospitable that the cancer shrinks."[36]

Explanatory style may have enough influence over the immune system to affect even infectious disease resistance. In one study, psychologist Stanislav Kasl and his colleagues at Yale University followed the development of infectious mononucleosis among a group of West Point cadets.[37] During a four-year period, all cadets entering West Point were given blood tests that screened for the presence of antibodies to the Epstein-Barr virus, the agent that causes mononucleosis. The cadets were also given interviews that included questions about their outlook, their expectations, and their family backgrounds.

About one in five of the susceptible cadets was infected—but only about one-fourth of those actually got sick. The ones who did get sick had a number of threads in common, including a pessimistic explanatory style, high expectations (usually centered in pressure from parents), and poor academic performance.

In a separate set of studies, researchers conducting studies at Yale University and the University of Pennsylvania compared immune function and explanatory style among a group of elderly people. According to the researchers, people with a pessimistic explanatory style had suppressed immune function.[38]

Specifically, said the researchers, the ratio of T-helper cells and T-suppressor cells was low, as was the number of lymphocytes, which arm the body for waging war against infection or disease.

To sum up the research, scientists have found direct evidence that a pessimistic style and a sense of helplessness may depress the immune system and decrease resistance. An optimistic style that allows for a sense of control boosts immunity. The end result does indeed depend on whether you see the glass as half full or half empty.

# ENDNOTES

1. Morton Hunt, "Don't Worry, Be Happy," *Longevity,* December 1991, 80.
2. Example is from Joan Borysenko, *Minding the Body, Mending the Mind* (Reading, Mass.: Addison-Wesley Publishing Company, 1987), 120.
3. Christopher Peterson, George E. Vaillant, and Martin E. P. Seligman, "Pessimistic Explanatory Style Is a Risk Factor for Physical Illness: A Thirty-Five-Year Longitudinal Study," *Journal of Personality and Social Psychology* 55(1): 1988, 23.
4. Carolyn Jabs, "New Reasons to Be an Optimist," *Self,* September 1987, 170–73.
5. Jabs, "New Reasons."
6. "Good Stress: Why You Need It to Stay Young," *Prevention,* April 1986, 28–32.
7. Martin E. P. Seligman, *Learned Optimism* (New York: Alfred A. Knopf, 1991), 178.
8. Christopher Peterson and Lisa M. Bossio, *Health and Optimism* (New York: Free Press, 1991), 60.
9. Seligman, *Learned Optimism.*
10. "Mind over Cancer: An Exclusive Interview with Yale Surgeon Dr. Bernie Siegel," *Prevention,* March 1988, 59–64.
11. "Mind over Cancer."
12. Ibid.
13. Ibid.
14. William Lee Wilbanks, "The New Obscenity," *Reader's Digest,* December 1988, 23.
15. "Mind over Cancer."
16. Ibid.

17. S. E. Taylor and J. D. Brown, "Illusion and Well-Being: A Social Psychological Perspective on Mental Health," *Psychological Bulletin* 103(2): 1988, 193–210.

18. Nan Silver, "Do Optimists Live Longer?" *American Health*, November 1986, 50–53.

19. Peterson and Bossio, *Health and Optimism*, Free Press, 106.

20. Leslie Kamen-Siegel, Judith Rodin, Martin E. P. Seligman, and John Dwyer, "Explanatory Style and Cell-Mediated Immunity in Elderly Men and Women," *Health Psychology* 10(4): 1991, 229–35.

21. H. Asuman Kiyak, Peter P. Vitaliano, and Jeffrey Crinean, "Patients' Expectations as Predictors of Orthognathic Surgery Outcomes," *Health Psychology* 7(3): 1988, 251–68.

22. Larry Dossey, *Meaning and Medicine: A Doctor's Tales of Breakthrough and Healing* (New York: Bantam Books, 1991), 16.

23. Janice K. Kiecolt-Glaser and D. A. Williams, "Self-Blame, Compliance, and Distress Among Burn Patients," *Journal of Personality and Social Psychology* 53(1): 1987, 187–93.

24. Silver, "Do Optimists Live Longer?"

25. Dossey, *Meaning and Medicine*, 33.

26. Silver, "Do Optimists Live Longer?"

27. "Mind over Cancer."

28. Lesley M. Wilkes, Jenny O'Baugh, and Suzanne Luke, "Positive Attitude in Cancer: Patients' Pespectives," *Oncology Nursing Forum* 3 (May–June 2003): 412–16.

29. Peterson and Bossio, *Health and Optimism*. 99.

30. Joseph Lederer, "Surgery: A Mind-Body Event," *Mind/Body/Health Digest* 1(4): 1–4.

31. Dossey, *Meaning and Medicine*.

32. Seligman, *Learned Optimism*, 173–74.

33. Emily H. Lin and Christopher Peterson, "Pessimistic Explanatory Style and Response to Illness," *Behavioral Research Therapy* 28(3): 1990, 243–48.

34. Blair Justice, "Think Yourself Healthy," *Prevention*, May 1988, 27–32, 102, 107.

35. Justice, "Think Yourself Healthy."

36. Daniel Goleman, "The Mind over the Body," *New Realities*, March/April 1988, 14–19.

37. Robert Ornstein and David Sobel, "The Healing Brain," *Psychology Today*, March 1987, 48–52.

38. Kamen-Siegel et al., "Explanatory Style," 229–35.

# CHAPTER 19

# Locus of Control and Health

*How shall I be able to rule over others when I have not full
power and command over myself?*

—François Rabelais

## Learning Objectives

- Relate how locus of control has been recognized throughout history.
- Discuss the factors that impact locus of control.
- Describe how locus of control and hardiness are related.
- Understand the influence of locus of control on health.
- Describe how control mitigates the effects of stress.
- Understand the effects of control on immunity and healing.

Noted psychologist Martin Seligman paints for us what he calls the infant's "dance of development." In it, the good mother mirrors and responds to the actions of her infant son or daughter. The baby smiles, and the mother smiles. The baby coos or gurgles with delight, and the mother does the same. The baby cries with hunger, and the mother responds with the warm sweetness of milk. Through this "dance of development," Seligman says, infants learn that they have control. And through the sense of control that results, infants learn that they can ensure their own survival.[1]

## What Does Locus of Control Mean?

What, exactly, is a sense of control, and why is it so important to health? The concept of a locus of control originated several decades ago with the work of Julian Rotter; it involves the belief that our own actions will be effective enough to control or master the environment.[2] Control does not mean that we need to control everything around us—such as other people, the environment, or our circumstances, whether good or bad. Control does entail a deep-seated belief that we can impact a situation by how we look at the problem.[3] We can choose how we react and how we respond. If we regard a loss with gloom and doom, we allow it to hurt us; if we view it as a chance for growth and opportunity, we minimize its ability to hurt us.

Suzanne O. Kobasa and Salvatore Maddi, renowned for their research into what makes us "hardy" and able to resist disease, theorize that a sense of control is crucial to health. They say that those "high in control believe and act as if they can influence the events of their experience, rather than being powerless in the face of outside forces." That kind of attitude allows people to take responsibility and act effectively on their own.[4]

Researchers working in the field of psychoneuroimmunology theorize that a person lies somewhere along a continuum as far as a sense of control is concerned. At one end of the continuum is the "external locus of control"; at the opposite end is the "internal locus of control." Where a person is along the continuum relates to his or her health.

People with an external locus of control believe that the things that happen to them are unrelated to their own behavior—and, subsequently, beyond their control.[5] Likening the victim of external locus of control to a boxer in the ring, physician S. I. McMillen explains,

*When the stresses of life buffet them, they lay against the ropes of despair and wish that things would get better. They erroneously decide that their opponent, stress, is much too strong for them, so they don't even try to fight back. [They feel that] everything that happens to them is controlled by external forces and that their actions do not influence what happens to them. Like pawns in a chess game, externals believe that they are randomly moved about by the players of "luck, chance, fate, or predestination."[6]*

At the opposite end of the spectrum are the people with an "internal locus of control." These people believe that negative events are a consequence of personal actions, and can thus be potentially controlled.[7] As McMillen defines them, "Internals believe that their own actions have a large influence on what happens to them. If they get fired from a job, internals believe that when they go out to look for a job they will be able to find one. They do not give up; rather, they hope for a brighter future."[8] As researcher Phillip Rice so aptly put it, "If the theme song of the external is 'Cast Your Fate to the Winds,' the theme song of the internal is 'I Did It My Way.'"[9]

## A Brief History of Control

Philosopher and researcher Leonard Sagan believes that an external locus of control dominated many cultures throughout a significant period of the world's history. As he states,

> Almost universally, the social adjustment to poverty and helplessness has been the adoption of a fatalistic, authoritarian world view: "These events are out of our hands, they are in the hands of God." Children are taught that bad outcomes are the result of forces beyond their control, that life must be lived in the present, since, in an incalculable world, individual effort counts for naught.
>
> [This] pervading sense of helplessness dominated the human condition throughout history—until the Enlightenment. The Enlightenment encouraged the attitude that all natural phenomena operate in conformance with universal physical-chemical properties and are predictable, not the result of whimsical divine forces. If men could understand those principles, they could control their environment and their destiny. These were heady and revolutionary thoughts, unique in human history.[10]

Sagan—an epidemiologist at Stanford University—points out that these perspectives are more than merely revolutionary; they have tremendous impact on the health and life expectancy of all of us. Sagan maintains that life expectancy has leapt by thirty years during this century because we have more control over our lives. The control that acts as a buffer against disaster in this century, he says, includes things like police and fire departments, insurance against loss, and a steady and reliable food supply. Because "we can foresee, avoid, and mitigate problems," he points out, "we have more resources to adapt and cope with them."[11] We have a greater sense of control over our environments.

## What Is the Source of Control?

A sense of increased control can come from a variety of sources:

1. Gaining information. People who are informed about a situation feel an increased sense of control because the situation becomes predictable and manageable.
2. Adopting a less pessimistic outlook.
3. Placing faith in someone or something we deeply trust.
4. Learning new coping skills.
5. Building a stronger support system.
6. Being prepared. When people feel prepared for something, they perceive a much greater ability to control even a difficult situation.[12]

The latter point is illustrated beautifully by a study conducted on a Special Forces unit in Vietnam that was expecting an enemy attack.[13] An Army psychiatrist, researcher Peter Bourne, lived in the camp with the men and took blood samples daily. He measured the amount of an adrenal hormone present when a person is under extreme stress.

It's difficult to imagine any situation much more stressful than anticipating an enemy attack in a war zone—but, to Bourne's surprise, the hormone levels of the men indicated that they were not experiencing any elevated stress. Other tests showed that the men had lower levels of anxiety and depression than even the basic recruits who were entering training.

What enabled these soldiers to rally so valiantly in such difficult circumstances? Bourne believes it was their sense of control. They gained that sense of control, he believes, by being prepared. The soldiers coped with the threat of impending battle by engaging in "a furor of activity," maintaining their equipment and building their defenses.

Only three men in the unit showed elevated stress hormones. They were the two officers and the radio operator who had to receive—and respond to—orders from a distant command post over which they had no control.

## Hardiness and Control

Psychologists Suzanne Kobasa and Salvatore Maddi first developed the now well-accepted theory that people who are able to stay healthy even while under stress have behaviors and personalities marked by "hardiness." One of the key components of hardiness, say the pair, is a sense of control. Dr. Arthur Schmale, a University of Rochester researcher, was one of the first to identify the importance of control; his research, paired with the work of Kobasa and Maddi, demonstrates the importance of control as a factor in health and well-being.

As a classic example, Schmale cites the case of a woman who was diagnosed with leukemia.[14] Her diagnosis came shortly before her husband's death from tuberculosis. She told her physician that she hoped to live until her son—then aged ten—was grown up and settled.

The course of leukemia can be charted by measuring red blood cell count, an indication of how well the body is battling the disease. As her physician measured her red blood count over the years, he was interested to note a trend. At times when she felt in control, her disease lapsed into remission. At other times, when she felt that she was losing control, her disease intensified.

The leukemia soared, for example, as she entered menopause. It intensified, too, when she finally admitted that her second marriage was failing.

It even came and went during various times of the year. For example, her disease became much worse every year about the time her physician was scheduled to take his annual summer vacation. Possibly she felt a dangerous loss of control in contemplating his absence.

The worst period of her disease occurred when her son left home to join the Army. Her condition became so critical that, for the first time since becoming ill, she required blood transfusions to stay alive.

The four years while her son was in the military were extremely difficult for her. According to her physician, she required almost constant medical treatment and various hospitalizations just to keep the disease under control. When her son was released from the military, he announced that he was engaged to be married. Shortly afterward, she died. As her physician related, she would now have almost no control in her relationship to him.

Another example of the importance of control and the problems that arise in its absence was demonstrated by an executive whom Kobasa studied while she was doing her original research.[15] The patient showed strong alienation, a disconnectedness from people, and a lack of commitment to his job. For a man in his mid-thirties, he had a particularly dismal medical history, peppered with problems such as high blood pressure, peptic ulcer, and migraine headaches.

When he visited Kobasa's office, the executive gained great insight into the cause of his problems. As she describes it, the visit to her office was "a catastrophe. The executive rushed into the office forty-five minutes late, commandeered her secretary's phone, and began making business calls to alert his cronies to where he would be. Kobasa recalls preparing to approach the sensitive subject of his apparent lack of connection to people, but she barely finished a sentence because each time her phone rang, the executive jumped up, convinced that the call was for him." As Kobasa put it, he was obviously not a man in control; his telephones ruled him, and he could not shut them out of his life for a moment.

According to Kobasa and Maddi and the other researchers who have since studied hardiness, it is earmarked by a sense of control. The control that characterizes hardiness is a belief that we can influence events coupled with a willingness to act on that belief rather than just be a victim of circumstances. It is not a desire or a need to be in control of situations or to control other people.

## The Influence of Control on Health

The results of a host of studies show the importance of control. As a whole, people with a greater sense of control are at less risk of illness. Recent research shows that people who believe they have poor control over what happens in their lives are more likely to suffer from chronic illness.[16] A sense of control is an important predictor of health behaviors as well; those who have a strong "health locus of control" (who believe in their ability to influence their health) tend to be healthier, and those who receive information consistent with that locus of control have better health behaviors.[17] As new research is completed, scientists are realizing that an internal locus of control has an even more profound role in protecting health than we once thought.

Former *Saturday Review* editor Norman Cousins, renowned for his work linking attitudes and health, maintains that, in general:

> *Anything that restores a sense of control to a patient can be a profound aid to a physician in treating serious illness. That sense of control is more than a mere mood or attitude, and may well be a vital pathway between the brain, the endocrine system, and the immune system. The assumed possibility is that it may serve as the basis for what may well be a profound advancement in the knowledge of how to confront the challenge of serious illness.[18]*

Cousins cites as an example the case of a well-known actor referred to him with cancer of the larynx. The actor spoke in a hoarse whisper. "It was a particularly poignant case because his voice was his prime asset," Cousins remembers. The disease had understandably caused the actor to sink into a deep depression. Cousins worked with the actor to help him understand that his depression was defeating him physically—and together they worked on figuring out ways to control the depression. Once the patient regained a sense of control over what was happening to him, his physician was better able to work at his best. Three months later, the cancer was in remission and the actor's voice was being restored.[19]

A sense of control can affect health and well-being in a number of ways. Studies show that people with little sense of control—those who see their lives and futures controlled by luck or fate—suffer much greater psychological distress. These people, who believe that nothing they do will significantly change their circumstances or their reliance on "luck," have higher levels of depression and anxiety and are much less effective in dealing with chronic pain.[20]

A pilot study of long-term AIDS survivors conducted by Dr. George Solomon and his associates found that the survivors had a number of psychosocial characteristics in common—many of which pointed to an increased sense of control over their situation. The survivors were assertive, able to nurture themselves, actively involved with others who had the disease, and able to communicate openly about their needs, according to Caryle Hirshberg. In addition, says Hirshberg, the long-term AIDS survivors in the study took personal responsibility for the disease, but did not perceive it as a death sentence; felt they could influence the outcome of the disease; had a sense of purpose; and took control by altering their lifestyles. Finally, many of the long-term AIDS survivors had successfully overcome a previous life-threatening illness—something that would certainly impart a sense of control.[21]

## Studies with Animals

A number of animal studies have shown the devastating effects on health and life when a sense of control is lost. In one of them, Johns Hopkins Psychologist Curt Richter found that rats put in a situation over which they had no control would quickly die.[22] After immersion in a jar full of water, the rats died, but not from drowning: Their lungs were dry. Instead, they died because their hearts literally stopped beating. In summing up the study, Richter theorized that their situation was one characterized by total lack of control: "The rats are in a situation against which they have no defense. . . . They seem literally to 'give up.'"

In another study, discussed by Rice University Psychologist Blair Justice, squirrel monkeys were confined in pairs to chairs for eight hours a day. One of the monkeys in each pair had to turn off a light once a minute to prevent a shock from being delivered to the tails of both monkeys.[23] At the end of the experiment, researchers studied both sets of monkeys—the ones who had not been able to control the shocks, and those who had. The task of turning off a light every minute for eight hours was obviously stressful—and, as expected, researchers found that the monkeys who had to control the light had elevated blood pressure. But of the six monkeys who had no control over the light or the electric shock, five collapsed from excessively slow heart action; four of them died from irregular cardiac rhythm.

## Studies with Humans

Carried to the extreme, a loss of control can have the same physiological reaction in humans. Authorities on heart disease gathered in a forum on coronary-prone behavior; they concluded that slowing of the heart causes death, even though there are no apparently fatal physiological changes in the heart itself.[24]

Taking control, on the other hand, can have the opposite effect on health. According to a study reported in *Clinical Psychiatry News*,[25] researchers at the University of Connecticut School of Medicine observed a group of more than 200 heart-attack survivors for eight years. The researchers noted that the patients who accepted the responsibility for their attacks had fewer second attacks than patients who blamed their genes, their spouse, or other factors. According to study leader Glenn Affleck, "The value in accepting responsibility for a heart attack could stem from its being a sign of taking control. Passing the buck, on the other hand, could be indicative of the very sort of thinking that may contribute to heart attacks in the first place—namely, feeling a lack of control. This, in turn, could lead to a feeling of helplessness in making adaptive lifestyle changes."

## Biochemical Imbalances

One reason why control has such a profound influence over health is that a lack of control disturbs the biochemical balance in the brain and body. An internal locus of control has a significant influence over the body's release of hormones, which has been found to be a powerful determinant of health. Three of these hormones that are influenced by a lack of control are:

- **Serotonin,** which regulates moods, relieves pain, and helps control release of the powerful pain-killing brain chemicals, the endorphins.
- **Dopamine,** which is largely responsible for a sense of reward or pleasure.
- **Norepinephrine,** which causes depression when depleted.

Both norepinephrine and dopamine are critical to relaying nerve impulses from one neuron to another; they are essential to the nervous system's ability to "communicate" among its many cells. All three of these hormones are essential to activity, appetite, moods, sleep, sex, reinforcement, reward, and pleasure, and they play an important role in healthy mental functioning.[26]

When we feel little sense of control, the levels of norepinephrine, dopamine, and serotonin drop.[27] As a result, a disturbance in our sense of control can also seriously disturb our mental functioning, appetite, mood, sleep, sex drive, and senses of reinforcement, reward, and pleasure.

Furthermore, when we have little internal locus of control, the level of corticosteroids in our bloodstream soars. The corticosteroids, released by the body during stress, cause a variety of physical damage. They lower our resistance to disease and suppress the body's manufacture of norepinephrine, dopamine, and serotonin—making lack of control a double-edged sword.

## Lack of Control Versus Stress

A lack of control may have an even stronger influence over health than do high levels of stress. Turning to a situation where people often have little control—the workplace—researchers have found that those with little control suffer more severe health problems than do those with high levels of stress.

Researcher Rena Pasick, with the University of California School of Public Health, studied almost 800 working adults in Alameda County, California.

She found a "significant association" between the amount of control on the job and health status.[28]

The study bore out some seeming contradictions until researchers considered the issue of control. For example, upper-level management and other white-collar employees have been considered at highest risk because of the amount of stress and responsibility they have. But Pasick's study showed that they actually enjoy better health than those they supervise or than blue-collar workers in general. This is because they have more control.[29]

Various studies among work populations have shown that lack of control can be deleterious to health. People with little control but high demands have more than three times the risk of heart disease and chronically escalated blood pressure than people with few demands but a high level of control. Robert Karasek, an industrial engineering professor at Columbia University, has found that people who have little control over their jobs have higher rates of heart disease than people who can dictate the style and pace of their work. Worst off are those whose work makes substantial psychological demands but offers little opportunity for independent decision making—occupations such as telephone operators, waiters, cashiers, cooks, garment stitchers, and assembly-line workers. According to Karasek, the combination of high demands and low control appears to raise the risk of heart disease as much as "smoking or having a high cholesterol level."[30]

According to researchers with the Framingham Heart Study, women clerical workers and others with little control have twice as much heart disease as women in occupations with higher levels of control.[31] The Framingham researchers suggest that the clerical workers and others with a low sense of control "experience severe occupational stress, including a lack of autonomy and control over the work environment, underutilization of skills, and lack of recognition of accomplishments."[32]

In another study of the link between control and heart disease, researchers found that heart disease is greater among waiters and assembly-line workers than among managers who are faced with equally high stress and demands but who have more control and decision-making ability.[33]

## The Stress-Buffering Power of Control

A person in a stressful situation who believes that he or she has some control over the situation suffers far less physiological damage normally associated with stress. And control acts as a buffer against stress when we believe we have control, even if we really don't.

In one study,[34] individuals were placed in booths and asked to perform arithmetic problems in their head. To make the situation even more stressful, researchers piped noise into the booths. Half of the people in the study were able to control the noise level by turning a knob in the booth; the other half were dependent on the first half for volume control. Both groups were exposed to an identical level of noise; the only difference between the two was the ability to control the volume of noise. At the end of the experiment, researchers took blood samples and studied the level of stress hormones in the blood. The people who did not have a knob to turn had much higher levels of cortisol, a major stress hormone. According to the research authors, "The ability to control external stress has a large influence on how much internal stress we experience."

The stress-buffering effects of control have been observed in a wide variety of situations, and the ability of control to buffer stress has even been seen in the most stressful conditions, such as those endured by hostages and prisoners of war. Those who have been able to maintain hardiness and survive their ordeals, according to researchers, are those who have somehow been able to achieve some sense of control, even in prison. National Institute of Mental Health Psychologist Julius Segal found that one of the hostages in Iran "achieved this by saving a bit of food from his meals and then offering it to anyone who came into his cell. That simple coping strategy had the effect of turning the cell into a living room, the hostage into a host welcoming visitors."[35]

Finally, control has been known to work with the less severe, everyday problems of big-city noise and crowding. According to Rice University Psychologist Blair Justice, city dwellers combat the intrusion of unwanted noise by masking it with music from their own radios or tape players—something they can do to put the situation in their own control. Similarly, they combat the sense of crowding by "filtering" out the crowd—paying little attention to the people, sounds, and stimuli that surround them. Thus, they maintain a sense of control in a situation they otherwise can't control.[36]

# The Influence of Control on Immunity and Healing

One reason why a lack of control may lead to poor health lies within the immune system. According to research, control may have a significant effect on the function of the body's immune defenses. People who feel powerless, helpless, and out of control generally have compromised immunity, whereas those who feel a sense of control have healthier immune systems.

Physicians tested women with early-stage breast cancer. Those who felt some control over their lives and their disease were compared with women who felt a distressing lack of control. The women with control had a far greater level of natural killer cell activity—a much stronger immune system.[37]

In a related study, researchers did a thirty-year follow-up study of children who had received psychological counseling during a period of juvenile delinquency. The researchers were surprised to find that the children who had received help for their problems had far more health problems than those who had not received help. When they probed into the situation, the researchers found that the issue, again, was one of control:

> *The untreated group may have perceived the world as more under their control than the group that was given assistance. One of the effects of outside intervention may be to lessen patients' sense of control of life's events. It is as if they have adopted the idea that the counselor is taking care of their troubles, not they themselves. They are like the animals locked in the cage that cannot control the delivery of shocks. This attitude may in turn affect the immune system, with troublesome consequences for the patients' health.*[38]

A sense of control also appears to trigger the body's internal healing mechanisms. Several different studies with patients about to undergo surgery demonstrate that a sense of control can have a significant effect on the healing process. In one, psychologist Ellen Langer took a randomly selected group of surgical patients at Yale–New Haven Hospital and divided the patients into three groups. Members of the first group were simply asked questions about what they expected to happen. Members of the second group were given some basic information about the surgery, including probable after-effects and discomfort. Members of the third group were given what Langer called a "coping device," consisting of detailed information, help in placing the experience in an optimistic light, and instructions detailing how patients could exercise control over their bodies.

When the surgeries were completed and Langer compared the three groups, the first two weren't much different from each other. But the people in the third group—the ones who were given the coping primer—used half as many painkillers and sedatives and stayed in the hospital an average of two days less than the people who received just basic information. The difference in recovery, suggests Langer, "was due to the patients' learning that they could diminish postsurgical discomfort and in so doing feel that they were in control."[39]

A similar experiment conducted by psychologists at the University of Iowa School of Medicine involved patients about to undergo coronary bypass surgery. The researchers structured their study much like Langer's, using three separate groups of patients. The patients in the group that had received enough information to give a sense of control "fared significantly better on all counts. There was less hypertension, anxiety, and pain." A greater sense of control "proved to be the most powerful predictor of recovery without complication."[40]

Other studies at other hospitals have had the same result: Patients with a sense of control heal more quickly and with fewer complications. All of the studies together show us the power of an internal locus of control. With it, we may have improved immune function, have the ability to fight disease, and recover more quickly when illness does strike. Control may possibly be the weapon researchers were referring to when they told us, "You carry with you the most powerful medicine that exists. Each of us has it if we choose to use it, if we learn to use it."[41]

## ENDNOTES

1. Joan Borysenko, *Minding the Body, Mending the Mind* (Reading, Mass.: Addison-Wesley Publishing Company, 1987), 22.
2. Phillip L. Rice, *Stress and Health* (Monterey, Calif.: Brooks/Cole Publishing Company, 1987), 109.
3. Blair Justice, *Who Gets Sick: Thinking and Health* (Houston, Tex.: Peak Press, 1987), 61–62.
4. Aaron Antonovsky, *Unraveling the Mystery of Health: How People Manage Stress and Stay Well* (San Francisco: Jossey-Bass, 1987), 36–37.
5. H. M. Lefcourt, *Locus of Control: Current Trends in Theory and Research* (Hillsdale, N.J.: Erlbaum, 1976), 29.
6. S. I. McMillen, *None of These Diseases*, rev. ed. (Old Tappan, N.J.: Fleming H. Revell Company, 1984), 177.
7. Lefcourt, *Locus of Control.*
8. McMillen, *None of These Diseases*, 177–78.
9. Rice, *Stress and Health*, 109.
10. Leonard A. Sagan, *The Health of Nations* (New York: Basic Books, 1987).
11. Tony Eprile, "Longevity Tied to Self-Mastery," *Omni Longevity* 2(10): 1988, 109–11.
12. Justice, *Who Gets Sick*, 145.
13. P. G. Bourne, R. M. Rose, and J. W. Mason, "17–0HCS Levels in Combat: Special Forces 'A' Team Under Threat of Attack," *Archives of General Psychiatry* 19: 1968, 135–40.
14. Case cited in Steven Locke and Douglas Colligan, *The Healer Within* (New York: E. P. Dutton, 1986), 96.
15. Locke and Colligan, *The Healer Within*, 96–97.
16. W. Stelmach, K. Kaczmarczyk-Chalas, W. Bielecki, and W. Drygas, "The Association Between Income, Education, Control over Life and Health in a Large Urban Population of Poland," *Int J Occup Med Environ Health* 17, no. 2 (2004): 299–310.
17. Pamela Williams-Piehota, Tamera R. Schneider, Judith Pizarro, Linda Mowad, and Peter Salovey, "Matching Health Messages to Health Locus of Control Beliefs for Promoting Mammography Utilization," *Psychology and Health* 19, no. 4 (August 2004): 407–23.
18. Norman Cousins, *Head First: The Biology of Hope* (New York: E. P. Dutton, 1989), 120.
19. Cousins, *Head First*, 119–20.
20. J. E. Crisson and F. J. Keefe, "The Relationship of Locus of Control to Pain Coping Strategies and Psychological Distress in Chronic Pain Patients," *Behavioral Medicine* 35(2): 1988, 147–54.

21. Caryle Hirshberg, "Spontaneous Remission: The Spectrum of Self-Repair," The Psychology of Health, Immunity, and Disease, vol. B, 186, in *Proceedings of the Sixth International Conference of the National Institute for the Clinical Application of Behavioral Medicine.*

22. Carl Richter, "On the Phenomenon of Sudden Death in Animals and Man," *Psychosomatic Medicine* 19(3): 1957, 191–98.

23. K. C. Corley, H. P. Mauck, and F. O'M. Shiel, "Cardiac Responses Associated with 'Yoked Chair' Shock Avoidance in Squirrel Monkeys," *Psychophysiology* 12: 1975, 439–44.

24. National Institutes of Health, *Proceedings of the Forum on Coronary Prone Behavior,* Department of Health, Education, and Welfare Publication no. 78–1451 (Bethesda, Md.: National Institutes of Health), 162, June 1987.

25. Clinical Psychiatry News, as reported in "Health Briefs," *Executive Fitness,* November 1987, 8.

26. H. S. Akiskal and W. T. McKinney, "Overview of Recent Research in Depression," *Archives of General Psychiatry* 32: 1975, 285–305.

27. P. Ahluwalia, R. M. Zacharko, and H. Anisman, *Dopamine Variations Associated with Acute and Chronic Stressors,* presentation at the Annual Meeting of the Society of Neuroscience, Dallas, Texas, October 20–25, 1985.

28. W. Vale, J. Spiess, C. Rivier, and J. Rivier, "Characterization of a 41-Residue Ovine Hypothalamic Peptide that Stimulates Secretion of Corticotropin and Beta-Endorphin," *Science* 213: 1981, 1394–97.

29. Vale et al., "Characterization."

30. Claudia Wallis, "Stress: Can We Cope?" *Time,* June 6, 1983, 48–54.

31. S. G. Haynes, "Type A Behavior, Employment Status, and Coronary Heart Disease in Women," *Behavioral Medicine Update* 6(4): 1984, 11–15.

32. Haynes, "Type A Behavior," 13.

33. R. A. Karasek, T. G. T. Theorell, J. Schwartz, C. Pieper, and L. Alfredson, "Job, Psychological Factors, and Coronary Heart Disease," *Advances in Cardiology* 29: 1982, 62–67.

34. U. Lundberg and M. Frankenhaeser, "Psychophysiological Reactions to Noise as Modified by Personal Control over Stimulus Intensity," *Biological Psychology* 6: 1978, 51–58.

35. Wallis, "Stress."

36. Justice, 148–49.

37. Sandra M. Levy, *Emotional Expression and Survival in Breast Cancer Patients: Immunological Correlates,* paper presented at the Meetings of the American Psychological Association, August 1983, Anaheim, California.

38. Michael S. Gazzaniga, *Mind Matters* (Boston: Houghton Mifflin Company, 1988).

39. Locke and Colligan, *The Healer Within,* 210–11.

40. Justice, *Who Gets Sick?* 310–11.

41. R. S. Eliot, *Cognitive and Behavioral Stress Management Considerations,* presentation at a Conference on Stress and the Heart of the American College of Cardiology, July 1986, Jackson Hole, Wyoming.

# CHAPTER 20

# Self-Esteem and Health

*We can secure other people's approval, if we do right
and try hard; but our own is worth a hundred of it.*

—Mark Twain

## Learning Objectives

- Define self-esteem.
- Understand what factors impact self-esteem.
- Describe the impact of self-esteem on the body.
- Define self-efficacy, and understand how it differs from self-esteem.

American humorist and author Samuel Clemens—the legendary
Mark Twain—believed that it's a hundred times more valuable to
approve of ourselves than to have the approval of others. A century after he
penned that advice, it is proving to be true.

In his book on *Honoring the Self,* psychologist Nathaniel Branden calls
self-esteem the reputation we have with ourselves; when we believe that we
are bad or unworthy, the reputation is poor, and low self-esteem is the result.

We stand in the midst of an almost infinite network of relationships: to
other people, to things, to the universe. And yet, at three o'clock in the
morning, when we are alone with ourselves, we are aware that the most
intimate and powerful of all relationships and the one we can never escape
is the relationship to ourselves. No significant aspect of our thinking, motivation, feelings, or behavior is unaffected by our self-evaluation.[1]

According to a growing body of evidence, a healthy self-esteem is one of
the best things a person can do for overall health, both mental and physical.
And a good, strong sense of self can boost the immune system, improve heart
function, protect against disease, and aid in healing.

## What Is Self-Esteem?

Self-esteem is a sense of positive self-regard, or the degree to which people like or dislike themselves.[2] It's a way of viewing oneself as a good person who is well in all aspects. It's a sense of feeling good about one's capabilities, physical limitations, goals, place in the world, and relationship to others. Self-esteem is a powerful element. The perceptions about oneself are what set the boundaries for what we can and cannot do. Self-esteem can be called the blueprint for behavior.

Self-esteem should not be confused with self-concept. Self-concept is a broad term used to encompass all the ways we compare and evaluate ourselves to those around us. It refers to the way we compare ourselves physically, mentally, and socially. Self-esteem contributes to, but is not the same as, self-concept.[3] Instead, self-esteem is characterized by a powerful source of inner strength—the willingness to cope with the basic challenges of life, knowing you are more than your problems, learning to discriminate, and having self-acceptance and self-responsibility.[4]

Self-esteem, the value we assign to ourselves, is generally based on five factors—two physical and three psychological. The physical factors that determine our self-esteem are (1) our appearance (the way we look) and (2) our physical abilities. The psychological determinants of self-esteem are (1) how well we do in school (our perceived intelligence), (2) how confident we are in social situations, and (3) how we regard ourselves.[5] Recent research by Finnish scientist Mirja Kalliopuska suggests that empathy—the ability to put oneself in the place of other people and appreciate their feelings—may also be linked to self-esteem.[6]

Esteem toward "self" necessarily encompasses more than one "person" because none of us is one unified person. We all are collections of multiple selves that have different minds, different intelligences, and different sets of emotions. Psychologist Robert Ornstein and physician David Sobel explain,

> You can see this when you remember a face but not a name, or when your intellect tells you that something is a good idea but your emotions disagree. Each of us acts differently and is genuinely a different person to lovers than to coworkers, to children and to the police, different to old, close friends and to new business acquaintances. We have a great range of abilities and talents within ourselves, and the more we use them, the healthier we are.[7]

Ornstein and Sobel continue, "An innovative study of 'self-complexity' finds that men and women who are complex and diverse, whose selves reach out in different directions, suffer fewer signs of life's stresses. They report less depression and fewer foul moods, colds, coughs, stomach pains, headaches, and muscle aches than their less complex counterparts."[8]

Researchers have been able to identify what constitutes a healthy self-esteem. One of the most focused definitions was presented by Leonard Sagan in his examination of the factors that influence health and wellness in the world's various nations. In his comprehensive work, *The Health of Nations,* Sagan writes that those with a high level of self-esteem also have an inner locus of control:

> *They are confident of their ability to make competent decisions. They do not rely solely on traditional authority for guidance, but are able to acquire and evaluate information and make decisions independently. In contrast with traditional people who believe that outcomes are determined by gods, chance, or persons of influence, healthy people believe that their decisions can be efficacious in determining outcomes—that is, they believe that what they think and do will matter.[9]*

In his definition of healthy people, Sagan pointed out a vital characteristic among those with high self-esteem. Although healthy people have high regard for themselves, he said,

> *They are not self-indulgent or preoccupied with their personal identity or welfare. Rather they are committed to goals other than their own personal welfare. Goals may be global in scope or quite modest; most important, however, they are not egotistical in nature but will benefit others. Healthy people are compassionate, they have a strong sense of community. I believe that these qualities are in a state of decline in the United States, and it may not be a coincidence that evidence of worsening health is appearing at the same time that Americans are preoccupied with "self-realization."[10]*

In summary, he says, those with a healthy self-esteem have confidence in themselves and their ability to control their own lives; those who have low self-esteem tend to view themselves as passive victims—and are much more prone to illness and the stress of difficult life situations. When you have a strong sense of self-esteem, the exhilarating feeling that you are worthwhile can have a positive influence on your health.

A variety of studies have shown a strong correlation between self-esteem and health. When the California Department of Mental Health surveyed 1,000 Californians, they found that the healthiest ones cared most for others—and for themselves. One reason for the finding, suggests researcher James Lynch, is that people with high self-esteem take better care of themselves. People who really care about themselves naturally take better care of their bodies.

People with positive self-esteem view themselves as good people who are well in all aspects of life. They have a physical, mental, social, emotional, and spiritual balance that enables them to achieve an equilibrium that acts as a buffer against stress and difficult life situations.

## Where Does Self-Esteem Come From?

The formation of self-esteem begins early in life. Some of the first ingredients that make up self-esteem are the messages we receive during childhood from our parents, our other relatives, our teachers, and our friends. It depends partly on physical limitations—whether we are overweight, hard of hearing, or incapable of speaking without stuttering. It is influenced by social class and by cultural restrictions. And it depends to a great extent on how much love we feel from those around us—how much acceptance, how much compassion, how much we are able to identify and feel identified with.

So far, the factors that influence self-esteem seem to be largely beyond our control. We can't determine how our third-grade teacher deals with us, for example, nor can we change the fact that a mother's problem pregnancy left us severely visually impaired. But each of us can control one large factor in self-esteem: It's the way we communicate with our self-esteem, the words we say about ourselves, which may have a powerful effect not only on our minds but also on our bodies.

Psychologist Susan Jeffers likes to use a demonstration to impress people with the importance of what they're communicating to their self-esteem.[11] Whenever she gives a talk, she invites a volunteer from the audience to come up to the front. She has the volunteer make a fist and extend his or her right arm in front of the body, angled down to the left for strength. She then asks the volunteer to resist as powerfully as possible while she tries to push down on the arm. She relates that she's never "won" this initial trial.

She then asks the volunteer to stand at ease, close his or her eyes, and repeat ten times aloud, "I am a weak and unworthy person." She encourages the volunteer to really feel the words while speaking them. She then asks the volunteer to open his or her eyes, assume the original posture, and resist her efforts to push the same arm down.

"I wish I had a camera to record the expression on my volunteer's face as I press his arm and it gives way," Jeffers exclaims. "A few object, 'I wasn't ready!' So I do it again."

Once again, Jeffers has the volunteer close the eyes, stand at ease, and repeat aloud a different set of words: "I am a strong and worthy person." Jeffers says that, to everyone's surprise, she once again cannot budge the arm.

She concludes that she can run this experiment backward and forward almost any number of times, and "it makes no difference if I leave the room while he speaks and I don't know what he has said: Weak words mean a weak arm; strong words mean a strong arm."

Jeffers explains this phenomenon by stating,

*It is as though the inner self doesn't know what is true and false, and believes the words it is told without judging them. . . . We can control our self-esteem by speaking to it. I think the conclusion is obvious: Stop feeding yourself negative words, and start building yourself up with positive ones.*[12]

## The Impact of Self-Esteem on the Body

Whether people do or do not get sick—and how long they stay that way—may depend in part on how strong their self-esteem is. A growing body of evidence indicates that low self-esteem is often a factor in chronic pain, for example. And several studies show that recovery from infectious mononucleosis is related to "ego strength"; the higher the self-esteem, the more rapid the recovery.[13]

The level of self-esteem one has appears to be a crucial factor in how people respond to stress, regardless of their personality type. Low self-esteem is a common denominator in stress-prone personalities, such as Type A and helpless-hopeless types.[14] Self-esteem may also be an important factor in the risk of heart disease. As discussed previously, scientists for years ascribed the highest risk of heart disease to the classic "Type A" personality. More recent in-depth research, however, has isolated two factors—anger and hostility—as the real culprits in the Type A personality pattern. A person can be a Type A personality and not have an increased risk of heart disease as long as he or she is not angry and hostile.

Self-esteem is so powerful an influence on health that it even impacts the way we react to life events. Some sources of stress can be categorized as "life events"—situations in life that researchers have determined cause stress. Many are negatives, such as the death of a loved one, divorce, a jail term, or assuming a new debt. But researchers have found that positive life events—such as getting married, getting a new job, or giving birth—are also sources of stress. Whether these stressors cause a person to become ill depends on many factors, including one's ability to cope with the stress.

In their research in life events, scientists have found that self-esteem has significant influence on how positive life events impact our health. If we've got strong self-esteem, the outlook is good: The more positive life events, the better our health. But if our self-esteem is poor, our health can decline in direct proportion as our life becomes peppered with more positive life events.[15] This may be because we believe we are not worthy of positive life events.

Results of various studies show that positive self-esteem helps protect health. One reason behind its protective nature may be its effect on the immune system. One study that gives a glimpse of the self-esteem/immunity link was conducted by psychiatrist J. Stephen Heisel and his colleagues at McLean Hospital. They studied 111 college students who had completed the Minnesota Multiphasic Personality Inventory (MMPI), a 566-item questionnaire that describes personality and other measures of mental health, such as level of depression. In analyzing the students' scores, he found that those with the highest self-esteem were also the ones with the strongest natural killer-cell activity. High self-esteem seemed to provide a boost to the immune system and give students stronger immunity against disease.[16]

Harvard Medical School Psychiatrist Steven Locke cites the work of psychoneuroimmunology pioneer Dr. George Solomon in making a further case for self-esteem as an influence on immunity.[17] According to Locke, Solomon gave the example of two homosexual men, both of whom had been diagnosed with AIDS. One was "a conservative, cultured college professor whose sex life was relatively monogamous," explains Solomon, but his self-esteem was battered because he had difficulty accepting his homosexuality and expressing negative emotions. The other man was a highly promiscuous individual who was heavily involved in sadomasochistic sex, drinking, smoking, drug abuse, and the frequenting of bars that catered to his whims. But "his self-esteem was excellent," Solomon notes. "He has a number of close friends and with a number of other sadomasochists he has formed a sadomasochist support group that meets every week to talk about their problems. He feels that his self-esteem in the past years is the highest it has ever been in his life."

When Solomon took blood tests and compared the immune systems of the two, the sadomasochist—the one who, by all rights, should have been in the poorest condition because of his deleterious health habits—had the strongest immune system. Solomon theorizes that his strong sense of self-esteem had kept his immune system in better shape.[18]

Researchers have also found a possible connection between poor self-esteem and premature death from coronary heart disease. Researchers from McGill University in Montreal gave thorough psychological questionnaires to 200 men recovering from heart attack. Over the next five years, the men who reported feeling "useless" or unable to "do things well" were nearly four times as likely to die from coronary disease as men with higher self-esteem. That association remained strong even after researchers adjusted for other factors.[19]

## Self-Efficacy: Believing in Yourself

An important part of self-esteem is what psychologists call self-efficacy, one of the components of self-esteem that apparently leads to both psychological and physical well-being. Self-efficacy is your perception of your own ability to do a specific task and to overcome the difficulties inherent in that specific task.[20] Dr. Albert Bandura of Stanford University says that self-efficacy is not related to your skills, but to what you think you can do with the skills you have.[21] It's your belief in yourself, your conviction that you can manage the adverse events that come along in your life.

People tend to pursue tasks they know they can accomplish and avoid those they believe exceed their capabilities.[22] In other words, your sense of self-efficacy generally influences what you will and will not try to do. For example, if you believe that you can learn a new software program recommended by an associate, you'll plunge in with gusto. If you believe that you have real problems learning software, you'll be unlikely to try—unless you're required to for a class or for your job. Self-efficacy also influences how much effort you'll make while trying something new and your persistence in overcoming any obstacles.[23]

Self-efficacy is measured by:[24]

- **Magnitude**—the judgment a person has about the ability to accomplish a number of things; a person with high magnitude believes she can accomplish everything on a list, for example, and will feel capable of doing even the most difficult things on the list.

- **Strength**—confidence about the ability to perform any single thing.

- **Generality**—how many areas the person feels confident in. The extent to which a person feels confident in the ability to do one thing will affect whether he feels confident in being able to do other related things.

Just as with self-esteem, various factors combine to determine how strong your self-efficacy is:

1. **Past performance.** If you've handled things well in the past, your faith in yourself is bolstered, and you are more likely to feel confident about facing any new situations.

2. **Vicarious experience.** This means keeping your eyes open and watching what goes on around you. You see how a friend deals with the death of her spouse. You watch what happens to a coworker when he loses several big accounts and then gets fired. You watch a television documentary about a midwestern farm family that faces seemingly insurmountable odds but emerges with spirit and courage after losing farm, home, and source of income. You read a magazine article about a young mother who faces with great courage the task of caring for her severely handicapped baby. You take all of that in, and the message comes through: If they can do it, so can I. You gain strength from their strength, courage from their courage. You make the unspoken commitment that when your time comes, you'll rally, too.

3. **The encouragement of others.** It's much easier to believe in yourself when the people around you are cheering you on.

Self-efficacy is an important component of self-esteem, because it can, in a very real way, predict your behavior. It determines your level of effort: If you really believe you can succeed, you're apt to keep on trying. It endows you with perseverance in the face of failure: If you really believe in yourself, you're less likely to give up. Your level of self-efficacy determines whether you will help yourself or hinder yourself. It determines, too, how well you will react to stress: If you are low in self-efficacy, you may become overwhelmed by stress because you become convinced that your life—or a particular situation—is unmanageable.

To sum it up, people with solid self-efficacy believe they'll come out on top—so they usually do. Bandura has identified three landmark characteristics of people with high self-efficacy:

1. They believe the intended outcome of a given behavior is of value to themselves.
2. They believe that performing the behavior will lead to that outcome.
3. They believe that they can successfully perform the behavior.[25]

As Bandura says, "When beset with difficulties, people who entertain serious doubts about their capabilities slacken their efforts or give up altogether, whereas those who have a strong sense of efficacy exert great effort to master the challenges."[26]

Psychologist Blair Justice gives an example of the difference that self-efficacy can make in one of the most stressful situations: the relocation of an elderly person from one place to another or from one institution to another. A marked increase in death rate often occurs, he says, usually within the first three months after relocation. When a home for the elderly in Chicago was closed, Justice writes, "The mortality rate was substantially lower for those who accepted the news of relocation philosophically but not with a sense of defeat or helplessness."[27] Those who became angry about the move fared almost as well—possibly because their anger mobilized them "to take care of themselves by eating, keeping as active as possible, and not giving up."

Self-efficacy is a potent predictor of health behaviors. For example, people who believe they can quit smoking are much more likely to actually quit. In one study of more than 800 smokers, those with the greatest self-efficacy moved most quickly—and most surely—from a stage of just *thinking* about quitting to actually quitting during the six-month period of the study.[28] Recent research also shows that self-esteem and self-efficacy are related to more positive health behaviors in young adults, and that healthy self-esteem acquired early in life can significantly impact key long-term preventive health behaviors.[29] Self-efficacy has also been positively related to many other health behaviors, including:

1. **Exercise.**[30] In one study involving more than fifty men who had suffered heart attacks, those with the highest self-efficacy did best on treadmill tests and were the ones who followed up most consistently at home.[31] In another study involving men and women with chronic obstructive pulmonary disease, those with the highest self-efficacy did best in following a program of walking, which helped control their disease symptoms.[32]

2. **Weight loss and nutrition.**[33] In one study of 179 men and women aged twenty to sixty, those with the highest self-efficacy followed through with a program of exercise and nutrition that led to weight loss.[34] In another study involving almost 200 men and women from three different ethnic groups (white, Hispanic, and black), self-efficacy was the highest predictor of who would follow exercise and nutrition guidelines and actually lose weight.[35]

3. **Persistence in following physician orders** following heart attack and other cardiac disease.[36] Interestingly, one study of 411 men and women from different ethnic groups found that those with the highest self-efficacy also had the lowest *risk* for cardiac disease, probably because of positive health behavior.[37]

4. **Consistency in using contraceptives.**[38]

Self-efficacy can actually cause physiological changes in the body. When under stress of any kind, the brain releases chemicals called catecholamines, which trigger a complex set of physiological reactions enabling a person to meet the challenge of the stress—the classic fight-or-flight syndrome. By measuring the levels of catecholamines in the blood, researchers can determine the degree of stress.

Bandura and his colleagues selected twelve women who had arachnaphobia and measured the level of catecholamine secretion when the women were faced with situations that frightened them—looking at a spider, putting a hand in a bowl with a spider, or allowing a spider to crawl on a hand. When women felt that they could handle a situation, catecholamine levels were low; when they felt that a situation was more than they could handle (in other words, when their self-efficacy was low), catecholamine levels shot up.

Bandura and his colleagues at Stanford worked with the women to bolster their level of self-efficacy regarding spiders. The women gained confidence, and some began to believe that they could manage an encounter with a spider. When that happened, says Bandura, catecholamine levels stayed low. Stress was eased, and the women did not suffer the physiological reactions as before.[39]

The real power of self-efficacy on health is demonstrated quite simply. If you want to get a fairly accurate prediction of how healthy someone is or will be, ask people how healthy they think they are. Researchers have found that "self-rated" health—much the same as self-efficacy—determines to a large extent how healthy a person will actually be. Some studies have even shown that asking that simple question will tell you more about a person's health than an entire battery of sophisticated laboratory tests.

Ornstein and Sobel report on a seven-year study carried out in Manitoba, Canada. More than 3,500 elderly people were asked, "For your age would you say, in general, your health is excellent, good, fair, poor, or bad?" Researchers conducting the study also sought health reports from physicians that gave detailed records on illnesses, surgeries, hospitalizations, and other medical problems. When researchers correlated actual health at the end of the study with self-ratings and medical observations seven years earlier, they found the self-ratings to be more accurate and predictive than the health measures from the physicians. Even more surprisingly, "Those who were in objectively poor health by physician report survived at a higher rate as long as they believed their own health to be good."[40] The only thing more powerful than self-rated health, in fact, was increasing age.

Belief in oneself is one of the most powerful weapons we have in protecting our health and living longer. It has a startling impact on wellness. And we are able to harness it to our advantage. As Madeline Gershwin said, "What wise people and grandmothers have always known is that the way you feel about yourself, your attitudes, beliefs, values, have a great deal to do with your health and well-being."[41]

## ENDNOTES

1. Joan Borysenko, *Guilt Is the Teacher, Love Is the Lesson* (New York: Warner Books, 1990), 45.
2. M. Rosenberg and H. B. Kaplan, *Social Psychology of the Self-Concept* (Arlington Heights, Ill.: Harland Davidson, 1982).
3. Phillip L. Rice, *Stress and Health: Principles and Practice for Coping and Wellness* (Monterey, Calif.: Brooks/Cole Publishing Company, 1987), 111.
4. National Branden, "Living with Self-Esteem," *Lotus,* Fall 1992.
5. Rice, *Stress and Health.*
6. *Psychological Reports* 70: 1119–22.
7. Robert Ornstein and David Sobel, *Healthy Pleasures* (Reading, Mass.: Addison-Wesley Publishing Company, 1989), 189.
8. Ornstein and Sobel, *Healthy Pleasures,* 190.
9. Leonard A. Sagan, *The Health of Nations* (New York: Basic Books, 1987), 187.
10. Sagan, *The Health of Nations.*
11. Described in Susan Jeffers, "Building Your Self-Esteem: Your Positive Words Will Make You Strong," *Success,* October 1987, 72.
12. Jeffers, "Building Your Self-Esteem."

13. S. Michael Plaut and Stanford B. Friedman, "Biological Mechanisms in the Relationship of Stress to Illness," *Pediatric Annals* 14(8): 1985, 563–67.
14. Brian Luke Seaward, *Managing Stress* (Boston: Jones and Bartlett Publishers, 1994), 104.
15. Barbara R. Sarason, Irwin G. Sarason, and Gregory R. Pierce, *Social Support: An Interactional View* (New York: John Wiley & Sons, 1990), 164.
16. "Research Strengthens Link Between Poor Mental and Physical Health," *Sexuality Today Newsletter,* November 24, 1986, 4.
17. Steven Locke and Douglas Colligan, *The Healer Within* (New York: E. P. Dutton, 1986), 131–32.
18. Locke and Colligan, *The Healer Within.*
19. "Danger from Depression," *Consumer Reports on Health,* August 1992, 63.
20. Rayane AbuShabha and Cheryl Achterberg, "Review of Self-Efficacy and Locus of Control for Nutrition- and Health-Related Behavior," *Journal of the American Dietetic Association* 97(1):1122–32, October 1997.
21. Albert Bandura, *Social Foundations of Thought and Action* (Englewood Cliffs, N.J.: Prentice Hall, 1986).
22. AbuShaba and Achterberg, "Review of Self-Efficacy," 1997.
23. Ibid.
24. Ibid.
25. Aaron Antonovsky, *Unraveling the Mystery of Health: How People Manage Stress and Stay Well* (San Francisco: Jossey-Bass Publishers, 1988), 59.
26. "Self-Efficacy," *University of California Berkeley Wellness Letter* 3(8): 1987, 1–2.
27. Blair Justice, *Who Gets Sick: Thinking and Health* (Houston, Tex.: Peak Press, 1987), 144–45.
28. J. O. Prochaska and C. C. DiClemente, "Self-Change Processes, Self-Efficacy and Decisional Balance Across Five Stages of Smoking Cessation," in A. R. Liss, ed., *Advances in Cancer Control: Epidemiology and Research* (New York: Alan R. Liss, 1984).
29. Erik T. Huntsinger and Linda J. Luecken, "Attachment Relationships and Health Behavior: The Mediational Role of Self-Esteem," *Pyschology and Health* 19, no. 4 (August 2004): 515–26.
30. R. Desharnais, J. Bouillon, and G. Gordin, "Self-Efficacy and Outcome Expectation as Determinants of Exercise Adherence," *Psychological Reports,* 59:1155–59, 1986.
31. AbuShaba and Achterberg, "Review of Self-Efficacy," 1997.
32. R. M. Kaplan, C. J. Atkins, and S. Reinsch, "Specific Efficacy Expectations Mediate Exercise Compliance in Patients with COPD," *Health Psychology* 3:223–48, 1984.
33. AbuShaba and Achterberg, "Review of Self-Efficacy," 1997; N. Bernier and J. Avard, "Self-Efficacy Outcome and Attrition in a Weight Reduction Program," *Cognitive Therapy Research* 10: 319–38, 1986; and R. S. Weinberg, H. H. Hughes, J. W. Critelli, R. England, and A. Jackson, "Effects of Pre-Existing and Manipulated Levels of Self-Efficacy on Weight Loss in a Self-Control Program," *Journal of Research Perspectives* 18: 352–58, 1984.
34. M. H. Weitzel, "A Test of the Health Promotion Model with Blue-Collar Workers," *Nursing Research* 38: 99–104, 1989.
35. M. H. Weitzel and P. R. Waller, "Predictive Factors for Health-Promotive Behaviors in White, Hispanic, and Black Blue-Collar Workers," *Family and Community Health* 13(1): 23–34, 1990.
36. AbuShaba and Achterberg, "Review of Self-Efficacy," 1997; C. K. Ewart, C. B. Taylor, L. B. Reese, and R. F. Debusk, "Effects of Early Postmyocardial Infarction Exercise Testing and Self-Perception and Subsequent Physical

Activity," *American Journal of Cardiology* 51: 1076–80; and C. B. Taylor, A. Bandura, C. K. Ewart, N. H. Miller, and R. F. Debusk, "Raising Spouse's and Patient's Beliefs Perception of His Cardiac Capabilities Following a Myocardial Infarction," *American Journal of Cardiology* 55: 635–38, 1985.

37. M. A. Winkleby, J. A. Flora, and H. C. Kraemer, "A Community-Based Heart Disease Intervention: Predictors of Change," *American Journal of Public Health* 84(5): 767–72, 1994.

38. Albert Bandura, "Social Cognitive Theory and Exercise of Control of HIV Infection," in J. Peterson and R. DiClemente, eds., *Preventing AIDS: Theory and Practice of Behavioral Interventions* (New York: Plenum Press, 1993).

39. Robert Ornstein and David Sobel, *The Healing Brain* (New York: Simon & Schuster, 1987), 249.

40. Cited in Ornstein and Sobel, *The Healing Brain*, 246–48.

41. Ibid., 249–50.

CHAPTER 21

# The Healing Power of Humor and Laughter

*With the fearful strain that is on me night and day,*
*if I did not laugh I should die.*

—Abraham Lincoln

## Learning Objectives

- Discuss professional trends toward using humor in healing.
- Understand the physical and psychological benefits of humor.
- Discuss the physiology of laughter.
- List the ways in which laughter is a form of exercise.
- Discuss the physical and psychological benefits of laughter.
- Understand how laughter contributes to pain relief.

**M**ark Twain once penned the sentiment that "against the assault of laughter nothing can stand." What the great American humorist and author believed more than a hundred years ago is being proven true today by some of our most gifted scientists: A sense of humor, and the laughter that accompanies it, can actually banish pain and keep us well.

Laughter as medicine is probably as old as humankind. One of the earliest written accounts recognizing the healing power of humor is found in the Bible, in which King Solomon remarked that "a merry heart doeth good like a medicine."[1] Members of royal courts around the world and throughout the ages have valued the court jester—the colorful clown who provided the humor that made governing a palatable job.

Henri de Mondeville, a thirteenth-century surgeon, told jokes to his patients as they emerged from operations. Sixteenth-century English educator Richard Mulcater prescribed laughter for those afflicted with head colds and melancholy; a favorite "cure" was being tickled in the armpits. Humor was even used by ancient Americans: Ojibway Indian doctor-clowns, the Windigokan, used laughter to heal the sick.[2]

They may not have had the scientific proof to back up their suppositions, but even early physicians recognized the healing power of humor. The famous seventeenth-century physician Thomas Sydenham said that "the arrival of a good clown exercises more beneficial influence upon the health of a town than twenty asses laden with drugs."[3]

Webster's dictionary defines humor as the quality that appeals to a sense of the comical or absurdly incongruous. What we generally refer to as a "sense of humor" is the ability to bring happiness both to your own life as well as to the life of others. (It's important to understand that there is also bad—or unhealthy—humor as well: Any time humor is used to hurt someone, lower another person's self-esteem, or bring tears of sadness, it is not a healthy kind of humor.)[4] According to Loretta LaRoche of Boston's Deaconess Hospital, good humor is "the ability to feel inner joy, peace, and harmony within yourself and your surroundings—to discover that we are all part of a divine comedy."[5] Humor is a way of looking at things that helps to dissipate stress and accentuate the positive. "When we become too serious," says LaRoche, "we help create the components for stress, rigid thinking, helplessness, cynicism, and hardening of the attitude."[6] Again, the type of humor that is positive does not involve ridicule, derision, sarcasm, or a caustic tongue—and is not leveled at someone else's expense.

Humor has been used across the span of cultures to make people feel better. A number of American Indian tribes—the Zunis, Crees, Pueblos, and Hopis among them—had ceremonial clowns whose sole purpose was to provide humor for their tribesmen. According to accounts, they were called in "to entertain and heal the sick with their hilarity, frightening away the demons of ill health."[7]

Humor has been widely used in traditional medicine in a number of cultures. Dr. Rosita Arvigo, who practiced in Belize under the tutelage of the great Mayan healer Don Elijio Panti, remembers that he was the "funniest man I ever knew," a man who referred to himself as "the doctor clown." Given the choice between being a doctor and a clown, he said, he would choose a clown. He believed laughter was extremely important in medicine—and greeted his patients by teasing them, doing hilarious dances, and performing crazy gestures until they were wild with laughter. She remembers that one of his lessons for contemporary physicians would be

> that a person's spirit needs to be uplifted as much as the body needs to be healed. And without an uplifted spirit I don't think there is enough energy within the body, enough vital force or what the Maya call ch'ulel [known as prana or chi in other cultures] for a person to properly and completely experience healing.[8]

One of the most renowned uses of laughter in our own day occurred when former *Saturday Review* editor Norman Cousins incorporated it in a program to treat ankylosing spondylitis, a debilitating connective tissue disease. Cousins employed funny movies and books to relieve the pain of the disease.

"Ten minutes of genuine belly laughter had an anesthetic effect and would give me at least two hours of pain-free sleep," Cousins relates. "When the pain-killing effect of the laughter wore off, we would switch on the motion picture projector again and, not infrequently, it would lead to another pain-free sleep interval."[9] Indeed, claims Cousins, of "all the gifts bestowed by nature on human beings, hearty laughter must be close to the top. The response to incongruities is one of the highest manifestations of the cerebral process."

C. W. Metcalf, an international consultant who helps people use humor to cope with stress, says, "Humor, then, is a set of survival skills that relieve tension, keeping us fluid and flexible instead of allowing us to become rigid and breakable, in the face of relentless change."[10]

The renowned novelist Dostoevski wrote, "If you wish to glimpse inside a human soul and get to know a man, don't bother analyzing his ways of being silent, of talking, of weeping, or seeing how much he is moved by noble ideas; you'll get better results if you just watch him laugh. If he laughs well, he's a good man. . . . All I claim to know is that laughter is the most reliable gauge of human nature."[11]

## Professional Trends Toward Humor

Researchers are now providing scientific proof that laughter (along with a sense of humor) can literally make a person feel better. Based on the most recent batch of scientific evidence proving laughter's health benefits, hospitals and medical clinics have started to utilize laughter in unique ways to promote the health of patients.[12]

One of the prototypes for "humor centers" in the nation's hospitals is the Living Room of the William Stehlin Foundation for Cancer Research at Houston's St. Joseph's Hospital. The room is filled with greenery and furnished with comfortable, overstuffed pieces. Patients are free to go to the room as often as needed for "comic relief" from the severity of their illness.

The "humor room" at Schenectady's Sunnyview Hospital and Rehabilitation Center boasts a poster reminding patients to take a "humor break" from illness. In the room, patients can check out funny movies, humorous tapes, and funny books. They are also given access to proven "mirth makers," such as balloons, clown noses, and bottles of bubble soap. At DeKalb General Hospital in Decatur, Georgia, patients can spend part of their recovery time in a brightly painted "Lively Room" stocked with funny games, tapes, and movies. Laurel and Hardy movies are shown in the Living Room of Orlando's Humana Hospital Lucerne.

Leslie Gibson, creator of the Comedy Cart Connection at Morton Plant Hospital in Clearwater, Florida, points out that being hospitalized puts people at the highest level of stress—and that humor is a natural remedy. "The loss of control often places patients in fearful, compromising situations. Besides promoting healing, humor is an excellent diversionary tool for keeping their minds off their pain."[13]

At the Detroit Medical Center's Children's Hospital of Michigan, clowns from the hospital's Clowns-on-Call program wander the halls, lobbies, and waiting rooms several days a week. These volunteers—mostly people from the community who volunteer on a regular basis—transform themselves into Dr. Ha Choo, Nurse Stefy Scope, and Dr. ICU Giggle. They make their rounds, visiting those patients who need a "clown consult" or a prescription for laughter. Founders of the program say that children with chronic diseases need to know it's okay to laugh—and so do their parents. "We try to make children forget about the hospital and focus on the fun," says Dr. Barry Duel, a pediatric urology fellow also known as Dr. Bee Dee who started the program. "If they're laughing, they're having fun and they can't focus on the pain."[14]

Another innovative program is the Clown Care Unit at Babies and Children's Hospital at Columbia-Presbyterian Medical Center in New York. Researchers there were awarded three pilot research grants to study the value of clown therapy for pediatric heart and cancer patients. Finding that the clowns helped decrease both the physical and psychological distress of patients who were undergoing medical procedures for heart disease and cancer, the program brought in specially trained clowns to work with the children. Researchers found that "the joyful distraction provided by the clowns would increase patient cooperation, decrease parental anxiety, and decrease the need for sedation during anxious moments in the hospital."[15]

The trend toward humor as a way of boosting both physical and mental health has spread to private practice. Increasing numbers of physicians throughout the nation have begun using humor and laughter as a way of easing tension, promoting healing, and even boosting immunity among their patients. Nurses, too, have caught the vision: More than 1,000 nurses joined forces several years ago to organize Nurses for Laughter (NFL). The members, who try to make humor a part of their bedside manner, boast the motto "Caution: Humor may be hazardous to your illness." The nurses work to help patients see some humor in their situations, and to bring some life and laughter to the hospital setting, which can too often be sterile and solemn.

Humor is also being used successfully in long-term care facilities. At Regency Healthcare and Rehabilitation Center, a 300-bed nursing facility in

Niles, Illinois, staff members act out whodunit mysteries, residents do imitations of John Wayne, and everyone at the facility comes together to put on their own Academy Awards show—with Clark Gable continuing to be a big winner. "Residents face so many challenges and losses—and when things get rough, humor is a coping mechanism," says Kevin M. Kavanaugh, director of community relations for Regency.[16]

Humor is even being used in a setting not normally considered at all funny—hospice care, where people are assisted in the death process. At the VNA Community Hospice in Arlington, Virginia, workers help the patients focus on *life*—on *living* each day until they die. At weekly Tuesday night meetings, people gather, have a cup of coffee, and share their experiences—and the room very often fills with laughter as people acknowledge the elements of humor in their stories, struggles, and memories. It's not unusual, say the organizers, to hear people describe uncontrollable laughter at times not usually thought of as funny, because humor is often a mechanism that frees them from emotional bondage.

The benefits of laughter on physical and mental health are being noted even in the corporate world. According to a report published in *Newsweek,*[17] some of the nation's largest corporations have instituted humor programs to help develop a sense of humor in employees—and the results include an increased employee capacity to deal with stress and an overall improvement in job performance. Management for Safeway Stores, in fact, reports a sharp decrease in the number of debilitating accidents since the stores began holding humor clinics in 1984. Other major entities that hold humor clinics or programs for employees include Manville Corporation, Southwestern Bell, IBM, Hewlett-Packard, the U.S. Air Force, Monsanto, the Internal Revenue Service, General Foods, and the Hartford Insurance Group.

## The Impact of Humor on Health

The physiological changes that occur from laughter are so effective that laughter may be classed as aerobic activity. And the outlook characterized by a good sense of humor is beneficial to both physical and mental wellness, according to the most recent evidence.

Educator and author John-Roger was traveling with some friends on the lecture circuit. When they arrived at one destination, the plane was late. To make matters worse, everyone else's luggage arrived first. When their luggage finally appeared, one piece of luggage was obviously damaged. Another suitcase had sprung open, and clothing and personal items were spread all over the conveyor belt. The people traveling with John-Roger were becoming increasingly upset.

Finally he turned to the group and said, "Relax, this is funny. In a few weeks we'll be telling stories about tonight and laughing about it. If it'll be funny then, it's funny now."

According to John-Roger, the focus changed. They started looking at the situation "as if it were a Woody Allen movie. When some of the luggage didn't arrive, we smiled. When the car rental agency didn't have our reservation (or cars), we laughed. When we heard there was a taxi strike, we howled."[18]

American actress Ethel Barrymore echoed the experience of the stranded travelers: "You grow up the day you have the first real laugh—at yourself." Some of the biggest crises we experience turn into some of our funniest moments. The mere passage of time transforms them. Top stand-up comic Judy Carter maintains that "there's a little bit of stand-up comic in everyone; the performance comes not when you're having a fight, but in telling a friend afterward."[19]

Antioch University Professor Harvey Mindess, an expert in humor, points out, "Humor at its best encourages a broad perspective on life. It provides a view of the ironies that abound, of the fact that nobody and nothing is as it seems. And recognizing life's zaniness encourages flexibility and adaptability, rather than rigidity and brittleness."[20]

One of the most healing things about humor, say some, is that it acts as a bond between people. Comedy writer Emily Levine suggests,

> *Humor is extraordinary for making connections with people. Everyone has such a separate reality, and it's alienating to feel you'll never really be understood because nobody sees the world the same way you do. But when you make a joke and someone else gets it, it means for that moment, your mind worked exactly the same, you were totally in sync. That's divine grace.*[21]

## The Physical Benefits of Humor

Humor has been shown to have a positive effect on people with heart disease. In one study, two groups of people who had experienced heart attacks were followed throughout their cardiac rehabilitation; one group was allowed to view humorous videos or television programs for half an hour a day as part of their standard therapy. That group, the research revealed, suffered fewer arrhythmias, had lower levels of harmful catecholamines in their blood and urine, required less medication, and had fewer heart attack recurrences.[22]

Because the Type A personality has been implicated in heart disease, one study looked at the relationship between humor and the Type A personality. Researchers found that 40 percent of people with coronary heart disease laughed less frequently and used humor less often during adversity. Basically, said the researchers, the people who laughed more were healthier.[23]

The results of recent research also show that a sense of humor—a point of view that sees the comical in things, and an attitude of merriment—can actually promote good health by strengthening the immune system. Studies have shown that people who tend to have a humorous outlook have greater immunity against a variety of diseases as well as increased ability to fight off infection.

In one study, researchers had a group of men watch a sixty-minute humor video, they then measured various immune indicators. After watching the video, the men had greater activity among their natural killer cells—the cells that assist in immune surveillance—that lasted for at least twelve hours after watching the video. Researchers determined that because the effect lasted for twelve hours, daily exposure to humor could prolong the elevation of natural killer cells, adding powerful immune protection.[24]

In another study, people were randomly assigned to watch either a humorous or a distracting video. Those who watched the humorous video had greater stress reduction and elevated natural killer cell activity. The investigators who conducted the study observed that "the amount of mirthful laughter was the major contributing factor for the increased immune function seen in these subjects, rather than the reduced stress levels."[25]

Finally, research has shown that healthy people who watch a sixty-minute humorous video have elevations in growth hormones and important decreases in stress hormones—including cortisol, dopamine, and epinephrine. The implication of these findings is that humor could reverse some of the classical physiological changes that occur during stress.[26]

## The Psychological Benefits of Humor

A sense of humor has tremendous psychological benefits as well, and correlates positively to quality of life. In one study, humor was shown to boost a number of factors that are related to psychological health, such as optimism and self-esteem. The same study found that those who did not score well on a scientific scale that measures humor were much more likely to show signs of psychological distress, such as depression.[27]

Researchers conducting a wide array of studies have found that, in addition to enhancing self-esteem, a humorous outlook on life can have far-reaching benefits, including promoting creativity, improving negotiating and decision-making skills, maintaining a sense of balance, improving performance, bestowing a sense of power, relieving stress, and improving coping abilities.

***Promoting creativity.***   People with a good sense of humor are generally more creative—and tend to have much more creativity in the way they approach life's problems. Edward de Bono, the world's leading authority on creativity, says that humor and the creative process are actually one and the same thing. With both, he says, the brain recognizes the value of the absurd or the creative idea only in hindsight, because, before that, both seem "crazy." The hallmarks of creative thinkers, then, are the willingness to play with ideas and to risk foolishness without fear.[28]

***Improving negotiating and decision-making skills.***     A good sense of humor apparently improves the ability to negotiate and to make decisions. Researchers who wanted to measure the impact of humor on negotiating situations set up a role-playing situation in which paired volunteers played the roles of buyers and sellers of appliances.[29] The volunteers were given a range of alternatives and were told to achieve the highest profit (the sellers) or the best deal (the buyers).

The pairs who read funny cartoons—of the *B.C.* and *New Yorker* variety— did best. During the face-to-face negotiation involved in the role playing, they were less anxious, had fewer contentions, and were better able to reach a solution that pleased both the "buyer" and the "seller."

***Maintaining a sense of balance.***     Renowned American clergyman Henry Ward Beecher wrote that a person without a sense of humor "is like a wagon without springs—jolted by every pebble in the road." Indeed, a sense of humor helps us achieve and maintain that delicate balance that puts life in perspective. We all suffer stress; we all endure heartache; we all struggle with situations that are less than perfect. Viewed through a sense of humor, it all seems okay. We don't take things too seriously, and we are able to coast through situations that would otherwise tip us precariously off balance.[30]

***Improving performance.***     Humor helps to improve both group and individual performance. The greatest benefits occur, says University of Tennessee Psychologist Howard Pollio, when the humor is directly related to the task at hand.[31]

***Bestowing a sense of power.***     A sense of humor can give us a sense of power. According to "jollyologist" Allen Klein, laughter helps us to transcend our predicaments.[32] He gives the example of Anatoly Sharansky, the Russian human rights advocate who was confined for nine years in Soviet prisons. His prison sentence included sixteen months of solitary confinement and the constant threat of the death penalty.

Klein relates that Soviet police constantly threatened Sharansky with the *rastrel* (the "firing squad"), knowing that Sharansky's greatest battle was against fear. Sharansky managed to win the war against fear through humor. He started actually joking about the firing squad and talking about it on a daily basis.

"You make jokes fifteen to twenty times," Sharansky remembers, "and the word becomes like any other word. The ear gets accustomed to it, and it no longer prompts fear."

Klein relates a second example involving eighteenth-century philosopher Moses Mendelssohn. While walking down the streets of Berlin one day, he accidentally collided with a plump Prussian officer. "Swine!" the officer bellowed. Mendelssohn, knowing that a reprisal would invite punishment from the officer, decided on a different approach—one laced with humor. He smiled, tipped his hat, and replied, "Mendelssohn." As Klein points out, humor can turn any situation around—and can give us a feeling of power over our circumstances.

***Relieving stress.***    Numerous studies have shown that people who withstand even tremendous stress without becoming brittle, bitter, and broken have several traits in common: They are altruistic (they actively care about the welfare of others), they get plenty of support from friends and the community, and they gain control over difficult situations with humor.[33]

Humor has been demonstrated in a wide variety of studies to help alleviate the effects of stress. In one, researchers showed that people with a good sense of humor don't get as stressed to begin with. They placed an old tennis shoe, a drinking glass, and an aspirin bottle on a table and asked volunteers to make up a three-minute comedy routine using the objects on the table. Results of the study showed that the volunteers who wrote the funniest routines were those who were least likely to become tense, depressed, angry, fatigued, or confused when stress occurred in their lives.[34]

Other studies produce the same results. In one, researchers obtained measures of stress, anxiety, coping, and appreciation on 101 volunteers. The scores revealed that the ones with the greatest appreciation of humor were also the ones who were most effective in coping with stress. The ones who were least effective in coping with stress were also the ones who had a very dismal outlook when it came to humor.[35] In a similar study involving fifty-six volunteers, researchers showed that a good sense of humor relieved stress and moderated the volunteers' physical responses to stressors.[36]

In one study, volunteers were shown a film about an industrial accident—a decidedly unfunny topic. Half the volunteers were asked to come up with a comical dialogue during the film; the other half were asked to give a straightforward report about the film afterward. Researchers were able to measure far less of the stress response in the bodies of those who came up with the comical dialogue—even among those who researchers characteristically would have categorized as "not funny."[37]

Results of that survey show not only that humor helps relieve stress, but also that it can be learned, even by those who may not consider themselves to have a great sense of humor. Study author Michelle Newman says that the study "suggests that the way we perceive ourselves may not necessarily reflect how capable we are of using humor to cope. It challenges the notion that using coping humor is an unchangeable trait rather than an acquired skill." According to Newman, the study results show that you can "rethink the situation to decide if it's really a big deal or if you can handle it. And it may help you distance yourself enough from a situation to calm down."[38]

In another study, researchers split a group of volunteers in half. One group watched an hour-long humorous video; the other group participated in a neutral activity. All members of both groups knew ahead of time which group they were being assigned to.

As researchers had expected, several stress hormones were significantly lower in the group that watched the humorous video. But here's where the surprise came in: Those who anticipated watching a humorous video had lower levels of stress hormones even before they actually started watching the video. Those who anticipated the neutral activity didn't.[39]

Humor has been shown repeatedly to be a tool that helps relieve the stress of illness, terminal disease, and hospitalization. Lenore Reinhard, coordinator of the humor program at Schenectady's Sunnyview Rehabilitation Hospital, says she has seen repeated evidence that humorous books and tapes really help relieve the stress of being confined to a hospital. She remembers one patient in his forties who was under significant stress and who was not helped by relaxation tapes.

"I suggested that he check out some of our humor tapes—we have Woody Allen, Bill Cosby, 'Father' Guido Sarducci, George Burns, Rodney Dangerfield, Mel Brooks, and others," she relates. "Several weeks later, after he left, I checked the sign-out book—he'd borrowed nine tapes. They really helped him relax and get his mind off the very difficult situation he was in."[40]

Norman Cousins points out that humor neutralizes emotionally charged stress and is especially helpful for people who are facing serious or terminal illness. He says that humor "accomplishes one very essential purpose. It tends to block deep feelings of apprehension and even panic that all too frequently accompany serious illness." In addition, he says, it frees concentration on the body and enables healing to begin.[41]

***Improving coping abilities.***    Lawrence Mintz, a professor of American studies at the University of Maryland, believes that "humor is the way we cope with living in an imperfect world with imperfect selves. When we can't win, the best thing to do is to laugh about it."

Antioch University Professor Harvey Mindess agrees that humor is "a great coping mechanism. When a client of mine is very anxious about something, I try to get him to break out of his anger or fear by laughing at himself."

As early as the turn of the twentieth century, eminent psychoanalyst Sigmund Freud touted humor as one of the only socially acceptable ways to release pent-up frustration and anger, and he hailed it as a way to preserve the emotional energy that would normally be required to cope with a stressful situation. "The essence of humor is that one spares oneself the effects to which the situation would naturally give rise," he explained, "and overrides with a jest the possibility of such an emotional display."

Humor increases coping capacity in a number of ways. Deborah Burton Leiber, founder of the nationally organized Nurses for Laughter, says study results verify that humor helps us avoid feelings that are too frightening to face; this kind of humor, known as "gallows humor," was first noted among prisoners in Nazi concentration camps who were about to face death. Leiber points out that humor also has a "normalizing" effect, helps reduce the severity of tense situations, and can actually reduce nervous tension to help us cope.[42]

Alison Crane, a registered nurse who founded the American Association for Therapeutic Humor, maintains that humor can help people cope even in the most harrowing situations. She remembers a thirty-one-year-old man who had been admitted to the hospital with a serious heart condition. One morning he began experiencing severe chest pains, and the cardiologist decided that the patient needed immediate surgery. The patient was frightened and panicked, and the cardiologist felt that he would do better in surgery if his wife and child—who lived an hour away—could visit with him before he went into surgery.

Crane says that the patient's condition rapidly deteriorated, and there was no way the team of surgeons could wait for the patient's family any longer. She and the others who attended the patient had to find a way to allay his fear and panic (and to keep a lid on their own sense of rising panic). Crane says that her coping mechanism is humor, and that she had a gut instinct that it would work for the patient, too.

"I tried to joke around—not as in gales of laughter, but just a little lightness to break the tension," she remembers. "For example, when hanging his IVs I put a baseball cap on his IV pole and said, 'This will be your friend for awhile.'" The humor was a success in breaking up the panic and tension of the situation. Surgery was successful; the patient's family attributed his survival to the staff's ability to squelch his sense of panic.[43]

A study among patients waiting for medical treatment showed that a good sense of humor could, indeed, relieve tension and reduce anxiety, helping the patients to better cope. Researchers chose seventy-five patients who were waiting for medical procedures at a hospital; one-third saw a nonhumorous film, one-third saw a funny film, and the other third did not see a film. When researchers measured each group's level of anxiety, those who saw the funny film were the least anxious and the best able to cope with the upcoming medical treatment.[44]

Allen Klein cites the examples given by psychologist Samuel Janus and scientists Seymour and Rhoda Fisher of famous "funny people" who used humor to cope with deep psychological pain. In Klein's book, *The Healing Power of Humor,* he points out that Totie Field's mother died when she was five, David Steinberg's brother was killed in Vietnam, Jackie Gleason's father deserted him, W. C. Fields ran away from home because his father was going to kill him, Dudley Moore was born with a clubfoot, Art Buchwald's mother died when he was very young, and Carol Burnett's parents were both alcoholics who fought constantly.

"Charlie Chaplin, too, found solace in humor," Klein writes. "Raised in one of the poorest sections of London, he was five years old when his father died of alcoholism; after that his mother went mad. Chaplin used these gloomy memories in his films and turned them into comedic gems. Who could forget the scene in *Gold Rush,* for example, where he eats a boiled leather shoe for dinner because no other food is available?"[45]

## Laughter: The Best Medicine

Psychologist Robert Ornstein and physician David Sobel recite the scientific definition of a laugh as "a psychophysiological reflex, a successive, rhythmic, spasmodic expiration with open glottis and vibration of the vocal cords, often accompanied by a baring of the teeth and facial grimaces."[46]

### The Physiology of Laughter

Laughter may seem simple, but it's actually a complex physical process. According to studies reported in the *Journal of the American Medical Association,* laughter does the following:

- Breathing: increases the breathing rate, increases the amount of oxygen circulated through the blood, and clears mucus from the lungs
- Muscles: provides limited muscle conditioning, provides muscle relaxation, and breaks the pain/spasm cycle common to some muscle disorders
- Cardiovascular system: temporarily increases the heart rate and blood pressure, increases circulation, and increases the amount of oxygen delivered to all body cells[47]

Stanford Medical School Psychiatrist William Fry, Jr., says that laughter is valuable for strengthening the heart muscle and, he says, just 20 seconds of laughter is the cardiovascular equivalent of three minutes of strenuous rowing.[48]

Consider this description, published in a scientific journal around the turn of the twentieth century:

> *There occur in laughter and more or less in smiling, clonic spasms of the diaphragm in number ordinarily about eighteen perhaps, and contraction of most of the muscles of the face. The upper side of the mouth and its corners are drawn upward. The upper eyelid is elevated, as are also, to some extent, the brows, the skin over the glabella, and the upper lip, while the skin at the outer canthi of the eye is characteristically puckered. The nostrils are moderately dilated and drawn upward, the tongue slightly extended, and the cheeks distended and drawn somewhat upward; in persons with the pinnal muscles largely developed, the pinnae tend to incline forwards. The lower jaw vibrates or is somewhat withdrawn (doubtless to afford all possible air to the distending lungs), and the head, in extreme laughter, is thrown backward, until (and this usually happens soon) fatigue-pain in the diaphragm and accessory abdominal muscles causes a marked proper flexion of the trunk for its relief. The whole arterial vascular system is dilated, with consequent blushing from the effort on the dermal capillaries of the face and neck, and at times of the scalp and hands. From this same cause in the main the eyes often slightly bulge forwards and the lachrymal gland becomes active, ordinarily to a degree only to cause a "brightening" of the eyes, but often to such an extent that the tears overflow entirely their proper channels.*[49]

## Laughter as Exercise

Laughter is one of the best exercises around. And one of the nicest things about it is its simplicity. It requires no special training. It requires no special equipment. You don't have to do it at the gym or on the track or on a Nautilus machine. All you need, in fact, is a sense of humor.

Stanford Medical School's William Fry likens laughter to a form of physical exercise—it causes huffing and puffing, speeds up the heart rate, raises blood pressure, accelerates breathing, increases oxygen consumption, gives the muscles of the stomach and face a workout, and relaxes the muscles that aren't used in laughing. Twenty seconds of laughing can double the heart rate for three to five minutes, he adds.[50]

Laughter provides what some experts have called "a total inner body workout"—and more and more researchers are finding out exactly what it is about a laugh that is so good for us.

In brief, he says that something you see or hear or think of sets off "a massive brain reaction." Nerve fibers in the involuntary nervous system trigger a snowballing cycle of discharges in the brain stem. "Your neural circuits reverberate with the news: something is funny."

Your humor is then converted into electrical and chemical impulses that wash through the frontal lobes of the brain, go over the motor centers of the brain, and land smack in the center of the cerebral cortex. The cortex then hands out an order to the body: Laugh!

"A laugh," Brody writes, "can run anywhere from a half-second giggle or guffaw to a sixty-second belly burster, a memorable earthquake down in your abdomen, with many variations in between." Fry, who has studied laughter extensively, estimates that people in good spirits let loose with as many as 100 to 400 laughs a day.

Once you're ready to laugh, the muscles in your face that control expressions start to contort, says Brody. Muscles throughout your body contract like fists. Your vocal cord muscles, designed for intelligible sound, cannot coordinate. Your glottis and larynx open, relaxed and ready to vibrate. Your diaphragm tenses up in anticipation of respiratory spasms. According to Brody, "Air in your body billows until you feel pressure building in your lungs. Trying to hold in a laugh is no less than a violation against nature—rarely successful."

Once the laugh gets into full gear, writes Brody, "your breathing is interrupted for a station break. Your lower jaw vibrates. A blast of air gusts into your trachea, flinging mucus against the walls of your windpipe. Pandemonium! Out comes your laugh, in some cases clocked at 170 miles an hour. You issue a strange machine-gun sound, almost a violent bark."

Once in the throes of a full-bodied laugh, your body bucks. Your torso is flexed. Your arms flail, your hands slap your thighs. "Your lacrimal glands squeeze out tears, giving your eyes a mirthful sheen. You puff and rasp with symphonic regularity. You can hardly stand so much glee coursing through you. You're wobbly in the knees, wheezing like an asthmatic. Pleading for mercy, you collapse on the nearest sofa. Sounds like fun, no?"

The complicated combination of physiological reactions makes laughing what some researchers have called "inner jogging." Your metabolism steps up, and calories are burned off. Your body temperature increases. And your entire system is showered with adrenaline, making you feel good all over. Best of all, the physical effects of laughter endure for up to two hours after you stop laughing.

Laughter is essentially an act of respiration—and the lungs immediately fill with air. Air volume is dramatically increased, and your breathing rate goes up. Because of increased air volume and breathing rate, much more oxygen is delivered to the body than with normal breathing. You also breathe out more carbon monoxide and water vapor, which can encourage bacterial growth if it stays in the lungs. Once you finish laughing, you usually cough—a reaction that finishes clearing out the lungs.

Second, your heart rate increases during laughter, and the increase is in direct proportion to how long and hard you laugh. The entire cardiovascular system is stepped up, and the circulation increases; as a result, the entire cardiovascular system is toned. Fresh nutrients and oxygen go coursing through your arteries. Your blood pressure goes up. When you finish laughing, your heart rate and blood pressure drop to levels below those when you started laughing.

Laughter improves your digestion and may even stimulate enzymes that act as natural laxatives. It stimulates your central nervous system. And it first contracts, and then relaxes, almost all the muscles in your body. When you begin to laugh, at least five major muscle groups begin a rhythmic movement; when you finish laughing, your muscles—especially those of the abdomen, diaphragm, shoulders, neck, and face—are more relaxed than when you started laughing. Laughter not only improves muscle tone, but also enables total relaxation of all major muscle groups in your body.

## The Health Benefits of Laughter

In describing the health benefits of laughter, Norman Cousins—who laughed his way back to health from a painful and debilitating disease—likes to relate the story of an encounter he had in a veterans' hospital. Concerned about the glum spirits of the men on the cancer ward at the hospital in Sepulveda, California, physicians asked Cousins to impress the men with how optimism and good cheer could actually help them feel better and maybe even help them heal. Cousins met with fifty or sixty of the veterans and discussed the role of humor and cheer. Then he told them he hoped they would work together to create an atmosphere conducive to the best medical treatment available.

When Cousins returned to the hospital a few weeks later, he noted that the men had accepted the challenge. He could see the changes immediately. In their meeting that morning, each veteran was asked to tell about something good that had happened to him since the previous meeting. Each one in turn told about something good, with intermittent cheers bursting forth from the others. When each had taken a turn, they all turned to face Cousins. Obviously, they expected him to relate a story as well.

In his book *Head First,* Cousins relates the following experience, which he feels demonstrates the power of laughter:[51]

> *"What I have to report is better than good," I said. "It's wonderful. Actually, it's better than wonderful. It's unbelievable. And as long as I live, I don't expect that anything as magnificent as this can possibly happen to me again."*

*The veterans sat forward in their seats.*

*"What happened is that when I arrived at the Los Angeles airport last Wednesday my bag was the first off the carousel."*

*An eruption of applause and acclaim greeted this announcement.*

*"I had never even met anyone whose bag was first off the carousel," I continued.*

*Again, loud expressions of delight.*

*"Flushed with success, I went to the nearest telephone to report my arrival to my office. That was when I lost my coin. I pondered this melancholy event for a moment or two, then decided to report it to the operator.*

*"Operator," I said, "I put a quarter in and didn't get my number. The machine collected my coin."*

*"Sir," she said, "if you give me your name and address, we'll mail the coin to you."*

*"I was appalled."*

*"Operator," I said, "I think I can understand the reason behind the difficulties of AT&T. You're going to take the time and trouble to write down my name on a card and then you are probably going to give it to the person in charge of such matters. He will go the cash register, punch it open and take out a quarter, at the same time recording the reason for the cash withdrawal. Then he will take a cardboard with a recessed slot to hold the coin so it won't flop around in the envelope. Then he, or someone else, will fit the cardboard with the coin into an envelope, first taking the time to write my address on the envelope. Then the envelope will be sealed. Someone will then affix a twenty-cent stamp on the envelope. All that time and expense just to return a quarter. Now, operator, why don't you just return my coin and let's be friends."*

*"Sir," she repeated in a flat voice, "if you give me your name and address, we will mail you the refund."*

*"Then, almost by way of afterthought, she said, 'Sir, did you remember to press the coin return plunger?'"*

*"Truth to tell, I had overlooked this nicety. I pressed the plunger. To my great surprise, it worked. It was apparent that the machine had been badly constipated and I happened to have the plunger. All at once, the vitals of the machine opened up and proceeded to spew out coins of almost every denomination. The profusion was so great that I had to use my empty hand to contain the overflow.*

*"While all this was happening, the noise was registering in the telephone and was not lost on the operator.*

*"Sir," she said, "what is happening?"*

*I reported that the machine had just given up all its earnings for the past few months, at least. At a rough estimate, I said there must be close to four dollars in quarters, dimes, and nickels that had just erupted from the box.*

> *"Sir," she said, "will you please put the coins back in the box."*
>
> *"Operator," I said, "if you give me your name and address I will be glad to mail you the coins."*

According to Cousins, the veterans "exploded with cheers. David triumphs over Goliath. At the bottom of the ninth inning, with the home team behind by three runs, the weakest hitter in the lineup hits the ball out of the park. A mammoth business corporation is brought to its knees. Every person who has been exasperated by the loss of a coin in a public telephone booth could identify with my experience and share both in the triumph of justice and the humiliation of the mammoth and the impersonal oppressor."

One of the doctors in the room, noticing how relaxed and mobile the men were, asked how many had been experiencing their usual amount of pain when they arrived at the meeting. More than half of the veterans in the room raised their hands. The doctor then asked how many noticed that their pain had receded or completely disappeared. The same hands went up.

The example given by Cousins is just one of the many that doctors and researchers studying laughter are hearing. Because of the physiological changes that take place during laughter, it packs a punch in terms of physical benefits, pain relief, boosts in immunity, and psychological benefits.

## Physical Benefits of Laughter

As discussed on page 571, Stanford University researcher William Fry concluded that laughter is like a form of physical exercise. According to Fry, laughter also stimulates the sympathetic nervous system, the pituitary gland, the cardiovascular system, and the hormones that relieve pain and inflammation—making it a possible benefit in conditions like arthritis and gout. Laughter has also been shown to reduce allergic reactions, especially allergen-induced skin hives; the results of one study suggest that laughter "may play some role in alleviating allergic diseases."[52]

Psychologist Jeffrey Goldstein of Temple University credits laughter with contributing to longevity, and says that results of his research show that laughter works physiologically to reduce stress, hypertension, depression, heart attacks, and stroke. Laughing, says Goldstein, is much like jogging as a physical exercise—and its benefits are just as great.

Researchers have even found that the tears you shed during a good laugh have the same chemical composition as the tears you shed during a good cry. Both have been scientifically proven to carry away toxins and the hormones manufactured during stress.

## Pain Relief Benefits of Laughter

The most well-known example of laughter as an anesthetic is provided by Norman Cousins. When his symptoms of achiness, fatigue, and fever worsened instead of getting better, he sought medical help. The diagnosis was devastating: a potentially life-threatening collagen disease that affected all the connective tissues of the body. Involvement was already so extreme that he was having difficulty merely moving his joints. His physician told him that recovery was not probable.

Instead of merely accepting the prognosis that would have sentenced him to pain and then death, Cousins decided to take things into his own hands. He designed a program of positive thinking, nutritious food—and, as a painkiller, laughter.

Cousins found that laughter was the most effective painkiller he could find. Ten minutes of hearty laughter (usually prompted by old *Candid Camera* reruns) provided two hours of pain-free sleep. Even more remarkably, he found that inflammation in the tissues was reduced after each laughter session.

A decade later—fully recovered and functioning as a vital, vigorous man—he wrote of his experience. He gave laughter part of the credit for his miraculous recovery. Following his claims, a number of scientists set out to test his theory that laughter could act as an analgesic.

According to the most recent research, laughter probably relieves pain for several different reasons. Renowned author Raymond Moody, Jr., says one of those reasons has to do with muscle relaxation. Pain often involves muscle tension—the same kind of muscle gripping and spasm you would experience if you tried to stand on one leg for a long time. When you laugh, the tension dissipates—the spasms relax.

Laughter also stimulates the brain to release endorphins.[53] These potent natural chemicals have painkilling power estimated to be 200 times that of morphine; they also reduce inflammation and can stimulate the immune system. These are the chemicals responsible for the famed "runner's high"—and researchers believe there may be a very real and similar "laugher's high" that results when these chemicals leave laughers feeling relaxed and good all over.

Laughter and humor can relieve not only physical pain, but emotional pain, too. By providing a new perspective and lightening the emotional tension of a situation, laughing can relieve emotional stress and ease psychological pain.

A number of studies are underway throughout Europe and the United States in an effort to duplicate the experience of Norman Cousins. The results of one study, published in the *Journal of American Medical Association*, involved only a small group of patients but shows great promise for the role of "humor therapy" in relieving pain.

Dr. Lars Ljungdahl and his colleagues at Sweden's Lyckorna Primary Health-Care Centre chose six women who were incapacitated with an extremely painful muscle-bone disorder. The physicians administered psychological tests to the women before beginning the experiment to determine general psychological well-being.

The women were then given "humor therapy" for thirteen weeks. The patients used humorous books, records, and videotapes daily; they also met once a week with nurses who gave lectures on humor and helped the women understand how to better use humor in their everyday lives. The patients were asked to regularly record on separate scales how amused they were and how much pain relief they had.

Ljungdahl said that the women who participated in the study enjoyed "significant relief" from their painful symptoms—and those with the greatest degrees of amusement were also the ones who had the greatest pain relief. Tests administered at the end of the thirteen-week period also showed that the women had a greater overall sense of well-being.

"Their self-confidence also seemed to increase, they coped more ably with their symptoms, and allowed themselves to be happy and enjoy life regardless of their medical problems," he said. Ljungdahl noted that pain relief was greater during the last seven weeks than during the first six weeks (during the first six weeks, the women learned how to use humor to relieve pain), indicating that laughter had the greatest benefits.

## Immunity-Enhancing Benefits of Laughter

All of the research on laughter has revealed what may be one of laughter's most important benefits: It apparently enhances the immune system. Researchers believe that the immune-enhancing powers of laughter are due to two separate aspects of laughter: (1) It boosts the production of immune enhancers, and (2) it suppresses the production of stress hormones that weaken immunity. Dr. Lee Berk, an immunologist at California's Loma Linda University Medical Center, has conducted studies involving both of these effects of laughter on the immune system. In experiments with students, those who watched humorous videotapes compared with those who didn't had the highest concentrations of lymphocytes, greater natural killer cell activity, and significantly better measures of overall immune system activity. "The changes in the white cell counts and hormones," he says, "have been more surprising than we ever realized."[54]

The other way laughter may improve immunity is by reducing the stress hormones secreted in the body, which generally suppress the immune system. According to psychologist Robert Ornstein and physician David Sobel, "When confronted with a threatening situation, animals have essentially two choices: to flee or fight. Humans have a third alternative: to laugh."[55]

One series of studies measuring the effects of laughter on stress hormones was carried out by Berk and his Loma Linda University Medical Center colleagues. Berk had five men watch an hour-long comedy video of the comedian Gallagher; he then took blood tests and compared them to test results from five men who did not watch the video.[56]

The five who watched the funny film had lower levels of the stress hormone epinephrine. They also had significantly lower levels of DOPAC (which indicates dopamine activity) and the stress hormone cortisol, which can shut down the body's production of the immune substance interleukin 2. Berk and his colleagues concluded from the studies (and others they conducted on laughter) that laughing definitely has beneficial effects on the immune system—and may even help combat certain diseases.

The message for us is clear. As psychologist Gordon Allport suggested, "I venture to say that no person is in good health unless he can laugh at himself, quietly and privately."

## Psychological Benefits of Laughter

Among the psychological benefits of laughter are its ability to diminish fear, calm anger, and relieve depression. But perhaps the most pronounced psychological benefits of laughter are its ability to relieve stress and its tendency to improve our perspective—on everything from pain to life itself.

*Laughter as stress relief.*    Steve Allen, Jr.—the physician son of comedian Steve Allen—believes that "laughter is not only as good a method of stress relief as a massage, a hot bath, or exercise, it's essential to stress relief." Some of the reasons are tied to the physical outcomes: The body doesn't produce stress hormones as efficiently during laughter, and laughter itself physically breaks up tension.

Lawrence Peter, author of *The Laughter Prescription,* considers laughter to be an important safety valve. When you laugh, Peters maintains, you get rid of stress-related tension that can otherwise accumulate and damage health.

The stress-relieving effect of laughter doesn't last just while you're chuckling, either. Experts agree that the ability of laughter to dispel stress lasts long after the laugh—and can even help the person who laughs to build an actual immunity to stress. That's the opinion of *Laughing Matters* magazine editor Joel Goodman, who believes that laughter can "provide immediate relief from life's daily pressures" as well as "build up an immunity to stress for the long haul."

**Laughter as new perspective.**   According to Yale surgeon Bernie Siegel, renowned for his work in helping patients heal themselves,

> *Humor's most important psychological function is to jolt us out of our habitual frame of mind and promote new perspectives. Psychologists have long noted that one of the best measures of mental health is the ability to laugh at oneself in a gently mocking way—like the dear old schoolteacher, a colostomy patient of mine several years ago, who named her stomas Harry and Larry.*[57]

Apparently laughter can give us a new perspective on almost anything—even something as real and so distressing as pain. Psychologists Rosemary and Dennis Cogan of Texas Tech University in Lubbock designed an experiment to see whether laughter would help change the perspective of pain. They randomly assigned students into one of four groups: one listened to a humorous audiotape, one listened to a relaxation tape, one listened to an informative narrative, and the fourth group did not hear a tape.

The Cogans then fastened automatically inflating blood pressure cuffs around the students' arms and subjected the students to the highest level of discomfort that the cuffs could produce.

The students who were able to withstand even the highest pressure without becoming distressed were those who had listened to the humorous tape. Laughter, the Cogans theorize, changes our perspective of discomfort or distress and enables us to withstand many times what we normally could.

Harvard University Psychologist Gordon Allport maintained four decades ago that laughter provides new perspective on our place in society—much as climbing a mountain or activity in a religion does. Dozens of researchers following up on Allport's theory have proved the same thing—and millions of people who laugh merrily at life's circumstances can confirm the truth of it, too.

Ornstein and Sobel tell us,

> *Most of us don't take laughter seriously enough. Too often, laughter is regarded as child's play. To be adult is to be hardworking, responsible, and serious. We need to revive our natural sense of humor. If laughter is as contagious as it is said to be, then let's start an epidemic. Or perhaps we need doctors by the thousands to prescribe regular doses of humor. Though this Great Laughter Cure may not be a panacea, it is reassuring to learn, in these days of painful and expensive medical therapies, that laughter is medicinal and the only side effects are pleasurable.*[58]

As mentioned earlier, it's not too late to "learn" to have humor, even if you feel you don't have that great a sense of humor now. If you want to have more fun in your life, try following these suggestions of Leigh Anne Jasheway, coordinator of health promotion at the University of Texas Health Science Center at Houston:

- Make a pledge to laugh out loud or to make someone else laugh at least ten times every day.
- Once a week, set aside time to call someone who always adds fun to your day.
- Read your favorite comics in the newspaper every day.
- Make regular dates with a friend or your spouse to do any recreation that you both enjoy.
- Do something silly at least once a week.
- Start a humor collection—go for jokes, clippings, cartoons, cards, mugs, books, or videos.
- Share funny items with others, and use stick-on notes that have humorous messages.
- Rent funny movies.
- Try to find the humor in every predicament.
- Keep a "fun first-aid kit"—cram it full of things like modeling clay, bubbles, puzzles, brain teasers, and other things you love to do.
- Finally, recall all the fun you had as a child!

Perhaps one of the best suggestions is to create what Loretta LaRoche calls a "humor survival kit"—and one of her best tools, she says, always gets a laugh:

> *Buy something silly you can put on (a pair of Groucho Marx glasses are my favorite). Put them on in situations where you tend to awfulize. I wear mine driving through Boston, especially when I have to merge. People always let me in. Food shopping is another favorite. Among others, going to the dentist, the doctor, staff meetings, talking to your mate, the children, a coworker. When things have really reached the limits of your endurance, go into a bathroom, look into the mirror, put on your glasses, and ask yourself this question: "How serious is this?"*[59]

## ENDNOTES

1. Proverbs 17:22.
2. Loretta LaRoche, "Fully Human, Fully Alive with Humor, Compassion, and Love," The Psychology of Health, Immunity, and Disease, vol. A, 326, in *Proceedings of the Sixth International Conference of the National Institute for the Clinical Application of Behavioral Medicine*.
3. Barbara Powell, *Good Relationships Are Good Medicine* (Emmaus, Pa.: Rodale Press, 1987).

4. Mary Christelle Macaluso, "Humor, Health, and Healing," *ANNA Journal* 20, no. 1 (February 1993): 14–16.
5. LaRoche, "Fully Human."
6. Ibid.
7. Powell, *Good Relationships*.
8. Michael J. Balick and Roberta Lee, "The Role of Laughter in Traditional Medicine and Its Relevance to the Clinical Setting: Healing with Ha!" *Alternative Therapies* 9, no. 4, (July/August 2003): 88–91.
9. Norman Cousins, "The Laughter Connection," *East/West*, February 1990, 58.
10. C. W. Metcalf and Roma Felible, *Lighten Up: Survival Skills for People Under Pressure* (Reading, Mass.: Addison-Wesley Publishing Company, 1992), 9.
11. Fedor Mikhailovich Dostoevski, *The Adolescent* (1875 reprint, W. W. Norton, 1981).
12. Nick Gallo, "Lighten Up: Laugh Your Way to Good Health," *Better Homes and Gardens*, August 1989, 31.
13. Barbara Graham, "The Healing Power of Humor," *Mind/Body/Health Digest* 4(2): 1990, 2.
14. Laurie Dayton, "Healing with Humor," *Michigan Health and Hospitals* 33, no. 5, (1997): 16.
15. Balick and Lee, "The Role of Laughter."
16. Dorothy Foltz-Gray, "Make 'Em Laugh," *Contemporary Long-Term Care* 2, no. 9, (September 1998): 44–50.
17. Penelope Wang, Karen Springen, Tom Schmitz, and Mary Bruno, "A Cure for Stress?" *Newsweek*, October 12, 1987, 84–85.
18. Peter McWilliams and John-Roger, *You Can't Afford the Luxury of a Negative Thought* (Los Angeles, Calif.: Prelude Press, 1989), 277.
19. Caryl S. Avery, "Lighten Up," *Self*, September 1988, 150–57.
20. Avery, "Lighten Up."
21. Ibid.
22. Balick and Lee, "The Role of Laughter."
23. Ibid.
24. Lee S. Berk, David L. Felten, Stanley A. Tan, Barry B. Bittman, and James Westengard, "Modulation of Immune Parameters During the Eustress of Humor-Associated Mirthful Laughter," *Alt Ther Health Med* 7, no. 2 (2001): 62–67.
25. M. Bennet, J. Zeller, and L. Rosenberg, "The Effect of Mirthful Laughter on Stress and Natural Killer Cell Activity," *Alt Ther Health Med* 9, no. 2 (2003): 38–43.
26. Balick and Lee, "The Role of Laughter."
27. James A. Thorson, F. C. Powell, Ivan Sarmany-Schuller, and William P. Hampes, "Psychological Health and Sense of Humor," *Journal of Clinical Psychology* 53(6): 605–19, 1997.
28. Metcalf and Felible, *Lighten Up*, 9–10.
29. Susan Lang, "Laughing Matters—At Work," *American Health*, September 1988, 46.
30. Allen Klein, *The Healing Power of Humor* (Los Angeles, Calif.: Jeremy P. Tarcher, 1989), 16–17.
31. Lang, "Laughing Matters."
32. Klein, *The Healing Power*, 4.
33. Metcalf and Felible, *Lighten Up*, 26.
34. Robert Ornstein and David Sobel, *Healthy Pleasures* (Reading, Mass.: Addison-Wesley Publishing Company, 1989), 218.
35. R. Fay, "The Defensive Role of Humor in the Management of Stress,"

*Dissertation Abstracts International* 44: 1983, 1219B.

36. R. A. Martin and H. M. Lefcourt, "Sense of Humor as a Moderator of the Relation Between Stressors and Moods," *Journal of Personality and Social Psychology* 45: 1983, 1313–24.

37. *Annals of Behavioral Medicine,* November 2, 1996.

38. *Annals of Behavioral Medicine.*

39. Loretta LaRoche, "Laughter and Healing," presented to the Fourth National Conference on the Psychology of Health, Immunity, and Disease, and published by the National Institute for the Clinical Application of Behavioral Medicine.

40. Cathy Perlmutter, "Comic Relief," Prevention, March 1988, 107.

41. Norman Cousins, *The Healing Heart* (New York: W. W. Norton and Company, 1983).

42. Deborah Burton Leiber, "Laughter and Humor in Critical Care," *Dimensions of Critical Care Nursing* 5(3): 1986, 163.

43. Perlmutter, "Comic Relief," 106–107.

44. Jolene M. Simon, "Therapeutic Humor: Who's Following Who?" *Journal of Psychological Nursing* 26(4): 1988, 11.

45. Klein, *The Healing Power,* 5–6.

46. Ornstein and Sobel, *Healthy Pleasures,* 216.

47. "Laughter—Can It Help Keep You Healthy?" *Mayo Clinic Health Letter,* March 1993, 6.

48. Metcalf and Felible, *Lighten Up,* 11–12.

49. Source unknown.

50. LaRoche, "Laughter and Healing."

51. From Norman Cousins, *Head First* (New York: E. P. Dutton, 1989), 143–45.

52. Judy Tidwell, "The Healing Power of Humor," *Allergies,* November 2004.

53. Karen Rutter, "The Healing Power of Humor," *Family Services of Western Pennsylvania Employee Assistance Program,* November 2004.

54. Berk et al., "Modulation."

55. Ornstein and Sobel, *Healthy Pleasures,* 218.

56. "Laughter and Immunity," *Advances* 6(2): 5.

57. Bernie S. Siegel, *Love, Medicine and Miracles* (New York: Harper & Row Publishers, 1986).

58. Ornstein and Sobel, *Healthy Pleasures,* 219.

59. LaRoche, "Laughter and Healing," 331.

# Part VI

# The Intervention of Behavioral Medicine

This section addresses the questions "What is behavioral medicine?" and "How effective is it?" The positive effects of healthy nutritional intake, behavioral interventions, and the development of stress management skills are discussed. The chapters and topics presented in this section are:

**Chapter 22**    *The Importance of Nutrition to Mind and Body Health*

**Chapter 23**    *Behavioral Medicine Treatment*

**Chapter 24**    *Methods of Intervention and the Principles of Stress Resilience*

# The Importance of Nutrition to Mind and Body Health

*All physicians are involved with nutrition,*
*for it is not the disease that is important,*
*but the person who has the disease,*
*and each person is the product of his nutrition.*
*What is nutrition?*
*It is the cornerstone of preventive medicine,*
*the handmaiden of curative medicine*
*and the responsibility of every physician.*

—Symposium on Nutrition for Physicians[1]

## Learning Objectives

- Understand the basic principles of nutrition and how to apply them in making daily food choices.
- Identify the major problems with the typical American diet and lifestyle as they relate to adequate nutrition.
- Understand how nutrition affects the brain and the mind, and how the process increases the evidence of a connection between the mind and the body.
- Discuss how nutrition affects physical and mental health.

While it is true that we depend on energy from our thoughts, feelings, and consciousness to fuel the functions of our body, it is also true that we need energy from oxygen and from the nutrients in the food we eat. It is clear that our mental, spiritual, and emotional processes depend on a healthy physical body.

Candice Pert, the Georgetown University researcher who wrote *Molecules of Emotion*,[2] demonstrated that every thought and emotion is also a

**585**

chemical molecule that has very concrete functions in the network of cellular messengers that course throughout the neurological, endocrine, and immune systems. In other words, you feel emotions like anger and compassion because their molecules have a chemical effect on the 100 trillion cells of your body. That body, in return, must be kept healthy if you hope for optimal expression of your thoughts and emotions—and one of the best ways to keep it healthy is by fueling it with the right nutrition.

Most of your *cognitive* functions occur in the brain—but the research of Dr. Pert and others shows that another form of consciousness is made up of the "molecules of emotions" that are found throughout your body. Your entire body, then, helps support the functions of your mind and spirit. Physicians from Mount Sinai School of Medicine believe, in fact, that consciousness occurs in the cell membrane of each cell in the body, not just in the neurons in the brain.[3] Your brain and each cell of your body depend on the functions of all organs of the body to provide the energy, oxygen, and means to detoxify each cell after the process of metabolism. What that means is that the digestive tract, the circulatory system, the liver, the kidneys, and practically every organ system of the body is involved in supporting the higher functions of the brain.

Cell communication is achieved through a network of messengers that act on interrelated receptors on the cell membrane. It's a network that acts as a single functioning unit and is best understood as a whole. In the same way, the mind—what we call the psyche—is tightly interwoven with the neurological, immune, and endocrine systems; it, too, can be regarded as a single functioning network that is best understood as a whole. The hormones produced by these systems not only impact the functioning of the system but also are significantly impacted by what we eat.[4]

## The Basic Principles of Nutrition

Before discussing the basic principles of nutrition, it's important to understand *why* diet and nutrition are so important. Simply, proper and balanced nutrition keeps the body functioning as it should, enabling the various systems of the body to perform as they were designed to. As we also know from important research done during the last several decades, good nutrition supports the mind and the emotions, allowing us to experience total wellness.

What we eat is also important because it is a major determining factor in how well we are able to resist disease. Some disease conditions have been directly linked to dietary factors; one of the best examples is the link between cardiovascular disease and total serum cholesterol levels—especially low-density lipids in the blood. Obviously there are other factors that contribute to high total serum cholesterol (and high low-density lipoproteins), but diet is a major one, and diet has been strongly implicated in both coronary heart disease and high blood pressure. A diet high in sodium (salt) has also been linked to high blood pressure. Dietary factors have even been implicated in some cancers; some have estimated that the degree to which diet contributes to the incidence of cancer exceeds 40 percent.[5] Cancers that have been especially linked to diet include cancer of the breast, colon, pancreas, and stomach. Diet can be a particular factor in contributing to disease when combined with other risk factors, such as stress.

## The Process of Converting Food into Energy

Before food can be used by the body to provide energy for cells and repair tissues, it has to be *metabolized*—changed into a form that can be absorbed into the blood and used by the body's cells. This portion of metabolism is called digestion.

Digestion begins when food is chewed; various enzymes in the saliva start the actual process of breaking down the food; starches and some fats (such as milk fats) are the first to be broken down. Large, solid pieces of food are shredded and ground into a more manageable form that can be swallowed without causing choking. The process of chewing also breaks open seeds, pods, and kernels (such as kernels of corn) that would otherwise travel undigested throughout the digestive system. Chewing and the saliva that is secreted also help soften sharp or rough foods that could otherwise tear the esophagus, and make each bite of food slippery enough to be swallowed easily. As chewed food is swallowed, it passes into the esophagus, where rhythmic, squeezing muscular action called *peristalsis* moves the food toward the stomach. A powerful circular muscle called the sphincter separates the esophagus from the stomach and prevents food from moving back into the esophagus from the stomach.

The stomach produces a mixture of water, enzymes, and gastric acids that further break down the food; the main nutrient that is broken down in the stomach is protein. A thick coating of mucus protects the stomach and other parts of the digestive system from being corroded by the acids that are produced for digestion. The secretion of these acids and enzymes is controlled by the vagus nerve, which is stimulated by the sight, smell, or even thought of food—so by the time food reaches the stomach, it already contains the gastric juices needed to help digest the food.

Food is stored in the highly muscular stomach for as long as several hours, where gastric juices and water help change the food into a fine, paste-like substance. At first, food is stored in the upper part of the stomach; it is then moved a little at a time into the lower section of the stomach, where powerful muscular contractions grind and mix the food thoroughly into a substance called *chyme*. Because the digestive process is well underway, chyme no longer resembles the food that was eaten—fats have been separated, proteins have undergone changes, and starches have started to be split.

The stomach acts as a type of holding tank; it releases only small amounts of food at a time into the duodenum, the first part of the small intestine. Another powerful muscle, the pyloric valve, controls how much chyme is secreted into the duodenum at any given time. It normally takes several hours for the food from a typical meal to be emptied completely from the stomach.

Enzymes from the pancreas and liver are secreted into the duodenum; pancreatic juices help break down fats, proteins, and carbohydrates, and the bile secreted by the liver helps break down fats. The bile produced by the liver is stored in the gallbladder, and is secreted from the gallbladder into the duodenum in response to foods that contain fats.

Most of the absorption of food into the bloodstream takes place in the small intestine, where its enzymes finish breaking down the food into amino acids. Every molecule of nutrient must move through one of the cells of the intestinal lining and into the blood and lymph. The intestinal lining is made up of millions of finger-shaped projections called villi, which are covered with microscopic hairs that trap particles of nutrients; each villi has its own lymph vessel and capillary network, which enables the nutrient to move into either the bloodstream or the lymphatic system. The surface of the small intestine—which is wrinkled into thousands of folds—is actually enormous: spread flat, it would cover almost one-third of a football field, though the total weight of the small intestine is only about five pounds.

The same kind of peristalsis that moves food through the esophagus moves it through the small intestine; the parasympathetic nervous system speeds up the movement of food through the small intestine, while the signals from the sympathetic nervous system slow it down.

Finally, what is left of the food moves into the colon. As the matter (made up of fiber and undigested materials) moves through the three sections of colon—ascending, transverse, and descending—minerals and extra water are absorbed into the bloodstream, and only those parts of the food that cannot be digested by the body remain. Fiber is an important element in the diet, because it provides the bulk against which the muscles of the colon push to move the waste along. That solid waste (called *feces*) then moves into the rectum and causes the urge to defecate, which removes the waste from the body.

## Achieving Balance in the Diet

Good health, both mental and physical, depends in part on getting the right amount and balance of nutrients in the diet. Generally, aim for a diet that is low in fat (especially saturated fat) and cholesterol and moderate in sugar, sodium, and salt. Your diet should contain plenty of fruits, vegetables, and grains and a variety of sources of proteins. Generally, there are four characteristics that make up a nutritious diet:

- **Amount**—the body requires different amounts of different nutrients, such as vitamins and minerals; recommended daily allowances are a good guideline that help determine how much of each nutrient (such as calcium, iron, or vitamin C) is needed to maintain optimal health.

- **Balance**—there are approximately forty nutrients that are needed for good health, and it's necessary to eat the right balance of foods to get all the necessary nutrients.

- **Moderation**—some nutrients (such as sugars, fats, and salts) are required for proper functioning of the body but can be detrimental in high amounts.

- **Calorie control**—the energy (fuel) your food provides should be balanced by the amount of energy you expend in a day; if you eat more energy than you expend, the excess is deposited as fat.

Make sure that any nutrition information you get is from a credible source—such as the American Dietetic Association, the Food and Drug Administration, or the U.S. Department of Agriculture. Volunteer health agencies—such as the American Cancer Society, the American Heart Association, or the American Diabetes Association—are also considered credible sources of nutrition information. You can generally also rely on your physician or reliable consumer groups, such as the National Council Against Health Fraud or the American Council on Science and Health.

# The Typical American Diet

Health objectives for Americans are established every ten years by the U.S. Department of Health and Human Services; one of the sections of the resulting document, *Healthy People 2010*, specifically addresses nutrition-related health objectives. Some of the objectives set for this decade include, but are not limited to, the following:

- Reducing coronary heart disease deaths
- Reducing cancer deaths
- Decreasing the incidence of Type 2 diabetes (adult onset diabetes, which is generally caused by diet)
- Reducing the incidence of osteoporosis (primarily related to lack of calcium)

- Increasing the prevalence of healthy weight and decreasing the prevalence of obesity
- Reducing growth retardation among low-income children
- Increasing the proportion of people aged two and older who meet the dietary guidelines for fat and saturated fats in the diet
- Increasing the intake of fruit and vegetables to at least five servings a day
- Increasing the intake of grain products to at least six servings a day
- Increasing the proportion of people who meet the recommendation for calcium
- Reducing iron deficiency in children, adolescents, women of childbearing age, and low-income pregnant women
- Increasing the proportion of children and adolescents whose intakes of meals and snacks at school contribute to overall dietary quality
- Increasing the proportion of schools teaching essential nutrition topics

So, how are we measuring up against these goals? According to the USDA, American children eat far too much fat and too few fruits and vegetables,[6] which has led to an epidemic of obesity among the nation's children. Americans in general also eat too much sugar and far too many animal fats.[7] In the past two decades, Americans have increased the amount of sugars, fats, and oils they eat and have sharply increased the soft drinks they consume. Most American adults—especially women and the elderly—get too little calcium, vitamin $B_6$, vitamin E, magnesium, and zinc.

In the United States today, 55 percent—230 million Americans—are obese, a number that will climb to an estimated 366 million in twenty-five years. The Centers for Disease Control report that American children now have a 33 percent lifetime risk of becoming diabetic—and by 2050, the incidence of diabetes will increase by 165 percent. It is estimated that one-fourth of all American children and one-third of the population at large have a prediabetic condition.

On the bright side, the same statistics show that during the past two decades, Americans have increased the amounts of fruits, vegetables, grains, and cereals they are eating and have replaced some of the red meat they eat with poultry and fish.

## How Nutrition Affects the Brain

The specific nutrients that help the brain to work well are found in high concentration in the Mediterranean diet, which has shaped our genes and determined what fuel we need for optimal function. The new field of *nutrigenomics* highlights these important concepts,[8] providing exciting opportunities in the field of nutrition.[9]

There is a tendency to think of medical problems, like depression, as being caused by "chemical imbalances" that are due to genetic factors. While it is true that such genes do exist, it is also true that genetic conditions can be moderated by getting proper nutrition, living in clean environments, learning good coping skills, having healthy intimate relationships, and developing a spiritual connection with our fellowpeople.[10]

As an example, Dr. Linus Pauling showed in the 1960s that nutritional intervention could help most people suffering from depression and schizophrenia,[11] research that has since been corroborated by many other publications. Some speak on the role of nutrition in general, while others address specific micronutrients in the diet. The basic finding is that there is more depression and mental dysfunction when there is poor diet.[12]

For example, vitamin C has been found to help in the treatment of schizophrenia and bipolar disorder.[13] Vitamin E can help in the treatment of stress-related mental dysfunction.[14] Chromium picolinate has been shown to improve depression,[15] as does magnesium, which facilitates more than 400 reactions of enzymes.[16]

These findings may create the impression that nutrition and micronutrients can be used to "treat" a medical or behavioral problem. Instead, it's better to conceptualize disease—mental or physical—as being triggered by a *lack* of these nutrients. Consequently, the beneficial effect of restoring these nutrients is not a "pharmaceutical" one, but the result of correcting the deficiency that triggered the problems in the first place.

## Essential Fatty Acids

Not surprisingly, essential fatty acids and B-complex vitamins are the nutrients most studied in relation to psychology, the function of the mind, the function of the nervous system, and the moderation of genetic conditions. While genetic predispositions have been implicated in behavioral conditions, it has been shown that nutrients can significantly reduce genetic tendencies, making disorders such as depression less likely.[17]

Essential fatty acids are those fatty acids that the body needs but cannot make in sufficient amounts to meet its physiological needs; two of them—linoleic acid and linolenic acid—are critical for the body's basic functions but cannot be made in any amount by the body, so they must be supplied completely by the foods we eat. Essential fatty acids are found in plant oils (corn, safflower, cottonseed, sesame, canola, soybean, and sunflower), cold-water fish (salmon, mackerel, tuna, sardines, herring, anchovy, bluefish, lake trout, mullet, sablefish, and menhaden), green leafy vegetables, and seeds, nuts (especially walnuts), grains, and breast milk.

Essential fatty acids are critical to cell membrane structure, and phospholipids (fats) in the cell membrane are essential for cell communication. These nutrients keep cell membranes fluid and in good repair, and because they are necessary to the function of neurotransmitters, they help in treating mental illness.[18] Essential fatty acids are also needed to build the fatty sheath around the tail of neurons, which conducts electrical impulses along the neurons.[19] Keep in mind, too, that 60 percent of the brain is "white matter," or phospholipids. Based upon this research, it is important to include essential fatty acids in the diet.

The following main points about essential fatty acids have been established:[20]

- The ideal ratio of omega-3/omega-6 fatty acids should be 1:1, but the typical American diet is 1:20 because we consume too much corn, sunflower, safflower, and cottonseed oils.
- The less fish in the diet, the greater the incidence of depression.
- There is a lower incidence of seasonal affective disorder (SAD) with a diet higher in fish.
- Depressed people have less omega-3 in their blood, and 35 percent less DHA (an essential fatty acid) in their adipose (fat) tissue, which is a reflection of long-term intake.
- Depression is an inflammatory disease; both antidepressants and essential fatty acids reduce inflammation.
- A diet deficient in essential fatty acids causes a number of serious problems in cell communication in the tissues of the brain and nervous system.
- Ten grams of omega-3 per day help in the treatment of bipolar disorder; the 2004 Meeting of the American Psychiatry Association determined that only 1 gram of essential fatty acid is the best dose to treat depression.
- Depression in premenstrual syndrome and postpartum depression are helped with 4 grams of the marine oil Krill.
- Social phobia is helped with 4 grams of Ecosapentanoid Acid (EPA), an omega-3 fatty acid.
- Antidepressant drugs work better when mixed with omega-3.
- Borderline personality disorder improves with 1 gram of EPA.

The best study on the antidepressant effects of essential fatty acids consisted of a twelve-week randomized, double-blind, placebo-controlled study of seventy patients. There was 50 percent improvement in the depression scores in 53 percent of the patients who took 1 gram of EPA (omega-3). They reported less depression, anxiety, sleep disturbances, lassitude, libido problems, and suicidal ideation.[21]

## B-Complex Vitamins

B-complex vitamins are just as important for function at every level as are essential fatty acids. The B-complex vitamins facilitate the work of every cell in the body, working to help metabolize fats, proteins, and carbohydrates. B-complex vitamins help the enzymes do their job in the body; some also help generate energy, while others help make proteins and build new cells. Because of its effect on proteins in the liver, B-complex vitamins affect not only detoxification in the liver but also our genes and how our neurotransmitters function.[22]

Of the B-complex vitamins, thiamin (vitamin $B_1$) is found in whole grains, legumes, nuts, pork, and liver. Riboflavin (vitamin $B_2$) is found in meat, leafy green vegetables, whole-grain enriched breads and cereals, milk, yogurt, cheese, and cottage cheese. Rich sources of niacin (vitamin $B_3$) include milk, eggs, meat, poultry, fish, whole-grain breads and cereals, and nuts. Vitamin $B_6$ is found in green leafy vegetables, legumes, fruit, whole grains, meat, fish, poultry, and shellfish; vitamin $B_{12}$ is found in animal products. Rich sources of folate include leafy green vegetables, legumes, seeds, liver, and enriched whole-grain products. Pantothenic acid and biotin are found in most foods.

Under normal conditions, the *blood-brain barrier* prevents many toxins in the blood from permeating the brain. A lack of thiamine causes the blood-brain barrier to leak, allowing toxins to penetrate the brain more readily. For this reason, some theorize that a lack of vitamin B can cause one's mental health to deteriorate. There is a twofold increase in risk of severe depression with vitamin $B_{12}$ deficiency.[23] Postpartum depression is often due to low levels of vitamin B, and premenstrual syndrome worsens when women are low in B-complex. The elderly are particularly vulnerable to decreased levels of B-complex: Their diets are notoriously poor, and a decrease in digestive enzymes as they age results in poor absorption of this key nutrient.[24]

Further research into the treatment of depression supports the idea that a B-complex deficiency may be partially responsible for depression. A metabolite of B-complex, S-Adenosyl-Methionine (SAMe)—also called "methyl magic"—became a drug in Europe used to treat depression. A symposium on SAMe held in Santa Barbara, California, made the following points:[25]

- 1,600 mg/day of SAMe is equal to 150 mg of the antidepressant Imipramine, but it causes fewer side effects and starts to work more quickly.

- SAMe may protect against Alzheimer's disease by making cell membranes more fluid (cell membranes appear to be stiffer in Alzheimer's disease patients).

- In order for SAMe to be used by the body, there needs to be enough vitamin $B_{12}$, folate, and L-methoinine. This explains why people who are deficient in those nutrients develop depression at an earlier age, and why the depression is relieved by administering those nutrients. Anti-depressant therapy is also potentiated by these nutrients.

## Amino Acids

Amino acids, the building blocks of protein, are needed for many functions, including the structuring of the brain and the production of neurotransmitters. The body produces in adequate amounts about half of the twenty amino acids it needs; the others, called essential amino acids, must be obtained from the foods we eat.

Amino acids are found in beef, pork, poultry, fish, shellfish, eggs, milk, yogurt, cheese, cottage cheese, broccoli, leafy green vegetables, seeds and nuts (walnuts, cashews, sesame seeds, sunflower seeds, and nut butters), and whole grains (oats, rice, cornmeal, barley, and bulgur).

One of the most publicized essential amino acids is L-tryptophan. People who cannot process L-tryptophan well in the brain have lower levels of serotonin; L-tryptophan supplementation has also been shown to be as potent as antidepressant drugs in the treatment of depression.[26] Additionally, L-tryptophan has been found to boost the effectiveness of tricyclic antidepressants.[27]

There were early concerns about L-tryptophan supplementation when it was initially linked to a condition called Eusinophilic syndrome. However, scientists have subsequently discovered that the syndrome was caused by the way the amino acid was processed in Japanese laboratories, not by the L-tryptophan itself.[28]

Other amino acids are also helpful in treating and preventing depression. The amino acids glutamine and glycine activate receptors in the brain, in collaboration with specific proteins.[29] In other words, amino acids and proteins are key to the proper functioning of the brain.[30] This, in turn, affects the entire body and its ability to function to its best potential.

## Vitamin D and Sunlight

Among the vitamins, vitamin D is unique because it can be produced by the body: When sunlight interacts with one of the cholesterol compounds in the skin, the compound is transformed into a precursor of vitamin D, which is then absorbed directly into the blood. The liver and the kidneys finish converting the substance into vitamin D. As such, vitamin D acts as a hormone—a substance that is produced by one organ (the skin) and that then acts on other organs and tissues. It is a member of a large interacting team of nutrients and hormones that work together in ensuring the function of the bones, intestines, pancreas, kidneys, skin, reproductive organs, and brain. It is also essential in helping the body properly absorb calcium, which is needed for the proper function of all cells and tissues of the body. Vitamin D draws calcium for the body to use from the blood, digestive tract, and kidneys.

Early pioneers in medicine used to treat depression by giving patients cod liver oil. Those pioneers have been vindicated through our findings about essential fatty acids and additional research[31] showing that light therapy works by restoring serotonin levels in the brain. And it turns out that vitamin D is also involved, acting more like a hormone with nearly the same nuclear receptors as thyroid hormone.[32]

Most Americans don't consume foods high in vitamin D (cod liver oil, salmon, mackarel, sardines, liver, and eggs). They also don't get vitamin D from sunlight: Americans spend 98 percent of their time indoors—and when they do go out they tend to use sunblockers, which limit vitamin D synthesis. Furthermore, people who live in higher latitudes don't get enough sunlight, compromising many bodily functions and contributing to diabetes, arthritis, lupus, thyroiditis, psoriasis, and possibly multiple sclerosis.

## How Nutrition Affects Physical and Mental Health

Not all diseases are equally influenced by the things we eat: We know that some diseases are not related to nutrition at all, while others are strongly related to nutrition. For example, genetic diseases—such as Down syndrome or sickle-cell anemia—are not caused at all by the foods we eat. On the other hand, a condition like iron-deficiency anemia is directly related to how much iron is in the diet. In between those two extremes, along a sort of continuum, are conditions that are related to some extent or another to nutrition—including diseases like cancer, diabetes, and coronary artery disease.

Along that continuum are conditions that have been established to have some sort of connection to nutrition. We know, for example, that

- Too few essential nutrients (especially proteins) can cause some forms of birth defects, low birth weight, some kinds of physical and mental retardation, growth deficits, poor resistance to disease, susceptibility to some kinds of cancer, and deficiency diseases (such as scurvy and cretinism).

- Too many fats—especially saturated fats—can cause coronary artery disease and certain kinds of cancers.

- Too much sugar can cause dental cavities and can lead to obesity and its related diseases (such as diabetes, high blood pressure, and certain kinds of cancers).

- Too much sodium (salt) may cause high blood pressure and related diseases of the heart and kidneys.

- Too little calcium can cause loss of bone tissue in adults, and may lead to high blood pressure and colon cancer.

- Too little iron causes iron-deficiency anemia.

- Too little fiber in the diet can cause some digestive diseases (including diverticulitis), can cause constipation, and can lead to the development of colon cancer and some other cancers.

- Too much alcohol can cause liver disease and may cause sudden death; because it has no nutrients, it can also cause the diseases associated with inadequate nutrition.

## Obesity

One of the greatest impacts of nutrition on health relates to *obesity*, an excessive accumulation of body fat. Generally, body fat should constitute about 15 to 22 percent of body tissues in men, and 20 to 27 percent of body tissues in women. Obesity is generally determined by a measurement called *body mass index* (BMI); you are considered overweight if your BMI is greater than 25, and you are considered obese if your BMI is greater than 30. (To determine your BMI, multiply your weight in pounds by 705, then divide twice by your height in inches.) People normally gain weight as they age; both metabolism and physical activity decline as people get older. Those who do not want to gain weight need to take in fewer calories, increase physical activity, or do both to avoid weight gain.

Obesity has become so commonplace that it has begun to replace malnutrition as the most important dietary contributor to poor health worldwide. In the United States, it has reached epidemic proportions. An estimated six in ten Americans is overweight, and almost one-third are obese; slightly more women than men are overweight or obese in the United States.

Obesity itself is a health risk, causing an estimated 300,000 deaths in the United States every year.[33] It can create conditions—such as high blood pressure and high cholesterol—that become their own risk factors for disease. Overweight and obesity have also been associated with diseases such as diabetes, arthritis, some kinds of cancer, gallbladder disease, high blood pressure, and coronary heart disease. Overweight and obesity can also cause potentially serious risks from childbearing, surgery, and the administration of anesthesia. Finally, many of the things that people attempt in the treatment of overweight and obesity—such as fasting, diet pills, and the use of other medications—can cause their own health risks.

Even mildly overweight women have an increased risk of heart disease and heart attack when compared to women of normal weight, studies show.[34] One study determined that women who are 30 percent overweight are more than three times as likely to develop heart disease as women who are of normal weight; that risk increased to five times if the women were also smokers.[35]

Interestingly, risks seem related to where the fat is deposited. Recent evidence suggests that the most dangerous is fat that is localized to the abdomen rather than the hips, buttocks, or thighs; localized abdominal fat is associated with a particular increase in high blood pressure, heart disease, diabetes, and some kinds of cancer. Also of interest is the apparent role of stress: People who carry their weight in the abdomen, rather than on the hips, tend to be more reactive to stress and show greater reaction of the cardiovascular[36] and nervous and endocrine[37] systems to stress.

The best solution for achieving and maintaining a healthy weight is one that is gradual and that involves *permanent* lifestyle changes. It's important to choose a realistic goal; most physicians advise losing no more than one to two pounds per week. The best approach is to eat a balanced diet consisting of plenty of whole grains, vegetables, fruits, and lean protein sources, reducing fats and refined sugars. Exercise is important—in addition to burning calories, it increases the body's metabolism, reduces body fat, and preserves lean tissue; the effects of exercise accumulate over time, so that the body's resting metabolism actually increases over time with exercise. Other approaches can include nutrition and exercise counseling, self-help or support groups, and various behavioral techniques (such as keeping a food diary, setting up a system of rewards, eating only while sitting down at the table, or putting the fork down after every bite). Those who have a high degree of confidence and who get support from family members and important others generally do the best in achieving permanent weight loss.

## Insulin Resistance

As stated in the *New England Journal of Medicine,* the "sweet death" associated with too much refined sugar "is a secret killer."[38] Too much refined sugar in the diet leads to insulin resistance, a situation in which the cell can't utilize insulin properly. Basically, the cell membrane becomes rigid and loses its ability to function normally. As mentioned earlier, cell membranes need to be flexible and fluid in order for molecules to move in and out of the cell successfully. Floating on the membrane layer are protein receptors, or "gates" where messengers of cell communication attach in a lock-and-key fashion. These protein receptors have undergone various modifications to maximize their structure and function through a process called *glycosylation.*[39]

In order for the protein receptors ("gates") to work properly, the correct kind of carbohydrates need to be attached to them. Protein receptors that have too much processed sugar become resistant to other glycoproteins that come to the cell membrane as messengers. The most classic example is insulin: A cell inundated with too much sugar resists insulin—a condition known as "insulin resistance," which causes diabetes. Other factors can cause insulin resistance as well—for example, too many transhydrogenated and saturated fats also cause the cell membranes to become rigid.

The correct glycosylation of proteins plays a major role in how both the body and the mind work. Studies have shown that improving glycosylation helps reduce the craving for tobacco and alcohol and can help in the treatment of Alzheimer's disease, attention deficit disorder, and dyslexia. And, according to research,[40] insulin resistance is also related to both depression and coronary artery disease.

## The Connection Between Insulin Resistance, Depression, and Cardiovascular Disease

Insulin resistance actually has a bidirectional relationship with depression. When cell membranes resist insulin, the pancreas starts to produce more insulin—creating a condition known as *hyperinsulinemia*. Insulin has also a central effect on the brain: Some of those effects include, but are not limited to, glucose metabolism by brain cells, stability of the blood-brain barrier, control of blood flow, and regulation of the autonomic nervous system. Insulin resistance combined with cardiovascular disease decreases blood flow to the brain, which in turn leads to more depression. And, as discussed elsewhere in this book, depression increases the risk of cardiovascular disease—as one example, depression is associated with pro-inflammatory cytokines, which contribute to both cardiovascular disease and insulin resistance.

It has been shown that antidepressants reduce insulin resistance; 60 mg per day of Fluoxetine/Prozac decreases insulin resistance by 20 percent. Antidepressants have also been shown to increase the amount of L-tryptophan in the brain; too little L-tryptophan not only can cause carbohydrate craving, binge eating, and obesity, but also has been associated with depression and insulin resistance. Finally, antidepressants help regulate serotonin—and we know that serotonin disturbances increase the platelet-binding sites associated with depression, which in turn may contribute to clotting and narrowed blood vessels, increasing the risk of cardiovascular events.[41]

Depression, insulin resistance, and cardiovascular disease have many risk factors in common: Stress, smoking, obesity, and alcohol lead the list. In other words, the same factors—mostly nutritional—that contribute to heart disease also contribute to depression.

The journal *Family Practice Recertification* says that the cause of depression "is still poorly understood, but it is probably not due to a simple deficiency of one neurotransmitter or another. Neuroscientists are coming to the realization that although many patients improve with a drug that inhibits the reuptake of a neurotransmitter (like Prozac does), that doesn't necessarily mean those patients were depressed because of a neurotransmitter deficiency. It now appears such thinking is akin to saying that a skin rash that improves with a steroid cream is due to a steroid deficiency."

Recent research suggests that depression, bipolar disorder, and many other mental illnesses might be related to cell membrane dysfunction—specifically inflammation of the cell membrane, particularly in the microglial cells, which are now recognized to be integral parts of the brain's "immune system."[42]

## The Connection Between Insulin Resistance and Brain Function

The same factors discussed above may well affect the brain in other ways. Researchers at the 2004 Annual Meeting of the American Neurology Association reported that the same factors that cause heart disease are at play in Alzheimer's disease, concluding that "what is good for the heart *may* also be good for the brain."

A diet low in refined sugars lowers the chance of cell membrane problems. According to research, hyperinsulinemia causes inflammatory plaques to form in the brain; MRIs of people with Type I diabetes show accelerated aging.[43] *Insulysin,* a chemical that breaks down insulin, has also been shown to be lacking in people with Alzheimer's disease.[44] Even patients who have insulin resistance—but not diabetes—show brain changes years before they are diagnosed with Alzheimer's disease. In other words, a sugar-laden diet leading to a prediabetic condition can have deleterious effects on the brain.

Normal levels of insulin and the insulin growth factor (IGF-1) clear inflammatory plaques from the brain. Both insulin and IGF-1 are secreted by the brain—and both hormones have a number of functions in protecting cells of the nervous system. When there is not enough insulin or IGF-1, the inflammatory plaques remain in the brain.[45] Because of that, researchers conclude that IGF-1 has promise in the treatment of degenerative nerve disorders, including multiple sclerosis. The connection underscores the importance of diet on brain function.

Diabetes has been clearly associated with an increase in degenerative nerve diseases of the brain, like Alzheimer's disease and Parkinson's disease, partly because of the formation of inflammatory plaques. These plaques play a role in diseases, such as Lou Gehrig's disease (ALS), multiple sclerosis, and Parkinson's disease, that we know to be inflammatory conditions.[46] But high-sugar diets also affect the brain directly: the blood-brain barrier, which normally weakens with age, also becomes weak from loss of insulin sensitivity.[47] Research shows that hyperglycemia makes the blood-brain barrier more porous, which allows toxins to penetrate the brain.[48] And sugar at high levels is itself toxic to the central nervous system.

People with diabetes have reduced cognitive functioning because they do not get as much blood flow to the brain, which can also increase the risk of stroke. They also have more neurological problems everywhere—feet, stomach, intestines, and eyes, for example—because of poor blood flow to the nerves wiring those areas. Even in people without diabetes, transient ischemic attacks (TIAs, or "mini-strokes") and strokes often result in insulin resistance.[49] Research shows that the elderly people who have impaired glucose tolerance or a prediabetic condition have greater cognitive dysfunction. And the reduction of blood sugar that occurs following an excessively large meal can cause emotional stress and hypersensitivity of the neurons even in healthy people.[50]

### Insulin Resistance and Thyroid Dysfunction

Hyperinsulinemia is the most common cause of thyroid dysfunction. And because the hormone produced by the thyroid gland is a powerful neurotransmitter, a poor diet high in sugar has yet another marked effect on the brain.

Treating thyroid dysfunction has been shown to be effective in the treatment of major depression.[51] Given the epidemic of depression in the United States, and the fact that traditional treatment with antidepressants is effective only about 50 percent of the time, thyroid treatment might be considered as a treatment for depression, even when thyroid dysfunction isn't obvious. Treatment with low levels of thyroid hormone, even in those with normal thyroid functions, has been shown to cause significant cognitive functions.[52]

## The "Second Brain": The Gastrointestinal Tract

A landmark symposium in Oxford, England,[53] reflects the increasing understanding that many nerve and psychiatric disorders actually begin in the gut—not surprising in light of the fact that 95 percent of the body's serotonin and other neurotransmitters are found in the gastrointestinal tract, not in the brain. After forty years of rejection by the medical community, the physician who authored *The Second Brain*,[54] about the role of the gastrointestinal (GI) tract, is now being hailed as a pioneer in neuroscience. A recent symposium held in Paris[55] resurrected similar ideas advanced by the winner of the 1908 Nobel Prize in Medicine. Unfortunately, these concepts have not received the attention they deserve, since we have developed a health care system that tends to deemphasize nutritional research. Fortunately, and thanks to these pioneers, this is slowly changing.

The Paris symposium—titled "The Intelligent Intestine"—also highlighted the concept that 60 percent of the immune system is in the GI tract, from which it exerts significant influence on the systemic immune system, where the other 40 percent is found. Thus, "The intestine is the primary immune organ of the body represented by the gut-associated lymphoid tissue . . . the microflora and the mucosal barrier." This is extremely important: When the mucosal barrier of the intestine is inflamed, toxic foods and food additives can leak through it, exerting significant influence on how our brains and minds work.

Several other significant ideas were discussed at the Paris symposium:[56]

- If the intestine is considered "intelligent," it must be able to send, receive, and understand messages.

- Carbohydrates line the membranes of the intestine and facilitate reception of messengers. Eating processed carbohydrates compromises this communication, resulting in problems such as adhesion of harmful bacteria, which slowly begin to gain power over the normal bacteria (flora) of the digestive tract.

- Loss of the gastric acid barrier results in altered intestinal bacteria.

- Mucosal cells produce antimicrobial peptides called "defensins."

- An unhealthy balance of intestinal flora will disrupt the immune system, causing inflammation throughout the body and brain. According to the symposium report, antibiotic treatment has a considerable effect on the equilibrium of bacteria in the intestinal tract. Regular doses of probiotics can help, as will a diet high in fiber and low in refined sugar.

An editorial in the journal *Gut* says that "the fathers of gastroenterology clearly recognized the relationship between the brain and the gut." But, the attitude that "if you can't measure something you don't know that it exists" banished recognition of the link between the brain and the gut. Fortunately, thanks to pioneers like those mentioned above and the laser doppler flow-meters that measure brain-gut activity, this knowledge is now considered to be sound science.[57]

Brain-gut activity goes both ways. An article in the *American Journal of Gastroenterology* pointed out that while irritable bowel syndrome (IBS) is very much associated with psychological issues and significant stress, it would be a mistake to think that the relationship is only one way (from mind to guts). There is ample evidence that IBS also works from gut to brain. That theory was also spelled out in the journal *Gastroenterology.*[58]

Furthermore, the vagus nerve, traditionally thought to be a nerve originating in the brain to send messages to the intestines and stomach, is composed of many neurons. One-third of those neurons do indeed travel from the brain to the stomach. But the other two-thirds originate in the stomach and travel to the brain. The journal *Lancet* explains that stimulation of the vagus nerve decreases inflammation, an effect generally attributed to the immune system.[59] Interestingly, vagus nerve stimulation has been used to treat problems such as seizures, schizophrenia, bipolar disorder, and depression.[60]

A landmark study reported in the *Journal of the American Medical Association*[61] pointed out that the clinical criteria for IBS diagnosis don't include symptoms outside the intestine, such as fatigue or pain. Instead, it says, these complaints are viewed as symptoms of other problems that coexist with IBS and fibromyalgia. In reality, 78 percent of patients with IBS have an overgrowth of bacteria in the small intestine, which can disrupt normal brain-gut interaction and prevent immune activation. The overgrowth of the bacteria is also responsible for intolerance to sugar, altered neurotransmitter levels, and disrupted brain responses—an effect that is made clear as a result of the two-way communication between the immune system and the autonomic nervous system of the intestines and the brain.[62]

The journal *Clinical Infectious Diseases* reported a very interesting case of a child with colitis who had psychological problems. When a flare-up of his colitis was treated with antibiotics, his psychosis disappeared! The researchers concluded that "maybe an opportunistic bacteria colonizing the colon produced a neurotoxin."[63] Exactly: Intestinal flora can mutate and become toxic to the body. Why do intestinal flora mutate? Wouldn't you try to adapt if you were constantly subjected to antibiotics, toxic foods, water chlorination, and who knows what else?[64]

This same process is probably why antifungal medication is effective in treating "atypical" depression.[65] Perhaps it wasn't so atypical after all, but a misdiagnosed problem of the "second brain." This point of view is supported by research showing that 5 HTP and L-tryptophan (dietary precursors of the neurotransmitter serotonin) have antifungal activity in the laboratory.[66] High-sugar diets encourage the growth of toxic organisms in the intestines, which taxes the brain-gut connection. This is compounded in carbohydrate-sensitive people, who lose serotonin more readily, especially when eating too much sugar.[67] Research shows that a diet too high in carbohydrates can cause depression,[68] and that migraine headaches and depression not only are bidirectionally associated, but also have gut connections.[69]

There may be other important ways that the intestinal tract impacts the brain. Half of all children with autism have gastrointestinal problems, such as bloating, diarrhea, and pain. Many are diagnosed after a course of antibiotics.[70] Most of them have enlarged lymph nodes in the intestines and a condition called "leaky gut."[71] Also, a significant proportion of children with developmental disorders have enterocolitis.[72]

An article in the *New England Journal of Medicine* further emphasizes the hormonal connection between the gut and the brain. Hormones other than insulin have been found to "talk" to the brain and subsequently alter behavior, including eating habits. The article concludes that "it is unlikely that any one molecule or derivative will provide a magic bullet to induce and maintain weight loss. Successful pharmacologic treatment for obesity may be possible only by simultaneously targeting the interlocking, redundant systems that drive food intake and act to resist the loss of body fat."[73]

The same theory explains why Parkinson's disease is associated with constipation. People who have fewer than one bowel movement a day have three times the risk of developing Parkinson's disease when compared to people who have more than one movement a day, and are four and a half times more likely to develop Parkinson's disease than men who have more than two movements a day. The reason? They cannot detoxify the agents associated with Parkinson's disease—mostly pesticides—and they have disrupted the brain-gut connection.[74]

A story published in the *Scientific American Journal* drives the brain-gut connection home; Robert Sapolsky, one of the foremost neuroscientists of our age, specializes in the psycho-neuro-immune-endocrine system and the mind-body-spirit concept. He describes a recent experience he had at the last Annual Meeting of the Society for Neuroscience,[75] where 28,000 scientists found themselves overwhelmed by how little they know about the workings of the human brain. Reflecting on this humble thought, he sat on the steps of the convention center, "bludgeoned by information and a general sense of ignorance."

He then noticed a murky stagnant puddle of water by the curb, which reminded him of a recent extraordinary paper he had read on how certain parasites control the brain of their host. He felt the bugs in the puddle knew more about the human brain than he did. He continues to cite many examples—perhaps the most remarkable being rabies and toxoplasma. Rabies has figured out exactly which neurons to infect to make the victim rabid and aggressive, which guarantees that rabies survives. *Toxoplasma gondii* is the parasite that pregnant women avoid in cat litter. Rats have developed a fear of cats to keep them alive, but this instinct is overridden in their brains by a chemical produced by toxoplasma. Losing their fear of cats, they get eaten, thus assuring toxoplasma's survival. Sapolsky concludes,

> *Many of us hold the deeply entrenched idea that primate mammals are the most evolved [organisms]. . . . If you [agree,] you are not just wrong but a step away from a philosophy that most evolved human beings are Northern Europeans. . . . So, remember, there are creatures out there that can control our brains . . . with even more power than Big Brother. . . . My reflection on a curbside puddle brought me to the opposite conclusion that Narcissus reached*

*in his watery reflection. We need humility. We are not the most evolved species, nor the least vulnerable. Nor the cleverest.*[76]

Changes in intestinal flora, caused mostly by poor nutrition, affect our minds. Is it any wonder why so many people are addicted to refined sugar?

## The Impact of Wheat Allergies on the Brain

Wheat allergies now afflict 1 in every 100 Americans, due mostly to wheat processing and poor reception by the intestines. The consequences of wheat allergies are far-reaching because of the increased leakiness of the guts, which is responsible for the increase in autoimmune disorders. In other words, the immune system gets so confused that it starts attacking the body. According to the *New England Journal of Medicine*, a wheat allergy adds to the development of diabetes, anemia, osteoporosis, chronic fatigue, autoimmune disorders, gastrointestinal cancer, dermatitis, miscarriages, irritable bowel syndrome, neurologic symptoms, and behavioral changes.

Wheat allergy causes such a wide variety of symptoms[77] that the *American Journal of Clinical Nutrition* recommends a very high level of suspicion when dealing with gastrointestinal symptoms of any kind. Gluten—a component of wheat, barley, and rye—is hidden in many products, including dairy products; it is in dextrins (sweeteners), natural flavors in potato chips and chewing gum, caramel coloring (in colas and soft drinks,) and the malt flavoring or extract found in corn flakes and rice cereals.

Wheat allergy can even occur without a trace of intestinal inflammation. Most people affected have mild symptoms, but with time, numbness, arthritis, and many other conditions may develop. In fact, gluten allergy has been associated with behavioral problems, changes in personality, and depression.[78] The journal *Lancet* reported that one-third of undiagnosed inflammation of the nerves is cause by wheat allergies.[79] Some of this is due to the antibodies made against the thyroid gland and possibly against insulin, since wheat allergy increases the risk of diabetes.

In addition to triggering behavioral problems, wheat intolerance can trigger migraines, a very common inflammatory condition of the brain.[80] Also, it has been shown that L-tryptophan, the amino acid that enables the body to use serotonin, is decreased in children with wheat allergy.[81]

## Conclusion

At a workshop in the Netherlands, practitioners were told,

> *It is essential that practicing physicians develop a working knowledge of herbs and stay abreast of these emerging findings in order to best advise their patients on the value of health promoting diets in disease and prevention. . . . These are*

*heady days for nutritional scientists as newer understandings of food and health promise to bring clinical nutrition to the forefront of clinical medicine. Practitioners must become nutritionally educated and oriented if they are to maintain their patients' confidence and stay abreast of this aspect of continuously evolving modern medicine.*[82]

These are indeed "heady days" when nutrition is coming to the "forefront of clinical medicine." It won't be long before we restore the principles that built the practice of medicine—that "food is the best medicine," as proposed by pioneers like Hippocrates, the founder of ancient medicine; Sir William Osler, the founder of modern medicine; Maimonides, a twelfth-century Arab-Spanish physician; and Hildegard of Bingen, a twelfth-century saint and health care worker.

Even though testimonials are not the mainstay of scientific validation, they are legitimate tools of expanding knowledge.[83] More than 90 percent of clinical problems can be corrected by empowering patients to live better lifestyles, including improvement in their nutrition, environment, and behavioral/spiritual well-being. Unfortunately, there are some physicians who may not agree, having not seen the research—possibly because of a "dumbing down" in clinical circles.[84]

A focus on nutrition and the mind/body connection is time consuming, and is as a result deemphasized by busy HMOs that continue to offer a "disease-care system." There is also a pervasive attitude in our society to treat symptoms quickly and pharmaceutically. The drug companies have capitalized handsomely on that attitude, perpetuating the use of drugs for medical problems, especially mental disorders. How else could we explain the fact that nutrition is now categorized as an "alternative" mode of providing care? Plato states in *The Republic* that "doctors who treat slaves prescribe medications, while doctors who treat free men teach health lifestyles to prevent disease."

Despite the fact that nine out of ten independent studies never found antidepressants to be any better than placebo in the treatment of depression, antidepressant drugs are now the "standard of care" for behavioral issues.[85] This has created a deeply rooted belief that nutrition, environmental toxins, and mind/body issues are not worth pursuing. Fortunately, recent books published by Harvard-connected doctors (*Overdosed America*),[86] a former *New England of Journal of Medicine* editor (*The Truth About Drug Companies*),[87] Pulitzer Prize winners (*Critical Condition*),[88] and the Institute of Medicine (*Crossing the Quality Chasm*)[89] are addressing these vital concerns.

## ENDNOTES

1. Symposium on Nutrition for Physicians, "What is Nutrition?" *American J. Clinical Nutrition* 77 (2003): 149.

2. C. B. Pert, *Molecules of Emotion,* Touchstone, 1999.
3. H. Hu and M. Wu, "Spin-mediated Consciousness Theory," *J. Medical Hypothesis* 63 (2004): 633.
4. M. A. Aller and J. L. Arias, "Neuro-Immune-Endocrine Functional System and Vascular Pathology," *J. Medical Hypothesis* 57 (2001): 561.
5. M. L. Fitzgibbon, M. R. Stolley, and D. S. Kirschenbaum, "Obese People Who Seek Treatment Have Different Characteristics Than Those Who Do Not Seek Treatment," *Health Psychology,* 12 (1993): 342–45.
6. USDA's Continuing Survey of Food Intakes by Individuals 1994–1996, 1999.
7. Ibid.
8. T. Peregrin, "The New Frontier of Nutrition Science: Nutrigenomics," *J. American Dietetic Association* 101 (2001): 1306.
9. D. Kritchevsky, "Diet and Cancer: What Is Next?" *J. Nutrition* 133 (2003): 386s.
10. J. Diamond, *Guns, Germs and Steel,* W. W. Norton & Company, 1999.
11. L. Pauling and D. Hawkins, "Orthomolecular Psychiatry," *J. Science* 160 (1969): 701.
12. C. Boult, U. B. Krinke, C. F. Urdangarin, "The Validity of Nutritional Status as a Marker For Future Disability and Depressive Symptoms Among High Risk Older Adults," *J. American Gerontology Society* 47 (1999): 995.
13. D. S. Kays, G. J. Naylor and A. H. Smith, "The Therapeutic Effect of Ascorbic Acid and EDTA in Manic Depressive Psychosis, a Double Blind Trial," *British Journal Psychiatry* 109 (1963): 294.
14. A. A. Shaheen, et al., "Effect of Pretreatment with Vitamin E or Diazepam on Brain Metabolism of Stressed Rats," *J. Biochemistry Pharmacology* 46 (1993): 194.
15. J. R. Davidson, K. Abraham and K. M. Connor, "Effectiveness of Chromium in Atypical Depression, a Placebo-controlled Trial," *J. Biology Psychiatry* 53 (2003): 261.
16. R. C. Hall and J. R. Joffe, "Hypomagnesemia. Physical and Psychiatric Symptoms," *JAMA* 224 (1973): 1749.
17. A. Lapillonne and S. D. Clarke, "Polyunsaturated Fatty Acids and Gene Expression," *J. Current Opinion Clinical Nutrition Metabolism Care* 7 (2004): 151.
18. P. M. Kidd, "Bipolar Disorder and Cell Membrane Function," *J. Alternative Medicine Review* 9 (2004): 107.
19. B. M. Cohen and A. L. Miller, "Lecithin in Mania," *American Journal Psychiatry* 137 (1980): 242; and S. Delion, S. Chalon, D. Guilloteau, "Age-related Changes in Phospholipid Fatty Acid Composition and Monoaminergic Neurotransmission in the Hippocampus of Rats Fed a Balanced or an N-3 Polyunsaturated Fatty Acid-deficient Diet," *J. Lipid Research* 38 (1997): 680.
20. A. C. Logan, "Neurobiological Aspects of Omega 3 Fatty Acids: Possible Mechanisms and Therapeutic Value in Major Depression," *J. Alternative Medicine Review* 8 (2004): 410.
21. M. Peet and D. F. Horrobin, "A Dose-ranging Study of the Effects of Ethyl-eicosapentaenoate in Patients with Ongoing Depression Despite Apparently Adequate Therapy with Standard Drugs," *J. Archives General Psychiatry* 59 (2002): 913.
22. R. A. Waterland and R. L. Jirtle, "Transposable Elements: Targets for Early Nutritional Effects on Epigenetic Gene Regulation," *J. Molecular Cell Biology* 23 (2003): 5293.
23. B. W. Penninx and J. M. Guralnik, "B-12 Deficiency and Depression in Physically Disabled Older Women: Epidemiologic Evidence from the Women's Health and Aging Study," *American J. Psychiatry* 157 (2000): 715.
24. S. E. Andres, E. Noel and N. H. Loukili, "Vitamin B12 Deficiency in Older Adults," *J. Geriatrics* 58 (2003): 12.

25. Symposium in Santa Barbara on SAMe, *American Journal Clinical Nutrition* 76 (2002): 1145s.

26. W. Poldinger and B. Calanchini, "A Functional-dimensional Approach to Depression: Serotonin 26 Deficiency as a Target Syndrome in a Comparison of 5-hydroxytryptophan and Fluvoxamine," *J. Psychopathology* 24 (1991): 53.

27. J. Walinder and A. Skott, "Potentiation of the Antidepressant Action of Clomipramine by Tryptophan," *J. Archives of General Psychiatry* 33 (1976): 1384.

28. M. Eubanks, "Allergies A La Carte. Is There a Problem with Genetically Modified Food?" *J. Environmental Health Perspectives* 110 (2002): A130.

29. V. Heresco-Levy, D. C. Javitt and M. Emilov, "Efficacy of High Dose Glycine in the Treatment of Enduring Negative Symptoms of Schizophrenia," *J. Archives General Psychiatry* 56 (1999): 29.

30. Z. Farfel and H. R. Bourne, "The Expanding Spectrum of G Protein diseases," *New England J. Medicine* 340 (1999): 1012.

31. G. W. Lambert, C. Reid and D. M. Kaye, "Effect of Sunlight and Season on Serotonin Turnover in the Brain," *J. Lancet* 360 (2002): 1840.

32. J. S. Bland, "Vitamin D update," *J. Functional Medicine Update,* (24) 8 (2004): 317.

33. D. B. Allison, K. R. Fontaine, J. E. Manson, J. Stevens, and T. B. VanItallie, "Annual Deaths Attributable to Obesity in the United States," *Journal of the American Medical Association* 282 (1999): 1530–38.

34. J. E. Manson, G. A. Colditz, M. J. Stampfer, W. C. Willett, B. Rosner, R. R. Monson, F. E. Speizer, and C. H. Hennekens, "A Prospective Study of Obesity and Risk of Coronary Heart Disease in Women," *New England Journal of Medicine* 322 (1990): 882–88.

35. Manson et al., "A Prospective Study."

36. M. C. Davis, E. W. Twamley, N. A. Hamilton, and P. D. Swan, "Body Fat Distribution and Hemodynamic Stress Responses in Premenopausal Obese Women: A Preliminary Study," *Health Psychology* 18 (1999): 625–33.

37. E. S. Epel, B. McEwen, T. Seeman K. Matthews, G. Catellazzo, K. Brownell, J. Bell, and J. Ickovics, "Stress and Body Shape: Stress-induced Cortisol Secretion is Consistently Greater Among Women with Central Fat," *Psychosomatic Medicine* 62 (2000): 623–32.

38. D. W. Foster, "Insulin Resistance: A Secret Killer?" *New England Journal of Medicine* 320 (1989): 733.

39. S. Hurtley, R. Service and P. Szumori, "Carbohydrates and Glycobiology," *J. Science* 291 (2001): 237.

40. R. Ramasubbu, "Insulin Resistance, a Metabolic Link Between Depressive Disorder and Atherosclerotic Vascular Diseases," *J. Medical Hypothesis* 59 (2002): 537.

41. Ramasubbu, "Insulin Resistance."

42. D. Ongur and W. C. Drevets, "Glial Reduction in the Subgenual Prefrontal Cortex in Mood Disorders," *J. Proceedings of the National Academy of Science* 95 (1998): 13290 and *J. Scientific American,* April 2004.

43. Z. Arvanitakis, R. S. Wilson, J. L. Bienjas, J. A. Evans and D. A. Bennett, "Diabetes Mellitus and Risk of Alzheimer's Disease and Decline in Cognitive Function," *J. Archives of Neurology* 61 (2004): 661.

44. B. C. Miller, E. A. Eckman, and K. Sambamurti, "Amyloid-Beta Peptide in Brain Are Inversely Correlated With Insulysin Activity In Iivo," *J. Proceedings of the National Academy of Science* 100 (2003): 6221.

45. L. Gasparini and H. Xu, "Potential Roles of Insulin and IGF-1," *J. Trends in Neuroscience* 26 (2003): 404.

46. G. Cohen, "Is the Brain on Fire?" *J. Annals of Neurology* 36 (1994): 333.

47. R. N. Kalaria, S. A. Gravina, J. W. Schmidley, G. Perry, and S. I. Harik, "The

Glucose Transporter of the Human Brain and Blood Brain Barrier," *J. Annals of Neurology* 24 (1988): 757.

48. J. M. Starr, J. Wardlaw, and K. Ferguson, "Increased Blood Brain Barrier Permeability in Type II Diabetes Demonstrated by Gadolinium Magnetic Resonance Imaging,"*J. Neurology Neurosurgery Psychiatry* 74 (2003): 70.

49. W. N. Kerman and S. E. Inzucchi, "Impaired Insulin Sensitivity Among Nondiabetic Patients with a Recent TIA or Ischemic Stroke," *J. Neurology* 60 (2003): 1447.

50. I. Berlin, A. Grimaldi, and C. Laundautt, "Suspected Post Prandial Hypoglycemia is Associated with Beta Adrenergic Hypersensitivity and Emotional stress," *J. Clinical Endocrinology and Metabolism* 79 (1994): 1428.

51. D. L. Ginsberg, "T4 Augmentation Effective in Partial Responders with Major Depression," *J. Primary Psychiatry* 9(7) (2002): 23.

52. S. Volpato and J. M. Guralnik, "Serum Thyroxine Levels and Cognitive Decline in Euthyroid Older Women," *J. Neurology* 58 (2002): 1055.

53. D. H. Raybould and F. Azpiroz, "2001; the Brain-Gut Odyssey," *J. Digestion* 63 (2001): 247.

54. M. D. Gershon, *The Second Brain,* Harper Collins, 1998.

55. The Danone Symposium, France, Paris, "The Intelligent Intestine," *American J. Clinical Nutrition* 78 (2003): 675.

56. The Danone Symposium, "The Intelligent Intestine."

57. D. G. Thompson, "Descartes and the Gut: I'm Pink, Therefore I am," *J. Gut* 49 (2001): 165.

58. H. Tomblom, G. Lindberg, B. Nyberg, and B. Veress, "Full Thickness Biopsy of the Jejunum Reveals Inflammation and Enteric Neuropathy in IBS," *J. Gastroenterology* 123 (2002): 1972.

59. R. A. Floto and K. G. Smith, "The Vagus Nerve, Macrophages and Nicotine," *J. Lancet* 361 (2003): 1069.

60. G. Elger, C. Gittopec and P. Falka, "Vagus Nerve Stimulation is Associated With Mood Improvement in Epileptic Patients," *J. Epilepsy Research* 42 (2000): 203.

61. H. C. Lin, "Small Intestinal Bacterial Overgrowth," *JAMA* 292 (2004): 852.

62. Lin, "Small Intestinal Bacterial Overgrowth."

63. N. E. Rosenstein, S. A. Stocker, and T. Popovic, "Relief of Psychiatric Symptoms in a Patient with Chron's Disease After Metronidazole Therapy," *J. Clinical Infectious Diseases* 30 (2000): 214.

64. E. Pennisi, "Close Encounters: Good, Bad, Ugly," *J. Science* 290 (2000): 1491.

65. R. Sovner and S. Fogelman, "Ketoconazole Therapy for Atypical Depression," *J. Clinical Psychiatry* 57 (1996): 227.

66. C. Lass-Florl, D. Fucks, and M. Ledochovski, "Antifungal Properties of 5-hydroxytriptamine (Serotonin) Against Candida in Vitro," *J. Medical Microbiology* 52 (2003): 169.

67. J. S. Bland, "Functional Medicine Update," (2)21 (2002): 199.

68. R. J. Wurtman and J. J. Wurtman, "Carbohydrates and Depression," *J. Scientific American* 260 (1989): 68.

69. N. Breslau, R. B. Lipton, and W. F. Stewart, "Comorbidity of Migraine and Depression: Investigating Potential Etiology and Therapy," *J. Neurology* 60 (2003): 1308.

70. A. J. Wakefield, "Ileal-lymphoid-nodular Hyperplasia and Nonspecific Colitis and Pervasive Development Disorder in Children," *J. Lancet* 351 (1998): 637.

71. P. D'Eufemia, M. Cell, and R. Finocchiaro, "Abnormal Intestinal Permeability in Children with Autism," *J. Acta Pediatrica* 85 (1996): 1076.

72.  A. J. Wakefield, A. Anthony, and S. H. Mursh, "Enterocolitis in Children with Developmental Disorders," *American J. Gastroenterology* 95 (2000): 2285.

73.  J. Komer and R. L. Leibel, "To Eat or Not to Eat: How the Gut Talks to the Brain," *New England Journal of Medicine* 349 (2003): 9236.

74.  R. D. Abbott, H. Petrovich, and L. R. White, "Frequency of Bowel Movement and the Future Risk of Parkinson's Disease," *J. Neurology* 57 (2001): 456.

75.  R. Sapolsy, "Bugs in the Brain," *J. Scientific American* 288 (2003): 94.

76.  Sapolsy, "Bugs in the Brain."

77.  R. McManus and D. Kelleher, "Celiac Disease, the Villain Unmasked," *New England Journal of Medicine* 348 (2003): 2517.

78.  A. De Rosa, A. Trocone, and M. Vacca, "Characteristics and Quality of Illness Behavior in Celiac Disease," *J. Psychosomatics* 45 (2004): 325, 336.

79.  M. Hadjivassiliou, A. Gibson, and G. A. Davies-Jones, "Does Cryptic Gluten Sensitivity Play a Part in Neurological Illness?" *J. Lancet* 347( 1996): 369 and *British Medical Journal* 318 (1999): 1710.

80.  M. Gabrielli, F. Cremonini, and G. Fiore, "Association Between Migraine and Celiac Disease," *American Journal Gastroenterology* 98 (2003): 625.

81.  A. Hernanz and I. Polanco, "Plasma Precursor Aminoacids of Central Nervous System Monoamines in Children with Celiac Disease," *J. Gut* 32 1991): 1478.

82.  Proceedings of the Third Heelsum International Workshop, Netherlands, December 2001. "Nutrition Guidance of Family Doctors Towards Best Practice," *American J. Clinical Nutrition* 77 (2003): 1001S.

83.  K. Malterud, "The Art and Science of Clinical Knowledge: Evidence Beyond Measures and Numbers," *J. Lancet* 2001, p 397.

84.  H. W. Horowitz, "A Piece of My Mind: Dumbing Down," *JAMA* 289 (2003): 1349.

85.  J. Abramson, *Overdosed America: The Broken Promise of American Medicine. How the Pharmaceutical Companies Distort Medical Knowledge, Mislead Doctors, and Compromise Your Health,* Harper Collins, 2004.

86.  Abramson, *Overdosed America.*

87.  M. Angell, *The Truth About Drug Companies: How They Deceive Us and What to Do About It,* Random House, 2004.

88.  D. L. Barlett and J. B. Steele, *Critical Condition: How Health Care in America Became Big Business and Bad Medicine,* Doubleday, 2004.

89.  Institute of Medicine, *Crossing the Quality Chasm: A New Health Care System for the 21st Century,* National Academy Press, 2001.

# Behavioral Medicine Treatment: Effects on Medical and Health Outcomes and Costs

*To a great extent, the very term psychosomatic has lost meaning. No longer can we talk about "psychosomatic illnesses," but we must acknowledge that most, if not all, disease is potentially influenced by psychosocial factors. Even dividing the body into systems—such as the immune system or the nervous system—has lost meaning as we observe the overlap and communication among systems.*

—Stanford B. Friedman, 1988 Presidential Address
to the American Psychosomatic Society

## Learning Objectives

- Understand how to best prove the mind-body connection, or the causal relationship between mental processes and physical illness.
- Examine medical outcome data when mental interventions are added in treating physical illness for high utilizers of medical care, for specific medical illnesses, or to reduce health costs.
- Explore the use of behavioral medicine interventions to fill the hole in current medical approaches.

Outcome research is a hot item these days. At the top of medical research priorities is the proof of whether a treatment or preventive measure significantly changes the incidence, costs, morbidity, or mortality of a disease—or, for that matter, of health in general. When we do something to change morbidity, we should not only reduce symptoms and disability but also improve a person's quality of life.

In the past, a main focus of research has been mortality rates. We now know that a powerful treatment that reduces the severity of the disease or that prolongs life may not be the best treatment if it creates even more misery for the patient or if it is tremendously expensive. A person who is ill may prefer a treatment program that improves quality of life more than a treatment that merely prolongs life. Optimally, of course, we would hope for an approach that does both.

Medical research has also focused on intermediate effects that were easy to measure and that were presumed to lead to beneficial outcomes. For example, researchers knew that high blood pressure (hypertension) is a risk factor in heart disease and stroke. The goal, then, has been to reduce blood pressure, with the assumption that lower blood pressure will result in a lower incidence of death from heart disease and strokes. One type of drug that works fairly well to lower blood pressure is a diuretic, or water pill. Higher doses of these worked even better to lower pressure than lower doses. As long as the focus was on intermediate steps, such as lowering blood pressure, everyone was happy with the diuretics. Once actual studies started looking at the outcome, however, researchers realized that high doses of diuretics were causing even *more* cardiac deaths than were caused by untreated hypertension. Why? Probably because they cause problems in the blood chemistry that subsequently lead to irregular heart rhythm.

Studies that look at the result of a specific treatment are called *outcome studies*. Outcome studies that look at the *bottom line* are often eye-openers. They can readjust our focus from the intermediate goals to the result that really counts, and can dispel mistaken myths that seem like common sense.

That's what we're starting to see with the outcome effects of several behavioral medicine interventions. These treatment programs are directed primarily at two things:

- Creating mental skills that are directed at lessening symptoms and disease processes
- Bringing behaviors and attitudes in congruence with those of optimal health, and with the patient's own deepest values

These are best done as an adjunct to, but not in place of, other proven medical treatments.

Saying that mental stress is the cause of a disease is a great oversimplification. But if mental factors really play a *role* in the evolution of an illness, then interventions that address mental factors should improve the outcome of treatment. It generally takes three things to document that a factor (such as mental distress) contributes to or helps cause a disease process:

1. You must show that when the factor is present, the disease is worse.

2. You must demonstrate that the factor worsens the pathophysiological processes that lead to the disease.

3. You must prove that interventions that reduce or remove the factor subsequently improve the disease incidence or the eventual outcome. Health outcomes are measured by reduced morbidity (*adverse disease effects*) and mortality and by improved quality of life and function.

Of these three requirements, the third—showing that active intervention to reduce the risk factor changes the outcome of the disease—is usually the most convincing and is the most important from a practical point of view.

A well-known example is the role of a high-cholesterol diet in contributing to coronary artery disease. Let's look at the three requirements as they apply to high cholesterol:

1. **If the factor is present, the disease is worse.** Early epidemiological studies, such as those in Finland, showed that people who eat a high-fat diet have a higher incidence of heart attacks and strokes.

   This association did not yet prove fatty diets as a cause, however, because people who eat high-fat diets may also have other undetected factors that lead to heart disease. One tongue-in-cheek researcher responded by showing a correlation between wearing a pocket watch—as the elderly then did—and increased heart attacks; then, with a grin, he suggested outlawing pocket watches as a major public hazard. An old saw called Mersky's second rule states, "More people die in bed than out of bed. So keep the patient out of bed!" While a high rate of an illness is associated with a certain factor, clearly more is needed to show cause and effect.

2. **The suspected factor worsens pathophysiological processes.** High fat intake was then shown to increase the cholesterol that formed plaques on the walls of the arteries. Those plaques narrowed the arteries that supplied blood to the heart and the arteries that supplied blood to the brain, leading to the occlusions that eventually caused heart attack and stroke.

   There are, however, other parts of the pathological processes (such as blood vessel spasm and clotting) that are not known to be prominently affected by fat intake.

3. **Interventions that reduce the suspected factor improve disease outcomes.** Active programs to lower dietary fat intake, with the subsequent lowering of blood cholesterol levels, were shown to reduce the incidence of cardiovascular events by about 12 percent. Medications that lowered cholesterol brought about an even higher reduction in heart attacks—about 40 percent.

Despite the somewhat modest benefits, this intervention effect was really the proof of the pudding, triggering major public education efforts to reduce cholesterol levels.

Demonstrating the role of mental factors in disease has followed a similar pattern. In the case of cardiovascular disease, improved mental states had even more profound effects on outcomes than did reducing dietary cholesterol alone. First came the studies correlating mental distress (or loneliness, or hopelessness) with higher incidences of various illnesses. For example:

- Half or more of general medical outpatients have physical ailments significantly related to psychosocial factors—25 percent have major psychiatric diagnoses, such as major depression or anxiety disorders. Many additional patients feel excessively distressed or have high-risk behaviors.[1]

- Sixty percent of all medical visits are primarily for stress-related symptoms;[2] among high utilizers of health care services, this percentage increases substantially.

- One-third to one-half of hospitalized medical patients have a psychiatric diagnosis in addition to their medical problem.

## The Connection Between Mental Stress and Medical Symptoms

In a classic study in primary care medical clinics, Kurt Kroenke and his colleagues evaluated the most common physical symptoms that patients presented. After *three years* of testing and follow-up, they found that, on average, less than 17 percent had a clear-cut organic diagnosis to explain those symptoms! That is, 84 percent were "unexplained" pathologically.

Certain bothersome medical symptoms, particularly if otherwise unexplained, are likely to have a high percentage of underlying mental anxiety or depression.[3] These include the following:[4]

- Persistent fatigue (55–58 percent)[5]
- Insomnia (87 percent)
- Headaches (44 percent)
- Chest pain (28 percent)
- Shortness of breath (33 percent)
- Palpitations (40 percent)
- Constipation (46 percent)

- Diarrhea (29 percent)
- Fainting (47 percent)
- Dizziness (48 percent)[6]
- Numbness (28 percent)
- Menstrual problems (56 percent)
- Multiple allergies (62 percent)[7]
- Prolonged convalescence from viral infections (such as influenza)[8]
- Irritable bowel syndrome (91 percent)[9]
- Premenstrual syndrome[10]

Patients with *combinations* of such symptoms, especially those that involve different body systems, are *highly* likely to have underlying anxiety, depression, or other mental distress.[11] For example, of those who have a *combination* of both dizziness and numbness/tingling, 93 percent have an anxiety disorder. And of those with *both* a pain symptom and also an unrelated symptom of autonomic dysregulation (such as palpitations, nausea, bowel problems, or shortness of breath), over 80 percent have an anxiety problem.

The above correlations still did not prove that mental distress can cause physical illness, however, because numerous other risk factors could easily be present. For example, anxious and depressed people smoke at a much higher rate, often tend to eat a richer diet, and use more alcohol and illicit drugs. Also, since many of these correlation studies were retrospective—that is, they looked at the person after the illness had already appeared—some might argue that the mental distress was brought on by the illness, rather than the other way around. Because understanding mind-body connections involved some new ways of viewing the world medically (new health paradigms), skeptics about the importance of those connections were, of course, abundant.

Next came many studies correlating mental distress, or mental conditioning, to the pathophysiological processes that lead to disease. Significant mental distress results in dysregulation of protective immune and hormone balance, as well as discoordinated autonomic nervous system control. The three systems most affected by mental factors—the hormone, immune, and nervous systems—form the communication networks that provide the *homeostatic* balance that maintains good health. That is, when health is challenged, these systems allow for a response that is neither too much nor too little, but just enough to keep the challenge in control and to maintain well-being. If emotional responses are too much (as with anxiety) or too little (as with severe depression), the bodily responses tend to follow suit. Even the process of damage to the blood vessels that eventually causes heart attack can be traced in part to disruptions in these three systems that are caused by mental factors such as hostility or depression.

Once again, however, the truly convincing evidence will come with intervention outcome studies. For example, does a treatment program that reduces hostility or depression also reduce heart attacks, cardiac death, or the costs and disability associated with them?

Much effort is now being directed at these mental intervention issues, with interesting and often impressive results. The treatment interventions have been behavioral, spiritual, psychological, psycho-educational, and even psychopharmacological in nature, with measurement of resulting medical and health outcomes. An example of such an intervention would be a program to create stress resilience.

What does participating in such a program do to subsequent health outcomes and costs? How does treating depression impact the physical diseases shown to be more associated with it—and the pathophysiological processes that cause those diseases? Or what does a psycho-educational program designed to help a person manage the full impact of specific serious diseases (such as breast cancer or rheumatoid arthritis) do to the activity and prognosis of the disease itself, as well as the quality of life of the person with that illness?

Although behavioral medicine is still in its childhood, and such intervention studies are really just beginning, some highly interesting results are beginning to emerge. One fact is becoming increasingly clear: Using the strict disease model to treat the many people with stress-related medical illness (or *psychosomatic* dysfunction) is not only costly, but also ineffective and frustrating to all involved. Only a few of the better known of many psycho-behavioral intervention studies, and those pertaining to some of the larger medical issues, will be considered to create a perspective and give a flavor of future potentials.

## Outcome Data from Behavioral Medicine Interventions

In the near future, a question like this might appear on a National Board exam for physicians in training:

Which one of the following has *not* clearly been shown to have an improved medical prognosis by adding stress management to the usual medical care?

1. Myocardial infarction

2. Metastatic breast cancer

3. Hip fracture repair in the elderly

4. Obstetrical delivery

5. Hypertension

6. High medical care utilization and costs

7. Psoriasis

Such a question is not likely to appear for some time, however, because most who take the exam are probably not familiar with the data. The correct answer right now is hypertension—treating mental stress has substantially and consistently improved the medical aspect of all of the above conditions except high blood pressure. Some stress interventions have been useful for hypertension and others have not, but when they are taken all together—in a *meta-analysis*—no persistent clear-cut benefit for lowering blood pressure was found from treating mental stress. (Reducing the *effects* of hypertension, such as heart attacks, has been another story, however.)

Some who conducted the successful hypertension trials might, of course, argue that the *type and style* of the stress reduction program may be crucial. For example, was the intervention purely *didactic*—talking about better ways to deal with stress, as many older stress management programs have been—or was it predominantly *experiential,* which involves mentally living the changes and feeling them in the body? Experiential approaches are increasingly being shown to be far more effective in improving outcomes, both behavioral and medical.

Another question: Did the intervention simply elicit the relaxation response alone, or did it also couple such relaxation with the reframing of upsetting thinking and the reprogramming of habitual, distressed responses? The answers to these questions appear to play an important role in the effectiveness of behavior medicine interventions. Moving beyond the relaxation response alone to include changing behaviors provides better outcomes.

Behavioral medicine as a "specialty" probably began formally with the 1978 Yale conference called to form the Academy of Behavioral Medicine Research. "Specialty" is in quotes because, by its nature, behavioral medicine goes in the opposite direction of specialties. By delving deeper into the function of a specific organ system, specialization in medicine has been of great value in creating special expertise. Behavioral medicine, on the other hand, goes up to higher levels of integrating all systems in an interdisciplinary way, explicitly reuniting the body systems and mind, and even the spiritual issues, that make up the whole person. As you can see from the data provided in this book, the past few years have brought a flood of research following those beginnings—some very solid, but some uncontrolled or with too few patients to draw broad conclusions. Behavioral medicine attempts to determine what is reliable in that research for creating new clinical methods to diagnose, treat, and prevent many of the problems that have been somewhat perplexing in the past. While the field is still new, some very real possibilities for changing our approach to patient care and health prevention are surfacing.

Some examples of treatment studies leading to these conclusions follow. Perhaps one bottom line that speaks loudest, and may reflect overall benefits the most, is the effect on medical costs and the need to utilize health care services.

# High-Volume Users of Medical Care and Resources

Overall, people who use more medical care and who have multiple medical maladies tend largely to have much more stress-related medical illness. As noted, they are also much more likely to have depression and/or anxiety disorders.[12] For example, over half of specialty visits and hospitalizations come from those in the top 10 percent of health care utilization. In this same top 10 percent, 68 percent have major depression and 32 percent have chronic low-grade depression. Many more have anxiety disorders.

Certain groups of medical problems are more likely to cluster in patients with mental or stress disorders, such as gastrointestinal problems, atypical chest pain, chronic pain, or unexplained neurological symptoms. These are all very common problems seen in primary care medicine as well as in specialty clinics. For example, of all patients entering a gastroenterology clinic, one-third were depressed (33 percent), one-third had panic disorder (34 percent), and one-third had anxiety-related somatization disorder (38 percent)—obviously with some overlap. The most common diagnosis coming out of a gastroenterology clinic is irritable bowel syndrome (IBS). Over the lifetime of gastroenterology patients with IBS, more than 90 percent will have a diagnosed anxiety or depression disorder.[13]

Another example is the high rate of multiple-system symptoms seen in patients with low back pain. Among those, anxious somatization is four to six times the usual rate in the population.[14]

Despite the fact that huge numbers of medical patients have stress and mental disorder problems, a large percentage go unrecognized and untreated. Only about one-fifth of those with diagnosable depression and anxiety disorders get help from mental health professionals. And despite considerable recent improvement, medical physicians, even those in primary care, usually only make such diagnoses about half the time.[15] The missed mental diagnosis is more understandable as we observe that most patients (and physicians) focus largely on the associated physical problems, and patients are often reluctant to bring up the mental issues, even if they are causing the most suffering. Even when diagnosed with a mental component, patients are reluctant to "see a shrink," and medical physicians often are not taught the needed skills to deal well with such psychosomatic problems. All this adds up to the fact that there is a huge hole in our total health delivery system, leaving many medical patients untreated for the real underlying issues. These patients are likely to return repeatedly and chronically with more stress-related medical problems. Some new treatment options are, however, beginning to emerge.

## Medical Outpatients

With the above realizations in mind, researchers in the Harvard Community Health Plan (a large HMO-managed care program in the Boston area) decided to see if stress reduction programs, which patients *do* tend to accept, would benefit high utilizers and reduce health care needs and costs.[16] Patients who utilized health services more than twice as often as average were randomly assigned to one of three different stress reduction programs available in the Harvard system:

1. An informational, "talk only" group discussing the role of stress in illness and methods for managing stress (much like many older stress management classes).

2. An intervention centered around "mindfulness meditation," experiencing deep relaxation and focused attention in the present moment, with daily practice.

3. An intervention that combined cognitive and language restructuring (new ways of thinking about the stressor) with both relaxation and the mental experience of visualizing responding more effectively in areas of recurrent struggle.

Note that both the second and third methods are "experiential" interventions, using mental practice in the group, compared to the first method, which only talks about how to manage stress without actually practicing stress reduction. The experiential programs were reasonably brief, holding ninety-minute sessions once a week for six weeks.

Researchers measured changes in physical and mental symptoms as well as how frequently the patients utilized health care systems over the subsequent six months. The results, as shown in Table 23.1, are as follows:

1. The "talk only" group did not experience any change in physical or mental symptoms, and did not change the frequency of using health care systems.

**Table 23.1**   Utilization of Health Care Systems

|  | **Mental Distress**<br>**(Bi-POMS Test Score, 0–36)** | **Physical Symptoms**<br>**(25-Symptom List)** | **Utilization**<br>**(In 6 Months)** |
|---|---|---|---|
| Mindfulness meditation | −4.7 | −6.2 | −1.6 visits |
| Combining cognitive change with meditation and imagery | −4.0 | −14.7 | −3.9 visits |

2. The experiential groups both significantly reduced both symptoms and utilization.

But does such an intervention just add more cost?

Most behavioral medicine intervention programs are very low in cost, particularly when done in groups. And for the majority (those without severe mental issues), group participation is usually even *more* effective than individual approaches. (Some of the reasons why will be addressed in Chapter 24.) Usually, people are much more ready to accept such psycho-educational programs—to learn how to become more stress resilient—than they are to start individual psychotherapy, as valuable as that would likely be for them.

For the Harvard treatment programs discussed above, overall cost savings were evident in addition to the health and life quality benefits to the patients. For the number of patients attending the two experiential programs, averaging their effects, the estimated net cost savings (after costs for the interventions were included) were $6,900 per year. With ten such programs offered per year, the Harvard Health Care Plan saw potential first-year savings of $69,000 (with compounding savings if the beneficial effects held in subsequent years).

## Hospitalized Medical Inpatients

The Department of Behavioral Medicine at Hohf Clinic and Hospital in Victoria, Texas, studied 235 hospitalized patients referred for stress-related disorders.[17] Using a more intensive intervention averaging eleven full inpatient days, they analyzed the subsequent need for hospitalization compared to before the intervention. The intervention program was multimodal, was somewhat tailored to individual patient needs, and used modalities such as biofeedback training, self-management activities, and outpatient psychotherapy if needed.

Comparing the subsequent two years to the five years before the intervention, hospitalization days dropped dramatically: from 22.8 days per year to 7.3 (a 68 percent reduction). Also note that the 7.3-day average over two years *included* the eleven days of inpatient behavioral medicine treatment program. Total calculated savings were more than $3 for each $1 invested in the intervention. Additionally, the program improved the overall well-being and health risk of those participating.

## Some Implications

Such behavioral medicine interventions represent an effective but nontraditional approach to some of our most common and perplexing medical problems. Rather than simply attempting to control physical symptoms with medications (as helpful as that might be), patients are taught to quiet their overarousal and to become aware of their thinking and bodily responses to typical stressful situations. They are then taught how to consciously recreate new, more healthy automatic responses that are in line with their reflective values about how they would most like to be in such situations. The processes involved are empowering to patients, giving them a sense of personal control to react to stress as they most deeply would want to respond. When the relationships between thoughts, values, and behaviors are thus experientially addressed, the physical health (and economic) benefits follow naturally.

# Outcomes for Specific Medical Illnesses

## Coronary Artery Disease

After a heart attack, in order to prevent recurrent heart attacks or cardiac death, many approaches to reducing risk factors are undertaken. These include low-fat diets, treatment of high blood pressure, exercise, smoking cessation, aspirin (to reduce clotting), and other certain medications. These interventions reduce the risk of a second heart attack by 8 to 20 percent. Stopping smoking or taking aspirin can result in close to a 30 percent reduction, and beta-blocker medication can result in a 25 percent reduction. It now appears, however, that group behavioral programs are even better, particularly those designed to reduce stress and transform hostile and socially isolating behaviors into the protective behaviors described earlier in this book. (See Chapter 4.)

Among heart attack survivors, over eight well-controlled studies have been described that compare those who were provided this behavioral modification approach in addition to the above standard preventive measures; these studies compared such patients to those who receive standard prevention without the behavioral program. These results are summarized in Table 23.2. Taken together, the studies reveal a 39 percent decrease in recurrent heart attacks and a one-third reduction in cardiac death. Some of the interventions were more effective than others. (The key elements are described in Chapter 24.) The large Friedman study showed a 46 percent reduction in heart attacks.

Adding treatment of depression when appropriate further improves on these outcomes. (See Chapter 6.) One trial demonstrated that treating depression after myocardial infarction reduced cardiac mortality by 61 percent compared to those who were depressed but not treated.[18]

In a similar second study, medically treated depression after heart attacks resulted in a 41 percent reduction in coronary death (which was substantially better than using stress reduction alone in these clinically depressed patients).[19]

A more recent study at Duke University compared the effects of stress reduction versus a good exercise program in reducing second heart attacks. The results showed recurrent attacks in 30 percent of those having the usual preventive care, 20 percent if exercise alone was added to usual care, but only 7 percent if stress reduction alone was added to usual care.[20]

On the other hand, for people with high-risk psychobehavioral styles (such as cynical hostility and social alienation, as described in Chapter 4), one might wonder if using a similar behavioral program would effectively prevent the *first* heart attack. One controlled European study, if reproducible, suggests the answer is clearly yes—and in spades. Of a group of middle-aged people with a high personality risk profile for coronary disease, half were treated with a behavioral modification program over several weeks and half were not. Thirteen years later, *twice* as many of the treated people were still alive.

Do such mental interventions actually affect the arterial wall pathology that leads to heart attacks and strokes? The answer appears to be yes. For example, meditation has been shown to reverse several of the processes by which mental stress and depression were shown to cause increased arterial plaque, spasm, and clot (detailed in Chapter 6). Excess peripheral norepinephrine, which contributes to vessel wall damage, and low central nervous system serotonin, which contributes to spasm and increased clotting, are both improved by meditative techniques and gaining a sense of personal control. Do those neurochemical changes actually reduce vascular lesions? A study of African Americans with high blood pressure looked at their carotid artery thickness in response to either practicing transcendental mediation or following good instruction for reducing other cardiovascular risk factors.[21] Those meditating regularly had significant reduction in carotid artery thickness, while those in the education-only group had progression of the artery thickening. Carotid artery thickening also closely correlates with that going on in the coronary arteries as well. Thus, we see these mental interventions documented as providing benefits for both the disease mechanisms and the clinical outcomes as well.

It should be noted, however, that such intervention for coronary patients (after an infarction) may need to be done differently for women than for men. A stress reduction program that showed a striking benefit for men (50 percent reduction in cardiac mortality)[22] did not work at all well for women. The authors concluded that men prefer to have a task given that they can work on, while women do not like being told what to do but have much better outcomes when they are listened to and emotionally supported.

There is some evidence as well that such behavioral interventions may be the best chance we have for changing other risk factors (such as smoking or overeating) as well. Is it possible that these kinds of behavioral interventions, coupled with the usual measures, could become our most important cardiac prevention?

## Hypertension

Earlier chapters documented the associations of mental stress (and lack of social support) with:

- Persistent elevations of hormones that cause high blood pressure (catacholamines, aldosterone, vasopressin, and cortisol)

- Observations of blood pressure elevations in anxious people being examined

- Development of hypertension

These associations have logically led many to conceive of treating the problem with stress management methods instead of with medication. Relaxation techniques, occasionally including biofeedback, have been the principles methods used. A review of twenty-five controlled trials (including more than 1,400 patients total, but most trials were small in number) showed significant benefit in twelve of the twenty-five studies, but not in the others.[23] The benefits, however, tended to be lost over time, and were better at three months after the intervention than at one year. This emphasizes the fact that experiential stress reduction techniques need to be continued over the long term. This is not a "quick fix."

One might wonder if adding substantially more than just relaxation or refresher sessions periodically would improve the results. However, a meta-analysis that also included some cognitive (thinking-change) methods also showed no benefit.[24]

Overall, state-of-the-art stress management methods alone cannot be fully endorsed for treatment of high blood pressure. At the same time, the reason for treating hypertension is the prevention of heart attacks, strokes, and kidney failure. So if cardiac outcomes are considered, rather than simply blood pressure reduction per se, adding hostility reduction and improved social connectedness to the relaxation methods that have been shown to prevent the heart attacks may be wise in people at high risk for hypertension anyway. So, once again, the mixed results may depend on the details of the intervention goals and methods. It may be difficult to interpret analyses that lump many different types of interventions together as "stress management."

## Noncardiac Chest Pain

People who have chest pain but who have normal coronary arteries (as shown on arteriograms) are well-known to have high rates of associated depression, anxiety disorders, and stress[25] (as much as seven to nine times the normal incidence of depression and panic disorder.) Spasm of the esophagus, coronary arteries, and/or chest wall muscles may be involved in creating the pain, but usually it is best managed when seen as a complex interaction between mind and body. More than half of new patients referred to cardiac clinics for chest pain fall in this group, and often they are simply reassured and discharged. Follow-up studies show that most continue to have the pain, have considerable anxiety about the pain, continue to use medical resources to reevaluate it, and usually limit their activities because of it.[26]

   In a controlled study of thirty-one patients with resistant atypical chest pain, clinical psychologists at Oxford used a program (averaging seven sessions) that sensitively explained how "real" chest pain can be caused by stress factors. They then used progressive muscle relaxation, breathing

**Table 23.2**  Secondary Coronary Prevention: Studies of Behavioral Medicine Interventions

|  | N | Years of Follow-Up | % Risk Reduction Nonfatal MIs | Cardiac Death |
|---|---|---|---|---|
| Friedman (1986–1987) | 862 | 4.5 | −46 | −28 |
| Frasure-Smith (1985) | 453 | 1.0 |  | −50 |
| Frasure-Smith (1989) | 355 | 7.0 | −33 | −15 |
| Ibrahim (1974) | 105 | 1.5 |  | −3 |
| Rahe (1979) | 44 | 3.5 | −100 | −100 |
| Patel (1985) | 169 | 4.0 | −54 | −100 |
| Fielding (1979) | 45 | 1.0 | −100 |  |
| Horlick (1984) | 116 | 0.5 |  | +60 |
| Stern (1983) | 64 | 1.0 | +149 |  |
| **Weighted risk reduction** |  |  | **−39%** | **−33%** |

control, distraction, thought checking, and skills for responding differently to triggering cues. The results were striking: Significant reductions were achieved not only for chest pain (one-third became pain-free) but also for other physical symptoms—dizziness, breathlessness, nausea, and palpitations. Psychological benefits included reductions in diagnosable depression, anxiety, and functional limitations. The improvements continued to be fully maintained four to six months later.

The treatment program was effective for patients both with and without diagnosable anxiety disorders. Pain medication use was eliminated by all but one patient. Cost savings were not calculated, but with these degrees of improvements in patients traditionally high in medical resource utilization, the savings were probably substantial. Whether the savings would exceed the cost of the intervention, as it usually does in such studies, is not known here, but the patient morbidity savings are considerable.

## Arthritis

Kate Lorig at Stanford University studied arthritis patients who were taught self-management skills at very low cost by a trained layperson who also had arthritis.[27] Four hundred patients with both osteoarthritis and rheumatoid arthritis participated in the controlled study, holding six two-hour sessions to learn how to have more self-efficacy—that is, how to increase their sense of control and capability despite the arthritis. The results:

- Self-efficacy was improved.
- Pain was reduced by 20 percent.
- Inflammation was reduced, and there were fewer swollen joints (actual decrease in disease activity).
- Medical office visits were reduced by 43 percent.
- Costs were reduced an average of $648 for each rheumatoid arthritis patient and $189 for each osteoarthritis patient over a period of four years.

How could even the inflammation and disease activity be reduced by a "mental" intervention? Remember the discussions in Chapters 1 and 2 about how the nervous system impacts the pain and immune systems. Improved "control" in the nervous system is reflected in improved control immunologically as well.

## Chronic Obstructive Pulmonary Disease

People who have asthma, chronic bronchitis, emphysema, and other problems in breathing are frequently anxious—and understandably so. But their anxiety usually compounds the airway spasm, making symptoms worse. In one study, only 39 percent of medical outpatients complaining of shortness of breath were able to get relief with medications.[28] And medications that relax the airway can be dangerous in the face of serious lung disease.

It would seem that learning mentally to relax—particularly to relax the airways (which it now appears possible to learn)—could potentially provide great relief, and perhaps improved breathing. Despite active breathing-education programs nationally, well-controlled treatment studies in this area have been few, and usually involve small numbers of patients.

One very economical approach used four weekly sessions of learning progressive muscle relaxation from a recorded audiotape (measuring the relaxation effectiveness by Bensen's criteria),[29] then practicing at home daily with the tape. Compared to controls who just sat quietly for twenty minutes, this simple intervention achieved significant reductions in anxiety and in the subjective feeling of shortness of breath, and a mildly improved peak expiratory flow rate—a measure of ease of airflow (6 percent, compared to worsening 7 percent in the controls).[30] There was no long-term follow-up, but the taped intervention could presumably be continued at home indefinitely. Asthmatics would likely have better improvements in measurable airway flow from relaxation than those with emphysema.[31]

Other similar behavioral interventions in children showed reduction in medication and lost school days. For asthmatics however, the stress issues vary greatly, and the mental interventions may need to be individually tailored. Interventions that work well for one individual may not be so effective for another.

## Menopausal Symptoms

The discomforts of going through menopause can be pervasive—and while not always dangerous (unless depression sets in), they can be very uncomfortable and disruptive. Taking estrogen replacement therapy is often helpful, but what about women who can't use these medications, or prefer not to do so?

One study described a program of simple relaxation methods using deep, quieting breathing and mindfulness training over eight one-hour training sessions. Symptoms significantly relieved included:[32]

- Hot flashes
- Night sweats
- Disturbed sleep
- Distressed emotions

This simple approach illustrates an interesting characteristic about behavioral medicine approaches that are different (and perhaps easier for physicians to understand) from many other psychological therapies. They involve specific techniques that can, if desired, be directed at changing unwanted symptoms (such as insomnia), unwanted observable behaviors (such as anger outbursts or lighting a cigarette when stressed), or even physiological reactions (such as hot flashes) in much the way a medication might be used. Results are often observable and measurable. In these regards, behavioral medicine is much closer to traditional biophysical medical approaches than are most other psychological interventions.

These techniques also, however, can often create a relaxed, disengaged state where the patient is able to see more clearly the real solution to his or her underlying distresses and "reprogram" habitual responses to be those most desired (such as might also be obtained in other forms of psychotherapy).

## Chronic Insomnia

One-third of the population has sleep problems. In addition to a significant increase in accidents and loss of social and performance function, sleep deprivation can produce some significant health problems. Longevity is reduced, pain worsens, and depression or anxiety exacerbates. (People with chronic insomnia have forty times the normal risk for developing depression, together with an increased family history of depression, suggesting a common neurochemical link between the two.)[33] As with depression, immune function and autonomic nervous system regulation are decreased when a person is deprived of sleep. These effects of sleep loss were detailed in Chapter 7.

If insomnia is not caused by treatable depression, anxiety, or medical disorders, treatment with medication alone has in the past been somewhat suboptimal because of a tendency to lose effectiveness after a month or so. Older sleeping pills can also adversely affect the parts of sleep that are most restorative for the body, often leaving some fatigue the next day. However, most persistent sleeplessness has a strong conditioned component to it; that is, the brain learns that what happens on going to bed is that one struggles to try to sleep, often frustrated and anxious about the next day's consequences. Trying to do anything is arousing. After that has been practiced a while, then just approaching the bed elicits that aroused response, resulting in a self-fulfilling prophecy.

A number of behavioral treatment approaches have been developed to specifically address the particular components of sleep that are disturbed. These were detailed in Chapter 7. For example, progressive relaxation before bedtime improves deep sleep, while stimulus control (some countermeasures for the mentioned conditioned part) can be more useful for initially getting to sleep. Medication used over the short term (particularly those that don't interfere with deep or dreaming sleep) can be helpful to recondition the expectation of what happens when one climbs into bed. The health improvement can be substantial.

A meta-analysis of twenty-one studies compared the effects of cognitive-behavioral treatment (CBT) to medication for insomnia. Both were equally effective in the short term.[34] A recent trial in young to middle-aged people compared CBT for insomnia to medication over eight weeks. The CBT was superior to medication and nearly as good as combining both.[35] In general, however, over a longer period, combining behavioral techniques with at least short-term medication works better than either alone.[36] Treating these sleep problems *early* is much more helpful in preventing the associated medical problems than is treating sleep difficulty later on.

## Irritable Bowel Syndrome and Related Disorders

As discussed earlier, IBS is the most common problem seen in the gastroenterologist's office. It is diagnosed when a person has abdominal pain and dysregulated bowel movements unrelated to damaged bowel tissue. In the medical setting, it is highly related to stress, depression, and anxiety. Usual methods of treatment involving antispasmodic medications and fiber are often unsatisfactory. Studies of the effects of stress reduction and behavioral methods on the physical symptoms are quite interesting.

A combination of relaxation techniques and mindfulness meditation exercises taught during four to six sessions produced a good response in two-thirds of the participants—considerably better than with antispasmodic medication.[37] Results were maintained one year later.

Another study using eight sessions of progressive muscle relaxation plus thermal biofeedback and cognitive coping training produced 73 percent improvement in IBS symptoms.[38] The response was not as good if anxiety was chronic and severe.

Hypnosis has also been effective for IBS, even one year later.[39]

Two studies have shown that psychotherapy—particularly that focusing on interpersonal and forgiveness issues—has also been effective.[40] Eight sessions of such psychotherapy produced good results, particularly for pain and diarrhea, in patients resistant to medical treatment. The benefits were maintained one year later.

IBS is a "hyperalgesic" or "hypersensitivity" disorder, that is, it has a neurochemical abnormality that causes excessive responsiveness to a bowel stimulus. Similar overresponsiveness to a stimulus is seen in two very common problems: nonulcer dyspepsia (stomach sensitivity) and fibromyalgia (muscle hypersensitivity). While these are not psychiatric problems per se, stress can clearly make them worse, and stress reduction approaches are highly beneficial. At least six studies have shown significant improvement in fibromyalgia using behavioral medicine (cognitive-behavioral) methods.

## Cancer

In considering the use of psychobehavioral interventions for medical diseases, few areas have been met with as much emotion and controversy as that of applications for cancer patients. While few would argue with the need for psychological support for most people with a diagnosis of cancer, claims that psychological treatment might improve a patient's medical prognosis have been met with skepticism.

David Spiegel at Stanford University was such a skeptic, but he believed that a group program to create an opportunity for personal expression, comfort, loving support, and finding meaning in and healing of one's life would be of value to women with metastatic breast cancer regardless of the effects on the disease itself. He set out in a well-designed and controlled study to determine the outcome effects of such a humanistic program. He was surprised. The women receiving the support lived almost twice as long as those without the program.[41] Part of the reason why such improved outcome could happen in the "healing" and psychologically supported group might be explained by improved immunity.

Better immune responses were seen during a similar intervention involving malignant melanoma patients: After only six weeks in the behavioral program, patients showed increases in lymphocytes and natural killer-cell activity that help suppress cancer activity.[42] The intervention—which included stress management, relaxation techniques, enhancement of problem-solving skills, and psychological support—resulted in significantly lower levels of distress and greater use of positive coping skills in the treated group members (compared to the controls). These benefits were even more pronounced six months later.

In addition to physical effects, psychological treatments for cancer patients can provide tremendous overall well-being even while they are going through the significant stress of such a disease. A review of twenty-two studies on the effects of such psychological and behavioral treatment programs for those with cancer showed that the programs resulted in less distress, better sense of control, less pain and anxiety, and less nausea.[43]

# Cost and Medical Care Utilization Issues

## Surgical Patients

Having surgery can be a frightening prospect. Much research interest has developed around how best to deal with that, and what happens to surgical outcomes when you do. A meta-analysis of psycho-educational interventions for surgery patients combined the findings of 191 controlled studies designed to create a positive expectation.[44] The average training required thirty minutes, and most training was provided by a registered nurse using audiovisual aids.

Eighty percent of the studies showed significant benefit for the following:

- Faster recovery
- Reduced length of hospital stay (an average of 1.5 days shorter)
- Fewer surgical or medical complications
- Improved breathing
- Less pain and reduced need for pain and sedative medications
- Less psychological distress

An earlier thirteen-study review of even modest psychosocial interventions for surgery and coronary care patients showed similar results, including a two-day reduction in hospital time. Of note, however, is the fact that the move to outpatient, same-day surgery has limited the logistics of providing these kinds of mental preparations.

Other studies of semihypnotic suggestion during anesthetic induction, when the unconscious mind is more receptive, have shown similar beneficial results (suggesting, for example, that pain would be minimal, that bowel function would return fairly quickly, and that healing would proceed well).[45] Some of the studies appear to confirm that such suggestion can be subconsciously incorporated even during deep anesthesia, leading to a conditioned automatic response following surgery. (Inadvertent negative remarks made in passing while the person is anesthetized may also be internalized.)

Even the aesthetics of the setting (such as color, light, and nature scenes) after surgery can play an important role in outcome and recovery rates. One study compared surgery patients who recovered in a room with a nature view to those in a room viewing a brick wall.[46] The average patient with a nature view required less pain medication, had less postoperative distress, and left the hospital one day earlier than those with the brick wall. Sounds strange, perhaps, but try staring at a dull wall for a while, and then compare the feelings of savoring a look at trees and meadows. Perhaps the "healing" influence is not so strange after all.

## Labor and Delivery

Like surgery, childbirth can be bewildering and frightening. In Latin American countries, this anxiety is sometimes dealt with quite well with the help of a *doula*—a gentle woman experienced in childbirth who is essentially a hand-holder, who informs the mother-to-be about what to expect, and who provides caring reassurance. When Latin American physicians and patients

**Table 23.3**    Doula Support Compared with Usual Care (Control)
in First-Time Mothers

| Outcome Reduced | Control | Supported | Percent Reduction |
|---|---|---|---|
| Caesarean section rates | 18% | 8% | Reduced 56% |
| Duration of labor | 9.4 hours | 7.4 hours | Reduced 25% |
| Epidural anesthesia | 55% | 8% | Reduced 85% |
| Oxytocin to increase labor | 44% | 17% | Reduced 61% |
| Forceps delivery | 26% | 8% | Reduced 70% |
| Baby hospitalized more than forty-eight hours | 24% | 10% | Reduced 58% |

Note: The group simply observed by a person in the room had about half the improvement.

anecdotally observed that mothers with a doula seemed to have better birth outcomes, a group in Texas decided to run a controlled study.[47] They randomly assigned 600 first-time mothers in labor to one of three groups: one with a doula, one with an uninvolved observer in the room, and one with usual care (a nurse who periodically came in to check monitoring and respond to questions). The cost of having a doula in the room was less than $200. See the results, shown in Table 23.3, above.

Dr. David Sobel, an internist who analyzes such outcome studies for the Kaiser-Permanente health plans in California, has observed that if we had a perfectly safe pill or device that could result in those kinds of reductions in obstetrical complications, every delivering woman would likely be on it. With the cost of the doula less than $200, large overall savings were also projected from reductions in operating room and hospital time, medications, and nursing staff time.

## Hip Fracture in the Elderly

Hip fracture can have surprisingly devastating effects on an elderly person's life, and the costs of surgical repair are substantial. James J. Strain and his colleagues wondered what effect psychological consultation might have not only on disability, but also on treatment outcomes and costs. They studied 452 patients admitted for surgical repair of fractured hips at two different hospitals in New York and Chicago.[48] They screened patients for their psychological needs, and then, if clearly indicated, referred them for psychological care. Sixty percent had a significant psychological diagnosis, and psychological consultations increased from 5 percent before the screening to 70 percent after screening, suggesting that psychological need may be significantly overlooked in the usual care. Medical costs were affected by the psychological referral in the following ways:

- Hospital stays were reduced by 1.7 to 2.2 days per patient.

- Overall costs were cut by $270,000 (the interventions cost $40,000).

- There was little difference in hip healing characteristics or location of placement after discharge.

These results confirm the findings of Levitan and Kornfield: They found that general orthopedic patients who had psychiatric care reduced their hospital length of stay by 29 percent, saving five times the cost of the psychological interventions.[49]

## Overall Medical Cost Reduction

As noted in some of the examples above, in addition to the quality of life (and often medical) benefits afforded by adding behavioral and psychologic interventions to the usual medical care, the costs of those interventions are usually low compared to the often substantial savings in medical costs and use of resources. A number of other examples might be cited. For example, a Harvard study of 109 chronic pain patients, often a costly and frustrating group, found that adding behavioral medicine approaches reduced clinic visits by 36 percent and produced savings of $35,000 over two years, including the cost of the intervention.[50]

Emily Mumford and her colleagues provided a much more global summary of the cost issues in two large-scale analyses. The first was a meta-analysis of fifty-eight controlled studies of medical and surgical patients comparing results when mental issues were addressed compared to when they were not. The studies were similar to some of those cited above, and included some well-controlled, unpublished doctoral dissertations to eliminate any bias toward positive results that might occur by including only published reports. Those results were then compared to the insurance files of 32,450 federal employees' families, looking to see if there were any differences in the changes in medical costs of those who received outpatient (but not inpatient) mental health services compared to those who did not.[51]

Once again, the savings were quite remarkable. The major savings came with reduced hospitalization. The meta-analysis revealed that attention to mental health gave a 73.4 percent reduction in inpatient costs and a 22.6 percent reduction in outpatient costs—impressive particularly when noting that only one of the fifty-eight studies was an exception to that pattern. They noted that despite a higher need for psychological support in the elderly, they were not psychologically treated as often as younger people.

The four-year insurance data for federal employees calculated the change in medical utilization before mental health treatment to those costs afterward, and compared the same trends in patients who did not receive mental interventions.[52] Before mental treatment, those later needing it had medical costs substantially (50 percent) higher than those not needing mental treatment, a finding consistent with what you might suspect from the evidence in this book. The costs after mental health treatment fell substantially below the inflation rate for those years, while costs for those not treated rose well above the inflation rate. After four years, the costs for the two groups nearly equalized—that is, the higher utilizers treated for their mental health were no longer higher utilizers. Again, the major savings came with less hospitalization, implying less severe medical illness after mental treatment. Older people showed greater savings after mental health treatment than younger people. The medical savings roughly equaled the cost of twenty mental health visits,[53] though seldom are that many visits used.

In the group behavioral medicine programs, the costs are usually considerably lower than with individual therapy, and provide more interactive time and feeling of group support. And sometimes, for the person stressed out without severe psychological issues, the experiential nature of these group approaches can change behavioral responses even more quickly.

Another entire area with great potential for expanded treatment possibilities (but somewhat beyond the scope of this book) is that of use of the antidepressant medications in stress-related medical illnesses that do not meet the full criteria for depression. Much of the physiological dysregulation we have explored in this book is mediated by changes in the mesolimbic brain neurochemistry that also underlies depression and anxiety disorders. For example, pain systems share striking neurochemical similarities with mood and stress systems.[54] We might use the analogy of a computer. The behavioral and psychotherapy approaches we have been considering here are much like reprogramming the software of a computer to elicit a new response. However, if the hardware of the computer is not working well, the software changes don't work well either, or may not even be possible to create. Antidepressants are not just symptom-relieving pills that cover up the learned responses. They work by correcting the underlying brain dysfunction, which then allows for much more effective "software reprogramming" to get the results for which a person hopes—or even just to allow for the possibility of the relaxed state that allows for the discovery of needed healing. Once the brain has done well for a period of time (often with temporary medication), nonpharmacological approaches work to keep it that way much better than they do to try to get that well-functioning state in the first place. When nonpharmacological treatment approaches are not enough, medical improvement of these overlapping neurochemical abnormalities can often be highly useful. Some illustrations are captured by the many studies shown in Table 23.4, where "antidepressant" medications are found highly effective in many medical problems, even when depression is not present. For example, one study found an 80 percent reduction in noncardiac chest pain treated with an antidepressant, even though no one in the study had depression or anxiety disorders.[55] Some of these medications, which often also work well for some kinds of pain, are called antidepressants because that was the disorder for which they were first studied. But the fact that not only the mind but also the body respond once again illustrates the tight interaction between the two.

Curiously, when treatment is discussed, even among many interested in mind and body integration, there still tends to be the old divisions between the "mind people" and the "body people." Rather than being forced to choose either the "mind" approaches (such as psychotherapy or behavioral therapy) or the body chemistry (medication) approach, it is likely that well-timed integration of both will provide the best solutions. This has been proven, for example, with both depression (with its physical problems) and sleep disturbances.

The bottom line suggested by most of the studies is that some of our best possibilities for reducing health care costs, while substantially improving quality, may lie in conscious and organized attention to the mental aspects of medical illness.[56]

## Filling the Hole in the Health Care Delivery System?

Earlier in this chapter, we noted the large numbers of general medical patients (over half) that have documented stress-related medical problems, and the small percentage of those in which the mental component is being actually diagnosed and treated. Large numbers of patients with some of the most common problems of pain, fatigue, gastrointestinal disorders, and strange neurological symptoms fall into this category. This leaves a big hole in the health care delivery system: About 40 percent of primary care patients have stress-related medical illness that is not receiving help from mental health professionals, and most of the physicians they are seeing are not being trained in behavioral interventions. A lot of people are not feeling well and are uncertain how to get help.

One solution may lie in providing low-cost group behavioral medicine and psycho-educational intervention programs—a solution that is patient-friendly, generally well received, and usually even enjoyable. Perhaps more practical in day-to-day clinical life (but with more cost), these methods can also be learned individually. And perhaps the treatment approaches that integrate mind and body will be even more effective—especially in the long run—than some of the traditional ways we have approached these perplexing problems.

**Table 23.4**    The Use of Antidepressant Medications for Medical Disorders Other than Pure Depression

**Of Demonstrated Benefit:**

1. Chronic pain disorders[57]
   a. Myofascial pain disorder and fibromyalgia[58]
   b. Migraine and tension headaches[59]
   c. Some types of arthritis[60]
   d. Trigeminal neuralgia
   e. Diabetic neuropathy[61]
   f. Herpes zoster neuralgia[62]
   g. Idiopathic pelvic pain[63]
   h. Temporomandibular joint syndrome[64]
   i. Chronic facial pain[65]
   j. Back pain[66]
   k. Fibromyalgia[67]
   l. Noncardiac chest pain[68]
2. Other psychiatric disorders[69]
   a. Panic disorder[70]
   b. Eating disorders: anorexia nervosa and bulimia[71]
   c. Obsessive compulsive disorder[72]
   d. Addiction and alcoholism control[73]
   e. Pseudodementia of the elderly[74]
   f. Appetite and weight loss in the elderly[75]
   g. Hypochondriasis[76]
   h. Posttraumatic stress disorder[77]
   i. Attention deficit disorder[78]
   j. Personality disorders[79]
3. Dementia[80]
4. Chronic fatigue syndrome[81]
5. Premenstrual syndrome[82]
6. Irritable bowel syndrome[83]
7. Sleep disorders (including sleep apnea)[84]
8. Urinary incontinence[85]
9. Peptic ulcer[86]
10. Recurrent hives, dermatitis, eczema, and pruritus[87]
11. Preventing heart attacks[88]
12. Preventing strokes[89]
13. Functional bowel disorders[90]

**Table 23.4**   *(continued)*

**Of Probable Benefit:**

1.  Medical illnesses to which stress contributes substantially[91]
    a.  Some asthma patients
    b.  Multiple allergies[92]
2.  Other endorphin deficiency states
3.  Somatization disorder (particularly in the aged)[93]
4.  HIV dementia[94]

## ENDNOTES

1.  J. D. Stoeckle, I. K. Zola, and G. Davidson, "The Quantity and Significance of Psychological Distress in Medical Outpatients," *Journal of Chronic Disease* (1964): 959–70; R. A. Crum, L. Cooper-Patrick, and D. E. Ford, "Depressive Symptoms Among General Medical Patients: Prevalence and One-Year Outcome," *Psychosomatic Medicine* 56 (1994): 109–17; and H. C. Schulberg and B. J. Burns, "Mental Disorders in Primary Care: Epidemiologic, Diagnostic and Treatment Research Directions," *Gen Hosp Psychiatry* 10 (1985): 79–87.
2.  N. A. Cummings and G. R. VandenBos, "The Twenty Years Kaiser-Permanente Experience with Psychotherapy and Medical Utilization: Implications for National Health Policy and National Health Insurance," *Health Policy Quarterly* 1 (1981): 159–75.
3.  S. Kroenke K, et al., *American Journal of Medicine,* 1989; (86) 266–68.
4.  K. Kroenke and R. K. Price, "Symptoms in the Community: Prevalence, Classification and Psychiatric Comorbidity," *Arch Int Med* 153 (1993): 2474–80.
5.  D. W. Bates, et al., "Prevalence of Fatigue and Chronic Fatigue Syndrome in a Primary Care Practice," *Arch Int Med* 153 (1993): 2759–65.
6.  M. Sullican, M. R. Clark, W. J. Katar, et al., "Psychiatric and Otologic Diagnosis in Patients Complaining of Dizziness," *Archives of Internal Medicine* 153 (1993): 1479–84.
7.  Terr, *Arch Int Med* 146 (1986): 145–49.
8.  J. B. Imboden, *Arch Int Med* 108 (1961): 393ff.
9.  R. B. Lydiard, M. D. Fossey, W. Marsh, and J. C. Ballenger, "Prevalence of Psychiatric Disorders in Patients with Irritable Bowel Syndrome," *Psychosomatics* 34 (1993): 229–34.
10.  J. Bancroft, D. Rennie, and P. Warner, "Vulnerability to Perimenstrual Mood Change: The Relevance of a Past History of Depressive Disorder," *Psychosomatic Medicine* 56 (1994): 225–31.
11.  N. L. Smith, "Physical Symptoms Highly Predictive of Depression and Anxiety Disorders," Paper presented at the American Psychosomatic Society Annual Meeting, 1996.
12.  W. Katan, M. Von Korff, E. Lin, et al., "Distresses High Utillizers of Medical Care," *General Hospital Psychiatry* 12 (1990): 355–62.
13.  R. B. Lydiard, et al., "Prevalance of Psychiatric Disorder in Patients with Irritable Bowel Syndrome," *Psychosomatics* 34 (1993): 229–34.
14.  N. M. K. Bacon, S. F. Bacon, J. H. Atkinson, et al., "Somatization Symptoms in Chronic Low Back Pain Patients," *Psychosomatic Medicine* 56 (1994): 118–27.

15. P. Freeling, B. M. Rao, E. S. Paykel, L. I. Sireling, and R. H. Burton, "Unrecognised Depression in General Practice," *Brit. Med J* 290 (1985): 1880–83; and S. M. Anderson and B. H. Harthorn, "The Recognition, Diagnosis and Treatment of Mental Disorders by Primary Care Physicians," *Med Care* 27 (1989): 869–86.

16. C. J. C. Hellman, M. Budd, J. Borysenko, D. C. McClelland, and H. Benson, "A Study of the Effectiveness of Two Group Behavioral Medicine Interventions for Patients with Psychosomatic Complaints," *Behavioral Med* 16 (1990): 165–73.

17. U. L. Gonik, et al., "Cost Effectiveness of Behavioral Medicine Procedures in the Treatment of Stress Related Disorders," *Journal of Clinical Biofeedback* 4 (1981):16–24.

18. A. H. Glassman, "Sadhart Trial: Sertraline Treatment of Depression After Myocardial Infarction," *Journal of the American Medical Association* 289 (2002): 701–9.

19. S. M. Czajkowski, *Journal of the American Medical Association* 289 (2003): 3106–16.

20. J. A. Blumenthal et al., *Archives of Internal Medicine* 157 (1997): 2213–23.

21. Richmond A. Castillo, *Stroke* 31 (2000): 568–73.

22. N. Farsure-Smith, et al., *Psychosomatic Medicine* 47 (1985): 431–45; and 51 (1989): 485–513.

23. D. W. Johnson, "The Behavioral Control of High Blood Pressure," *Current Psychological Research Review* 6 (1987): 99–114.

24. D. M. Eisenberg, T. L. Delbanco, C. S. Berkeley, et al., "Cognitive Behavioral Techniques for Hypertension: Are They Effective?" *Annals of Internal Medicine* 118 (1993): 964–72.

25. L. J. Lantinga, R. P. Sprafkin, J. H. McCroskery, et al., "One Year Psychosocial Follow-up of Patients with Chest Pain and Angiographically Normal Coronary Arteries," *American Journal of Cardiology* 62 (1988): 209–13.

26. R. A. Mayou, "Invited Review: Atypical Chest Pain," *Journal of Psychosomatic Research* 33 (1989): 393–406; and R. C. Pasrenak, G. E. Thibault, et al., "Chest Pain with Angiographically Insignificant Coronary Arterial Obstruction," *American Journal of Medicine* 68 (1980): 813–17.

27. K. Lorig, et al., "Outcomes of Self-Help Education for Patients with Arthritis," *Arthritis and Rheumatism* 28 (1985): 680–85.

28. K. Kroenke, M. E. Arrington, and A. D. Manglesdorf, "The Prevalence of Symptoms in Medical Outpatients and the Adequacy of Treatment," *Archives of Internal Medicine* 150 (1990): 1685–89.

29. Relaxation is measured by skin temperature, heart rate, and breathing rate. H. Bensen, J. F. Beary, and M. P. Carol, "The Relaxation Response," *Psychiatry* 37 (1974): 37–45.

30. A. G. Gift, T. Moore, and K. Soeken, "Relaxation to Reduce Dyspnea and Anxiety in COPD Patients," *Nursing Research* 41 (1992): 242–46.

31. P. D. Freedberg, L. A. Hoffman, W. C. Light, and M. K. Kreps, "Effect of Progressive Muscle Relaxation on the Objective Symptoms and Subjective Responses Associates with Asthma," *Heart and Lung* 16 (1987): 24–30.

32. R. R. Freedman, *Am J Obstet Gynecol* 167 (1992): 436–39.

33. D. E. Ford and D. B. Kamerow, *Journal of the American Medical Association* 263 (1989): 1479–84.

34. M. L. Perlis, M. T. Smith, D. D. Cacialli, et al., "On the Comparability of Pharmacotherapy and Behavior Therapy for Chronic Insomnia," *Journal of Psychosomatic Research* 54 (2003): 51–59.

35. G. D. Jacobs, E. F. Pace-Schott, R. Stickgold, and M. W. Oho, "Cognitive Behavior Therapy and Pharmacotherapy for Insomnia," *Archives of Internal Medicine* (2004):1.

36. C. Morin, *Sleep Research* 22 (1993): abstract 21.
37. G. Shaw, *Digestion* 50:36–42.
38. E. B. Blanchard, *Behavioral Research Therapy* 24 (1985): 215–16.
39. P. J. Whorwell, *Lancet* 2 (1984): 1232–34.
40. E. Guthrie, *Gastroenterology* 100 (1991): 450–57; and J. Svedlund, *Lancet* 2 (1983): 589–91.
41. D. Spiegel, H. C. Kraemer, J. R. Bloom, and E. Gottheil, "Effect of Psychosocial Treatment on Survival of Patients with Metastatic Breast Cancer," *Lancet* 2 (October 14, 1989): 888–91.
42. I. F. Fawzy, "A Structured Psychiatric Intervention for Cancer Patients: Changes over Time with Methods of Coping and Affective Disturbance and in Immunological Parameters," *General Hospital Psychiatry* 13 (1991): 361–62.
43. R. W. Trijsburg, F. C. E. van Knippenberg, and S. E. Rijpma, "Effects of Psychological Treatment on Cancer Patients: A Critical Review," *Psychosomatic Medicine* 54 (1992): 489–517.
44. E. C. Devine, "Effects of Psychoeducational Care for Adult Surgical Patients: A Meta-Analysis of 191 Studies," *Patient Education and Counseling* 19 (1992): 129–42.
45. R. P. Blankfield, "Suggestion, Relaxation and Hypnosis as Adjuncts in the Care of Surgery Patients: A Review of the Literature," *American Journal of Hypnosis* 33 (1991): 172–86.
46. R. Ulrich, "View Through a Window May Influence Recovery from Surgery," *Science* 224 (1984): 420–21.
47. J. Kennel et al., "Continuous Emotional Support During Labor in a U.S. Hospital: A Randomized Controlled Trial," *Journal of the American Medical Association* 265 (1991): 2197–201.
48. James J. Strain, J. S. Lyons, et al., "Cost Offset from a Psychiatric Consultation Liason Intervention with Elderly Hip Fracture Patients," *American Journal of Psychiatry* 148 (1991): 1044–49.
49. S. J. Levitan and D. S. Kornfield, "Clinical and Cost Benefits from Liason Psychiatry," *American Journal of Psychiatry* 138 (1981): 790–93.
50. M. Caudill, R. Schnable, P. Zuttermeister, H. Benson, and R. Friedman, "Decreased Clinic Use by Chronic Pain Patients: Response to a Behavioral Medicine Intervention," *Clinical Journal of Pain* 7 (1991): 305–10.
51. E. Mumford, H. J. Schlesinger, G. V. Glass, C. Patrick, and T. Cuerdon, "A New Look at Evidence About Reduced Cost of Medical Utilization Following Mental Health Treatment," *American Journal of Psychiatry* 141 (1984): 1145–58.
52. E. Mumford, H. J. Schlesinger, and G. V. Glass, *American Journal of Public Health* 72 (1982): 141–49.
53. H. J. Schlesinger et al., "Mental Health Treatment and Medical Care Utilization in a Fee-for-Service System: Outpatient Mental Health Treatment Following the Onset of a Chronic Disease," *American Journal of Public Health* 73 (1983): 422–29.
54. P. L. Delgado, "Common Pathways of Depression and Pain," *J Clin Psychiatry* 65, suppl 12: 16–19; M. Briley, "Clinical Experience with Dual Action Antidepressants in Different Chronic Pain Syndromes," *Hum Psychopharmacol.* 19 suppl 1 (October 2004): S21–5; and S. K. Brannan, C. H. Mallinckrodt, E. B. Brown, M. M. Wohlreich, J. G. Watkin, and A. F. Schatzberg, "Duloxetine 60 mg Once-Daily in the Treatment of Painful Physical Symptoms in Patients with Major Depressive Disorder," *J Psychiatr Res.* 39 no. 1 (Jan–Feb 2005): 43–53.
55. I. Varia, "Sertraline Treatment of Noncardiac Chest Pain," *Am Heart Jl* 140 (2000): 367–72.

56. We are indebted to David S. Sobel, M.D., MPH, editor of *Mental Medicine Update* (special report, 1993), for bringing several of these studies to our attention.

57. Briley, "Clinical Experience"; I. G. Egbunike, and B. J. Chaffee, "Antidepressants in the Management of Chronic Pain Syndromes," *Pharmacotherapy* 10, no. 4 (1990): 262–70; K. R. Krishman and R. D. France, "Antidepressants in Chronic Pain Syndromes," *Am F Physician* 39, no. 4 (1989 Apr): 233–37; M. Valdes et al., "Psychogenic Pain and Depressive Disorders: An Empirical Study," *J Affective Disorders* 16, no. 1(1989): 21–25; R. D. France, "The Future for Antidepressants: Treatment of Pain," *Psychopathology* 20, suppl. 1 (1987): 99–113; and Z. Herman, "Enkephalins and the Action of Psychotropic Drugs," *Pol J Pharmacol Pharm* 39, no. 5 (1987): 633–39.

58. D. H. Finestone and S. K. Ober, "Fluoxetine and Fibromyalgia," *JAMA* 264, no. 22 (1990): 2869–70; and D. L. Goldenberg (Tufts University School of Medicine, Boston), "Diagnostic and Therapeutic Challenges of Fibromyalgia," *Hosp. Pract.* 24, no. 9A (1989): 39–52.

59. A. Bonazzi, "Fluoxetine vs. Amitriptyline in the Prophylaxis of Tension Type Headache," *Cephalagia* 11 suppl. 11 (1991): 341–42; S. Diamond and F. G. Freitag, "The Use of Fluoxetine in the Treatment of Headache," *Clin J of Pain* 5 no. 2 (1989): 200–1; H. G. Markley et al., "Fluoxetine in Prophylaxis of Headache: Clinical Experience," *Cephalgia* 11, suppl. 11 (1991): 164–65; G. Sandrini et al., "Antalgic and Antidepressant Activities of Fluoxetine in Daily Chronic Headache," *Cephalgia* 11 suppl. 11, (1991): 280–81; and P. J. Orsulak and D. Waller, "Antidepressant Drugs: Additional Clinical Uses," *J. Fam Pract* 28, no. 2 (February 1989): 209–16.

60. M. Gringas, *Jl Int Med Res* 4, suppl. 2: 41; M. Scott, *Practioner* 202:802; Krishman and France, "Antidepressants," 233–37; and France, "The Future for Antidepressants," 99–113.

61. M. B. Max, R. Kishore-Kumar, et al., "Efficacy of Desipramine in Painful Diabetic Neuropathy: A Placebo-Controlled Trial," *Pain* 45, no. 1 (April 1991):69, discussion 1–3; K. A. Theesen and W. R. Marsh, "Relief of Diabetic Neuropathy with Fluoxetine," *DICP* 23 nos. 7–8 (July–August 1989): 572–74; Krishman and France, "Antidepressants," 233–37; and France, "The Future for Antidepressants," 99–113.

62. F. A. Bucci, Jr. and R. A. Schwartz, "Neurologic Complications at Herpes Zoster," *Am Fam Physician* 37, no. 3 (March 1988): 185–92; and C. E. Argoff, N. Katz, and M. Backonja, "Treatment of Postherpetic Neuralgia: A Review of Therapeutic Options," *J Pain Symptom Manage.* 28, no. 4 (October 2004): 396–411.

63. M. B. Hahn et al., "Idiopathic Pelvic Pain," *Postgrad. Med.* 85, no. 4 (March 1989): 263–66, 268, 270.

64. M. Harris, "Medical Versus Surgical Treatment of Temperomandibular Joint Pain and Dysfunction," *Br J Oral Maxillofae. Surg.* 25, no. 2 (April 1987): 113–20.

65. Krishman and France, "Antidepressants," 233–37.

66. France, "The Future for Antidepressants," 99–113.

67. L. M. Arnold, Y. Lu, L. J. Crofford, M. Wohlreich, M. J. Detke, S. Iyengar, and D. J. Goldstein, "A Double-Blind, Multicenter Trial Comparing Duloxetine with Placebo in the Treatment of Fibromyalgia Patients with or without Major Depressive Disorder," *Arthritis Rheum.* 50, no. 9 (September 2004): 2974–84; and O. Vitton, M. Gendreau, J. Gendreau, J. Kranzler, and S. G. Rao, "A Double-Blind Placebo-Controlled Trial of Milnacipran in the Treatment of Fibromyalgia," *Hum Psychopharmacol.* 19, suppl 1 (October 2004): S27–35.

68. W. M. Wong and R. Fass, "Noncardiac Chest Pain," *Curr Treat Options Castroen-terol.* 7, no. 4 (August 2004): 273–78; and I. Varia, "Sertraline Treatment of Noncardiac Chest Pain," *Am Heart Jl* 140 (2000): 367–72.

69. R. J. Baldasserini, "Current Status of Antidepressants: Clinical Pharmacology," *J Clin Psychiatry* 50, no. 4 (April 1989): 117–26.

70. J. M. Gorman, M. R. Liebowitz, A. J. Fyer, et al., "An Open Trial of Fluoxe-tine in the Treatment of Panic Attacks," *J Clin Psychopharmacol* 7, no. 5 (1987): 329–32; K. Brady, M. Zarzar, and R. B. Lydiard, "Fluoxetine in Panic Disorder Patients with Imipramine-Associated Weight Gain," *J Clin Psychopharmacol* 9, no. 1 (1989): 66–67; F. R. Schneier, M. R. Liebowitz, S. O. Davies, et al., "Flu-oxetine in Panic Disorder," *J Clin Psychopharmacol* 10 no. 2 (1990): 119–121; P. J. Orsulak and D. Waller, "Antidepressant Drugs" 209–16; and L. Solyom, C. Solyom, and B. Ledwidge, "Fluoxetine in Panic Disorder," *Can J Psychiatry* 36, no. 5 (June 1991): 378–80.

71. H. G. Pope, Jr., et al., "Bulimia Treated with Imipramine," *Am J Psychiatry* 140 (1983): 554–58; R. G. Granet, "Fluoxetine Treatment of Obsessive Compul-sive Disorder," *J. Clin. Psychiatry* 50, no. 11 (1989): 436; H. E. Gwirtsman, B. H. Guze, J. Yager, and B. Gainsley, "Fluoxetine Treatment of Anorexia Ner-vosa: An Open Clinical Trial," *J. Clin. Psychiatry* 51, no. 9 (1990): 378–82; D. B. Herzog, A. W. Brotman, and I. S. Bradburn, "Treating Eating Disorders with Antidepressants," *Aust. Paediatr. J.* 24, no. 3 (1988): 169–70; S. H. Kennedy and D. S. Goldbloom, "Current Perspectives on Drug Therapies for Anorexia Nervosa and Bulimia Nervosa," *Drugs* 41, no. 3 (1991): 367–77; M. R. Trim-ble, "Worldwide Use of Clomipramine," *J. Clin. Psychiatry* 51 suppl. 8 (1990): 51–54; P. L. Hughs et al., Treating Bulimia with Desipramine," *Arch Gen Psy-chiatry* 43 (1986): 182–86, C. P. L. Freeman and M. Hampson, "Fluoxetine as a Treatment for Bulimia Nervosa," *Int J Obes* 11, suppl 3 (1987): 171–77; M. Fava, D. B. Herzog, P. Hamburg, et al., "Long-Term Use of Fluoxetine in Bulimia Nervosa: A Retrospective Study," *Ann Clin Psychiatry* 2, no. 1 (1990): 53–56; and Solyom et al., "The Fluoxetine Treatment," 421–25.

72. Orsulak and Waller, "Antidepressant Drugs,"209–16.

73. C. A. Naranjo, K. E. Kadlec, P. Sanhueza, D. Woodley-Remus, and E. M. Sell-ers, (Clinical Pharmacology Program, Addiction Research Foundation Clinical Institute, 33 Tusse St, Toronto, Ont. M5S 2S1 Canada), "Fluoxetine Differen-tially Alters Alcohol Intake and Other Consummatory Behaviors in Problem Drinkers," *Clin. Pharmacol. Ther.* 47, no. 4 (1990): 490–98; D. A. Gorelick, "Serotonin Uptake Blockers and the Treatment of Alcoholism," *Recent Dev Alcohol* 7 (1989): 267–81; and J. Rosecan: *World Congress of Psychiatry,* 1983.

74. J. T. Moore, "The New Antidepressants," in R. Ham, ed., *Geriatric Medicine Annual 1986,* 3–23.

75. J. Talley, "Geriatric Depression: Avoiding the Pitfalls of Primary Care," *Geria-trics* 42, no. 4 (1987): 53–60, 65–66.

76. D. V. Sheehan, J. Ballenger, and G. Jacobsen, "Treatment of Endogenous Anxi-ety with Phobic, Hysterical and Hypochondriacal Symptoms," *Arch Gen Psychia-try* 37 (1980): 51–59; and N. Fernando, "Monosymptomatic Hypochondriasis Treated with a Tricyclic Antidepressant," *Br J Psychiatry* 152 (June 1988): 851–52.

77. C. J. McDougle, S. M. Southwick, D. S. Charney, and R. L. St. James, "An Open Trial of Fluoxetine in the Treatment of Posttraumatic Stress Disorder," *Journal of Clinical Psychopharmacology* 11, no. 5 (1991): 325–27; and J. David-son, S. Roth, and E. Newman, "Fluoxetine in Post-Traumatic Stress Disorder," *Journal of Traumatic Stress* 4, no. 3 (1991): 419–23.

78. Orsulak and Waller, "Antidepressant Drugs," 209–16.
79. M. J. Norden, "Fluoxetine in Borderline Personality Disorder," *Progress in Neuro-Psychopharmacology & Biological Psychiatry*, 13, no. 6 (1989): 885–93; and J. R. Cornelius, P. H. Soloff, J. M. Prel, and R. F. Ulrich, "A Preliminary Trial of Fluoxetine in Refractory Borderline Patients," *J. Clin. Psychopharmacol.* 11, no. 2 (1991): 116–20.
80. W. M. McDonald et al. "Pharmacological Management of the Symptoms Dementia," *Am Fam Phys* 42, no. 1 (1990 Jul): 123–32.
81. M. Sharpe (Department of Psychiatry, Oxford University, Oxford United Kingdom), "Psychiatric Management of Post Viral Fatigue Syndrome," *Br. Med. Bull.* (United Kingdom) 47, no. 4 (1991): 989–1005; D. A. Matthews, P. Manu, and T. J. Lane (Division of General Medicine, University of Connecticut Health Center, Farmington, CT 06030 USA), "Evaluation and Management of Patients with Chronic Fatigue," *Am. J. Med. Sci.* (USA) 302, no. 5 (1991): 269–77; P. J. Goodnick, "Bupropion in Chronic Fatigue Syndrome," *Am J Psychiatry* 147, no. 8 (1990 Aug): 1091.
82. R. Rickles, E. W. Freeman, S. Sondheimer, et al., "Fluoxetine in the Treatment of Premenstrual Syndrome," *Curr Ther Res* 48, no. 1 (1990): 161–66; and A. B. Stone, T. B. Pearlstein, and W. A. Brown, "Fluoxetine in the Treatment of Late Luteal Phase Dysphoric Disorder," *J Clin Psychiatry* 52, no. 7 (1991): 290–93.
83. D. S. Greenbaum, J. E. Mayle, et al., "Effects of Desipramine on Irritable Bowel Syndrome Compared with Atropine and Placebo," *Dig Dis Sci* 32, no. 3 (March 1987): 257–66; J. I. Hudson and H. G. Pope Jr., "Affective Spectrum Disorder: Does Antidepressant Response Identify a Family of Disorders with a Common Pathophysiology?" *Am J Psychiatry* 148, no. 2 (February 1991): 280; also 148, no. 4 (April 1991): 548–49.
84. J. C. Ware and J. T. Pittard, "Increased Deep Sleep after Trazodone Use: A Double Blind, Placebo Controlled Study in Healthy Young Adults," *J Clin Psychiatry* 51, suppl. (1990 Sep): 18–22; R. L. Manfrede and A. Kales, "Clinical Neuropharmacology of Sleep Disorders," *Semin Neurol* 7, no. 3 (1987): 286–95.
85. Orsulak and Waller, "Antidepressant Drugs," 209–16.
86. Orsulak and Waller, "Antidepressant Drugs," 209–216; and D. S. Singh, S. Sunder, and K. K. Tripathi, "Tricyclic Antidepressant Therapy in Duodenal Ulcer," *J Indian Med Assoc* 85, no. 9 (September 1987): 265–67.
87. M. A. Gupta, A. K. Gupta, and C. N. Ellis, "Antidepressant Drugs in Dermatology: An Update," *Arch Dermatol* 133, no. 5 (May 1987): 647–52; and B. A. Harris, E. F. Sherertz, and F. P. Flowers, "Improvement in Neurotic Excoriations with Oral Doxepin Therapy," *Int J Dermatol* 26, no. 8 (October 1987): 541–43.
88. Glassman, "Sadhart Trial"; and Czajkowski, *JAMA.*
89. A. Rasmussen, M. Lunde, D. L. Poulsen, K. Sorensen, S. Qvitzau, and P. Bech, "A Double-Blind, Placebo-Controlled Study of Sertraline in the Prevention of Depression in Stroke Patients," *Psychosomatics* 44, no. 3 (May–June 2003): 216–21; and K. R. Krishnan, "Depression as a Contributing Factor in Cerebrovascular Disease," *Am Heart J.* 140, 4 suppl. (October 2000): 70–6.
90. Antidepressants in the Treatment of Irritable Bowel Syndrome and Visceral Pain Syndromes. *Curr Opin Investig Drugs.* 5, no. 7 (July 2004): 736–42.
91. Hudson and Pope, "Affective Spectrum Disorder," 548–49.
92. J. S. Seggev and R. C. Eckert, "Psychopathology Masquerading as Food Allergy," *J Fam Pract* 26, no. 2 (February 1988): 161–64.

93. R. G. Ruegg, S. Zisook, and N. R. Swerdlow, "Depression in the Aged: An Overview," *Psychiatry Clin No Am* 11, no. 1 (March 1988): 83–99; and R. H. Gerner, "Geriatric Depression and Treatment with Trazodone," *Psychopathology* 20, suppl. 1 (1987): 82–91.
94. J. K. Levy and F. Fernandez, "Neuoropsychiatric Care for Critically Ill AIDS Patients," *J Crit Illness* 4, no. 3 (1989): 33–42.

# CHAPTER 24

# Methods of Intervention and the Principles of Stress Resilience

*He who cannot change the very fabric of his thought will never be able to change reality.*

—Anwar Sadat

## Learning Objectives

- Explain the principles of stress resilience.
- Describe the central core of what mental, physical, and even spiritual well-being are about.
- Examine a synthesis of the research and thought described in previous chapters.

Life is stress . . . in fact, it's one stressor after another. Finding life meaningful involves finding the stress meaningful. Having fun with life requires having some "fun" with the challenge of solving problems—or at least seeing the personal opportunity that comes along with them. That holds true even for depression; noting that all episodes of depression are not bad, Scott Peck speaks of the "healthiness of depression."[1]

Much of the effect of stress depends on how you respond to it. One response is, "I want to get back to where I was before." Quite another is a response of humility: "I need to change. I think I'm wiser now."

Times of great stress or crisis provide a catalyst for change—and, at times, quantum leaps in growth. We joke about smaller trials being for our growth, but the fact is that problems do indeed provide the opportunity to become wiser. For millennia the Chinese have recognized that fact in their language: The pictogram character for crisis combines those for danger and opportunity.

Three simple factors define whether stress is productive or destructive:

- The way you see and regard stress—is it an opportunity or an intolerable burden?

- Whether you can see both the pros and the cons—and whether you can create solutions (simply stated, whether you have a healthy brain).

- Whether you have mental or behavioral tools and principles that enable you to deal well with the stress.

The first of these factors—the way you choose to regard the stressful situation—is the basis of cognitive therapy. It may be the most rapidly effective of the traditional psychotherapy approaches we have. This factor is heavily influenced by one's propensity to see the world in positive (optimistic) terms or in pessimistic ways.

The second—a healthy brain—requires normally functioning tissues and neurochemistry. Reversible neurochemical abnormalities, such as depression and anxiety disorders, are actually more common barriers than is organic brain tissue disease. Both the pleasure and pain centers in the midbrain need to be adequately functioning if you're to deal well with stress; for that reason, medication may have a role, at least temporarily. Nutrition, exercise, and sleep are also highly important here.

The third requirement—the tools and principles—form the central focus of this final chapter. With this perspective, we'll describe some tools for transforming thought, behavior, and physiology into a condition congruent with the principles of total health.

## Lessons from Cancer Studies

As mentioned in the previous chapter, few areas of behavioral medicine have been as emotionally charged and controversial as the treatment of cancer patients. In *The Type C Connection: The Mind-Body Links to Cancer and Your Health*, Lydia Temoshok and Henry Dreher perhaps best summarize the studies in this field. An enormous paradigm shift is required to see behavioral and mental interventions as a form of "adjuvant" cancer therapy that improves prognosis (*adjuvant* refers to a substance that enhances the action of another substance in the body); such new concepts are bound to be met with resistance. Less controversial is the attempt to use behavioral interventions as "supportive measures" to help a person emotionally deal optimally with the immense stress of confronting cancer and all its specters.

As discussed, the following associations exist between mental factors and cancer risk, morbidity, and mortality:

**Good Prognosis**

- Feeling a sense of personal control
- Hope of survival
- Trust in one's ability to deal with crisis

- Determination to live, sense of purpose
- Connectedness
- Good coping ability
- Ability to express distressed feelings

**Worse Prognosis**

- Helplessness/hopelessness
- Lack of assertiveness
- Lack of meaning in life; apathy
- Unsatisfactory personal relationships
- Ineffective at solving problems
- Clinical depression or anxiety
- Stoicism; inability to discuss problems

Temoshok and Dreher concluded that the most important of the mental risk factors listed above—and the pathological core of their risky "Type C behavior"—were the suppression of anger and other negative feelings in an attempt to be "nice." This suppression involves passively giving up important parts of your own values so you'll be acceptable to others—a violation of integrity. Such a behavior pattern may be more associated with the progression and mortality of some existing cancers than it is with getting cancer in the first place. It should also be noted that certain mental factors have been associated with certain kinds of cancers, such as melanoma, lymphoma, or breast cancer—and it's not certain whether they apply to cancer in general. In general, cancers affected more by hormones and immunity (such as genital and breast cancers, lymphomas, and skin cancers) seem to be impacted more by the central nervous system issues that modulate those hormones and immunity.

Even with these caveats in mind, would clinical programs that help cancer patients develop "better-prognosis" mental states also improve outcomes—at least in those cancer types we know to be associated with such psychological factors? We believe that the immune factors of protective cancer surveillance (such as natural killer-cell activity) may be involved because those immune responses are influenced beneficially by some of the same mental factors that benefit cancer patients (see Chapter 1).

Dr. Sandra Levy at the Pittsburgh Cancer Institute has shown that prognosis in breast cancer can be improved with an optimistic rather than a pessimistic expectational style; she extended that knowledge to a therapeutic program designed to boost optimism in colon cancer patients. It worked—and it helps confirm hope as one of the principles we are looking for.

This same principle was confirmed by Greer's fifteen-year follow-up on British breast cancer patients. Those with a sense of hope and personal control had four times the survival rate of those who felt hopeless and helpless (80 percent versus 20 percent).[2] Derogatis similarly documented what physicians have sensed for hundreds of years: that an increased will to live, and having a purpose for that living, increased breast cancer survival.[3]

You must, however, tread lightly when creating hope therapeutically. Why? Although large numbers with positive expectation may survive longer, a particular individual with a great deal of hope may die early. To have a sense of control, you need to accept responsibility—but it can be devastating to imply that a person is to blame for either developing cancer or failing to survive longer. What are we "responsible" for? The answer is simple: We're not so much responsible for the cancer as for how we choose to respond to the cancer. David Spiegel's support intervention that doubled life expectancy in breast cancer patients (see Chapter 23) was based not so much on expectations, but rather on providing a sense of personal control in dealing with caregivers, a sense of meaning and purpose, a sense of connectedness to others struggling with the same crisis, the ability to deal wisely with the stress, and an opportunity to express and explore distressed feelings. (It also involved a longer period of time—a full year—than the usual psychobehavioral group intervention.)

Caroline Bedell Thomas's landmark study of physicians over a period of twenty-five years confirmed the importance of close, meaningful relationships as a protection from cancer. She found a four times greater incidence of cancer in those who lacked that connectedness.[4] She also found optimistic expectations to be important to overall health.

The same lessons about healing and protective principles we learned from cancer apply as well to other diseases.

# Four Core Principles Underlying Stress Resilience and Well-Being

If we pull together the healing principles outlined in the previous chapters, we might construct the following "stress-resilient" qualities around which behavioral interventions might best be directed:

1. **A sense of empowerment and personal control** (Chapters 2 and 19)
   - Control over one's responses, not necessarily over the environment
   - The ability to live by one's deepest values (integrity)
   - Feeling heard and valued

2. **A sense of connectedness and acceptance** (Chapter 4 and Part III)
   - To one's deepest self
   - To other people
   - To the earth and the cosmos
   - To all regarded as good, and to the sources of one's spiritual strength

3. **A sense of meaning and purpose** (Chapters 14 and 15)
   - Giving of self for a purpose of value; a caring sense of mission
   - Finding meaning and wisdom in here-and-now difficulties
   - Enjoying the process of growth
   - Having a vision of one's potential

4. **Hope** (Chapters 14, 16, 17, and 18)
   - Positive, optimistic expectation
   - The ability to envision what one wants before it happens

This group of core principles arises not only from the multitude of medical and health studies reviewed in this book, but also from careful studies of highly healthy and effective people. The key characteristics of such people include:

- The seventeen common characteristics of Maslow's self-actualizers (see Appendix A)[5]
- The three components of Kobasa's and Maddi's "stress-hardy" people (see Chapter 8)
- The seven habits of Covey's highly effective people (see Appendix B)[6]
- The characteristics of Garfield's peak performers
- The characteristics of Friedman's "cardio-protected" Type B's (see Appendix C)
- Seligman's optimistic expectational style (see Chapters 17 and 18)

If you synthesize the underlying "ways of being in the world" by which these people function, you find that the four core principles listed above tie all of them together. And the studies discussed throughout this book show that they underlie optimal physical health as well.

Also common to all these groups of healthy people are the values that led them to the above ends. When people in a relaxed, introspective state in a clinical setting are asked to reflect on who they really are—on the values they most deeply cherish—a small set of what seems to be nearly universal core values keeps appearing. Interestingly, they're the same core values by which well-functioning, healthy people actually operate—the core values that motivate them to do what they do.

What are those deeper, more universal values?

- **Caring love:** the kind that lifts and empowers both that which is loved and they who love

- **Responsible free will:** feeling in charge of one's own experience and responses to what happens in life

- **Integrity:** being the way we want to be; acting out of our clearly defined core values and wisdom

- **Growth:** enjoying a challenge, the love of continually getting wiser and more capable

Nearly all of what we've discovered about well-functioning people are variants of these four core values, and these "universal" values are obviously closely linked with the four core principles above that have been proven to bring better health. Interestingly, even the most "healthy" companies (those whose success lasts longest) tend to operate through these same principles.[7] These principles seem to be basic qualities of well-being; there is a remarkable universality about them, and they seem to be the deeper longings of most people who find them absent.

Professionals who do the hands-on work with patients struggling over mind-body issues often comment that stress finally resolves when "the spiritual issues resolve." They sense, in other words, that spiritual well-being underlies much of both mental and physical well-being (see Chapter 14). The World Health Organization defines health as "a state of complete well-being in all the aspects of one's life: physical, mental, social, and spiritual—not just the absence of disease."

What is meant by "spiritual well-being"? The answers are varied, and the condition is difficult to measure in a study. We can measure with considerable precision optimal physical health and function. We can even measure with fair accuracy what mental well-being is. But, even though spiritual well-being escapes the precise measurement of these others, practitioners claim that it may be possible to demonstrate the essence of spiritual well-being. How? In essence, the four core principles listed above make up overall wellness. They are also the ends toward which many spiritual traditions are working: empowerment, deep integrity, connectedness, a sense of purpose and meaning, and hope. It is no coincidence that these principles are also what many in the world are hungering for.

It's important to note that the "spirituality" that undermines these principles is likely to be a misconception. For example, being angrily judgmental of "imperfect" people doesn't empower; it puts down. It doesn't foster connectedness; instead, it causes alienation. It doesn't promote hope, instead, it promotes discouragement. With this in mind, are such misguided attempts to be spiritual more likely to advance physical health or to cause physical illness?

How, then, do these stress-resilient principles work? Table 24.1 gives a handful of examples.

A person may also need treatment of the neurochemical abnormalities that cause much of the depression and anxiety—even, at times, in the absence of significant situational stress. It can be almost impossible to make the kind of mental change required with these four principles if the mental instrument needed to do it isn't working properly. When that's the case, medication—even on a temporary basis—can be of immense benefit. Medication is usually required for major clinical depression or anxiety accompanied by symptoms of mesolimbic brain dysfunction (see Chapters 5, 6, and 23).

## A Sense of Empowerment and Personal Control

Creating a personal sense of control in the face of stress is no trivial matter. But it appears to lie at the heart of stress resilience, because the bottom line about feeling distressed is that the stressful situation feels beyond control. In fact, all four core principles of stress resilience contribute to a natural sense of control. And all of them create the mental structure that fosters a sense of personal control—of how to be in the world. Some further observations about a sense of personal control will help demonstrate why some of the behavioral treatment approaches work.

**Table 24.1**   Stress-Resilient Principles

| Major Issues Causing Distress | Core Values and Principles That Can Resolve the Distress |
| --- | --- |
| Issues of personal worth: low self-esteem, aloneness, uncertain identity, perfectionism | Integrity to unconditional love, acceptance, connectedness, a sense of purpose, and continued growth |
| Blaming—feeling "forced" | Responsible free will, bringing a sense of control |
| Demanding that things be different than they are | Acceptance of self and others; understanding cause and effect, and working with it (wisdom) |
| Threat, worry, and negative expectation | Hope, caring love, and positive expectation |

## Stressed Animals and Control

A mental state of being "out of control" is accompanied by physiology that's "out of control"—a dysregulation of autonomic, hormonal, and immunological balance that protects from disease. An example comes from the work of Martin Seligman and his colleagues.

In Seligman's studies, animals were placed in a classical stress setup: They were confined in a box, and an electrode was attached to their tails that delivered intermittent shocks. Each shock was preceded by a warning bell. Each animal was assigned to one of three groups:

1. The first group was given a wheel that, when turned, aborted the shock, as the animals quickly learned. The bell rang, the animals spun the wheel, and no shock occurred. They were captains of their destiny. They were in control, despite the stressor.

2. The second group had no wheel. They were truly victims, cowering at the bell that signalled the imminent misery.

3. The third group acted as controls; they were not given shocks.

The animals were then injected with cancer cells to see which were most likely to develop cancer and which were best able to immunologically reject the cancer and stay healthy. Those in the group who had control over the stress were able to reject sarcoma cells 63 percent of the time compared with only 28 percent of the victims. Interestingly, the group who had control over stress did even better than the group that had no stress at all: Only 60 percent of the unstressed animals rejected the cancer cells. When researchers measured the immune responses in the different groups, those with control over stress had the best immune response; the victims had the worst.

The same pattern holds up across many types of studies dealing with stress: It's not the stressor that matters as much as the ability to control the response to stress. Those who are stressed but who have a sense of control, in fact, are often even more healthy than those who are not stressed at all. Out of control, stress becomes distress; under control, it becomes eustress. And, as noted in Chapter 2, the neurochemical and physiological responses differ between the two.

It should be noted that a fascinating paradox exists about how to achieve a sense of control. The more you attempt to control the external situation (such as what others do), the more out of control things feel—because, simply, the external world can seldom be reliably controlled. On the other hand, the more you let go—the less you try to control the external world and the more you respond with wisdom and maturity—the greater the sense of personal control. When you accept that things exist as they are for a reason (whether good or bad), you can respond with creative, persuasive wisdom to draw others in a different direction.

## Brain Neurochemistry and the Sense of Control

Finding a sense of control also seems to improve the neurochemical abnormalities associated with extreme stress, depression, and anxiety. UCLA's Michael McGuire studied how gaining and losing social control affect serotonin levels.[8] (Serotonin is a key player not only in depression and anxiety, but also in keeping physical and emotional responses "in balance" and in control.) McGuire studied the different serotonin levels in dominant versus submissive males in three groups: vervet monkeys, fraternity men, and football players.

The results were fascinating. Serotonin levels were twice as high in the alpha male, the dominant ("in control") monkeys, as in the submissives. Then researchers "dethroned" the dominant monkey by placing him behind a one-way mirror where he could watch the submissive males eating his special food, getting their needs met, and cozying up to his harem of females, but none of the others could see or hear him. He ranted and raved, as he always did to maintain power, but—unheard and unseen—to no avail. As he began to give up, feeling helpless and hopeless, his serotonin levels dropped. Some dropped to the level of the formerly submissive males; some dropped even lower. Interestingly, as the previously submissive monkeys started to gain some control, their serotonin levels rose to those of the previously dominant male. Similar patterns were found among the fraternity men and the football players.

In the second part of the study, McGuire used drugs to change the serotonin levels, then watched the resulting behaviors. When drugs were given to raise serotonin levels in passive males, they acted dominant. When drugs were given to inhibit serotonin in dominant males, they acted subordinate—and were anxious over tests they had previously done with confidence. Another fascinating observation was that researchers could predict which monkey would soon dominate by watching which monkey the females were cozying up to—regardless of which monkey was winning all the battles. The brain serotonin levels in the male being sought by the females increased, and within two weeks, he dominated.

Social dominance also affects the immunity of animals. In response to stress, dominant animals show a more optimal antibody response; that of submissive animals is decreased.[9] Dominance increases not only brain serotonin levels, but also natural painkillers (opioids), such as endorphins. These opioids, in turn, affect immunity; animals with high endorphin levels have increased resistance to cancer. On the other hand, higher cortisol levels—seen with chronic submission and "helplessness"—are correlated with decreased immune competence. It all plays into why people who feel depressed or helpless have more difficulty clearing infections and a worse prognosis for certain treated cancers (see Chapters 1 and 6).

Boston University researcher David McClelland showed that when frustrated, students with a need to exercise power over others had significantly increased blood epinephrine levels and decreased salivary IgA antibody levels. The effect? More upper respiratory infections when under academic stress.[10] Students under the same stress but not under the same need for control didn't have the same rate of infections or the same drop in antibodies. Interestingly, the brain tends to elicit behavior to help get the chemicals it needs.

McClelland's study illustrates another paradox about a sense of control: Those people lower in brain serotonin function are often driven to seek control—maybe in an attempt to get levels back up. That is, a strong need for control can be a symptom of deficient brain serotonin. Examples are seen in people with compulsive behaviors, perfectionism, or hostility toward competitors. Seeking power and control is often a symptom of the underlying insecurity that accompanies diminished serotonin function (as may also be seen in some Type A behavior).

So, if you find yourself with an excessive need to control, consider doing other things to increase serotonin function: get good sleep, meditate mindfully, and eat high-tryptophan foods. And best of all, recognize the paradox of control: Let go of trying to control the external world; take back your power to be the way you want to be, regardless of external forces. Refuse to blame others for making you feel or behave in ways you don't want to. Then a personal kind of control begins to settle in, and serotonin function naturally improves.

## Cognitive Structuring and Therapy

Many intervention approaches are built around giving a greater sense of integrity and personal control. One of the most rapidly effective forms of psychotherapy for converting distressed responses into those more healthy is cognitive (thinking) therapy. Cognitive restructuring underlies both cognitive therapy and some of its spinoffs (such as rational behavioral therapy or rational emotive therapy).[11] These therapies are based on the realization that stressful situations do not really cause our feelings and physiological responses nearly as much as does the way we choose to think about those situations.

The sequence creating feelings and behavior is this:

1. The perceived situation
2. Our thinking about the situation
3. Our responses:
   - Feelings
   - Physical responses
   - Behavior

The situation leads to the way we choose to think about the situation—how we regard the situation and its meaning for us. The way we think about the situation leads to our response: feelings, physiological responses, and behavioral responses. Each time this process occurs for a specific situation, it becomes more automatic.

Note that feelings and behavioral responses are not caused directly by the situation at all, but rather by the way we choose or learn to think about the situation. The situation is only the event around which the thinking forms. It is the thinking, rather than the event, that creates the reality for that person. That's why one person feels "blown away" by the same situation that another person sees as a creative challenge. When you blame the situation for your feelings and behaviors, you become a victim—you give up your sense of control. On the other hand, if you recognize that most situations aren't as distressing as the way you've chosen to think about them, you open up many possibilities for regarding the situation in more mature and wise ways. If the response is destructive and distressful, almost invariably a more rational way of thinking can be found that fits much better with one's deeper values and wisdom. This new thinking will create a more productive response, will result in less distress, and will bring back a sense of control.

The following is an example. If a father felt upset and angry when his teenaged daughter rebelled with provocative remarks, instead of trying to control her, he could regain personal control by refusing to blame the teen's behavior (the situation) for "making" him feel bad or for "causing" him to react in certain destructive ways toward his daughter. By realizing that he himself created the thinking about his daughter that in turn caused the disturbing reaction, he can—in a more reflective, disengaged moment—create new ways of thinking and dealing with a struggling teenager. This could include ways to lift and encourage his daughter—the way he actually wants to be as her dad—instead of putting her down. Then he could mentally practice his new skills repetitively, helping his new reaction become more automatic. Instead of being extremely distressful and alienating, his new reaction could be creatively empowering—and even bonding.

At first, the way you think about a situation may seem like the only way to regard it. At that point, it's easy to be misled about what the most rational thoughts are. But there's a key guideline as to whether thinking is maturely rational: Look at the feelings and behavior it engenders. *If the feelings or behavior are destructive, then the thinking that caused it has two characteristics:*

- It is in some way irrational (that is, it's not totally reliable—if you examine it closely, you'll find you don't totally believe it).

- It in some way violates your deepest values.

By destructive feelings and behavior, we mean that which makes you miserable, hurts relationships or other people, or keeps you from doing or becoming what you more deeply want.

Let's look again at the example of the father who was struggling with his teenaged daughter. What's so irrational about getting angry over his daughter's rude remarks? It's irrational to think that the father *has* to be angry and upset. Instead, the father may try to understand his daughter's struggle with identity and independence—which is what is really causing her behavior—and may respond with gentle wisdom that encourages his daughter instead of trying to put her down. In the long run, that kind of reaction is probably more in harmony with his deepest values, anyway: He wants to lift and encourage his daughter rather than make her feel diminished. There's an important caveat here, too: The father isn't suppressing his anger. Instead, when he thinks about his daughter differently, his anger simply dissipates. His new feelings toward her may even be compassionate for her struggle to find independence.

Remember: If feelings are destructive, there is always a wiser, more rational way of thinking that is more in harmony with your deeper values—and that will result in a very different response to the same situation. The first step to gaining control of your responses is giving up blame—fully realizing that you create your own thinking and responses. Accepting that responsible free will is the first step to control.

Typical ways of thinking about distressful situations have to do with:

- The shoulds (How does the situation fit with what "should" be true?)

- Issues of worth (What does this situation mean about my worth and value?)

- Threat (Am I likely to lose something of value because of this situation?)

- Force (Am I feeling forced to do something I don't want to do?)[12]

Then what is the most effective way of dealing with a distressful situation? First, reexamine your way of thinking. Second, discover a more rational way of regarding the situation (something more in line with your deeper values and wisdom). And, finally, use visualization or some other technique to help your new way of thinking and responding become automatic. The result? A sense of personal control—in harmony with your values. And your new response will become as automatic as the way you tie your shoes: You've done it so many times that you do it without any conscious thought.

Notice also how this process begins to create hope: an expectation that you can deal well with both this situation and others like it.

## Basic Elements of Behavior Change

To change distressed behaviors, whether emotional or physiological:

1. Clarify the present state.
2. Clearly determine in explicit, specific terms what you wholly desire your behavioral outcome to be.
3. Experientially practice your new behavioral response (for example, by relaxing and visualizing it).

Research has shown that it's very difficult to mentally "reprogram" yourself if you're aroused—which is likely if you're also distressed. The key is to become deeply relaxed and receptive through "meditative methods"—behaviors that help you relax, become calm, disengage from destructive thinking, and create and practice new mental models. This usually involves becoming centered in the present moment (which is the only moment in which you can feel a personal sense of control).

There are some meditative methods that elicit the relaxation response, that help you become calm and mentally disengage from old ways of thinking. Other meditative methods help you change to a new, better behavior. You'll need to use both.

## Methods of Eliciting the Relaxation Response

### Meditative Breathing

Using your breath can be a very effective method for calming the mind. This is a body-to-mind technique, because the mind automatically associates certain patterns of breathing with either anxiety or calm. For example, if you right now breathe in very, very deeply and hold it, then breathe shallowly high in the lungs, with nearly a full breath still held in, you are likely to start feeling anxious. That's because this kind of breathing is anxious breathing. Check it out next time you are very stressed: Notice how you are breathing; it's likely to be shallow and high in the chest.

Now, shift gears and breathe slowly in such a way that a hand on your abdomen rises and falls, as though you were breathing gently down into your belly (diaphragmatic breathing). You likely will find your mind calming and becoming more focused: This type is relaxed breathing.

Practice simply following your relaxed breathing for a few minutes. Sense breathing in energy and life (which, after all, is exactly what you are doing), and breathing out the unnecessary things (which is also physiologically true). Sense the metaphor in this: energy (and even insight) flowing out to your extremities and mind, and letting go of that which no longer needs to be held. Perhaps you will even find yourself being grateful for this remarkable, automatic process that has kept you alive for so long. As you focus on the bodily feelings of letting go with the breath, you will find an interesting paradox: As your body and mind calm, you become more keenly aware of what is going on. In some cultures, this simple breathing practice has been used for millennia to facilitate spiritual insight.

After getting good at this by practice, during your day when you notice anxious breathing, simply change it to relaxed breathing, and your mind and body will follow.

## Progressive Muscle Relaxation

With this method, you tense specific muscles as you inhale, become aware of the feeling of tension, then totally "let go" to relax those same muscles as you exhale, closely noticing the difference between tension and relaxation. You usually involve all the muscles in the body in a systematic way—starting with your foot and leg, for example, and then moving up the body to the buttocks, trunk, chest, shoulders, arms, hands, neck, and face. Once you know the difference between feeling tense and relaxed, you can recognize situations ("cues") that make you feel tense. You can then practice relaxing, using an "anchor"—a certain kind of breath, body position, or touch—to trigger the relaxation response. After regular practice, the anchor then becomes your cue to quickly elicit deep relaxation.

## Autogenic Training

This technique has been used for over a century, particularly among European athletes to enhance performance. It creates a trance much like self-hypnosis. You simply sense different parts of your body, such as your hands and feet, getting heavy and warm (and tell yourself so), and then the bowel getting relaxed and calm, and the heartbeat slowing and becoming more regular. When this state is reached, gentle suggestions or visualizations about optimal performance can be more fully realized.

## Mindfulness Meditation

This method involves living fully in the present moment, giving complete, caring attention to whatever you choose.[13] You focus attention on one thing at a time, allowing intruding or distracting thoughts to pass; as a result, you feel a quiet sense of control instead of a frazzled attempt to concentrate on several thoughts at once. To practice, you can devote complete concentration and attention to simple things like breathing or eating, the sensations of these, and the increased awareness that accompanies such attention. The frequent self-monitoring that helps you know what's going on from one moment to the next has been used very effectively in a number of stress reduction programs, including those at the University of Massachusetts, Harvard, and the University of Utah.

## Imagery

Imagery involves mentally going to a safe, beautiful place—then you totally experience it with all your senses: the visual beauty, the smells, the sounds, the touch, the feelings of being there. With practice, you can take a "mental trip" every day to the mountains or the seashore—and not only experience the sensations, but also experience the mental detachment, perspective, and focus that come from actually traveling to a similar place for a few days.

## "Body Work"

Techniques like yoga usually involve "relaxed stretching"—putting the body under stress while you relax your mind. Like progressive muscle relaxation, body work can act as a kind of gauge that helps you get quiet and relaxed—even while under stress or in pain. Other useful relaxing body work methods include tai chi, qi gong, and Feldenkrais.

Which of these techniques is best? It really doesn't matter so much which you use, as long as it best matches your preferred way of mental processing. Those who are auditory—liking words and dialogue—may prefer to mindfully meditate on a meaningful word or phrase, letting the sound and its meaning resonate within. A visual processor may prefer imaging a beautiful place or meditating on an image. Someone who likes physical feelings and touch may do best with breathing and muscle relaxation methods. Someone geared spiritually may enjoy a deeper experience such as transcendental meditation.

Some (particularly men) sometimes like to do the breathing and muscle relaxation first, because it feels more tangible (like a biofeedback gauge). But then, with more experience, other methods become more attractive.

# Methods of Changing Behavior

Several meditative methods help to clarify your core values and solutions and, as a result, help you change your behavior.

## Quiet Contemplation

In a peaceful, quiet environment free of distraction, you think and record about what has deepest meaning in your life. It's a key way of clarifying your values. The more sensory detail you put into your written record, the more effective it will be for change. Record what you would be seeing, feeling, hearing, and sensing when your desired outcome is in place. This will make it easier to visualize.

## Guided Imagery

There are two kinds of guided imagery[14] that help you reprogram your thoughts and change your behavior. The first, imagery to the "inner child,"[15] helps you mentally visit yourself as a child who is going through a disturbing event. You then reprogram the meaning of that event through mature eyes—you nurture and heal by giving the child new ways of dealing well with the event.

In the second kind of guided imagery, imagery to the "inner advisor,"[16] you personify your inner wisdom and values into an "inner advisor." Then, while picturing interacting, that advisor then provides you rapid access to solutions congruent with your own values.

## Visualization

Through visualization,[17] you actually practice "seeing" yourself performing or functioning the way you want to. It's a highly effective way of rapidly changing your behavior, and it hinges on four techniques:

- You need to define your desired goal or outcome in clear detail. The brain doesn't process "don'ts" very well; to be effective, you need to define the outcome only in terms of what you *do* want. Your outcome, of course, needs to be compatible with your deepest values—and all parts of you must intensely want that outcome.
- You must be totally relaxed.

- You must see and feel yourself achieving the desired result in great detail. In essence, you need to "experience" it completely—including the place, cues, who's there, your style of behavior, and your physical sensations. This goes beyond fantasizing; instead, you see yourself with enough feeling and trust that you generate the energy to actually carry out the vision. You may find it easier to first visualize this happening, like watching yourself in a movie. And then, when you are comfortable with that, shift to visualizing what's going on from within the event (seeing through your eyes, sensing the feelings of being actually in the event). This needs to be repeated at least three or four times.

- You need to practice regularly.

## Other Ways to Change Behavior

There are other keys to changing behavior—ways of achieving a personal sense of control. Although they've been discussed in greater detail earlier in this book, they deserve to be mentioned here.

### Increasing the Internal Locus of Control

Training in self-assertion helps you become aware of your own needs and values and then use the combined principles of honesty and kindness to express them. An internal locus of control engenders a proactive spirit— you refuse to choose helplessness or being hopeless as a response.

### Practicing Forgiveness

Entire treatment approaches have been built around the practice of forgiveness.[18] To some, forgiving someone who has been offensive or caused pain is like giving a gift to someone who doesn't deserve it. In reality, genuine forgiveness involves regaining personal control—refusing to blame someone else's actions for your feelings and behavior. Forgiveness involves choosing to act in ways that are wise and mature, regardless of how someone else has acted. Experiencing real forgiveness is at the heart of gaining personal control.

### Keeping a Journal

When you write about your feelings, you become aware of how you think and behave in response to stressful situations. When you capture the experience on paper, you "get a handle on it"—get some sense of how to deal with it. Keeping a journal has the added benefit of creating a sense of who you really are and the values for which you stand. Include a description of how you would have wanted to respond to a recorded situation. Also record what you hope to become.

## Building Social Support

Some key features of creating social support involve:

- Identifying a type of relationship that would be deeply satisfying for you
- Writing down the words that describe ways you would treat each other in such a great relationship
- Choosing to be that way no matter how the other is currently acting
- Practicing being that way (visualizing and in reality)
- Expecting others to respond in like manner, but not being unduly disturbed if they do not

Social support not only increases your quality of life, but also increases overall health and longevity (and reduces your risk of coronary disease).[19] For detailed information on the benefits of social support, see the chapters in Part III.

## Summarizing the Process for Rapid Change to Healthier, More Resilient Behavior

At times, we seem to have two minds. One is the mind by which we operate in the world, creating thoughts by which to function. Some of those thoughts cause us trouble. Then we also seem to have a deep, wise mind that knows the solutions and the values by which we want to live. The key in this process is how to transform the operating mind to be one with the wise mind, bringing behaviors to follow our own deep wisdom.

Using the above elements, changing old destructive habits and stress reactions might go something like this:

1. **Conscious awareness: "I can respond as I choose."**

   Half the solution is won with this realization: "I am no longer a victim."

2. **Develop and practice relaxation skills.**

   Letting go of old thoughts and getting centered.

3. **Clarify deep values and wisdom.**

   "How do I want to be?"—preferably written in great detail and in positive, not negative, terms.

4. **Visualize (experience) being the new way.**

This requires several repetitions for each situation where change is desired. The new style then becomes easier, almost like a habit.

Visualizing what to do is important, not what not to do. For example, it doesn't help to try to not be Type A hostile and cynical. Rather, defining what is wanted instead (for example, the healthy Type B described in Appendix C) can then be visualized. Behaviors are created by mental pictures. The visualizing brain cannot visualize not doing something (it needs to know what to do instead). One might, for example, explore whether some of the characteristics of Maslow's Self Actualizers in Appendix A resonate with your values as solutions, and if so, then picture yourself responding in similar ways that suit you.

## Mind-Body Treatment: Can It Change the Course of Disease?

With all of our knowledge about behavioral techniques, we come to a sobering question: If someone starts practicing the techniques described in this chapter at an early age, will it actually prevent or alter the course of disease?

The answer lies in results of pioneering studies in the field of mind-body treatment. For example, Jon Kabat-Zinn at the University of Massachusetts Medical Center Stress Reduction Clinic takes on patients with difficult medical problems that other physicians have given up on. In turn, he uses methods based on mindfulness meditation. Among more than 4,000 patients he treated over ten years, that simple technique reduced medical illness in these difficult cases by 35 percent.[20] Even diseases as specific and resistant as psoriasis have responded positively.[21] Among the elderly, other forms of meditation have had even greater health benefits.[22] Chapter 23 gives the medical outcome effects of many such interventions.

As noted in Chapter 1, distressed thinking can adversely affect the immune system—with an obvious link to disease. Behavioral interventions that have been shown to improve immune response include:

- Clinical biofeedback
- Meditation
- Autogenic training
- Progressive relaxation
- Visualization
- Hypnosis
- Behavior modification[23]

Although the results of such studies have been encouraging, they have also been somewhat inconsistent; the field of achieving stress resilience is filled with paradox. A good example is the controversial use of imagery for "healing" cancer. Many years ago, Ainsley Mears used two different types of imagery with cancer patients. The first created a state of relaxed peacefulness and acceptance; patients used the crisis to focus on their deepest values and heal their lives. The result? Cancer progression slowed; more patients actually went into remission.

For the second part of his study, Mears instructed patients to use imagery to imagine the active destruction of the cancer cells by white blood cells and macrophages. His aim was rejection of the tumor by the immune system. That didn't happen, though; for a majority of the patients, tumor recurrences began to increase. What went wrong? Maybe it was just a function of time—because the second part of the study took longer, there was time for recurrences to happen. But a greater issue involves whether creating an aroused, hostile state aimed at destroying the tumor may actually be counterproductive; instead of creating a sense of inner peace, it involves a threat to one's sense of control.

The first approach—creating a state of relaxed peacefulness—allowed patients to accept things as they are, to respond with wisdom, maturity, and love to the situation. It let patients use the crisis to get focused on healing the parts of their lives that had been neglected or had gone unresolved. That kind of approach, argue researchers, creates a greater sense of personal control even if the tumor goes uncured.

Other methods of mental control, such as biofeedback that changes body temperature, have been beneficial in the treatment of autoimmune diseases, such as rheumatoid arthritis.[24] Treatments that have included social support, guided imagery, and progressive relaxation have also helped rheumatoid arthritis patients; the psychological interventions have been more effective than social support alone.[25] In one study, 81 percent said that relaxation training was a major factor in reducing pain, reducing inflammation, and decreasing levels of serum rheumatoid factor. In another study,[26] patients were given a cognitive-behavioral treatment designed to boost self-efficacy in managing the disease; patients were taught self-relaxation, cognitive pain management, and goal setting. The more the patients enhanced self-efficacy (a measure of their sense of control), the more their pain and inflammation were reduced.

Ohio State University researcher Janice Kiecolt-Glaser has extensively studied the effects of mental distress on immune function. One such study involved forty-five nursing home residents who were taught progressive relaxation and guided imagery as a way to gain control over their world. This simple step resulted in significantly less mental distress, as well as better prognosis and greater longevity. And that's not all: Those who used progressive relaxation and guided imagery had significantly improved cellular immune response, including an increase in natural killer-cell activity.

We know that mental conditioning can affect immune response. In Chapter 1, we noted that University of Rochester researcher Robert Ader mentally conditioned a group of mice to suppress their immune response. Here's how he did it: He gave the mice a mixture of the drug Cytoxan—which suppresses the immune response—and saccharine. Later, he gave the mice saccharine but no Cytoxan. What happened? The taste of the saccharine triggered the memory of the Cytoxan, causing the immune response of the mice to be suppressed by that memory alone.

Ader then extended his experiment to a group of New Zealand mice that genetically get lupus erythematosus, an autoimmune disease in which an overactive immune system destroys the kidneys and causes death at a predictable age. The drug Cytoxan diminishes the extra immune function and, as a result, delays kidney failure and prolongs life. Ader gave the mice saccharine with the first few doses of Cytoxan; their immune suppression was linked in the brain to the saccharine taste, so giving them saccharine alone later suppressed the immune response. The result? Saccharine alone delayed kidney failure and prolonged life.

Perhaps as we learn more precisely to understand the fascinating interactions between the mind and the body and how to effectively work with them, we can embark on new and safe therapies in the future that we haven't even considered today.

## The Spiritual Connection

In Chapter 14, we described some polls of Americans in pain. They claimed that their pain was relieved as much by spiritual counseling and practices as by medical methods. How could this be? Perhaps the answer lies in what good spiritual practices bring about in an individual.

Why does spiritual counseling work so well? It is designed to:

- Give purpose and structure to life—transforming the *meaning* of life's events
- Empower people to live in accordance with that structure and to forgive (*personal control*)
- Help people identify and live by their deepest values and wisdom
- Provide support and caring (*connectedness*)
- Foster *hope*

Simply stated, spiritual guidance provides the sense of control, connectedness, meaning, and hope proven to bring about healing. These same four core principles, shown repeatedly through the studies in this book to foster good physical and mental health, thus seem to define true spiritual well-being also. When health interventions or spiritual practices are directed toward these four ends, the evidence suggests that total well-being (health) is a likely result. Markers of spiritual well-being would likely include a sense of gratitude for life, oneness, seeing beauty, and wholeness. Healing, after all, is about making separated things whole.

An interesting point is that the behavioral interventions described in this book are going in the opposite direction of the growing medical trend toward specialization. That specialization—reaching now to the molecular level—has reaped great benefits, but has also tended to separate the parts of a person and his or her care. The studies cited in this book call for a focused and concerted effort to treat the whole person and integrate each part of an individual's care. Combining both approaches will provide the most optimal outcome.

That integration requires the targeted use of not only behavioral and psychological interventions, but strong educational efforts as well—all preferably in both the medical and health prevention settings. Perhaps the most potent mind-body intervention of all is a deeply trusting and caring relationship with the medical caregiver who is sensitive to these issues and who truly understands how these interventions work.

We have seen some major medical revolutions in the past:

1. The surgical revolution (since ether anesthesia, about 1846)

2. The scientific revolution (proving results, began in earnest about 1870)

3. The chemical revolution (since penicillin, about 1936)

4. And now: the behavioral revolution (since about 1979)

This phase is seeing shifts from

- organ-based medicine toward person-based emphasis.

- technology toward humanely-based approaches.

- treatment toward prevention.

- paternalistic to cooperative care.

Revolutions do not come easily, but each of the revolutions above has been very valuable. We seem to be in a moment in time where new ways of thinking in mind-body terms are being proven to be very fruitful.

As we move into that future, we discover the truth of what mathematician Charles Muses proclaimed when he said, "The potentials of consciousness remain well nigh the last reachable domain for man not yet explored—the Undiscovered Country." We anticipate a realm in which we will, as French neurologist Frederic Tilney challenged us, "by conscious command evolve cerebral centers which will permit us to use powers that we now are not even capable of imagining."

## ENDNOTES

1. Scott Peck, *The Road Less Traveled*, 69.
2. S. Greer et al., "Psychological Response to Breast Cancer and 15-Year Outcome," *Lancet* (1990) 1: 49–50.
3. L. R. Derogatis, *Science*, 200: 1363ff.
4. C. B. Thomas et al., *Johns Hopkins Medical Journal* 151 (1982): 193ff.
5. Abraham Maslow, *Personality and Motivation*, ch. 11.
6. Stephen R. Covey, *The Seven Habits of Highly Effective People* (New York: Fireside–Simon & Schuster, 1989).
7. Thomas J. Peters and Robert H. Waterman, Jr., *In Search of Excellence: Lessons from America's Best-Run Companies* (New York: Harper & Row, 1982).
8. Michael McGuire, *The Biology of Power*.
9. Bessel A. van der Kolk, *Psychological Trauma* (Washington, D.C.: American Psychiatric Press, 1987), 47.
10. John Jemmott, 1982.
11. Some useful guides to cognitive therapy principles include Maxie C. Maultsby, *Rational Behavior Therapy* (Englewood Cliffs, N.J.: Prentice-Hall, 1984); Donald Meichenbaum, *Cognitive Behavior Modification: An Integrative Approach* (New York: Plenum Publishing, 1977); and Donald Meichenbaum, *Stress Inoculation Training: A Clinical Guidebook* (1985).
12. Maultsby, *Rational Behavior Therapy*.
13. Early books describing the clinical use of mindfulness meditation include Jon Kabat-Zinn, *Full Catastrophe Living* (New York: Delacorte Press, 1990); Joan Borysenko, *Minding the Body, Mending the Mind* (New York: Bantam Books, 1988); Herbert Benson, *The Relaxation Response* (New York: Morrow, 1975); Thich Nhat Hanh, *The Miracle of Mindfulness: A Manual of Meditation* (Boston: Beacon Press, 1976); and H. Benson and E. Stuart, *The Wellness Book* (New York: Carol Publishing Group, 1993).
14. William Fezler, *Creative Imagery: How to Visualize in All Senses* (New York: Fireside–Simon & Schuster, 1989).
15. Joan Borysenko, *Guilt Is the Teacher, Love Is the Lesson* (New York: Warner Books, 1990), chs. 3 and 4.
16. Martin L. Rossman, *Healing Yourself* (New York: Pocket Books, 1989).
17. Adelaide Bry, *Visualization: Directing the Movies of Your Mind* (New York: Harper & Row, 1978).
18. Robin Casarjian, *Forgiveness: A Bold Choice for a Peaceful Heart* (New York: Bantam Books, 1992).
19. W. Ruberman, "Psychosocial Influences on Mortality of Patients with Coronary Artery Disease," *Journal of the American Medical Association* 267 (1992): 559–60.
20. Kabat-Zinn, *Full Catastrophe Living*.
21. J. Bernhard, J. Kirsteller, and J. Kabat-Zinn, "Effectiveness of Relaxation and Visualization Techniques as an Adjunct to Phototherapy and Photochemotherapy of Psoriasis," *Journal of the American Academy of Dermatology* 19 (1988): 572–73.

22. *Journal of Personality and Social Psychology* 57: 950–64.

23. K. R. Pelletier and D. L. Herzing, *Advances* 5, no. 1 (1988): 27–56.

24. J. Achterberg, P. McGraw, and G. F. Lawis, "Rheumatoid Arthritis: A Study of Relaxation and Temperature Biofeedback as an Adjunctive Therapy," *Biofeedback and Self-Regulation* 6 (1981): 207–23; and K. A. Applebaum, E. B. Blanchard, and E. J. Hickling, "Psychological and Functional Measurement in Severe Rheumatoid Arthritis Before and After Psychological Intervention: A Controlled Evaluation [Summary]," in *Proceedings of the 17th Annual Meeting of the Biofeedback Society of America* (1986), 5–7.

25. L. A. Bradley, L. Young, K. O. Anderson, L. K. McDaniel, R. A. Turner, C. Agudelo, E. J. Pisko, E. L. Semble, and T. M. Morgan, "Effects of Psychological Therapy on Pain Behavior of Rheumatoid Arthritis Patients," *Arthritis and Rheumatism* 30 (1987): 1105–14.

26. A. O'Leary, S. Shoor, K. Lorig, and H. R. Holman, "A Cognitive-Behavioral Treatment for Rheumatoid Arthritis," *Health Psychology* 7 (1988): 527–44.

# EPILOGUE

*Everything can be taken from a man but one thing: the last of
the human freedoms—to choose one's attitude in any given set
of circumstances, to choose one's own way.*

—Viktor Frankl

Sophisticated executives who run this nation's largest cities as well as
quiet folks tucked into the rolling hills of America's heartland want
to know how to stay well and how to live longer. It's a quest that is as old as
humanity itself, and in some ways it continues to defy us as surely as it did
at the dawn of civilization. But in many other important ways we are
unraveling the mysteries and piecing together the clues that are making it
possible for us to enter the twenty-first century with the promise of better
health and a longer life.

During the last several centuries, attempts at keeping people well and
helping them live longer focused on the body—the complex bundle of cells,
the intricate network of blood vessels, the incredibly jointed framework of
bone wrapped in muscle and ligament and skin. It is there, reasoned scientists, that disease starts, and it is there that disease must be first diagnosed
and then cured. Only during the last two decades has the scientific community begun to look in earnest beyond the network of blood vessels, the clusters of lymph nodes, the peculiar and distinct characteristics of internal
organs. Only in the last handful of years has the scientific evidence come
pouring in to support what now seems so intuitive, as if we had known it all
along: that what we think and how we feel has tremendous impact on how
our physical body works. Only now, as we enter a new millennium, is the
volume of that evidence compelling enough to force even the most hard-
ened skeptics into taking a closer look.

Interest in behavioral health—in knowing how behavior and thoughts
and emotions affect our well-being—continues to capture the imagination
of the world's brightest minds. Building on the work of researchers who
were considered "on the fringe" just a few years ago, these visionary scientists are expanding the original studies, adding to the exploding volume of
information about a field of medicine that did not even exist thirty years
ago. What these scientists are investigating started as a movement back to
"holistic" health, a call to consider the whole person who presented himself
in a physician's office instead of separate, "diseased" entities waiting to be

examined. Hippocrates, the father of Western medicine, stated it eloquently when he said that the human being can only be understood as a whole. In commenting on his practice, he quipped, "I would rather know the person who has the disease than know the disease the person has." It is a view the ancients understood well: We as human beings are subject to the laws of nature, which govern the universe, and to the mental and spiritual laws that, though they are infinitely more difficult to measure, have an equally profound influence on our physical bodies.

What started as a return to this "holistic" background has come full circle to the ushering in of a scientific discipline that is at once as rooted in ancient tradition as it is balanced on the edge of a far-reaching frontier. The frenetic research that it entails—and the nation's interest in it—are hopeful signs that one day we as a people will conquer the diseases that now claim too many of us. It provides the possibility that we will finally solve the puzzle behind today's leading killers—not strictly under the scrutiny of a microscope, but also in the daily chronicles of how we live our lives. Anger and hostility may take their places next to bacteria and viruses as leading causes of disease; hope and optimism and forgiveness and prayer may line up with our most advanced antibiotics as antidotes to disease. What we are discovering is a way to live our lives so we not only avoid the danger of asbestos and tobacco smoke, but also the deadly effects of stress and cynicism and depression.

Everyone who leafs through the pages of this book will someday die. The Iowa farmer who wipes sweat from his brow with the back of his hand as he leans against his stilled combine will die. The mother in Alabama who hauls a basket of fresh laundry to the kitchen table while she keeps an anxious eye on her toddler, swinging under the magnolias, will die. The Fifth Avenue advertising executive who agonizes over a new corporate identity scattered on a pile of art boards will die. And the weathered fisherman who catches a sharp breath of salty air off the coast of Alaska as he pulls in a thrashing salmon will die.

The key is not in the dying; we are powerless against its inevitable approach. Norman Cousins tells us that "death is not the ultimate tragedy in life. The ultimate tragedy is to die without discovering the possibilities of full growth."

No matter what our chronological age, the realization of death's inevitability can bring us to the greatest appreciation for the life that still lies ahead. "Good-by world," writes Thornton Wilder. "Good-by to clocks ticking and Mama's sunflowers. And food and coffee. And new-ironed dresses and hot baths . . . and sleeping and waking up. Oh, earth, you're too wonderful for anybody to realize you."

The key is in the living, because in that we exercise tremendous power. "Life is the ultimate prize, and it takes on ultimate value when suddenly we discover how tentative and fragile it can be," Cousins warns us. We need, at this moment, to realize how wonderful it is.

We can't annihilate the world's population of disease microorganisms—but we can cut down our own chances of being felled by them. We may not see a triumphant technician hail the cure for cancer during this decade, but we can do plenty of things—today, tomorrow, and the day after that—to reduce our own chances of becoming a grim statistic.

There is no single factor in disease. If there were, cures would be simple. Instead, there are puzzles. Scientists unraveling the mysteries of the amazingly complex human immune system know that the presence of microorganisms doesn't always lead to infection. Researchers know that only some of the executives who lose their jobs during a hostile takeover will be crippled by ulcers or low back pain. And, while one child rising from the squalor of poverty and despair in a ghetto's broken home is tethered by physical and emotional illness, his brother shines with resilience.

We call that resilience *hardiness*, and it makes of us a healthier people. University of Chicago Psychologist Salvatore Maddi, who helped establish the concept of hardiness, sums it up nicely as a feeling of self-confidence:

> *The world is rather benign. You have commitment, or the knack of finding something important about whatever it is you are doing. You also have control, or the belief that you can influence what is going on around you. Further, you think your life is best led in pursuit of development. Pressures and disruptions, however painful, appear to be something you can learn from and grow from.*

"The world breaks everyone," Ernest Hemingway penned in *A Farewell to Arms*, "and, afterward, many are strong at the broken places." What determines who is strong at the broken places? Much of it may lie in the way we think and the way we behave. The power of thought—the literal power of the brain—is key to physical well-being. When those thoughts are negative, when depression and doubt and pessimism reign, "illness messages" are sent to every cell in the body. It doesn't take a Nobel scientist to figure out the result. But when those thoughts are positive, "wellness messages" emanate to the body—and literal chemical and physical changes take place that guarantee health and wellness.

The brain is the key. It houses chemical factories that can energize the immune system against bacteria, viruses, even cancer. What goes on in the brain literally determines health or illness—healing and resistance to disease.

The phenomenal power of the brain over the body is illustrated by imagery, the clarion mental visualization that enables a middle-aged secretary in the front office to mobilize her immune system against cancer. A man who visualized his white blood cells as killer white sharks devouring the floating shards of cancer tissue nearly doubled the number of active white blood cells—in just one week. Convincing research shows you can enhance your immune system with just ten minutes a day of imagery, and doing it just three times a week can multiply your natural killer cells. People trained in imagery have even been able to control their response to the chickenpox virus.

There's reason to believe that you can decide to fight a disease. Even cancer patients have used imagery to get the greatest benefit from treatment (imagining the radiation as healing rays of sun) and to defeat what was packaged and sold as a terminal disease (imagining immune cells as soldiers destroying the enemy cancer).

With current scientific interest in behavioral health and the power of the brain, volumes could be written. Libraries could be filled. If you're like most people, you don't have time to explore the rows of crowded shelves in even one of them. So we have tried between the covers of this book to give you enough of a glimpse to make a difference in your life.

In a nutshell, then, how can you achieve wellness?

Before we answer that question, consider what you mean by wellness. Can a seven-year-old victim of muscular dystrophy, twisted and helpless in his motorized wheelchair, be considered well? Can a chemotherapy patient in her last month of life be considered well? Can an AIDS patient languishing between bouts of savage pneumonia or covered with the lesions of Kaposi's sarcoma be considered well? Can a wheelchair-bound grandmother twisted by rheumatoid arthritis be considered well? Yes. The answer to all these is an emphatic *yes*. Sometimes these people, and countless other examples just like them, can achieve a higher level of wellness than the muscled competitive swimmer who breezes through repetitions on the weight machines and eats salads sprinkled with wheat germ.

Physical health is only one aspect of wellness. Wellness goes far beyond blood cholesterol levels and bone density. Psychology plays a role; wellness includes mental acuity, a zest for learning, and a tolerance of different ideas. Sociology plays a role; wellness brings with it empathy, compassion, and a sense of cohesiveness with the rest of humanity. Spirituality plays a role; wellness encompasses a fighting spirit, an optimistic outlook, an attitude of hope, and a sense of our own position in the universe in relationship to those who surround us on this intensely interesting planet of ours. Even religion plays a role: As Albert Einstein put it, "Everyone who is seriously involved in the pursuit of science becomes convinced that a spirit is manifest in the laws of the universe—a spirit vastly superior to that of man, and one in the face of which we with our modest powers must feel humble."

A zest for learning? A tolerance of differences? A sense of cohesiveness with the rest of humanity? The humble acceptance of a guiding spirit? Those qualities are all as much within the reach of a wheelchair-bound child or a cancer-stricken woman as they are a powerfully muscled athlete. In ways that are difficult to comprehend, they may be even *more* in reach of those with physical challenges, squarely confronting our longheld notions about what it means to be "well."

When the mental, emotional, and spiritual aspects of wellness are manifest, the physical aspects usually follow naturally. Renowned surgeon Bernie Siegel predicts that the chemicals we produce in our own brains—the chemicals stimulated in part by our feelings and attitudes—will become the basis of future medical treatment. If you are spiritually or emotionally healthy, you are likely to be physically healthy for your current circumstances, because as you have read on the pages of this book, our attitudes influence our bodies. Stepping outside your own realm of concern to help another person reduces blood pressure, but waving your fist in an explosive burst of rage as you sit in a traffic tie-up clogs your arteries. Charity builds immunity. Revenge literally eats you alive. Guilt enslaves. Forgiveness frees. "Among the prime assets of the human mind," writes Cousins, "is the ability to cut loose from vengeful or burdensome memories."

Essential, too, is the ability to keep things in perspective. Robert Ornstein and David Sobel write in *Healthy Pleasures,*

> *We need to restore some sensibility to the pursuit of health. Many of us increasingly view ourselves as fragile and vulnerable, ready to develop cancer, heart disease, or some other dreaded disease at the slightest provocation. In the name of health we give up many of our enjoyments. The important point is that worrying too much about anything—be it calories, salt, cancer, or cholesterol—is bad for you, and that living optimistically, with pleasure, zest, and commitment, is good. Medical terrorism shouldn't attack life's pleasures.*

Thanks to the battalions of scientists who have designed careful studies, these are no longer mere theories of a religious zealot or an isolated pioneer. They are scientifically proven prescriptions for better health and longer life. Best of all, they are here for the taking. As you approach, put off the shackles of your own blindness: They should not be wasted by blind rejection, nor should they be embraced by blind acceptance. Bring to the exercise your keenest perceptions, your boldest courage.

With that, what can you do?

*Pay attention to the basics.* Plato, one of the most respected of the ancients, called attempting to cure the body without the soul the great error of his day. It is an error that plagues us still. But Plato was not admonishing us to sacrifice the one at the expense of the other: We must attend to both body *and* soul. Attitudes can literally change the pressure of the blood coursing through your veins, but they can't do it all. Start with a good foundation. Use your common sense.

*Exercise regularly.* You don't have to run a marathon or swim the English Channel. In fact, exercise physiologists agree that regular moderate exercise, such as walking, packs greater benefits in the long run. Famed British poet William Wordsworth logged an estimated 180,000 miles during his lifetime, and claimed that walking along the forested lanes of his homeland inspired his poetic pen.

Wordsworth may have been right: Walking not only improves circulation but also literally stimulates the brain. It increases cerebral metabolism—the brain's ability to use oxygen. And many of the brain neurotransmitters—the critical circuitry that links the delicate wiring of the nervous system—depend on oxygen to function.

*Get enough sleep.*

*Eat well*—as much as you can, choose fresh foods that are low in fat, low in sugar, and high in dietary fiber. You don't need to concentrate on food charts, but do try to eat a wide variety of health-promoting foods every day. Avoid the things you know will hurt you such as tobacco, alcohol, and too much caffeine.

*Work hard, but not too hard.* If you can still make choices, opt for work you'll really enjoy; you spend too many hours at it to be miserable. Choose work that doesn't sacrifice the other important things in your life, and consider the impact your job has on those things. When you are mulling possibilities, remember that, in the long run, satisfaction and reward and congruence with our values outweigh a hefty bank balance. Hubbard reminds us, "We work to become, not acquire."

*In your work and in your play, avoid boredom.* The old adage that boredom is deadly may be hauntingly accurate. Some of the nation's leading researchers have shown that a brain that is bored will do almost anything to spark some interest—even create pain and illness, if that's what it takes. Boredom can even change the actual physiology of the brain—laboratory experiments with mice show that the number of neurons decreases among those who are stagnant.

*Vary your routine; break out of the rut.* Take educated risks. Boredom can exist even in the face of pressing responsibilities. Make room in your life for exploration and creativity. Develop new interests. Invite surprise. Relish the unexpected.

*Never stop learning.* Neurosurgeons tell us that new learning and information actually create new connections between the brain cells. Renew your library card. Enroll in a community or adult education class. Dust off the leather-bound collection of Civil War books you inherited from your grandmother; become an expert on little-known battles. Start a friendly office competition to see who can be the first to order a meal in French.

*Savor leisure time.* The chant of a nursery rhyme reminds us that "all work and no play makes Jack a dull boy." Learn to play as hard as you work—it can make a staggering difference in your life. Finishing a first-class client presentation complete with color overlays on crisply designed graphs can be euphoric, but so can the first trills of a distant bluejay, singing across the expanse of a mountain lake where you and the kids pitched your old Boy Scout tent last night. It's great to win a corporate game; it's even greater to help your grandson win his first horseshoe game.

*Do something creative.* Capture the first autumn leaves in a swirl of watercolors, tackle a Beethoven sonata on the old piano, or express your thrill at your child's first steps in a free-verse poem. Don't aim for perfection; instead, concentrate on expressing yourself and having fun.

*While you're playing—and even when you're not—laugh.* Laugh a lot. As Will Rogers advised, "We are here for a spell—get all the good laughs you can." Settle into a chair with a good humorous book. Rent a side-splitting video. It's been proven that laughter raises the level of immune cells that fight viruses. And it's also a great form of "internal jogging." Your whole body gets a workout—your heart, your lungs, your brain, the vast network of lymph and blood vessels that lace through even the most delicate internal organs. Cousins, who healed himself of a crippling and fatal disease in part with laughter, claimed that "of all the gifts bestowed by nature on human beings, hearty laughter must be close to the top."

*While you're at it, don't forget to cry when you need to.* Science tells us that human tears contain healing chemicals that are carried through the bloodstream to all parts of the body. If you think you feel better after a good cry, you're probably right. Sophisticated tests in laboratories even show that crying actually speeds the healing of skin wounds.

*With all your laughing and crying, take the time to build self-confidence.* Serve up a hefty dose of belief in yourself. Those who feel good about themselves are less likely to give up; they stay in the battle until the final scene. Your sense of self is strongly tied to your ability to cope—which is, in turn, linked without question to your body's immune response. Break big tasks into small ones, then pat yourself on the back when you accomplish it. Concentrate on the things you do well instead of flogging yourself for the things you haven't mastered. And, above all, treat yourself with patience and kindness.

*Get rid of all the stress you can.* There are almost surely splatterings of stress in your life that can be totally eliminated with a little strategy. Get up fifteen minutes earlier every day. Leave for appointments ten minutes earlier. Keep your gas tank at least a quarter full. Leave your car keys in the same place every time you come through the door. Unplug the phone if you need a warm bath, a nap, or a half hour of meditation.

*Moderate the stress you can't eliminate.* Try relaxation—moderate exercise, deep breathing, progressive muscle relaxation, or a warm bath. Another stress-buster is meditation; many believe that the deep breathing used in meditation and yoga not only relieves stress, but also has a powerful effect on the brain. Meditation can range from simple, quiet reflection under the spreading branches of a favorite tree to the full-fledged practice of an art that has gained increasing respect among medical practitioners.

*Get a pet.* One of the best strategies for dealing with stress doesn't spring from the printed pages of a book, but walks on four legs straight into your heart. It's called *pet therapy,* and it does much more than relieve stress. Scientists know that the act of merely stroking a pet stabilizes the heart rate and reduces blood pressure. Pet owners live longer, too, and their survival rates after heart attacks or surgery have made headlines in medical journals.

*Change the way you look at stress.* If you can't eliminate or moderate it, reshape it. It was Carl Jung who said that "it all depends on how we look at things, and not on how they are in themselves." We know that the most resilient people, the people who just don't seem to buckle under stress, are the ones who confront it head-on. Instead of seeing it as the enemy, they greet it as a friend. They see it as a challenge—one they're eager to meet.

*Attend church.* People who regularly worship at the church of their choice have less stress, better health, and longer lives.

*Get rid of anger and hostility.* And while you're at it, work on envy and hatred. Former U.S. President George Bush attracted kudos and criticism alike as he took office with the call to become a kinder, gentler nation. George Bush's call to his country may, in fact, be one of the most powerful keys to good health and long life. Why? We now know that hostility drives up blood pressure, clogs up arteries, batters the heart, and chokes the system with menacing hormones. And it kills. So does anger. In fact, anger and hostility are as lethal a combination as science could ever concoct in the laboratory.

*Love.* Romanticists claim that it makes the world go 'round. And one humorist revised that sentiment to say that "love doesn't make the world go 'round—love is what makes the ride worthwhile." Love is a powerful healer—a determinant of good health. Love is, according to Karl Menninger, "an element which binds and heals, which comforts and restores, which works what we have to call—for now—miracles." Bernie Siegel says it best: If you love, you can never be a failure.

*Get involved in service to others.* Escape from your own orbit. Charity, or altruism, or whatever you call it, works—not nearly as much for the recipient as for the giver. The act of helping someone else is wired directly to your brain, and it boosts your health and immunity. A powerful example is shown by World War II's concentration camp survivors. There, in the midst of the world's greatest atrocity, the ones who survived were the ones who reached out. Even in the meanest of circumstances that defeated millions, they swept the filth out of a corner, offered a covertly saved morsel of food, and invited friends to "visit."

The poignancy of their story is matched only by that of the brave Dutch people who risked life itself to help their hunted compatriots. In narrow attic rooms they hid the frightened Jews—whole families—desperate to escape the madman. They gave their own meat and bread, these simple Dutch families who valued human life above the comforts of compliance. Years later, their health and longevity stood as testament to their charity.

Other examples come to the forefront in every disaster that faces humankind—in tornadoes, floods, and furious storms that tear the roofs from houses and scoop children from their mothers' arms. In every case, newspaper reporters zero in on those who, despite their own loss, busy themselves to soothe the hurt of another.

*Involve yourself.* The philosopher warned that no man is an island. We weren't designed to be alone. We need each other. And being involved with each other is one of the best ways to protect health.

*Find social support.* Researchers the world over have analyzed it, dissected it, and quantitatively studied it. All you have to do is practice it. People who have good friends have better health. So do people who have even one trusted friend in whom they can confide. So do people who belong to churches and professional organizations and clubs. So do people who are married. So do people who make their families the top priorities in their lives.

*Find a confidant.* Find one person with whom you can truly communicate your innermost hopes, goals, dreams, fears, sorrows, and disappointments. And be a confidant for someone else.

*Keep a journal.* Record your emotions and attitudes toward events that happen in your life. If you need to, stretch back into the dank expanses of memory and pull out that one difficult thing you've never been able to talk about to anyone. Let your pen do the talking, dancing across the lined pages. You'll be amazed at how much better you feel after the secret's out.

*Face this world, with all its uncertainties and heartaches, with hope.* Hope can be more powerful than anything that confronts it.

*Learn to laugh at yourself.* Cultivate a sense of humor; find joy in the things around you—even the hard things.

*Face this world with a fighting spirit.* Confront whatever you will, but never, never give up.

*Pray.* Your spirit feels a prayer's healing balm . . . and even science has proven that it works.

*Finally, have faith.*

Norman Cousins summed it all up when he told us, "Hope, faith, love, and a strong will to live offer no promise of immortality, only proof of our uniqueness as human beings and the opportunity to experience full growth even under the grimmest circumstances."

# The Elements of Human Fulfillment

According to famed researcher Abraham Maslow,* human fulfillment is based on the following characteristics, which describe his studies of self-actualized people:

*Growth-motivated rather than deficiency-motivated.* As Maslow stated, "The motivation of ordinary men is a striving for the basic need gratifications they lack. But for self-actualizing people, motivation is just character growth, character expression, and maturation." Simply stated, fulfillment rests in the ability to distinguish between living and preparing to live.

*Good sense of reality.* Self-actualized people, says Maslow, have "an unusual ability to detect the spurious, the fake, and the dishonest in personality. . . . They are far more apt to perceive what is there rather than their own wishes, hopes, fears, anxieties, their own theories (prejudices) and beliefs or those of their cultural group . . . unfrightened by the unknown. . . . Doubt, tentativeness, and uncertainty, which are for most a torture, can be for some a pleasantly stimulating challenge, a high spot in life rather than a low."

*Acceptance of self and others.* Human fulfillment is characterized by a relative lack of crippling guilt, though self-actualized people do feel bad about the discrepancy between what is and what ought to be; the ability to see through unnecessary guilt and anxiety; the ability to accept the frailties and imperfections of human beings (in other words, the ability to see human nature as it is instead of as they would prefer it to be); a relative lack of disgust and aversion toward average people; a lack of defensiveness, and distaste for such artificiality in others; and an unusual lack of hypocrisy, game-playing, and attempts to impress others.

*Honest authenticity and naturalness.* Self-actualized people have a tendency toward unconventional thinking, though not necessarily unconventional behavior; an internalized code of high ethics (not necessarily the same as those around them); and a superior awareness of who they are, what they want, and what they believe.

*Commitment and problem centering.* Self-actualized people have a strong sense of purpose outside themselves—a "task they must do." They are concerned with the good of mankind, and work for that which they love; they have a great sense of care for others. They see problems as a stimulating challenge rather than an intolerable dilemma.

*Autonomy.* The self-actualized have a greater sense of "free will"; they are less dependent on or determined by their circumstances or other people. Self-movers, they are self-disciplined and have a sense of determining their own destiny through their personal choices.

*Independence and resistance to enculturalization.* Human fulfillment is characterized by relative independence from the need for approval, respect, and even love; the tendency to act conventionally in affairs regarded as important or unchangeable; and patient entrepreneurialism in wanting to change the status quo for the better.

*An element of detachment and privacy.* Self-actualized people practice objectivity; they are able to withstand personal misfortunes without reacting as violently as most would.

*Continued freshness of appreciation.* The self-actualized have, as Maslow states it, "the wonderful capacity to appreciate again and again (with newness), freshly and naively, the basic goods of life, with awe, pleasure, wonder, even ecstasy, however stale these experiences have become to others." They avoid taking things for granted; instead, they "retain a constant sense of good fortune and gratitude for it."

*High energy levels, peak experiences.* "Their energy is not supernatural," Maslow says of the self-actualized; "it is simply the result of loving life and all the activities in it. They don't know how to be bored. . . . They are aggressively curious. They never know enough. They search for more and want to learn each and every present moment of their lives. . . . They are mystic, with peak experiences of transcendence of self; they have a sense of limitless horizons opening up to vision, coupled with ecstasy and a transforming feeling of strength."

*Deep interpersonal relations.* Human fulfillment is characterized by the capability of more fusion, intimacy, and obliteration of ego boundaries than seen in most people. The self-actualized tend to be kind to—or at least patient with—almost everyone, particularly children, yet they often have few profoundly close relationships because of the time required to maintain them. When they express hostility, it is not toward someone's character, but to achieve some good end.

*Democratic character structure.* The self-actualized are oblivious to barriers of class, education, politics, or race; they possess a certain sense of humility that allows them to learn from anyone and to be aware of how little they know when compared with what could be known.

*Discrimination between ends and means.* Ethically, the self-actualized believe that means are subordinated to ends, but means are usually enjoyed as ends in themselves. Simply, the self-actualized appreciate the process of doing for its own sake.

*Philosophical, unhostile sense of humor.* Humor for the self-actualized is usually directed at self or at people who are trying to be big when they are small; humor extends to work—which, though taken seriously, is approached with a sense of play. They find that humor often has an educational function beyond the simple value of laughter.

*Creativity.* The self-actualized are often not creative in the usual artistic forms; their creativity is more a process and attitude than a product. Their creativity extends to a way of approaching all of life; they find fresh, direct solutions with naive newness.

*Guiltless acceptance of sexuality.* For the self-actualized, sex is fused with love and full of underlying intimacy; they do not usually seek sex for its own sake. Theirs is a paradox: They seem to enjoy their sexuality far more than average, yet consider it much less important.

*Resolution of complementary opposites.* Finally, the self-actualized seem to enjoy—even thrive on—differences rather than fear them. They creatively seek overarching principles that make seeming opposites synergic (complementary) rather than antagonistic; peak experiences often occur during the resolution.

*Abraham Maslow, *Motivation and Personality* (New York: Harper & Row, 1954).

# The Seven Habits of Highly Effective People

According to Steven R. Covey,[*] the seven habits of highly effective people are as follows:

1. *Be proactive.* Use the responsible free will to act as you desire, with integrity.

2. *Begin with the end in mind.* Have clearly defined values; cultivate a sense of purpose and mission; and visualize the results ahead of time.

3. *Put first things first.* Be able to distinguish core values from lesser values and act with integrity toward the deeper ones (with discipline and sacrifice as necessary).

4. *Think win/win.* Aim for mutual acceptance and empowerment; strive for connectedness; and build on integrity, maturity, and an abundance mentality.

5. *Seek first to understand, then to be understood.* Use caring love and acceptance and a sense of connectedness when dealing with others.

6. *Synergize.* Accept, and even appreciate, differences; try creative cooperation and connectedness; work from a common sense of mission and purpose; and have a positive expectation.

7. *Renew yourself.* Experience a sense of purpose and mission (commitment); continued growth; and meditative reflection and visualization.

---

[*]Stephen R. Covey, *The Seven Habits of Highly Effective People* (New York: Fireside—Simon & Schuster, 1989).

# The Misunderstood Alternative: Effective Type B Characteristics of Those Proven to Be Protected from Heart Disease*

People with Type B characteristics are often peak performers and hold many top positions. Below are protective traits that need fostering:

## No time urgency

- More mindful in giving attention to the central task at hand
- Not easily bored or eager to move on to something else
- Usually keeps on schedule, but without frenzy or rage
- Patient (no habitual haste)
- Contemplative: enjoys beauty and metaphor, tends to see the whole more than the parts
- Able to value and enjoy the things already done, or being now done, as much as those things to be done in the future

## Able to relinquish control

- Good at delegation, team players—comfortable with this
- Tolerant of differences—even enjoys them
- Often good at inspiring creative involvement with others—good leaders

## An internal locus of high self-value

- Appreciates self for what he or she *is* as much as what he or she *does*
- Accepts and values self as is
- Understands that self-identity and worth are far more important than numbers
- Feels valued and of worth regardless of achievement (often derived from parents)

- Often works as hard at something as Type A's, but failure does not collapse self-esteem
- Loves growth, getting better (often through mistakes)
- Competes with self, not with others

## No free-floating hostility

- No need to find fault to bolster own ego
- Can accept with equanimity the trivial errors of subordinates ("They practice the art of being wise by knowing what to disregard.")
- Enjoys empowering and lifting others
- Uncommonly feels tense or induces tension in others
- Their self-confidence allows objectivity and ability to see through another's eyes
- Capable of both feeling and expressing affection—enjoys intimate relationships

*See the discussion of the characteristics of noncoronary prone individuals in M. Friedman and D. Ulmer: *Treating Type A Behavior and Your Heart* (New York: Fawcett, 1984), ch. 3.

# Name Index

*Note:* A general Subject Index follows this Name Index.

Abel, Jennifer L., 174, 187
Achterberg, Jeanne, 512
Ackerman, Diane, 304
Ader, Dr. Robert, 4, 8, 22, 662
Affleck, Glenn, 540
Ainsworth, Dr. Mary D. Salter, 367
Akiskal, Hagop, 199
Alexander, Dr. Franz, 88
Allen, Karen M., 335
Allen, Steve, 578
Allen, Steve, Jr., 578
Allport, Gordon, 578, 579
*Altruistic Personality,* 459
*American Health,* 380
*American Housing Survey,* 510
*American Journal of Clinical Nutrition,* 604
*American Journal of Gastroenterology,* 601
*American Journal of Health Promotion,* 162
*American Journal of Public Health,* 219
Anda, Robert, 211
Andrews, 462
Angell, Marcia, 93, 94
*Anger,* 148, 150
Arnold, Kay, 461
Arvigo, Dr. Rosita, 560
Auslander, Wendy, 382

Bahnson, Claus, 120
Bandura, Dr. Albert, 553, 554, 555
Banks, R., 423
Barasch, Marc, 266, 422
Barbach, Lonnie, 510
Barefoot, John, 162
Barrymore, Ethel, 564
Baum, Dr. Andrew, 21
Baumrind, Diana, 367, 368
Beaumont, Dr. William, 127
Beecher, Henry Ward, 566

*Behavioral and Brain Sciences,* 457
Bell, Iris R., 31
Bellow, Saul, 276
Benor, Daniel, 484
Benson, Dr. Herbert, 114, 432, 433, 462, 477, 478, 483, 494
Berg, Dr. Alfred, 492
Berk, Dr. Lee, 577, 578
Berkman, Lisa, 295
Bernard, Claude, 29
Bernikow, Louise, 319
Bingham, Davis, 473
Biorck, Dr. Gunnar, 296, 297
Blalock, Ed, 514
Blascovich, James J., 335
Blass, Elliott, 13
Bloom, Floyd, 12
Blumberg, Eugene, 27–28, 116, 117
Borysenko, Joan, 280, 311, 425, 434, 474
Bosworth, H. B., 440
Bourne, Peter, 536–537
Braiker, Harriet B., 372
Branden, Nathaniel, 547
Breitbart, William, 301
Brenner, M. Harvey, 61
Breznitz, Shlomo, 479
*British Heart Journal,* 61
*British Journal of Medical Psychology,* 95, 113
Bro, Harmon, 469
Brody, 572
*Broken Heart, The,* 454
Brooks, Marjorie, 156
Brown, Dr. George W., 197
Brown, Jonathan, 503
Brown, Timothy A., 187
Buchwald, Art, 570
Buddha, 428–429
Buechner, Frederick, 139
Bukowski, Charles, 52
Bulloch, Karen, 514
Burn, 525

Burnett, Carol, 570
Byrd, R. B., 434
Byrne, Don, 111

Cannon, Walter, 7
Caporall, Linda R., 457
Carney, Robert M., 213
Carroll, 73
Carver, Dr. Charles S., 505, 510, 511
Casarjian, Robin, 434, 435, 437
Cassileth, Barrie R., 93, 123
Chaplain, Charlie, 570
Chesney, Margaret A., 104, 140, 151
Chiriboga, David A., 312
Chopra, Deepak, 476
Churchill, Winston, 195
Circulation, 158
Clemens, Samuel, 547
Clinical Psychiatry News, 540
Clinical Infectious Diseases, 602
Cobb, Dr. Sidney, 277, 368
Cogan, Dennis, 579
Cogan, Rosemary, 579
Cohen, Lorenzo, 123
Cohen, Sheldon, 74, 507
Corson, Samuel A., 332
Cortis, Bruno, 418, 426
Cousins, Norman, 5, 184, 488, 505, 506,
    512, 518, 538, 539, 561, 568, 573, 575,
    576, 667, 668, 672, 674
Covey, Steven R., 678
Cox, Michael, 76
Crane, Alison, 569
Cummings, Nicholas, 177

Daaleman, Dr. Timothy P., 473
Dabbs, James, 530
Daldrup, Roger J., 146, 147
Darko, Denis, 514
Davidson, Glen, 391, 392, 393
Davis, Dr. J. Mostyn, 493
Davis, Maradee, 357
Dawson, Geraldine, 221
de Bono, Edward, 565
de Mondeville, Henri, 559

de Saint-Pierre, Michel, 523
DeFrain, John, 383
DeGarmo, Scott, 515
DeLap, Robert, 489
Dembroski, Theodore M., 144
Demos, John, 363
Derogatis, Leonard, 21, 645
Descartes, Réne, 6
Diagnostic and Statistical Manual, 213
Domar, Alice, 69
Dossey, Dr. Larry, 291, 432, 458
Dostoevski, Fyodor, 561
Draus, Hans, 31
Dreher, Henry, 129, 643, 644
Duff, Robert W., 441
Duszynski, Dr. Karen, 320, 321

Eagleton, Thomas, 195
Eddy, Mary Baker, 483
Edwards, Patrick, 372, 373
Einstein, Albert, 417, 446, 452, 669
Eisenberger, Naomi I., 30
Eliot, Robert S., 43, 48, 70, 71, 72, 77, 181
Emerson, Ralph Waldo, 3, 472, 515
Engle, Dr. George, 404, 406
Epstein, Gerald, 428
Eysenck, Hans J., 88, 89

Family Practice Recertification, 598
Farewell to Arms, A, 668
Fassel, Diane, 61, 62
Fathman, Robert, 32
Fawzy, Fawzy I., 301
Feldman, Dr. Mark, 32, 127
Felten, David L., 4
Ferman, Louis, 53
Field, Totie, 570
Fields, W. C., 570
Fischer, Joey, 511
Fisher, Rhoda, 570
Fisher, Seymour, 570
Fosdick, Harry Emerson, 192
Fowles, Richard, 61
Francis, Martha E., 283
Frank, Jerome D., 475, 480, 481, 485

Frankl, Victor, 427, 666
Frautschi, Nanette, 104
Freud, Sigmund, 569
Freudenberger, Herbert J., 94
Friedman, Howard S., 87, 251, 261
Friedman, Meyer, 96, 97–98, 101, 102, 103, 107, 130, 153, 267
Friedman, Stanford B., 610, 621
Friedmann, Erika, 332, 333
*From Stress to Strength* (Harvey), 70
Fry, William, Jr., 570, 571, 575
*Full Catastrophe Living*, 187

Galen, 6, 116
Gandhi, Mohandas K., 262
Garfield, James A., 172
Gartner, John, 443
*Gastroenterology*, 601
Gawain, Shakti, 424
Gaylin, Willard, 456
Gershon, Elliot S., 195–196
Gershwin, Madeline, 556
Gersten, Dennis, 221
Gibson, Leslie, 562
*Gift from the Sea*, 312
Gill, James, 142
Girgus, Joan, 527
Glaser, Ronald, 347
Glass, David, 154
Gleason, Jackie, 570
Gold, Phillip, 202, 205
Goldberg, Joan, 14
Goldstein, Jeffrey, 575
Goldston, Stephen, 392
Goleman, Daniel, 480, 518
Goliszek, Andrew, 71
Good, Robert, 531
Goodkin, Karl, 218, 263
Goodman, Ellen, 166
Goodman, Joel, 578
Goodwin, Frederick, 193
Goodwin, James, 354
Graves, Pirkko L., 28, 91, 121
Green, W. H., 52
Greenberg, Michael, 509, 510

Greene, Dr. William, 210, 402
Greer, Dr. Steven, 512, 645
Grossarth-Maticek, Ronald, 88, 89
Grossbart, Ted, 150
Gurin, Joel, 518
*Gut*, 601
Guy, William, 207

Haggerty, Robert, 253
Haley, Alex, 380
Hall, G. Stanley, 150
Hall, Nicholas, 513
Hammerskjold, Dag, 471
Hammett, Frederick, 304
Hanh, Thich Nhat, 187
Harlow, Dr. Harry F., 303, 364
Harlow, Margaret, 303
Harper, Michael, 431
Harvey, William, 70, 96, 97
*Head First*, 573
*Healing Brain, The*, 463
*Healing Power of Humor*, 570
*Health and Optimism*, 525
*Health of Nations*, 549
*Healthy People*, 589
Heisel, J. Stephen, 552
Helgeson, Vicki, 348
Hemingway, Ernest, 195, 430, 668
Hildegard of Bingen, 605
Hinkle, Lawrence, 256
Hippocrates, 6, 9, 88, 96–97, 418, 605
Hirshberg, Caryle, 539
Hitler, Adolf, 91
Holmes, Thomas, 49
*Honoring the Self*, 547
Horne, Dr. R. L., 29
Horowitz, Dr. R., 488
House, Dr. James, 278, 321, 322, 454, 455, 467
Houston, Kent, 145
Howard, 462
Hubbard, 671

Idler, Ellen, 441, 443, 528
Irwin, Dr. Michael, 215, 403, 514

Janus, Samuel, 570
Jasheway, Leigh Anne, 579
Jeffers, Susan, 550, 551
Jefferson, Thomas, 362
Jewell, Kealan, 504
John-Roger, 505, 563, 564
Johnson, Dr. Jeffrey, 325
Johnson, Samuel, 340
*Journal of Applied Social Psychology,* 111
*Journal of Community and Applied Social
    Psychology,* 312
*Journal of Nervous and Mental Disease,* 25
*Journal of the American Medical Association,* 121,
    196, 214, 218, 295, 488, 570, 576, 602
*Journal of the National Cancer Institute,* 38
Julius, Mara, 158
Jung, Carl, 443, 673
Justice, Blair, 540, 543, 554

Kabat-Zinn, Dr. Jon, 187, 660
Kahn, Robert L., 278
Kalliopuska, Mirja, 548
Kaplan, George A., 320
Kaplan, Helen Singer, 33
Karasek, Robert, 62, 79, 542
Kasl, Stanislav, 441, 528, 531
Katcher, Aaron, 332
Katoff, Lewis, 515
Katz, Lynn Fainsilber, 348
Kavanaugh, Kevin M., 563
Keller, Steven, 403
Kemeny, Margaret, 216, 217, 324
Kennel, Arthur, 434
Kennell, John, 322
Ketterer, Mark, 162
Kiecolt-Glaser, Janice, 299, 347
Kiefer, Christie, 459
King, Martin Luther, Jr., 362
Kissen, David, 29, 120
Kissinger, Henry, 104
Klein, Allen, 566, 570
Klopfer, Dr. Bruno, 483, 484
Knapp, Peter, 45
Kobasa, Suzanne Ouellette, 253, 255, 256,
    260, 261, 266, 267–268, 535, 537, 538

Koch, Robert, 6–7
Koenig, Harold, 439, 477
Kohn, Alfie, 459
Koocher, Gerald, 392
Korneva, Elena, 18
Kornfield, D. S., 631
Kreiger, Dolores, 485
Kroenke, Kurt, 177
Kronfol, Dr. Ziad, 217
Kübler-Ross, Elisabeth, 392

*Lancet,* 488, 602, 604
Landfield, Philip, 68
Langer, Ellen, 544
LaRoche, Loretta, 560
Larson, Alfred N., 460
Larson, David, 439
Laudenslager, Mark, 323
*Laughing Matters,* 578
*Laughter Prescription, The,* 578
Lawlis, Dr. G. Frank, 512
*Lawrence of Arabia,* 477–478
Lazarus, Richard, 506
Lee, David, 335
Leiber, Deborah Burton, 569
Lerner, Michael A., 531
LeShan, Lawrence, 28, 119–120, 300, 496, 512
Levav, Itzhak, 410
Levenson, James L., 25
Levenson, Robert W., 348
Levin, Jeffrey S., 479
Levin, Lowell, 460
Levine, Emily, 564
Levinson, Boris, 331
Levitan, S. J., 631
Levitt, Shelly, 332
Levy, Sandra, 511, 529, 644
Lincoln, Abraham, 195, 417, 559
Lindbergh, Anne Morrow, 312
Ljungdahl, Dr. Lars, 577
Locke, Dr. Steven, 14, 552
Longfellow, Henry Wadsworth, 388
Louis, Emperor, 185
Lown, Bernard, 186
Luks, Allan, 454, 461, 462, 463

Lynch, Dr. James, 285, 296, 319, 321, 323, 334, 454, 549

Machlowitz, Marilyn, 108
MacMahon, Brian, 407
MacNutt, Francis, 434
Maddi, Salvatore, 256, 266, 535, 537, 538
Maimonides, 605
Mann, John, 197
Manov, Gregory, 207
*Man's Search for Meaning,* 427
Mark, Dr. Daniel, 530
Maslow, Abraham, 675, 677
Masten, Ann, 261, 341
Matthews, Andrew, 172
Matthews, Dr. Karen, 100
McClelland, David, 467, 482, 651
McKinney, William, Jr., 199
McMillen, S. I., 535
McWilliams, Peter, 505
*MD,* 94
Mears, Ainsley, 661
*Medical Journal of Australia,* 20
Mendelssohn, Moses, 567
Menningers, 97
Merva, Mary, 61
Metcalf, C. W., 561
Meyer, Roger, 253
Miller, Brian, 113
Miller, Bruce, 209
Miller, Dr. Theodore, 9
Milton, John, 251
*Mind/Body Medicine,* 518
Mindess, Harvey, 564, 568
Minkler, Meredith, 464
Mintz, Lawrence, 568
Mittleman, Dr. Murray, 158
*Molecules of Emotion,* 585
Monroe, Kristen, 457
Moody, Raymond, Jr., 576
Moore, Dudley, 570
Moos, Rudolf, 125
Mulcater, Richard, 559
Mumford, Emily, 631
Mundy, William L., 446

Nebuchadnezzar, 195
*New England Journal of Medicine,* 93, 157, 251, 597, 603, 604
*New York Times,* 440, 517
Newman, Michelle, 567, 568
*Newsweek,* 363
Nickel, J. Curtis, 489
Nilson, Linda, 454
Nixon, Richard, 104
Nolen-Hoeksema, Susan, 527
Norris, Patricia, 513

Oliner, Pearl M., 457, 458, 459
Oliner, Samuel P., 457, 458, 459
*Opening Up,* 281
Ornish, Dr. Dean, 5, 113, 114, 455
Ornstein, Robert, 141, 259, 264, 463, 502, 503, 548, 556, 570, 578, 579, 670
Orth-Gomer, Dr. Kristina, 325
Osler, Sir William, 97, 605

Paffenbarger, Dr. Ralph, 326
Paget, Sir James, 116
Panksepp, Jaak, 30, 453
Panti, Don Elijio, 560
Pare, Ambrose, 473
Pargament, K. I., 427
Pasick, Rena, 541
*Path of Transformation, The,* 424
Pattishall, Evan G., 251
Paul, Steven, 193
Pauling, Dr. Linus, 591
Payne, Peggy, 463
Pearsall, Paul, 109, 391, 426, 428, 429, 478
Peck, Scott, 642
Pelletier, Dr. Kenneth, 276, 294, 427, 454
Pendleton, Brian, 433
Pennebaker, James W., 281, 282, 283, 284, 330
Peplau, Dr. Anne, 398, 399
Pert, Candace, 4, 13, 514, 585, 586
Peter, Lawrence, 578
Peterson, Christopher, 503, 506, 507, 508
Pett, Marjorie A., 341
*Philadelphia Inquirer,* 517

Picard, Dr. R. S., 29
Pizzamiglio, Pearl, 185
Plath, Sylvia, 195
Plato, 605, 670
Pollio, Howard, 566
Poloma, Margaret, 433
Post-Gorden, Joan C., 263
Powell, Lynda H., 151
*Primary Care*, 37
Pruzinsky, Thomas, 173
*Psychological Bulletin*, 527
*Psychology Today*, 13, 95, 105, 199, 503
Pugh, Thomas, 407

Quinn, Janet, 485

Rabelais, François, 534
Rahe, Richard, 50
Ramey, Estelle, 164
Reece, John, 406
Reinhard, Lenore, 568
Reite, Martin, 216
Remen, Rachel Naomi, 79, 446
Renoux, Gerard, 18
*Republic, The*, 605
Reyes, Barbara, 185
Reynolds, Peggy, 320
Rice, Phillip, 535
Richardson, Dr. Charles, 32, 127
Richter, Curt, 539
Roberts, Alan, 496
Robinson-Whelan, Susan, 516
Rockefeller, John D., 456–457
Rogers, Will, 672
Rosch, Paul, 44, 60, 525
Rosen, Robert, 109
Rosenfield, Israel, 11–12
Rosenman, Ray, 73, 96, 97–98, 99, 104, 107, 140, 153
Roskies, Ethel, 115
Rossman, Marty, 177
Rotter, Julian, 534
Ruberman, Dr. William, 314–315
Rubin, Lillian B., 330
Ruff, Michael, 514

Russell, Bill, 63
Russell, Dr. Jon, 206

Sadat, Anwar, 642
Sadoughi, Wanda, 33
Sagan, Leonard, 76, 276, 368, 443, 535, 536, 549
Salber, Dr. Eva, 281
Salk, Jonas, 9
Sand, George, 471
Sapolsky, Robert, 67, 68, 603
*Saturday Review*, 5
Saul, 195
Schachter, Dr. Stanley, 286
Scheier, Michael, 504, 505, 511
Scherwitz, Larry, 455
Schleifer, Steven, 389, 402, 403
Schmale, Dr. Arthur, 389, 537
Schneck, Jerome M., 22
Schoeborn, Charlotte, 349
Schweitzer, Albert, 87, 452, 498
*Science*, 30, 467
*Science News*, 112, 218, 304
*The Sciences*, 276
Seagraves, Dr. Robert, 345
*Second Brain, The*, 600
Segal, Julius, 543
Seligman, Martin, 195, 456, 507, 514, 515, 516, 523, 525, 526, 529, 530, 534
Selye, Hans, 7, 42, 65–66, 252–253, 453
Shaffer, John, 121
Shakespeare, William, 228
Sharansky, Anatoly, 566–567
Shekelle, Dr. Richard, 209
Siegel, Bernie S., 21, 51, 52, 266, 389, 420, 422, 430, 431, 467, 486, 506, 517, 526, 527, 529, 531, 579, 670
Siegel, Judith M., 332
Siegler, Dr. Ilene C., 159
Silverman, Samuel, 323
Simon, Suzanne, 434
Simonton, O. Carl, 422, 512, 513
Simpson, Randolph, 185
Slaney, Mary Decker, 263
Smith, Dr. N. Lee, 255

Smith, Ken R., 398
Smith, Ruth, 258
Smith, Timothy, 105, 115, 143
Sobel, David, 141, 259, 264, 463, 502, 503, 548, 556, 570, 578, 579, 630, 670
Solfvin, Jerry, 493
Solomon, George, 125, 539, 552
Solomon, G. F., 7
Soubirous, Marie Bernarde, 480
Spiegel, David, 4, 7, 38, 300, 301, 628, 645
Spielberger, Charles D., 28, 89
Spitz, Dr. Rene, 365, 390
Staub, Ervin, 459
Stearns, Peter, 150
Stein, Marvin, 402
Stein, Sara, 4
Steinberg, David, 570
Stevenson, Robert Louis, 327
Stewart, Michael, 185
Stinnett, Nick, 383
Stone, Arthur, 34
Strain, James J., 630
Strauss, Dr. Stephen, 486, 487
Strube, Michael J., 145–146
*Success*, 515
Suomi, Dr. Stephen, 365
*Super Immunity*, 109, 478
Swaim, Loring T., 32
Sword, Richard, 202
Sydenham, Thomas, 560
Syme, Leonard, 285, 287, 294

Tavris, Carol, 140, 141, 147
Taylor, Robert, 290
Taylor, Shelly, 503
Temoshok, Lydia, 117, 118, 119, 120, 157, 643, 644
Terman, Lewis, 261
Theorell, Dr. Tores, 62, 63, 79
Thomas, Caroline Bedell, 27, 92, 320, 321, 645
Thompson, S. C., 262
Thoreau, Henry, 504
*Time*, 5, 42, 59

Tooby, John, 457
Torrijos, Omar, 185
Tripp-Reimer, Toni, 485
Twain, Mark, 547, 559
*Type C Connection, The*, 643

*U.S. News and World Report*, 12

Vaillant, George, 455, 506
van der Ploeg, Henk M., 28
Vanderpool, Hearold Y., 479
Vasey, Dr. Michael, 188
Vavak, Christine, 145
Virchow, Rudolf, 7
von Humboldt, Wilhelm, 91

Walker, Dr. Lenore, 148
Ward, Vince, 461
Werner, Emmy, 258
Whitehead, William E., 33
Wickramasekera, Ian, 53
Wilbanks, William, 526
Wilder, Thornton, 667
Williams, Redford, 101, 105, 106, 109, 114, 139, 141, 143, 146, 157, 159, 160, 161, 163
Williamson, Gail, 465
Willis, Thomas, 29
Wilson, Ian, 406
Wirth, David P., 486
Wise, Harold, M. D., 384
Wolf, Dr. Stewart, 211, 296, 487
Wolf, Katherine, 365, 390
Wolter, Dwight, 436
Wootton, Sir Henry, 388
Wordsworth, William, 671

Yalom, Irvin, 7
*You Can't Afford the Luxury of a Negative Thought*, 505

Zarren, Harvey, 115
Zonderman, Alan, 121, 218

Abortion, 403–404
Accident, 235, 395
Adolescent. *See* Children
Adrenal, 7, 26, 46, 217. *See also*
    Adrenaline
Adrenaline, 8, 10, 25, 110, 185
Affirmation, 376–377
Aggression, 146. *See also* Anger;
    Hostility
  hyperaggressiveness, 103
Aging, 58, 69. *See also* Elderly;
    Longevity
  affects on body, 17
AIDS, 294–295, 515, 539
Alameda County study, 275–277, 287,
    292–293, 320, 323, 327, 517, 541
Alcohol/drugs, 59, 64–65, 127, 232, 233,
    235, 319, 356
  affect on immune system, 8
  gender differences, 258
Alexithymia, 258
Allergy, 217
  discussed, 31
  wheat allergy, 604
Altruism
  altruistic personality, 457–460
  in general, 452–453
  health benefits, 453–457
  love
    animals, 468
    children, 468–469
    in general, 466–467
  volunteerism
    consistency, 464
    desire to volunteer, 463–464
    in general, 460–463
    liking the work, 464
    motive, 464–466
    one-on-one contact, 463
Alzheimer's disease, 69, 364, 593,
    598, 599

Amino acids, 245, 594. *See also* Nutrition
Amish, 196–197
Amygdala, 13
Anger, 24–25, 32, 92, 106. *See also*
    Emotions; Hostility
  angry heart, 157–162
  cancer and, 155–157
  definitions, 139–141
  expression
    healthy expression, 148–149, 149–152
    unhealthy expression, 146–148,
      156–157, 348
    vs. suppression, 163–165
  manifestations, 142–144, 257
  significance, 144–145
  suggestions, 165–166
Anhedonia, 200–201. *See also* Depression
Animals, 406. *See also* Pets
  love and, 468
  stress affecting, 649–650
Antibodies, 14
Antidepressants, 179–180, 199–200, 206,
    212, 218, 220, 221, 245. *See also*
    Depression
  Use of Antidepressants, 634t–635t
Anxiety. *See also* Worry
  anxiety disorder, 174–175, 179, 195
  mental illness and, 179–181
  obsessive-compulsive disorder, 176
  panic disorder, 175
    physical symptoms, 178t
  social anxiety disorder, 175–176
  somaticizing, 176–177
  what to do about it, 187–188
Appendix, 15
Arteriosclerosis, stress and, 73
Arthritis
  discussed, 31–32, 624
  rheumatoid arthritis, 32, 217–218
    rheumatoid arthritis personality,
      123–126

Aspirin, 127
*Astangahradaya Sustrastahana*, 6
Asthma. *See also* Asthma personality
  asthmatic children, 182, 209
  discussed, 31
  family and, 374
  worry and, 182–183
Asthma personality, discussed, 128–129
Attitude, 529–530
Autoimmune disease. *See also* Immune
    system
  discussed, 17, 19

B cells, discussed, 16
Back pain, 31, 59–60. *See also* Pain
Balance, 566, 614
Behavior. *See also* Behavior change;
    Behavioral medicine
  cognitive behavioral therapy, 240
Behavior change. *See also* Change
  elements, 654
  methods, 657–660
  summary, 569
Behavioral medicine, 5. *See also*
    Psychoneuroimmunology
  cost and utilization issues, 628–635
  filling hole in health care deliver system?,
    633–634
  in general, 610–613
  high-volume medical users, 617–620
  outcome data, 615–617, 620–628, 623t
  outcome studies, 611
  stress health effects, 613–615
Bereavement. *See* Grief and bereavement
Beta Blocker Heart Attack Trial, 488
Biofeedback, 20
Blame, 166, 437, 529
Blood pressure, 25, 47, 69, 70, 71, 108, 110,
    155, 159, 163, 181, 326, 331, 334, 347,
    348, 353, 530, 587
  discussed, 622–623
  marriage and, 352–353
Body work, 656–657
Bone marrow, 8, 15, 514

Boredom, 44, 64, 263, 506–507, 671
  loneliness and, 312
Brain, 218, 586, 643, 668
  blood-brain barrier, 593
  brain-immune system connection, 18–20
  chemicals produced by
    control and, 650–651
    endorphins, 13
    peptides, 13–14
  emotions produced by, 12
  in general, 9–10
  nutrition and, 599–600
  stress and, 67–68
  what it does, 11–12, 94
  what it is, 10–11, 592
Breathing, 187
  meditative breathing, 654–655
Bronchitis, 163–164
Burnout, 370–371

Caffeine, 127, 232, 233, 241, 264, 671
Cancer, 9, 17, 21, 88, 208, 320, 390, 511,
    512, 513. *See also* Type C personality
  anger and, 155–157
  breast cancer, 6, 88, 90, 116, 120, 156
    support groups, 7
  "cancer personality", 27–28, 88–89,
    91, 92
  depression and, 121, 218
  discussed, 628
  emotions and, 26–29, 529–530
    mind-body influences, 27–29, 93–94
  family affecting, 374
  "fighting spirit", 122, 129
  leukemia, 52, 537
  loneliness and, 327
  lung cancer, 29
  marriage and, 353–354
  melanoma, 117, 118, 529
  stress and, 26, 26–29, 51–52, 301–302
  stress resilience and, 643–645
  support groups, 7
Cardiovascular system. *See also* Heart
  stress and, 70–72

Catecholamines, 185–186, 555
  discussed, 153–154
Central nervous system (CNS), 8, 10, 212
  disorders of, 207, 238
Challenge, discussed, 263
Change. *See also* Behavior change
  lifestyle change, 597
  sensitivity to, 490
  stress and, 51, 53
Chest pain, 623–624. *See also* Pain
Children. *See also* Family; Women
  asthma affecting, 182, 209
  cancer affecting, 52
  depression affecting, 221
  diabetes affecting, 30
  diet, 590
  divorce affecting, 341–343
  effects on fetus, 302–303
  healthy children, 9, 14, 441–442
  hostility affecting, 145–146
  loneliness affecting, 316, 317, 321
  love and, 468–469
  marriage affecting, 352
  social support affecting, 280
  stress affecting, 65, 77–78, 382, 543–544
    discussed, 54–56, 253–254
    Hawaii study, 258–260
    prenatal stress, 53–54
  Type A behavior, 100–101, 112
Cholesterol, 47, 159, 586
  stress and, 72–73
Chronic pain. *See also* Pain
  discussed, 30–31
Circulation system, worry and, 181–182
CNS. *See* Central nervous system
Coherence, discussed, 264
Colds, 74, 150–151, 215, 507
  discussed, 34
Commitment, discussed, 262
Communication, 371, 376, 586
Community, 78, 279–280, 294, 311
Commuting, 77
Competitiveness, 102, 131, 154
Confidant, 78, 315, 351, 674
Confiding, 281–283, 330

Contemplation, 657. *See also* Meditation
Control
  brain chemistry and, 650–651
  cognitive structuring and therapy,
    651–654
  controlling behaviors, 176, 315, 371,
    436
  discussed, 262–263
  empowerment and, 645, 648–651
  hardiness and, 537–538
  health and
    animal studies, 539–540
    biochemical imbalances, 540–541
    in general, 538–539
    human studies, 540
    immune system, 543–544
  lack of control vs. stress, 541–542
  locus of control
    definition, 534–535
    history, 535–537
    source of control, 536–537, 658
  negative feelings about, 57–58, 315
  placebo control, 178, 490
  positive feelings about, 5, 27, 62, 65, 131,
    166, 436, 445, 463–464, 504, 526
  power and, 566–567
  as stress-buffer, 542–543
Cooke Medley Hostility Scale, 143, 145
Coping ability, humor and, 568–569
Coronary disease. *See* Heart disease
Coronary personality. *See* Disease-prone
  personality
Corticotropin-releasing hormone (CRH), 46,
  152, 197, 205
Cortisol, 26, 68, 69, 217, 324
  discussed, 154
Creativity, 28, 268, 672
  promoting, 565–566
CRH. *See* Corticotropin-releasing hormone
Crisis, spirituality and, 429–431
Crohn's disease, 208
Crying, 672
Cynicism, 106–107, 111, 143
  Cynical Distrust Scale, 151
Cytokines, discussed, 18

Dental cavities, discussed, 32
Depression, 20, 35, 54, 55, 60, 70, 92, 99,
    111, 143, 151, 174, 349, 593. *See also*
    Antidepressants
  cancer and, 121, 218
  causes, 196–200, 527
  characteristics, 200–202
  chemical depression, 199–200
  clinical depression, 192, 621
  costs, 196
  definition, 192–194, 213
  feeling sad, feeling bad, 219–220
  "healthiness of", 642
  heart and, 210–214
  immune system and, 214–218
  insomnia and, 235–236
  insulin resistance and heart disease,
      598–599
  kindling phenomenon, 198–199
  longevity and, 208–210
  medical conditions mimicking, 207–208,
      214
  mental illness and, 200
  Patient Health Questionnaire,
      193–194
  physiological changes, 205–206
  PMS and, 202–203
  prevalence and manifestations,
      194–196, 200t
  seasonal affective disorder,
      203–205
  stress and, 257–258
  vs. grief, 215
  what to do about it, 220–221
Diabetes. *See also* Diabetic personality
  emotions and, 29–30
  family and, 374–375
  nutrition and, 599–600
Diabetic personality, 30
Diet, 74, 78, 113, 130, 199–200, 220, 586.
      *See also* Nutrition; Obesity
  balance in, 588–589
  nutritional deficiency, 208
  typical American diet, 589–590
Digestion, 587–588. *See also* Nutrition

Digestive tract. *See* Gastrointestinal tract
Disease-prone personality. *See also* Disease-
    resistant personality; Personality
  asthma personality, 128–129
  controversy about, 93–94
  definitions and foundation, 87–90
  disease cluster view, 92
  disease-prone personality view, 92
  explaining the differences, 94–95
  in general, 90–91
  generic view, 91–92
  overcoming, 129–131
  personality cluster view, 93
  rheumatoid-arthritis-prone personality
      in general, 123–124
      identical twin study, 124–125
      immune system factor, 125–126
      Solomon/Moos study, 125
  Type A personality, 92, 160, 551, 564
      causes, 100–101
      characteristics of, 101–109
      controversy about, 115–116
      effects on women, 112–113
      emotional effects of, 110–113
      foundations of, 96–97
      in general, 92, 95–96
      harmless behaviors, 101–102
      heart disease risk, 111
      impacts of, 112
      insecurity of status, 102
      MRFIT study, 98–99
      role in other illnesses, 113–114
      studies, 297–298
      "toxic core" of, 104
      Western Collaborative Group Study,
          98–99, 99–100, 106, 113
  Type C personality
      depression, 121
      emotions, 120
      in general, 116–119
      LeShan's analysis, 119–120
      stress, 26–29, 51–52, 120–121
  Type D personality, discussed, 114–115
  ulcer, 32–33
  ulcer personality, 127

Disease-resistant personality. *See also* Stress
  in general, 251–252, 256, 258–261
    challenge, 263
    coherence, 264
    commitment, 262
    control, 262–263
    hardiness, 261–262, 264–268
    healthful choices, 264–268
  role of stress, 252–253
Divorce, 363. *See also* Marriage
  effects on adults, 343–346
  effects on children, 341–343
  in general, 340–341
  vs. unhappy marriage, 346–349
Dopamine, 155, 200
Dry mouth, 47
Dyspepsia, 179–180
Dysphoria, 528. *See also* Emotions

Eastman Kodak study, 210, 402, 404
Eating disorders, 176, 201
Education, 314–315
Elderly. *See also* Aging; Longevity
  divorce and, 341, 346
  grief affecting, 390, 395, 398
  hip fracture, 630–631
  hostility reduction, 161
  loneliness and, 317, 326
  pets and, 332, 333, 334
  religion and, 441, 660
  sleep patterns, 230
  social support, 279, 288–289
  stressors, 56, 288–289
Emotional support, 69. *See also* Social
  support
Emotions
  affect on health, 6, 8, 12, 19, 96, 257
  alexithymia, 258
  cancer and, 26–29
  diabetes and, 29–30
  dysphoria, 528
  expressing, 21, 120, 129, 394
  immune system and, 20–23, 514
  produced by brain, 12

  repressing, 21, 28–29, 32, 91, 114–115,
    120–121, 374
  Type A personality affecting, 110–113
"Emotions, Immunity, and Disease"
  (Solomon), 7
Empowerment. *See also* Control
  control and, 645, 648–651
Endocrine system, 18
  disorders of, 207
  stress and, 68–69
Endorphins, 8, 10, 126, 206, 454, 576
  discussed, 13
Enjoyment, 377–378
Epinephrine, 25, 153–154, 185
Epworth Sleepiness Scale, 230t. *See also* Sleep
Essential fatty acids, 591–592. *See also*
  Nutrition
Exercise, 74, 78, 113, 218, 237, 670–671
  discussed, 243, 555
  laughter as, 571–573
Expectations, 77–78, 234, 240. *See also*
  Goals
  Law of Expectations, 144, 173, 178, 187
  negative expectations, 184
  placebos and, 489–490
Explanatory style
  in general, 523
  health influences
    in general, 526–527
    immune system, 531–532
    mental health, 527–528
    physical health, 528–531
  what is it?, 523–525

Failure, 505
Faith, 400, 674. *See also* Religion; Spirituality
  definition, 472
  in general, 471–475
  healing power
    in general, 480
    Lourdes, 480–481
    other examples, 481–484
  health benefits, 476–480
  impact, 475–476

placebo
  defined, 487–488
  definition, 487–488
  in general, 486–488
  how do they work?, 489–490
  myths about, 490–492
  negative effects, 494–495
  physicians' expectations, 492–494
  power of, 495–498
  transfer of energy theory, 484–486
Family, 290, 328, 344. *See also* Children;
    Friends; Marriage; Social support;
    Women
  health benefits, 380–384
  household size, 313–314
  parental influence
    baby studies, 365
    in general, 363–364
    monkey experiments, 364–365
    neglect effects, 365–367
    parental loss, 369, 390–391
    parental styles, 367–368
  reunions, 384–385
  strong family
    affirmation/support, 376–377
    communication/listening, 376
    enjoyment, 377–378
    in general, 376
    leisure time, 378
    positive interaction, 378
    privacy, 379–380
    problem solving, 380
    religion, 379
    respect, 377
    right and wrong, 379
    service, 380
    shared responsibility, 378
    traditions, 379
    trust, 377
  weak/stressed family
    anorexia nervosa, 375
    asthma, 374
    cancer, 374
    diabetes, 374–375
    in general, 369–372
    learned pain, 372–373
    strep, 373–374
    what is it?, 362–363
Fatigue, 211, 229, 237
Fear, 12. *See also* Worry
  health consequences, 184–186
Fertility, 69
Fibromyalgia, 180, 237, 417–418, 602
  discussed, 206–207
"Fight-or-flight" response, 7, 22, 25, 45, 66,
    68, 105, 150, 152, 186
Fighting spirit, 122, 129
Food, 13. *See also* Diet; Nutrition
Forgiveness, 165, 670. *See also* Religion;
    Spirituality
  discussed, 434–437, 658
Fridays, 79
Friends, 78. *See also* Family; Loneliness;
    Social Support
  in general, 327–328
  health benefits, 329–331
  types, 328–329
    close friends, 329
    convenience friends, 328–329
    cross-generational friends, 329
    historical friends, 329
    special-interest friends, 329

GABA, 180
Gastrointestinal tract, 600–604. *See also*
    Nutrition
  depression and, 208
  factors affecting, 46–47
General adaptation syndrome, 66. *See also*
    Stress
Genetics
  behavior and, 101
  hostility and, 145–146
  longevity and, 34
  stress and, 43, 64–65
Germs, 6–7
Glucocorticoids, 8, 10, 67–68
Glycosylation, 597–598

Goals, 265–266. *See also* Expectations
  personal aspirations, 77
Granulocytes, discussed, 16–17
Grief and bereavement
  compared to depression, 215
  definition, 393
  in general, 388–389
  health effects
    in general, 393–401
    heart disease, 401–402
    immune system, 402–404
    mortality, 407–409
    risk reduction, 409–411
    spousal death, 393–401
    sudden death, 404–407
    suicide, 407
  loss effect, 391–393
  loss that leads to, 389–391
  stress and, 257–258
Guilt, 266, 435, 670

Happiness, 503
Hardiness, 668
  control and, 537–538
  discussed, 261–262, 264–268
Hassles, 126, 143, 163, 330, 417. *See also*
  Problem solving
  stress and, 52–53
Headache, 151, 179, 207
Healing, 291, 391, 420, 466. *See also* Health
  control and, 543–544
  definition, 420, 421–422
  faith healing, 485–486, 496
  optimism and
    in general, 510–512
    imaging, 512–513
    other measures, 513–514
  self-healing, 266–267, 526, 556
Health, 129. *See also* Healing
  choices for, 264–268
  control and, in general, 538–539
  definition, 444–445
  perception of, 91, 517, 528–529
  spiritual health, 424, 431, 647

*Healthy Work*, 62
Heart. *See also* Heart disease
  angry heart, 151, 157–162
  broken heart, 401–402
  depression and, 210–214
  loneliness and, 325–327
  social support and
    in general, 295
    Roseto study, 295–296
  stress affecting, 47, 70–72
  trusting heart, 105, 143–144, 377
Heart disease, 88, 105, 382, 542
  angina, 352–353
  depression and insulin resistance, 598–599
  discussed, 24–25, 111, 297–298
  grief and, 401–402
  marriage and, 352–353
  outcomes, 620–622
  social support and, 277–278, 296, 348
  Type B characteristics, 679–680
Herbs, 245
Herpes, 21–22, 150, 216–217, 324
Hibernation, 203, 204
Higher power, 78. *See also* Religion
Hip fracture, discussed, 630–631
Hippocampus, 68, 69
Hives, 217
Holmes-Rahe scale, 50–51. *See also* Stress
  discussed, 50–51
Homeostasis, 43
Homicide, 395, 396. *See also* Suicide
Hope, 445, 646
Hopelessness, 122, 129, 202, 301
Hormones, 8, 530
  hostility and, 152–155
  insomnia and, 238
Hospitalism, 280
Hostility, 92, 100, 116, 126. *See also* Anger;
  Emotions
  causes, 145–146
    hormones and neurotransmitters,
      152–155
  Cooke Medley Hostility Scale, 143, 145
  definitions, 139–141

expression, 148–149, 149–152
free-floating hostility, 101, 104–106, 131, 141
Hostility Scale, 142–143
manifestations, 142–144, 257
mortality and, 162–165
significance, 144–145
Human fulfillment, elements, 675–677
Humor, 78
    in general, 559–561
    health impact
        in general, 563–564
        physical benefits, 564–565
        psychological benefits, 565–570
    laughter
        in general, 570–573
        health benefits, 573–575
        immunity-enhancing benefits, 577–578
        pain relief benefits, 576–577
        physical benefits, 575
        psychological benefits, 578–580
    professional trends toward, 561–563
Hyperaggressiveness, 103. *See also* Hostility
Hyperinsulemia, 598
Hypertension, 622–623. *See also* Blood pressure
Hypnosis, 19–20, 510, 627, 629
    self-hypnosis, 242
Hypothalamus, 7, 18, 46, 109–110, 531

Identity, 390
Imagery, 242. *See also* Imaging; Visualization
    discussed, 656
    guided imagery, 514–515, 657
Imaging. *See also* Visualization
    discussed, 512–513
Immune system
    in action, 16–17
    autoimmune disease, 17, 19, 217–218
    brain-immune system connection, 18–20
    control and, 543–544
    depression and, 214–218
    emotions and, 20–23, 514

explanatory style and, 531–532
in general, 14
grief and, 402–404
influences upon, 8, 123, 283, 300, 330, 344, 347, 355–356, 508
insomnia and, 238
laughter and, 577–578
loneliness and, 323–325, 344
lymphoid organs, 15
malfunctions, 17–18, 69
optimism and, 514–515
stress and, 74–76, 299
Indians, 560
Inflammation, 208
Insomnia. *See also* Sleep
    chronic insomnia
        in general, 232–233, 239–240, 626–627
        mental conditioning, 233–234
    circadian rhythm disorders, 246
    conclusions, 246–247
    effects
        accidents, 235
        depression, 235–236
        in general, 235, 237
        hormones, 238
        immune system, 238
        mortality, 239
        nervous system, 238
        pain, 237–238
        quality of life issues, 236–237
    in general, 228–231
    sleep disorders, 245–246
    treatment
        chronic insomnia, 239–240
        exercise, 243
        medication, 244–245
        paradoxical intention, 243
        relaxation methods, 241–242
        short-term insomnia, 239
        sleep hygiene, 240–241
        sleep restriction, 244
        stimulus control, 241
        thought-stopping, 242–243
        transient insomnia, 239

types and causes
  daytime sleepiness, 232
  early awakening, 231–232
  initiatory insomnia, 231
  multiple awakening, 232
Insulysin, 599
Insurance, medical insurance, 351–352
Interferon, 69
Irritable bowel syndrome, 20–21, 70,
    179–180, 207
  discussed, 33, 627–628

Journaling, discussed, 79–80, 658–659, 674

Kindling phenomenon
  depression, 198–199
  fibromyalgia, 207
Kirlian photography, 485–486

Laughter. *See also* Humor
  as exercise, 571–573
  health benefits, 573–575
  immunity-enhancing benefits, 577–578
  pain relief benefits, 576–577
  physical benefits, 575
  physiology, 570–571
  psychological benefits, 578–580
Law of Expectations, 144, 173, 178, 187
Law of the Boomerang, 143–144
Leukemia, 52. *See also* Cancer
Lie detector, 47
Life events, 49, 184, 551
Lifestyle change, 597. *See also* Change
Light, 203, 204, 205, 241
  sunlight, 594–595
Linn, 179
Loneliness. *See also* Friends
  cancer and, 327
  causes, 315
  in general, 310–311
  health consequences, 319–322
  heart and, 325–327
  immune system and, 323–325
  longevity and, 323
  personal characteristics

bad relationships, 316–317
culture, 316
in general, 315
precipitating events, 317
situation, 316
social relationships, 316
  pets and, 331–335
  reasons for, 314–315
  risk factors, 317–319
  social support and, 292–293
  trends in being alone, 313–314
  UCLA Loneliness Scale, 324
  vs. aloneness, 312–313
  what is it?, 311–312
Longevity. *See also* Aging; Elderly;
    Mortality
  depression and, 208–210
  discussed, 34–36
  family and, 383
  loneliness and, 323
  optimism and, 517–519
Love, 255, 673. *See also* Social support
  animals, 468
  children, 468–469
  in general, 291–292, 466–467
Lupus, 208, 217
Lymphatic system, 8, 14. *See also*
    Lymphocytes
  lymphoid organs, 15
Lymphocytes, 8, 14, 15, 18
  discussed, 16

Macrophages, 18, 155
  discussed, 16
Marriage, 35, 53, 77, 105, 313, 317–319. *See
    also* Divorce; Family
  in general, 340
  health benefits
    cancer, 353–354
    in general, 349–350
    heart disease/blood pressure, 352–353
    immune system, 355–356
    injuries/medical insurance, 351–352
    mental health, 356–357
    social support, 350–351

life expectancy and, 357
negative/positive marriage, 346–349
Meaning, 58, 63, 80, 445, 646
Medical care. *See also* Surgery
  cost and utilization issues, 628–635
  filling hole in health care deliver system?,
    633–634
  high-volume medical users, 617–620,
    619t
  implications, 620
  inpatients, 619–620
  outpatients, 618–619
Medicine, 418. *See also* Behavioral
  medicine
Meditation, 20, 123, 165, 240, 242, 428,
    433, 656. *See also* Relaxation methods
  contemplation, 657
  meditative breathing, 654–655
Meetings, 79
Melanoma, 117, 118, 157. *See also*
  Cancer
Melatonin, 204, 245
Memory, 11–12
Menopause. *See also* Women
  discussed, 625–626
Mental health. *See also* Health; Mental
    illness
  explanatory style and, 527–528
  marriage and, 356–357
  optimism and, 515–517
  religion and, 439
Mental illness, 320, 491, 495
  anxiety and, 179–181
  depression and, 200
"Metabolic Syndrome", 211–212
Michigan study, 293, 454, 460
Mind-body connection. *See also*
    Psychoneuroimmunology
  contemporary considerations, 8–9
  criticisms of, 36–37
  discussed, 660–662
Mindfulness, 130–131, 187, 242, 428, 656
Minnesota Multiphasic Personality
    Inventory (MMPI), 142–143, 214, 324,
    552

MMPI. *See* Minnesota Multiphasic
    Personality Inventory
Monocytes, 514. *See also* Monokines
  discussed, 16
Monokines, discussed, 16
Mood, 527–528
Mortality. *See also* Longevity
  frightened to death, 185
  grief and bereavement, 407–409
  hostility and, 162–165
  insomnia and, 239
  sudden death, 404–407

Natural killer cells, 35, 215
  discussed, 16
Nature, 77, 247
Neuropeptides, 10, 514
Neuroplasticity, 198
Neurotransmitters, 8, 65, 218
  hostility and, 152–155
Niceness, 117
Norcpincphrine, 153–154
Nursing homes, 209
Nutrigenomics, 591
Nutrition, 671. *See also* Diet
  brain and, 599–600
  digestion, 587–588
  in general, 555, 585–586
  health effects
    amino acids, 594
    B-complex vitamins, 593–594
    essential fatty acids, 591–592
    gastrointestinal tract, 600–604
    in general, 590–591, 595–596
    insulin resistance, 597–598
    insulin resistance, depression, heart
      disease, 598–599
    thyroid, 600
    vitamin D/sunlight, 594–595
    wheat allergy, 604
  nutrigenomics, 591
  principles, 586–587

Obesity, 151, 590. *See also* Diet
  in general, 596–597

Optimism, 261. *See also* Optimist
  dispositional optimism, 507, 509, 516
  factors affecting, 441
  in general, 502
  healing and
    in general, 510–512
    imaging, 512–513
    other measures, 513–514
  health benefits, 505–510
  imaging, 512–513
  immune system and, 514–515
  longevity and, 517–519
  mental health and, 515–517
  pessimism and, 503–504
Optimist
  characteristics of, 504–505
  discussed, 502–504
Outcome studies, 611

Pain
  chest pain, 623–624
  chronic pain, 30–31
  insomnia and, 237–238
  laughter and, 576–577
  learned pain, 372–373
Panic disorder. *See also* Anxiety
  discussed, 175
  physical symptoms, 178t
Paranoia, 143
Parkinson's disease, 91, 599, 603
Patient Health Questionnaire, 193–194. *See also* Depression
Peptides, discussed, 13–14
Performance, 566
Personality. *See also* Disease-prone personality; Disease-resistant personality
  altruistic personality, 457–460
  as crystalline structure, 221
  depression-prone personality, 202, 221
  immune-prone personality, 93
  Minnesota Multiphasic Personality Inventory, 142–143
  negative personality traits, 25
  self-healing personality, 266–267

Pessimism. *See also* Optimism; Pessimist
  optimism and, 503–504
Pessimist, discussed, 524–525
Pet therapy, 673
Pets, 78, 322, 673. *See also* Animals
  in general, 331–332
  health benefits, 333–334
  pet-facilitated therapy, 335
  stress and, 335
Phobia, 175
  discussed, 186
Pituitary, 7, 109, 205, 280
Placebo
  in general, 486–487
  how do they work?, 489–490
    amplifiers, 489
    reducers, 489
  myths about, 490–492
  negative effects, 494–495
  physicians' expectations, 492–494
  power of, 495–498
PMS. *See* Premenstrual syndrome
PNI. *See* Psychoneuroimmunology
Possessions, 390
Poverty, 196, 318
Power, 566–567. *See also* Control
Prayer, 23, 674. *See also* Faith; Religion; Spirituality
  effects, 433–434
  in general, 431–432
  relaxation response, 432–433
Premenstrual syndrome (PMS), depression and, 202–203, 220
Priorities, 79
Privacy, 379–380
Problem solving, 187, 566. *See also* Hassles
  in family, 380
Productivity, 58–60
Prolactin, discussed, 154–155
Psychoneuroimmunology (PNI)
  challenge for twenty-first century, 37–38
  definitions, 4–6
  in general, 3–4
  history, 6–8

Psychotherapy, 627
Pulmonary disease, discussed, 624–625

Quality of life, 439

Refugees, 254–255
Relaxation, 130. *See also* Relaxation
    methods
Relaxation methods, 241–242, 672–673. *See*
    *also* Imagery
  autogenic training, 655–656
  body work, 656–657
  imagery, 242
  meditative breathing, 654–655
  mindfulness, 242, 656
  muscle relaxation, 242, 655
  self-hypnosis, 242
Religion, 400–401, 418, 420, 428. *See also*
    Faith; Spirituality
  church affiliation and
  attendance and affiliation, 440–442, 673
    church teachings, 442–444
    in general, 437–440
    specific illnesses, 444
  definition, 472
  family and, 379
  in general, 471–475
  health benefits, 476–480
  prayer, 23, 431–434
  role of, 23–24
Religious experience, 421
Relocation, as stressor, 254–255, 288–291,
    343
Respect, 377
Restless leg syndrome, 246
Retirement, 61
Rheumatoid-arthritis-prone personality. *See*
    *also* Arthritis
  in general, 123–124
  identical twin study, 124–125
  immune system factor, 125–126
  Solomon/Moos study, 125
Rorschach test, 28, 90, 321
Roseto study, 295–296

Saccharin, 22–23
SAD. *See* Seasonal affective disorder
Savings, 77
Seasonal affective disorder (SAD), 220. *See*
    *also* Depression; Light
  discussed, 203–205
Self-assertion, 149
Self-awareness, 129
Self-confidence, 577
Self-destruction, 103–104
Self-efficacy, 552–556
Self-esteem, 102, 103, 131, 197, 202, 315,
    317
  in general, 547
  impact on body, 551–552
  what is it?, 548–550
  where does it come from?, 550–551
Self-evaluation, 527
Self-harm, 176
Self-improvement, 267
Self-involvement, 108
Self-worth, 58, 202
Serotonin, 43, 65, 180, 182, 197, 203, 209,
    212
Service, 380
Seven Habits of Highly Effective People, 678
Sex hormones, 46
Sexual dysfunction, discussed, 33–34
Sexuality, contraceptives, 555
Skin. *See also* Skin disorders
  discussed, 304
Skin disorders, 150, 478
Sleep, 78, 163, 188, 220, 671. *See also*
    Insomnia; Sleep disorders
  Epworth Sleepiness Scale, 230t
  naps, 229, 241
  sleep deprivation, 229
  sleep needs, 229–230
  stages, 234–235
  why do we sleep?, 234
Sleep disorders
  discussed, 245–246
    restless leg syndrome, 246
    sleep apnea, 245–246

Smoking, 29, 99, 127, 212, 233, 264, 343, 554
Social support, 69, 105, 111, 123, 129, 151, 163, 165, 195, 268, 327, 344, 381, 393. *See also* Friends
  Alameda County study, 275–277, 287, 292–293, 320
  building, 659
  definition, 277–278
  in general, 275–277
  health and, 280–284, 299–303, 319
  heart and
    in general, 295
    Roseto study, 295–296
  Japan study, 294–295
  loneliness, 292–293
  marriage and, 350–351
  Michigan study, 293, 454
  North Carolina study, 293
  other studies, 298–299
  sources, 278–280, 674
  Sweden study, 293, 296–297
  ties that bind
    battle stress, 286–287
    in general, 284–286
    pregnant women under stress, 287–288
    relocation and disruption, 288–291
    unemployment, 287
  touch, 303–305
  Type A study, 297–298
Soldiers, 97
Solomon/Moos study, 125
Somaticizing, anxiety, 176–177
Spiritual counselor, 417
Spirituality. *See also* Religion
  crisis and, 429–431
  definition, 471, 647–648
  essence of, 444–446
  forgiveness, 434–437
  in general, 417–420, 471–475
  health benefits, 425–429, 476–480
  prayer, 23, 431–434
  spiritual connection, 662–664
  what is it?, 420–425

Spleen, 8, 15, 69
Strep, 373–374
Stress, 562. *See also* Disease-resistant personality; Stress buffers; Stress resilience
  affect on animals, 649–650
  affect on family, 369–372
  affect on health, 7, 8, 19, 35, 613–615
  age-related stressors
    adult, 56
    children/adolescents, 54–56
    miscellaneous, 56
    prenatal stress, 53–54
  arteriosclerosis and, 73
  brain and, 67–68
  cancer and, 26–29, 51–52, 120–121
  cardiovascular system and, 70–72
    arteriosclerosis, 73
    disease events, 73–74
  cholesterol and, 72–73
  coping with, 70, 75
    in general, 64–65
    general adaptation syndrome, 66
    pregnant women under stress, 287–288
    stress reduction techniques, 72
    weak links, 94–95
  costs and outcomes, 48–49, 253
  definition, 42–44
  distress and eustress, 44–45
  endocrine system and, 68–69
  factors leading to, 49–50
  gender and
    anger/hostility, 257
    depression/grief, 257–258
    in general, 65, 256–257
  in general, 42–44
  hassles and, 52–53
  Holmes-Rahe scale, 50–51
  humor and, 567–568
  immune system and, 74–76
  job stress
    costs, 59–60
    frequency of, 57
    in general, 56–57, 161

handling, 78–80
health effects, 60–61
how much is enough?, 63–64
how much work?, 61–62
job burnout, 57–59
job characteristics, 62–63
shift work, 73
laughter and, 578
mechanisms of, 253–255
mental/physical stress, 74, 75
perception of, 43–44, 53, 67, 68, 70, 254, 268
self-perception of, 76
physiological reactions to, in general, 65–67
post-traumatic stress disorder, 97
protecting yourself from, 76–78, 672
reconstructing stress, 267
relocation as, 254–255
role in health, 252–253
stress response, 45–48, 252
Survey of Medical Interns, 58t
types
physical stress, 45
psychological stress, 45
psychosocial stress, 45
Stress buffers
control as, 542–543
discussed, 255–256
friends, 330
optimism, 516
religion, 24
Stress resilience
cancer and, 643–645
empowerment and control, 648–651
in general, 642–643
principles, 645–648, 648t
Stroke, 302, 345
Substance P, 126, 199, 206
Sugar, insulin, 47, 211
Suicide, 69, 195–196, 208, 320, 335, 345, 363, 391, 394, 395. *See also* Homicide
grief affecting, 407
Sunlight, 594–595. *See also* Light
Support groups, 7. *See also* Social support

Surgery, 481–482, 528. *See also* Medical care
surgical patients, 628–629
Survey of Medical Interns, 58t
Suspicion, 107–108
Sweden, 325
studies, 296–297
Sweets, 13, 203

T cells, 126
discussed, 16
Ten Commandments, 428
Thought, 187
Thought-stopping, 242–243
Thymus, 8, 15, 17, 18, 35, 69, 514
Thyroid, 46
nutrition and, 600
Time, time-urgency, 103, 130
Time management, 77
Tonsils, 15
Touch, 303–305. *See also* Social support
Trauma, 176, 283
post traumatic stress disorder, 176
Trust, 105, 143–144, 429
discussed, 377
Tuberculosis, 49–50, 254–255
Type A personality, 92, 160
causes, 100–101
environmental factors, 100–101
characteristics of, 101–109
controversy about, 115–116
emotional effects of, 110–113
in general, 92, 95–96
harmless behaviors, 101–102
heart disease risk, 111
impacts of, 112
insecurity of status, 102
MRFIT study, 98–99
role in other illnesses, 113–114
studies, 297–298
"toxic core" of, 104
Western Collaborative Group Study, 98–100, 106, 113
Type B personality, 297
characteristics, 679–680

pe C personality. *See also* Cancer
  depression, 121
  emotions, 120
  in general, 116–119
  LeShan's analysis, 119–120
  stress, 26–29, 51–52, 120–121
Type D personality, discussed, 114–115

Ulcer, 70, 183–184
  discussed, 32–33, 127–128
  ulcer personality, 127
Uncertainty, worry and, 183–184
Unemployment, 383
  discussed, 61–62, 287
"Uplifts", 74–75

Vaccines, 14
Vigilance reaction, 48
Vigilant observation, 109
Visualization, 173–174, 178–179, 187. *See also* Imagery
  discussed, 657–658, 660
Vitamins. *See also* Diet; Nutrition
  B-complex vitamins, 593–594
  vitamin D, 594–595
Volunteerism. *See also* Altruism
  consistency, 464
  desire to volunteer, 463–464
  in general, 460–463
  liking the work, 464
  motive, 464–466
  one-on-one contact, 463
Voodoo, 181
*Vulnerable but Invincible*, 258, 468

Warts, 510
Western Collaborative Group Study, 98–100, 106, 113
Western Electric, 209
Women. *See also* Children; Family
  abortion and, 403–404
  anger and, 144, 151, 156, 158, 159, 162–164

breast cancer affecting, 6, 7, 52, 88, 90, 116, 120, 122, 156, 216, 256, 265, 300, 320, 403, 479, 529, 543, 587, 644–645
breast milk, 14
depression and, 194, 195, 197, 203, 214, 215, 219
diseases affecting, 20, 577, 596–597
divorce affecting, 342, 348, 355–356
effects on fetus, 302–303
faith and, 482–483
grief affecting, 395
identical twin study, 124–125
loneliness affecting, 318, 323
marriage and, 313, 351
menopause, 625–626
PMS affecting, 202–203, 220
pregnancy-related problems, 33, 69, 183, 221, 287–288, 322, 395–396
  labor and delivery, 629–630, 630t
  prenatal stress, 53–54
religion and, 441–442
sleep disorders, 231
social support, 279, 286, 301, 329
stress affecting, 42, 62, 67, 112–113, 257, 287–288, 328
widowhood, 395–398, 403, 408
Workaholism, 61–62, 108–109
Worker compensation, 48, 59
*Working Ourselves to Death* (Fassel), 61
Worry, 69. *See also* Anxiety
  asthma and, 182–183
  circulation system and, 181–182
  definitions, 173–174
  fear consequences, 184–186
  in general, 172–173
  physical effects, 177–179
  uncertainty and, 183–184
  what to do about it, 187–188
  worried well, 176–177
  worry period, 188
Writing, 283–284. *See also* Journaling